BRAIN EVOLUTION AND COGNITION

BRAIN EVOLUTION AND COGNITION

Edited by

GERHARD ROTH and
MARIO F. WULLIMANN

University of Bremen, Brain Research Institute and Center for Cognitive Science, Bremen, Federal Republic of Germany

A JOHN WILEY & SONS, INC. and SPEKTRUM AKADEMISCHER VERLAG CO-PUBLICATION

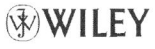 New York · Chichester · Weinheim · Brisbane · Singapore · Toronto

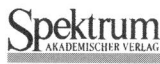 Heidelberg · Berlin

Copyright © 2001 by John Wiley & Sons, Inc. and Spektrum Akademischer Verlag

John Wiley & Sons, Inc.
605 Third Avenue
New York, NY 10158-0012
USA

Spektrum Akdemischer Verlag
Vangerowstrasse 20
D-69115 Heidelberg
Germany

Telephone: (212) 850-6000

Telephone: ++ 49 6221 91260

Address all inquiries to John Wiley & Sons, Inc.

Published simultaneously in Canada.

All rights reserved. No part of this publication may be reproduced, stored in a retrieval system or transmitted in any form or by any means, electronic, mechanical, photocopying, recording, scanning or otherwise, except as permitted under Sections 107 or 108 of the 1976 United States Copyright Act. without either the prior written permission of the Publisher, or authorization through Payment of the appropriate per copy fee to the Copyright Clearance Center, 222 Rosewood Drive, Danvers, MA 01923, (508) 750-8400, fax (508) 750-4744. Requests to the Publisher for permission should be addressed to the Permissions Department, John Wiley & Sons, Inc., 605 Third Avenue, New York, NY 10158-0012, (212) 850-6011, fax (212) 850-6008, E-Mail: permreq@wiley.com.

While the authors, editors and publishers believe that drug selection and dosage and the specification and usage of equipment and devices, as set forth in this book, are in accord with current recommendations and practice at the time of publication, they accept no legal responsibility for any errors or omissions, and make no warranty, expressed or implied, with respect to material contained herein. In view of ongoing research, equipment modifications, changes in governmental regulations and the constant flow of information relating to drug therapy, drug reactions, and the use of equipment and devices, the reader is urged to review and evaluate the information provided in the package insert or instructions for each drug, piece of equipment, or device for, among other things, any changes in instructions or indication of dosage or usage and for added warnings and precautions.

Library of Congress Cataloging-in-Publication Data

Brain evolution and cognition / edited by Gerhard Roth and Mario F. Wullimann.
    p. cm.
   Includes index.
   ISBN 0-471-33170-8 (cloth : alk. Paper)
   1. Cognition. 2. Brain-Evolution.
  I. Roth, Gerhard, 1942 Aug. 15- II. Wullimann, Mario F.
QP360.5. B734   2001
   573.8'6-DC21   00-023095

Die Deutsche Bibliothek – CIP-Einheitsaufnahme

Brain evolution and cognition / ed. By Gerhard Roth and Mario F. Wullimann. – New York ; Chichester ; Weinheim ; Brisbane ; Singapore ; Toronto: Wiley ; Heidelberg ; Berlin : Spektrum, Akad. Verl., 2001
   ISBN 0-471-33170-8

This book is printed on acid-free paper.

Printed in the United States of America
10 9 8 7 6 5 4 3 2 1

Contents

INTRODUCTION

Problems in the study of brain evolution and cognition 1
Mario F. Wullimann and Gerhard Roth

    Handicaps in the search for an evolutionary history of vertebrate brains 1
    Silent revolutions emerging 2
    The amniote telencephalon as a case in point 3
    A special position for humans? 5
    What is cognition? 6
    References 7

PART I   DEVELOPMENTAL AND ADULT BRAIN ORGANIZATION IN EVOLUTION

**1 Brain phenotypes and early regulatory genes:
The *Bauplan* of the metazoan central nervous system** 11
Mario F. Wullimann

    Introduction 11
    Comparative phenotypic analysis of metazoan central nervous characters 13
        The cladistic framework 13
        A can of worms: Plathelminths, nemathelminths, nemertines 14
        The molluscan controversy 20
        The arthropod CNS, rather than being ancestral to the vertebrate CNS,
        is equally remote from the basic bilaterian *Bauplan* as the craniate brain .. 22
        Deuterostome nervous systems 25
        Conclusion 28
    Early genes in neural development - Do they tell a different story? 30
        Development and *Bauplan* of the vertebrate CNS 30
        Early regulatory genes and neuromeres in the vertebrate brain 32
        Early regulatory genes and the insect CNS 32
        Phylogenetic interpretation of molecular genetic and phenotypic data 34
    Conclusion 36
    References 37

2 The echinoderm nervous system and its phylogenetic interpretation 41
Thomas Heinzeller and Ulrich Welsch

    Introduction 41
    Description of Nervous Systems 44
        Larval nervous system 44
        Postmetamorphotic nervous system: Common features 45

       Postmetamorphotic nervous system: Group-specific features 51
       Cryptosyringida 54
       Inter-class comparison of sensory versus motor function 60
Questions of Symmetry 60
       Central part of the body 60
       Bilateral symmetry and segmentation of the arms 61
       Are echinoderm arms homologous with bilaterian trunks? 62
       Echinoderm ectoneural cord versus chordate neural plate 62
       Additional body axes 64
       Hydrocoel and notochord - are they convergent or homologous? 65
Locomotion of Echinoderms 66
Phylogenetic Aspects 68
       Consistency versus flexibility of regulatory genes 68
       Garstang's hypothesis 68
       Systematics of echinoderms 69
       Missing brain 69
References 69

3   Evolution of vertebrate motor systems 77

Hans J. ten Donkelaar

Introduction 77
Basics of vertebrate locomotion 80
Prehensile extremities 84
Features of the ancestral vertebrate motor system 85
Neural control of quadrupedal locomotion 91
Supraspinal control 93
       Descending supraspinal pathways 93
       The cerebellorubrospinal limb control system 98
       The special case for birds 104
Summary 106
References 107

4   Sensory system evolution in vertebrates 113

William Hodos and Ann B. Butler

How many senses? 113
How many cranial nerves? 115
Trends in sensory system evolution 116
Ascending sensory pathways 119
Neuroembryology and the evolution of sensory systems 120
       Evolution of new sensory receptors 122
       Evolution of new primary, secondary, and higher order
       sensory nuclei 122

    The evolution of sensory specialists 123
    Evolution of central sensory pathways 124
    The evolution of new central sensory nuclei 125
    The evolution of sensory maps 126
    Loss of sensory receptors and central pathways 127
    Mechanisms of sensory system evolution 130
  References 131

5 Evolution of the forebrain in tetrapods 135
Toru Shimizu

Introduction 135
Evolution of tetrapods 137
    Early tetrapods - Ancestral amphibians 137
    Early amniotes - Ancestral reptiles 139
    Synapsids - Mammals 140
    Sauropsids - Reptiles 142
    Sauropsids - Birds 144
    Conclusion 145
Forebrain organization of living tetrapods 145
    Amphibian pattern 146
    Mammalian pattern 152
    Sauropsid pattern 156
    Conclusion 161
Evolutionary history of the tetrapod forebrain 162
    Early tetrapods 163
    Early amniotes 163
    Synapsids and sauropsids 165
    Conclusion 169
Environmental pressures on the tetrapod forebrain 170
    Anamniote pattern versus amniote pattern 171
    Sauropsid pattern versus mammalian pattern 172
    Conclusion 175
References 176

6 Neocortical macrocircuits 185
Rudolf Nieuwenhuys

Introduction 185
Major sensorimotor projections 186
Control systems 189
Reticular, greater limbic and general modulatory inputs to
neocortical circuitry 192
    The ascending reticular system 192
    The greater limbic system 193
    Monoaminergic and cholinergic modulatory systems 194

Cortico-subcortico-cortical association systems 195
    The thalamic association system 196
    The striatal association system 198
    The cerebellar association system. 199
Summary 201
References 202

7 Hunting in barn owls: Peripheral and neurobiological specializations and their general relevance in neural computation 205

Hermann Wagner

Introduction 205
Evolutionary position and geographical distribution of the barn owl 206
Hunting as a complex behavior 206
    General comments 206
    Formal description of the hunting situation 208
    Adaptations of barn owls to hunting in the night 209
The barn owl's brain 212
    Morphological adaptations of the owl's brain to hunting and
    life at night 213
    Physiological adaptations 216
    Coincidence detection 218
    Further brain adaptations subserving sound-localization behavior 225
    Differences in the representation of acoustic space in diurnal and
    nocturnal owls 228
General meaning of coincidence detection and across-frequency
integration 228
Conclusions 231
References 232

8 Evolution and devolution: The case of bolitoglossine salamanders 237

Gerhard Roth and David B. Wake

Introduction 237
The Bolitoglossini 238
The brain of salamanders and frogs 244
The visual system of bolitoglossines 249
    Retina and retinofugal system 249
    Tectum 250
The fate of other sensory systems 253
Causes and consequences of simplification in the context of
paedomorphosis. 254
What do bolitoglossines tell us about evolution in general and brain
evolution in particular? 258
References 260

9   Evolutionary constraints of large telencephala 265
Gerd Rehkämper, Heiko D. Frahm, and Michael D. Mann

    Evolution –What does that mean? 265
    Brain and brain part size as a heuristic tool 266
    What factors influence brain size or brain part size? 268
        There is no brain size alteration 269
        Brain size alterations are epiphenomena 269
        Brain size is influenced by individual learning 270
        Brain size and brain part size reflect adaptation 271
    Definition of "large telencephala"............................ 271
    Mammals.. 272
        Telencephala enlarged because of dominance of olfactory orientation ... 272
        Telencephala enlarged because of superior spatial cognition 272
        Telencephala enlarged because of a voluminous isocortex 275
        Isocortex (and therefore, telencephalon) enlarged because of
        elaborated somatosensory areas together with a necessity of motor
        coordination in a subterranean life 276
        Telencephala enlarged because of multimodal integration 278
    Birds 278
        Telencephala enlarged because of olfaction 278
        Telencephala enlarged because of spatial cognition 279
        Telencephala enlarged because of isocortical equivalents......... 280
    Domesticated animals...................................... 283
    Again: Theories of brain size and brain composition.............. 285
    Conclusions 288
    References 289

PART II   COGNITION: FROM NEURAL BASIS TO BEHAVIOR

10 Brain and cognitive function in teleost fishes 297
Leo S. Demski and Joel A. Beaver

    Introduction 297
    Studies on cognition in fishes 298
    Brain lesions and cognitive behavior in fishes................... 300
        Telencephalon: Nonspatial learning......................... 300
        Telencephalon: Spatial learning............................ 301
        Cerebellum 302
        Tectum 303
    Relative brain size and development: Implications for cognitive
    function in fishes 304
        Studies in minnows (Cypriniformes) 304
        Blind and sighted characins.............................. 306

    The cichlids of the African great lakes.............................306
    Coral reef percomorphs...307
Microcircuitry of telencephalic enhancements in selected percomorphs 311
    Area dorsalis telencephali pars lateralis (dorsal part)................313
    Area dorsalis telencephali pars centralis 317
    Area dorsalis telencephali pars medialis 319
    Behavioral studies on the enlarged telencephalon of percomorphs 321
Summary and conclusions 323
References 325

11 Cognition in insects: The honeybee as a study case...................333

Randolf Menzel, Martin Giurfa, Bertram Gerber, and Frank Hellstern

Introduction: Brain, behavior, and biology of honeybees.................333
    Behavior and biology of honeybees..............................333
    Design of an insect brain..335
Elementary and configural forms of learning in classical conditioning 338
    The preparation: Classical conditioning of the proboscis
    extension reflex 338
    A cognitive approach to memory dynamics......................340
    The elementary-configural distinction 342
    Cognitive aspects of elementary forms of conditioning? 342
    Configural forms of conditioning 345
Learning in the natural context 346
    Context-dependent learning and retrieval 346
    Serial order in a spatiotemporal domain 348
    The representation of space in navigation 350
    Visual discrimination learning in honeybees: Generalization,
    categorization, and concept formation 354
Conclusion 359
    Basic cognition with a small brain 359
    The ecological niche and basic cognition 360
References 362

12 Insect brain..367

Nicholas J. Strausfeld

Introduction 367
General features of segmental ganglia 368
The protocerebrum and the preoral brain 372
    Evolutionary considerations 372
    General organization of the protocerebrum 373
The mushroom bodies 375
    Structure 375
    Evolution of mushroom bodies in insects 377
    Relationship to primary sensory neuropils........................378

    Mushroom body physiology 381
        Roles of mushroom bodies 382
    The central complex 384
        Evolutionary considerations 384
        Organization of the central complex 384
        Central complex function 385
    Comparisons of brain regions amongst arthropods 389
        Mushroom bodies 389
        The central complex 390
    Insect and vertebrate brains compared 392
        Equivalence of insect and vertebrate embryonic forebrain ... 392
        The adult brain 393
    References 395

13 Conservation in the neurology and psychology of cognition in vertebrates 401
Euan M. Macphail

    Introduction: Complexity in brains and behaviour 401
    Species differences in intelligence 402
    Birds and mammals compared 403
    The basal ganglia 405
    Paleostriatal lesions and classical conditioning in the pigeon ... 407
    The archistriatum 409
        Posteromedial archistriatum: Fear and avoidance 409
        Anterior and intermediate archistriatum: Parallels with isocortex ... 411
    Cortex 411
        Olfactory cortex 411
        Hippocampal complex 412
        Isocortical analogues/homologues 416
    Conclusions 426
    References 427

14 Multimodal areas of the avian forebrain—Blueprints for cognition? 431
Onur Güntürkün and Daniel Durstewitz

    The theme 431
    Working memory and prefrontal cortex 432
    Avian brain and cognition 434
    Details of the machine 437
    The decline of a memory store 439
    Simulation of the machine 442
    Looking inside 449
    References 450

xii Contents

15 Cognition of birds as products of evolved brains 451
Juan D. Delius, Martina Siemann, Jacky Emmerton and Li Xia

Introduction 451
Categorization 456
Concepts 461
Transitivity 467
Numerosity 472
Epilogue 477
References 483

16 What can the cerebral cortex do better than other parts of the brain? 491
Almut Schüz

Introduction 491
Basic connectivity of the isocortex 492
The cerebral cortex and cognition 494
Comparative aspects 497
    Brain size and connectivity 497
    Allocortex and reptilian cortex 498
References 499

17 Evolution and complexity of the human brain: Some organizing principles 501
Michel A. Hofman

Introduction 501
Evolution of brain size 502
Encephalization in primates 505
General constraints on brain evolution 507
Evolution and geometry of the cerebral cortex 510
Design principles of neuronal organization 514
Biological limits to information processing 515
Concluding remarks 518
References 519

18 The evolution of neural and behavioral complexity 523
Harry J. Jerison

Introduction 523
Vigilance and attention: An old-fashioned view 525
Costs and attention 526
Costs and brains 531
Brain size in living vertebrates: Allometry and encephalization 533
Exceptions 535
Early avian and mammalian encephalization 539

Progressive encephalization in mammals 542
More on neural information 544
Neural and behavioral complexity 546
Why some brains are big: What do big brains do? 547
References 551

19 The evolution of consciousness 555

Gerhard Roth

Phenomenology of consciousness 556
The neurobiological basis of the different states and appearances
of consciousness 558
Cognition and consciousness in animals 564
Animal brains and human brain 568
Consciousness and language 577
Conclusions 579
References 580

Index 583

Introduction

PROBLEMS IN THE STUDY OF BRAIN EVOLUTION AND COGNITION

Mario F. Wullimann and Gerhard Roth, University of Bremen, Brain Research Institute and Center for Cognitive Science

Why a book about the evolution of brains and their cognitive functions? Although the evolution of nervous systems and brains has been much investigated, it still is a debated and unsettled topic, as is the question about the relationship between brains and cognitive functions. Therefore, we organized an international symposium entitled "Brain Evolution and Cognition" at the University of Bremen in December, 1994. Many scientists followed our invitation to present their current ideas on that topic in Bremen. In the wake of that meeting, the plan emerged to publish a book, and almost everyone involved agreed to make a contribution. A few more authors not initially involved with the symposium were asked to join the book project (and they kindly agreed to do so) and so here we are at last.

In our introductory remarks to the symposium, the contributors were encouraged to search for answers to the following questions: Can one draw principles of brain evolution? Why did some brains become large and complex, and others small and simple and still others remained as they were for hundreds of millions of years? Where, how, and why did cognition evolve? Is there any definable relationship between cognitive functions and brain structures and function? What are the forces that drove the evolution of cognitive functions (external, internal, or both)?

Before we let the chapter authors provide answers to these questions, we discuss some problems in the study of brain evolution and cognition.

HANDICAPS IN THE SEARCH FOR AN EVOLUTIONARY HISTORY OF VERTEBRATE BRAINS

The case of horses is one of the finest examples of what paleozoology, paleobotany, paleoclimatology, and paleoecology can do in reconstructing the phylogeny and evolutionary history of a certain animal group (Carroll, 1988). The reason why there is so much more known on the evolution of horses than on the evolution of vertebrate brains is obvious: There is an almost complete fossil record in the case of horses. This primary source of information is missing in the case of brains and represents the first handicap for the search for an evolutionary history of brains. The only paleontological information on fossil brains is available in the form of endocasts and has mostly been used in the context of brain weight/body weight analyses. Although this approach yields fascinating results in its own right—particularly in the primate and other mammalian cases (van Dongen, 1998; Jerison, this volume, Chapter 18)—it cannot go beyond the primary data and explain the emergence of particular cytoarchitectonic differences, let alone their related functional implications that arose in the course of vertebrate brain evolution. Unfortunately, as in the case of most soft organs, there is no paleontological record of the fine structure of brains. Thus, historical brain research is mostly left with neontological data from extant species and its analysis using the phyletic method. A second handicap becomes apparent when we look at the drastically different functional interpretations of, for example, the bird versus the mammalian brain that have been given during the past century based on comparative descriptive neuroanatomy. The sometimes breathtaking beauty of diverse histological and cytoarchitectonic patterns in various vertebrate brains (Nieuwenhuys et al., 1998) apparently has gone along with conflicting evolutionary explanations (i.e., these differences have an immense potential for divergent interpretation). Thus, it is clear that descriptive neuroanatomy alone is not a sufficient source for a stringent functional explanation of brain structures. One of the greatest problems in that respect has been that certain preconceived views—deeply rooted in the teleological preevolutionary concept of a *scala naturae* (i.e., nature's attempt at arriving stepwise to perfection going from lower to higher vertebrates)—were sought to be confirmed in the sometimes great apparent morphological differences in brain structure (e.g., between fishes and mammals). The idea was that of a successive addition of major brain parts and related increasingly complex functions going from fish to human in evolution (see critical reviews by Northcutt, 1981; Roth, 1994; Wullimann, 1997). Naturally, the study of behavior and cognition has been influenced by such preconceived notions coming from comparative neuroanatomy. However, research of the past three decades has increasingly shown that there are more commonalities in general brain organization and behavior of vertebrates than was previously believed.

SILENT REVOLUTIONS EMERGING

Three events had a substantial effect on a new understanding of vertebrate brain evolution in the second part of the twentieth century. First, the explosive development of neurobiological methodology (e.g., the invention of many new investigative tools such as immunohistochemistry, neuronal tracing agents, improved extracellular and intracellular neurophysiology, and refined protocols for controlled behavioral studies) marked massive progress for various disciplines of the neurosciences. At the same time, the quantity and diversity of data available for comparative evolutionary brain studies has been tremendously enlarged, and the validity of interpretations has been improved. Second, the introduction of Hennigian cladistics (Hennig, 1966; Northcutt, 1984; compare Wullimann, this volume,

Chapter 1) into the comparative discussion as a tool for analyzing neural characters altered the way one deals with the interpretation of evolutionary change in brains (compare, for example, a treatise on the evolution of the mammalian isocortex by Northcutt and Kaas, 1995). Finally, the immense new input coming from developmental molecular genetic studies led to the discovery of many early active regulatory genes and developmental pathways that directly bear on the vertebrate brain *Bauplan* and continue to have a tremendous effect on evolutionary brain studies (Heinzeller and Welsch; Strausfeld; Wullimann, this volume, Chapters 2, 12, and 1, respectively).

THE AMNIOTE TELENCEPHALON AS A CASE IN POINT

In browsing through many chapters of this book, it becomes clear that a central question in the discussion on vertebrate brain evolution is how the large and differentiated telencephalon of birds compares to that of mammals: Are there comparable structures and functions in their respective pallium and subpallium, and what, if any, is their common origin in phylogeny? There is a long and winding road of comparative neuroanatomy starting at the beginning of the twentieth century on that subject (nicely summarized by Striedter, 1997). However, by midcentury, the eminent American neurobiologist of that time, C. Judson Herrick, succinctly summarized the then accepted view (which became the traditional one for later decades) in 1956 in his book *The Evolution of Human Nature*: "The bird's cerebral hemispheres are composed almost entirely of the enormously enlarged corpora striata, which are concerned almost exclusively with stereotyped reflex and instinctive behavior." Thus, the suspected less well developed plasticity of behavior, learning capacity, and other cognitive abilities of birds compared to mammals was considered beautifully consistent with two neuroanatomical findings, the first one being that birds have a massive intraventricular telencephalic nuclear neural mass, the dorsoventricular ridge, resembling the relatively much smaller basal ganglia of mammals. Second, the situation seemed in reverse when the pallium (especially the isocortex or dorsal pallium) was considered: Birds have a rather small structure (Wulst) in comparison to the large isocortex of most mammals (Hofman; Nieuwenhuys; Schüz, this volume, Chapters 17, 6, and 16 respectively). However, views changed dramatically as new data became available on the intrinsic neurochemical, hodological, and neurophysiological organization of avian telencephalic areas during the 1960s. Harvey Karten, a pioneer of a new school of comparative neurobiology, proposed that most of the avian dorsoventricular ridge in fact functionally corresponds to isocortex of mammals and that the avian basal ganglia are equally represented by a limited territory at the base of the telencephalon, much like the situation in mammals (Karten, 1969; Shimizu, this volume, Chapter 5). This view is indeed more consistent with the mammal-like, fascinating learning and cognitive capabilites of the vocalizing African gray parrot Alex (Pepperberg, 1990). Cognitive abilities are partially equally well developed in pigeons (Delius, Siemann, Emmerton, and Xia; Macphail, both this volume, Chapters 15 and 13, respectively), which even display a suite of critical anatomical, neurochemical, neurophysiological, and behavioral features together composing an equivalent to a prefrontal cortex of sorts (Güntürkün and Durstewitz, this volume, Chapter 14; compare also Wagner, this volume, Chapter 7, for the special case of the barn owl).

However, as convincing as the neuroanatomical similarities and functional correspondences might be, the question of whether or not they are homologous rests on data to be gained in taxa outside birds and mammals (Northcutt and Kaas, 1995). Only a comparative evaluation, including an outgroup comparison, will eventually tell us which characters might be considered ancestral for amniotes and which are derived for birds or mammals. Not unexpectedly, the situation is complex. Clearly, the avian telencephalic morphotype (i.e., dorsoventricular ridge versus isocortex) is present in other sauropsids (Ulinski, 1983), and many of the diagnostic features that led to the recognition of basic pallial regions, such as a medial (hippocampus; Rehkämper, Frahm, and Mann, this volume, Chapter 9), lateral (olfactory) and dorsal pallium (isocortex), as well as of subpallial divisions (e.g., septum, caudatoputamen, pallidum), are seen in nonavian sauropsids as well (Butler and Hodos, 1996). Although many forebrain features typical of amniotes are recognized meanwhile in anamniotes as well (Wullimann, 1997; Demski and Beaver, this volume, Chapter 10), the search for the ancestral amniote condition remains a matter of controversy. On the motor side (basal ganglia), recent investigations point to a detailed correspondence of structure and function between the amniote and the amphibian brain (Marin et al., 1998; ten Donkelaar, this volume, Chapter 3). However, the ancestral condition for sensory and integrative systems is less well established, and there may be many independently derived features, such as dominance and detailed functional properties of visual subsystems in the bird and mammalian cases (Hodos and Butler, this volume, Chapter 4). An eminent problem for a comparative analysis is that amphibians—the outgroup of sauropsids and mammals—are paedomorphic in their brain morphology to various degrees and might not reliably be used for establishing the ancestral tetrapod condition (Roth et al., 1993; Roth and Wake, this volume, Chapter 8).

A third event that revived comparative neurobiology recently is the new alliance between molecular developmental and evolutionary studies. Many early active regulatory genes and developmental pathways clearly are common to all bilaterian animals and their brains even outside the vertebrates (for a critical review of the relationhip between genes and brain phenotype, see Wullimann, this volume, Chapter 1). There are equally amazing correspondences between invertebrate and vertebrate brains on the anatomical (Strausfeld, this volume, Chapter 12) and the behavioral level (Menzel, Giurfa, Gerber, and Hellstern, this volume, Chapter 11). To return to the vertebrate range, early regulatory gene expression patterns led to the proposition of a new (neuromeric) model of the vertebrate brain *Bauplan* (Puelles and Rubenstein, 1993) that has proven to be highly fruitful in a number of evolutionary questions. In particular, early forebrain gene expression patterns shed new light on the evolution of the amniote brain, challenging Karten's theory outlined previously: The dorsoventricular ridge may be homologous to part of the mammalian amygdala and claustrum rather than to isocortex (Puelles et al., 1999), as similarly proposed based on neural circuitry before (Bruce and Neary, 1995; compare Shimizu, this volume, Chapter 5).

Some of the discussed pervasive similarities between different vertebrate brains (and even between all bilaterian brains) should not be misunderstood to advocate a generality of animal brain organization. A true comparative neurobiology will finally explain not only the commonalities but also the various specializations of vertebrate brains (Nieuwenhuys et al., 1998). The search for the evolutionary emergence of those vertebrate nervous structures subserving complex behavior, including cognition, is far from being completed and the discussion about it continues. The present book lends vivid testimony to that notion.

A SPECIAL POSITION FOR HUMANS?

In traditional Western thinking, humans are situated well above the animal kingdom; they have qualities and capabilities that are either unique or greatly exceed those found in animals. However, during the nineteenth century, it became undeniable that at least with regard to their anatomy, human beings are representatives of one out of many evolutionary lines in the sense that in every aspect of their body they are vertebrates, mammals, primates, and great apes. This certainly was a shocking conclusion: Human beings are animals.

At the same time, most biologists (Charles Darwin being among the notable exceptions) continued to believe that at least with respect to spiritual or cognitive abilities, humans are still far superior to animals: Only humans have mind and consciousness, only humans can think and plan. However, unless these abilities were assumed to be supernatural qualities, they had to be derived from properties of the brain. Thus, a necessary conclusion was that—unlike the rest of the body—the human brain had unique properties in comparison to other vertebrate brains. Many candidates for such unique properties have been discussed, including the absolute or relative size of the entire brain, of the cerebral cortex, of the prefrontal cortex, the possession of speech centers, and the degree of lateralization.

However, even that view has been questioned by modern comparative and evolutionary neurobiology. The human brain appears to be a "typical" primate brain, and while in some respects (e.g., degree of encephalization) it exceeds most, if not all, other animals, no fundamental gap is apparent between the brains of nonhuman animals and *Homo sapiens*. Furthermore, in many lines of invertebrate and vertebrate animals, anatomically and functionally complex and large brains have evolved independently. Thus, the human brain is not even unique in that respect. If we stick to the assumption that the cognitive or spiritual abilities of humans derive from brain properties, three explanations remain: (1) The exact properties that are the basis for unique abilities of the human brain have not yet been discovered; (2) these abilities originate from a special combination of brain properties that taken by themselves are not unique; and (3) there are no unique cognitive or spiritual abilities of humans.

WHAT IS COGNITION?

The term cognition has a long and diverse tradition in philosophy and psychology. Until recent times, this term was often restricted to perceptual, mental, emotional, and volitional states as far as these were connected to awareness and consciousness. Later, the term cognition has been applied to all those psychological functions that exceed simple stimulus-response relationships (D.O. Hebb) and/or refer to the acquisition or generation of meaning (E.C. Tolman). According to a much-cited definition by Ulric Neisser, cognition "refers to all processes by which the sensory input is transformed, reduced, elaborated, stored, recovered and used" (Neisser, 1967). In terms of cognitive psychology, this includes faculties such as pattern recognition, attention, short- and long-term memory, the representation and organization of knowledge (visual images, categorization, semantic organization, etc.), and complex cognitive skills such as language, comprehension and memory for text, problem solving, expertise and creativity, and decision making (Reed, 1996).

In another much-read textbook of cognitive psychology by Anderson (1990), cognition—as the target of cognitive psychology—is identified with the "nature of human intelligence and how people think" and at the same time with "information processing." Of course, the latter interpretation is too narrow and not very useful in the context of comparative neuroscience. First, it is unclear, what is meant by "human intelligence," and it is even more unclear what could be meant by "information processing." There is no logically satisfactory distinction between information processing in the sense of signal processing and in the sense of processing and generation of meaning. While there is a well-elaborated information theory for the former (e.g., that developed by Shannon and Wever; 1949), no such theory exists for the latter. This is most regrettable, because what brains do is not just processing of neural signals, but the generation of meaningful states. One of the greatest challenges of cognitive sciences is the establishment of such a theory of meaning.

It is likewise clear that cognitive psychology concentrates exclusively on human cognitive functions and largely ignores the question of cognitive functions in nonhuman animals. Historically, most authors either believed that there are no cognitive functions in animals at all or that they are beyond consideration. However, in cognitive psychology, cognitive functions were not restricted to states characterized by awareness and consciousness. This approach was an important step forward when compared to a more philosophical understanding of cognition as "highest mental states" necessarily involving consciousness. The recent establishment of the field of cognitive neuroscience is best exemplified by the voluminous book edited by Michael Gazzaniga (1995). However, the book does not give an explicit definition of the term cognition, but the titles of book chapters are largely identical with those of Reed's (1996) book, (i.e., Sensory Systems, Stragegies and Planning, Attention, Memory, Language, Thought and Imagery, Emotion and Consciousness). Since a substantial amount of data presented in these chapters come from animal experiments—mostly from primates and other mammals, with some data from birds and amphibians—it is indirectly implied that cognition is something that is found in animals as well.

Accordingly, in this book the term cognition is used in a wide sense to designate brain functions that exclude only primary sensory and motor functions, autonomic brain functions, reflexes and reflexlike stereotyped behavior. Cognition thus includes such diverse functions as perception, learning, memory, imagination, thinking, expecting, and planning, be they accompanied by consciousness or not. From this follows that cognition is not necessarily restricted to human beings, nor does it presuppose the existence of consciousness.

REFERENCES

Anderson, J.R. (1990) *Cognitive Psychology and Its Implications*. Freeman, New York.
Bruce, L.L., and T.J. Neary (1995) The limbic system of tetrapods: a comparative analysis of cortical and amygdalar populations. *Brain Behav. Evol.* 46:224–234.
Butler, A.B., and W. Hodos (1996) *Comparative Vertebrate Neuroanatomy*. J. Wiley & Sons, New York.
Carroll, R.L. (1988) *Vertebrate Paleontology and Evolution*. Freeman, New York.
Gazzaniga, M. (1995) *The Cognitive Neurosciences*. MIT Press, Cambridge, MA.
Hennig, W. (1966) *Phylogenetic Systematics*. University of Illinois Press, Urbana.
Herrick, C.J. (1956) *The Evolution of Human Nature*. University of Texas Press, Austin.
Karten, H.J. (1969) The organization of the avian telencephalon and some speculations on the phylogeny of the amniote telencephalon. *Ann. N.Y. Acad. Sci.* 167:161–185.
Marín, O., W.J.A.J. Smeets, and A. González (1998) Basal ganglia organization in amphibians: evidence for a common pattern in tetrapods. *Prog. Neurobiol.* 55:363–397.
Neisser, U. (1967) *Cognitive Psychology*. Appleton, New York.
Nieuwenhuys, R., H.J. ten Donkelaar, and C. Nicholson (eds.): (1998) *The Central Nervous System of Vertebrates*. Springer, New York.
Northcutt, R. G. (1981) Evolution of the telencephalon in nonmammals. *Ann. Rev. Neurosci.* 4:301–350.
Northcutt, R.G. (1984) Evolution of the vertebrate central nervous system: patterns and processes. *Am. Zool.* 24:701–716.
Northcutt, R.G., and J.H. Kaas (1995) The emergence and evolution of mammalian isocortex. *Trends Neurosci.* 18:373—379.
Pepperberg, I.M. (1990) Cognition in an African gray parrot (*Psittacus erithacus*): Further evidence for comprehension of categories and labels. *J. Comp. Psychol.* 104:41–52.
Puelles, L., E. Kuwana, E. Puelles, and J.L.R. Rubenstein (1999) Comparison of the mammalian and avian telencephalon from the perspective of gene expression data. *Eur. J. Morphol.* 37:139–150.
Puelles, L., and J. Rubenstein (1993) Expression patterns of homeobox and other putative regulatory genes in the embryonic mouse forebrain suggest a neuromeric organization. *TINS* 16:472–479.
Reed, S.K. (1996) *Cognition. Theory and Applications*, 4th ed. Brooks/Cole Publishing Company, Pacific Grove, CA.
Roth, G. (1994) *Das Gehirn und seine Wirklichkeit, 5. Auflage 1996*. Suhrkamp, Frankfurt.
Roth, G., K.C. Nishikawa, C. Naujoks-Manteuffel, A. Schmidt, and D.B. Wake (1993) Paedomorphosis and simplification in the nervous system of samalanders. *Brain Behav. Evol.* 42:137–170.
Shannon, C.E., and W. Weaver, (1949) *The Mathematical Theory of Communication*. University of Illinois Press, Urbana.
Striedter, G.F. (1997) The telencephalon of tetrapods in evolution. *Brain Behav. Evol.* 49:179–213.
Ulinski, P.S. (1983) *Dorsal Ventricular Ridge. A Treatise on Forebrain Organization in Reptiles and Birds*. John Wiley & Sons, New York.
van Dongen, P.A.M. (1998) Brain size in vertebrates. In R. Nieuwenhuys, H.J. ten Donkelaar, and C. Nicholson (eds.): *The Central Nervous System of Vertebrates*. Springer, New York, pp. 2099–2134.
Wullimann, M.F. (1997) The central nervous system. In D. Evans (ed.): *The Physiology of Fishes*. CRC Press, Boca Raton, pp. 245–282.

PART I

Developmental and Adult Brain Organization in Evolution

Chapter 1

BRAIN PHENOTYPES AND EARLY REGULATORY GENES: THE *BAUPLAN* OF THE METAZOAN CENTRAL NERVOUS SYSTEM

Mario F. Wullimann, University of Bremen, Brain Research Institute and Center for Cognitive Science

INTRODUCTION

In this chapter, I discuss certain aspects of the relationship between cladistically oriented comparative neuroanatomy and developmental neurogenetics. These two fields meet in the scientific search for the biological roots of the metazoan nervous system, one focusing on the phenotypic reconstruction of the basic *Bauplan* and its subsequent evolutionary alterations, the other focusing on the fundamental developmental mechanisms creating that *Bauplan* and its variations. At first sight, one might get the impression that the conclusions reached in these fields are contradictory regarding the early evolution of the central nervous system (CNS). A closer look, however, reveals that this need not be the case. Cladistic methodology is used with great success in comparative biology to reconstruct evolutionary patterns (e.g., ancestral phenotypes and their subsequent alterations). As is detailed later, recent conclusions regarding the ancestral phenotypic condition of the nervous system (e.g., with respect to its segmentation) are often based on patterns of gene expression alone. The message purported here is simple: It may be fatal to ignore the results of an otherwise successful methodology of comparative biology (i.e., cladistics) in the special case of the nervous system because the genes appear to tell us a different story.

Revolutionary studies in molecular genetics during the past decade showed that very many genes relevant for early neural development have orthologues in animals as remotely related as fruit fly and mouse. The *pax-6* gene is a prominent example (Callaerts et al., 1997). Orthologues of this gene are present in most metazoans where they are involved in eye morphogenesis at a hierarchically high level. By gene technology means, *pax-6* can experimentally be interchanged interspecifically and still function within its host developmental program (Halder et al., 1995). This could be taken as proof that all phenotypes produced by the *pax-6* gene are homologous. Thus, despite the fact that developmental programs with the *pax-6* gene at the top have been altered during metazoan evolution and led to similar eyes (*Octopus* eye and vertebrate eye) and dissimilar eyes (insect compound eye and vertebrate camera eye), the resulting phenotypes all become homologous according to the logic outlined above. Thus, usage of the term *homology* apparently is very critical. Wiley (1981) offered a useful definition that excludes convergence and parallelism: *A character of two or more taxa is homologous if this character is found in the common ancestor of these taxa, or, two characters (or a linear sequence of characters) are homologues if one is directly (or sequentially) derived from the other(s)*. As far as their detailed similarity is concerned, the *Octopus* eye and the vertebrate eye represent neither case, but are in fact a case of parallelism. The novelty value of the *pax-6* story is, however, that the underlying developmental program is partly identical in all metazoans and that we can, thus, assume that the *Octopus* eye and the vertebrate eye are homologous to the eye of their last common ancestor.

Even more relevant to the discussion raised here are those regulatory genes (e.g., the homeotic genes of the *Hox* complex) that are expressed in similar spatiotemporal patterns in various developing metazoan animals and control regionalization in the anteroposterior axis, especially during head and CNS formation. Some of these genes involved in head and brain formation can also be functionally replaced among metazoan species (see later discussion). One might conclude that the ancestral condition of the metazoan brain must have been rather complex already, for example, including a multisegmental structure (Reichert and Boyan, 1997). Such direct inference from patterns of gene expression in recent species to an ancestral phenotype is not, however, unchallenged by researchers who find alternative explanations for the same facts (Akam, 1989; Slack et al., 1993). In the following, I attempt to reconcile interpretations resulting from neurogenetics with those resulting from cladistic analysis of the phenotype of the metazoan CNS.

Cladistically oriented neuroanatomy using phenotypic characters reveals that there is indeed a pattern of ancestral (plesiomorphic) neural characters. Some of those may not change during evolution and may be similar and homologous for that reason (non-neural example: many characters in the tetrapod foreleg). Other characters may, however, reach similarity independently (i.e., not inherited from a common ancestor), and they therefore represent *homoplastic* features as far as their similarity is concerned (e.g., bat and bird wings). Again, another class of characters may change (i.e., become divergent in their phenotype) but remain homologous (e.g., reptilian foreleg/bird wing). Note that if, hypothetically, all recent and extinct amniotes had wings, we would, based on the very same data, conclude that bat and bird wings *are* homologous.

Another enlightening example of the relationship of similarity and evolutionary descent is the evolutionary loss of teeth in birds. Developmentally, the formation of teeth can be experimentally induced in chicken (Kollar and Fisher, 1980). Thus, the genetic basis for teeth is retained in birds, although no recent bird species displays teeth in the phenotype. Were a future bird to redevelop teeth phenotypically, these could not be considered homologous to the teeth of other vertebrates. The critical point for an evolutionary biologist here would be the phenotypic absence of teeth in the ancestor of the hypothetical future toothed bird. Thus, vertebrate teeth would not have a continuous history, and the hypothetical *new* bird teeth would be considered a case of parallelism, despite the fact that the genetic basis was largely identical.

It is generally accepted in evolutionary biology that these distinctions are valuable and of great heuristic value. In the foreleg (and teeth) case, we can safely assume that the cascade of interactions of genes and their products is very similar in all vertebrates, and yet nothing is gained for the understanding of tetrapod foreleg evolution by proclaiming that the underlying developmental program and all its subsequent alterations are homologous. This would extend the definition of homology to the point of becoming meaningless (e.g., the fruit fly *Drosophila melanogaster* is homologous to humans because the same ancestral developmental program with certain modifications is at work).

In the following, I first use cladistic analysis on prominent neural characters of extant metazoans in order to identify major events in the evolution of the nervous system. Alternative cladograms are used to exemplify how such hypotheses critically depend on the choice (and, ultimately, the adequacy) of the cladograms used. In light of this analysis, I then, discuss the conclusions regarding the early metazoan head and brain proposed in some of the neurogenetic literature.

COMPARATIVE PHENOTYPIC ANALYSIS OF METAZOAN CENTRAL NERVOUS CHARACTERS

The Cladistic Framework

A common procedure chosen for textbook contributions on the evolution of nervous systems consists of describing these systems along a phylogenetic tree and to assume that, by doing so, a more or less adequate picture of nervous system evolution emerges. Often, two assumptions are implicit to this approach: (1) Animals, and with them nervous systems, evolve as whole organisms in certain directions, and (2) the direction of evolution is always toward increasing complexity (i.e., nervous systems range from simple/primitive to more complex/advanced states in a linear fashion). For example, the urodele CNS retains early ontogenetic character states into adulthood, (i.e., the CNS is *paedomorphic*). The resulting simple morphological appearance of the urodele CNS was often interpreted as representing the ancestral tetrapod condition. The urodele CNS can, however, be demonstrated to represent a case of secondary simplification (Roth et al., 1993; Roth and Wake, this volume, chapter 8), a phenomenon that must remain principally unconsidered as an evolutionary possibility if one uses the two assumptions outlined above.

In contrast to this traditional *scala naturae* approach, the cladistic approach of analyzing CNS evolution has explicit epistemological foundations. Cladistic methodology (Hennig, 1950, 1966), once introduced into comparative neurobiology (Northcutt, 1984), has been widely used to determine the evolutionary polarity of nervous system characters by establishing whether a certain neural character represents an ancestral feature (plesiomorphy) or a derived feature (apomorphy) (Wullimann and Northcutt, 1988; Striedter, 1991; Roth et al., 1993; McCormick,

1992; Wicht and Northcutt, 1992; Northcutt, 1995; Roth and Wullimann, 1996; Wullimann, 1997).

Brain characters, like all characters, are traits that can evolve independently of each other (i.e., brains [or organisms] are not ancestral or derived as entities but represent a mosaic of plesiomorphic and apomorphic characters). The composition of this mosaic can be investigated by determining the evolutionary polarity of neural characters. Before determining the evolutionary polarity of certain characters, one has to accept a phylogenetic hypothesis, commonly proposed in the form of a cladogram. Cladograms are branching diagrams of biological taxa and are based on the hierarchical occurrence of evolutionary novelties (i.e., new characters or *apomorphies*) that characterize one (*autapomorphy*) or several (*synapomorphy*) taxa. A synapomorphy unites two or more taxa relative to other taxa (i.e., *outgroups*). The cladogram requiring the least amount of convergent character transitions is given preference by an argument of parsimony. Consequently, suspected synapomorphies supporting alternative cladograms are interpreted as cases of convergence.

Some of the best corroborated cladograms based largely on *non-neural* characters are used below. Thus, circular reasoning is avoided when the simple tool of outgroup comparison (Hennig, 1966) is applied to analyze the evolutionary polarity of metazoan neural characters with the help of these cladograms. In short, if two taxa show a different character state of a homologous character (e.g., presence vs. absence of lamination in the mesencephalic tectum in frogs compared with salamanders), then the one occurring in the outgroup(s) is considered the plesiomorphic condition (e.g., lamination present in bony fishes and cartilaginous fishes). I cannot list here, but simply cite, the sources for the hierarchy of non-CNS synapomorphies that support the chosen cladograms or the sources for the dendrograms resulting from molecular systematic studies. In many cases, alternative dendrograms exist, and the consequences for phenotypic CNS evolution are discussed.

The backbone of information on the diverse metazoan CNS is the classic monograph by Bullock and Horridge (1965), in addition to a bulk of more recent literature. The following analysis delivers a rough picture of the order, in which new CNS characters (apomorphies) appear to have arisen during metazoan evolution and, thus, highlights some longstanding and controversial topics of CNS evolution.

A Can of Worms: Plathelminths, Nemathelminths, and Nemertines

Although coelenterates display many ancestral eumetazoan characters, they—in contrast to sponges—have neurons forming a peripheral nervous system (nerve plexus), which is by no means simple and is beautifully adapted to guide coelenterate behaviors (Mackie, 1990). Nevertheless, the absence of a CNS may be considered a plesiomorphic condition for eumetazoans. Ring-shaped condensations of neurons at the oral as well as at the aboral animal pole in hydrozoans and scyphozoans as well as longitudinal neuronal aggregations in siphonophores and ctenophores (Grimmelikhuijzen et al., 1996, T.H. Bullock, personal communication) occur as secondary specializations. If one considers ctenophores as a taxon not included in the ceolenterates, the former would already share longitudinal nerve cords as a synapomorphy with plathelminths (platyhelminths), which are conventionally viewed as the outgroup of the remaining bilaterians (see later discussion.).

What are the first steps in evolution toward a CNS in bilaterians? The hypothesis that a CNS evolved independently in each major bilaterian clade from a nerve plexus is extremly unparsimonious. Therefore, if we accept the cladogram of metazoans by Jefferies' (1986, Fig. 1.2), the ancestral condition for the bilaterian CNS (Fig. 1.1, lower panel) is characterized by a brain (supraesophageal or cerebral ganglion) and longitudinal medullary cords, which, by definition, contain nerve fibers as well as neuronal cell bodies. Respective medullary cords of each body side are interconnected by commissures. In many bilaterians, a more superficial nerve plexus (peripheral nervous system) exists in addition; this represents a symplesiomorphy shared with coelenterates. The CNS condition outlined above can be recognized as the plesiomorphic set of characters for bilaterians. In the plesiomorphic condition, the medullary cords may have been located dorsally, ventrally, and laterally as seen in at least some nemertean and plathelminth species, but many wormlike taxa need further comparative analysis. Molluscs retain the basic bilaterian *Bauplan* ancestrally (see later discussion), and so do tentaculates (including bryozoans, phoronids, and brachiopods), albeit in a simplified form. Within deuterostomes, especially chordates, changes in life history complicate the comparative interpretation, but the basic bilaterian *Bauplan* may be concluded to be retained, if somewhat simplified, in some stages of life history of at least some species (see below). In Jefferies, and other cladograms (Fig. 1.2; Fig. 1.7). annelids are the sister group of arthropods. It is, thus, parsimonious to assume that the cerebral and ventral cord ganglia forming a *strickleiter* nervous system originated once for the articulates (Figs. 1.1 and 1.2; see also Fig. 1.7). Within the articulates, only onychophorans must be interpreted as having partially regressed from the more complex *strickleiter* nervous system back to the described ancestral bilaterian condition, because these animals exhibit medullary cords.

An important alternative branching diagram based on a variety of molecular (18S rRNA sequences) and paleontological data has been proposed by Conway Morris' (1993) (Fig.1.3). Similar to Jefferies' cladogram (1986), the clade designated as nemathelminths in Figure 1.3 appears monophyletic and includes nematomorph, nematode, gastrotrich, rotiferan, as well as acanthocephalan species. Also, tentaculates—although only data from brachiopods and phoronids, but not bryozoans, were included—are considered monophyletic (S. Conway-Morris, personal communication), as are arthropods. Protostomes, if plathelminths are included, are polyphyletic. Different from Jefferies' (1986), however, articulates (arthropods and annelids) would represent a polyphyletic group. An outgroup comparison of major CNS characters leads to a similar set of characters typical of the basic bilaterian CNS *Bauplan* outlined above (Fig. 1.3). As in Jefferies' cladogram (1986), deuterostomes (in certain life history stages; see later discussion) would plesiomorphically retain— if somewhat simplified—the basic bilaterian CNS *Bauplan*. Assuming that the *strickleiter* nervous system evolved only once (x in Fig. 1.3), not only onychophorans but additionally the nemertines, the pogonophorans, and the taxon including molluscs

1 Brain Phenotypes and Early Regulatory Genes

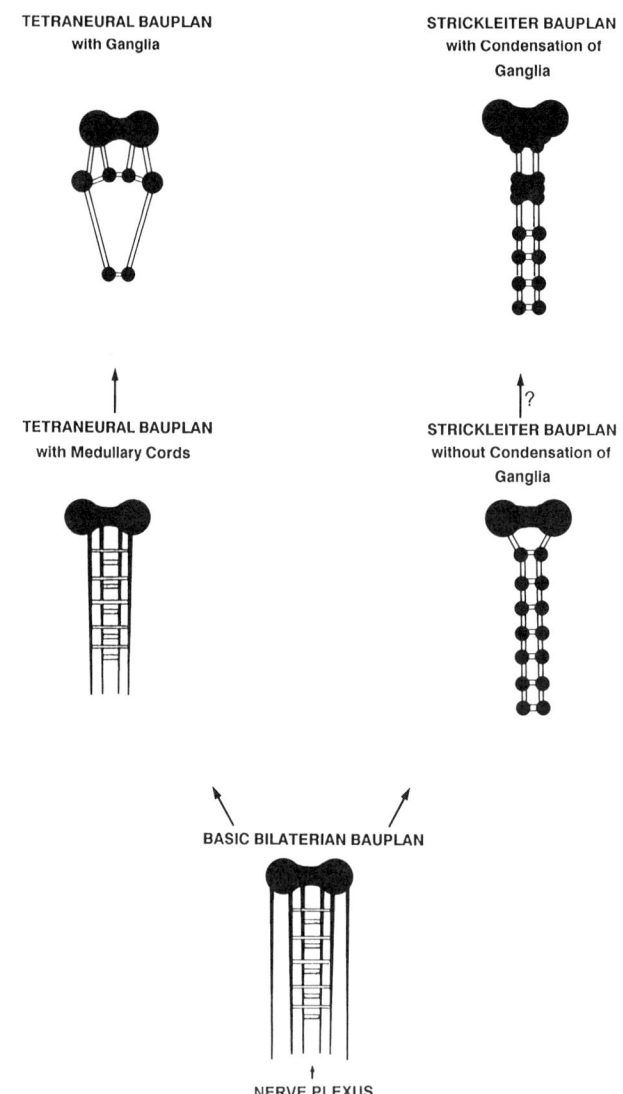

Figure 1.1. Schematic sketches of major invertebrate CNS *Bauplan* characters and an interpretation of the direction of evolutionary change in the molluscan and articulate lineages, respectively. The five drawings represent dorsal views (anterior is at the top) and show the set of likely ancestral CNS characters for certain metazoan taxa. The basic bilaterian *Bauplan* characterizes most nonsegmented wormlike taxa (e.g., plathelminthomorphs, nemathelminths, and nemertines) as well as onychophorans, and it may be ancestral for bilaterians. The tetraneural *Bauplan* with medullary cords is found in aplacophorans, polyplacophorans, and monoplacophorans and is ancestral for molluscs. The tetraneural *Bauplan* with discrete ganglia characterizes gastropods, bivalvians, scaphopods, and cephalopods. The *strickleiter Bauplan* without condensation of ganglia is seen in annelids, kinorhynchs, and tardigrades, and the *strickleiter Bauplan* with condensation of ganglia characterizes all remaining arthropods. Black: CNS contains neuronal somata. White: cords, commissures, or connectives without neuronal somata.

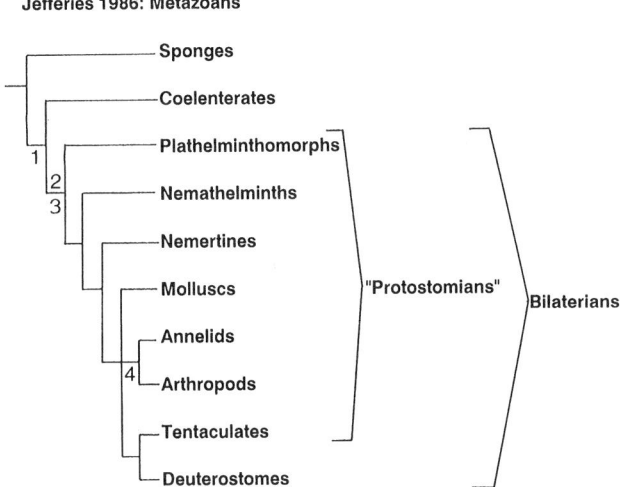

Figure 1.2. Legend on p.26.

(the latter only in their plesiomorphic condition), sipunculids, tentaculates, and the latter's sister taxon (including kinorhynchs and priapulids) would secondarily regress to the plesiomorphic bilaterian CNS state. The segmental organization of ventrally located ganglia in kinorhynchs would, however, be the retention of an ancestral feature. This scenario would, thus, involve at least four cases of secondary simplification. In contrast, the assumption that the *strickleiter* nervous system evolved independently in annelids and arthropods (4 in Fig. 1.3) clearly is more parsimonious in the dendrogram of Conway-Morris' (1993). Accordingly, nemertines, pogonophorans, as well as molluscs, sipunculids, tentaculates, priapulids, and kinorhynchs would retain the plesiomorphic CNS condition; kinorhynchs, however, would independently form segmental ventral cord ganglia. Only onychophorans would be a case of secondary simplification of the *strickleiter* nervous system, as was the case in the first scenario. Importantly, after considering the distribution of neural characters in two dendrograms as different as those of Jefferies' (1986) and of Conway-Morris' (1993), the major conclusion regarding the plesiomorphic condition for the bilaterian CNS remains the same.

Recently, another very different branching diagram for metazoans (Fig. 1.4) has been suggested based on phylogenetic analysis of 18S ribosomal DNS sequences (Halanych et al., 1995; Aguinaldo et al., 1997). In contrast to both Conway-Morris' and Jefferies' dendrograms, tentaculates are now considered to be polyphyletic, but protostomes (if plathelminths are included) are the sister group of deuterostomes and represent a monophyletic taxon here (Fig. 1.4), consisting of two sister taxa, the lophotrochozoans (including molluscs, annelids, inarticulate and articulate brachiopods, phoronids, bryozoans, rotiferans, and plathelminths) and the ecdysozoans (moulting animals; i.e., all arthropod groups plus nematodes, nematomorphs,

1 Brain Phenotypes and Early Regulatory Genes

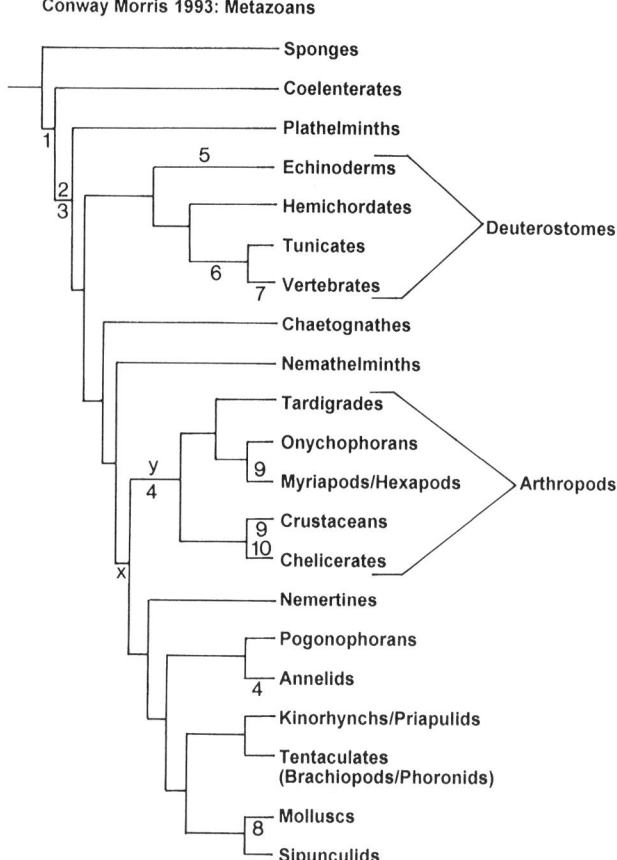

Figure 1.3. Legend on p.26.

kinorhynchs, and priapulids). Thus, nemathelminths are polyphyletic because rotiferans belong to the lophotrochozoa, while nematomorphs and nematodes are ecdysozoans. Furthermore, arthropods do not form a monophyletic taxon (see Fig. 1.4). Morever, the most drastic departure from other branching diagrams is that the plathelminths are not the outgroup of all other bilaterians, but are part of the lophotrochozoa (see Fig. 1.4).

What are the consequences for CNS evolution if neural characters are interpreted in light of this branching diagram? In applying the outgroup comparison, a rather simple set of neural characters resembling much the plesiomorphic metazoan CNS condition outlined above (i.e., an anteriorly located brain and at least some medullary cords) results at the basis of both the lophotrochozoa and the ecdysozoans. Thus, similar to the conclusion reached above, this *Bauplan* likely was present in the last common ancestor of all protostomes as defined in this dendrogram. No clear picture emerges, however, for the ancestral condition of the deuterostome CNS using this

Comparative Phenotypic Analysis of Metazoan Central Nervous Characters 19

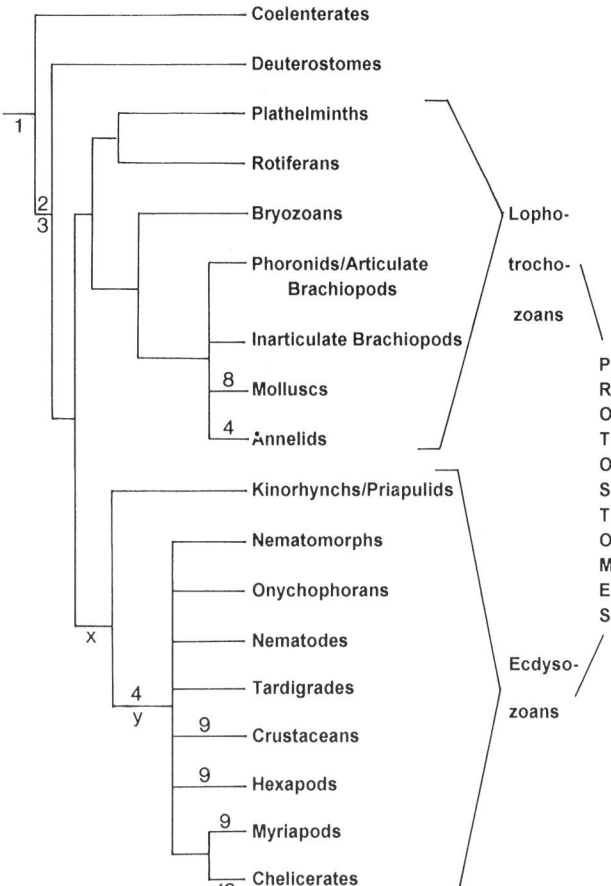

Figure 1.4. Legend on p.26.

dendrogram (see later discussion). A *strickleiter* nervous system—as in Conway-Morris' branching diagram—would have evolved twice, once in annelids and a second time at the base of the node, which includes all arthropods (4 in Fig. 1.4). Following this dendrogram, it is even more unlikely than in that of Conway-Morris' that annelids and arthropods share a segmented ancestor with a *strickleiter* nervous system. Furthermore, many of the ecdysozoan taxa remain cladistically unresolved in this dendrogram, and a *strickleiter* nervous system may well constitute a synapomorphy for tardigrades and arthropods only (Fig. 1.4). Interestingly, onychophorans would then simply retain the plesiomorphic CNS condition, but kinorhynchs would independently form a segmented ventral cord.

1 Brain Phenotypes and Early Regulatory Genes

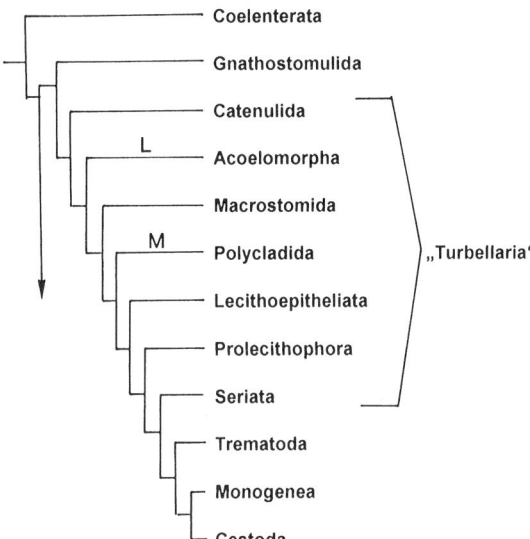

Figure 1.5. Legend on p.26.

Using the presently best corroborated cladogram for plathelminthomorphs (Ehlers, 1985) (Fig. 1.5), the basic bilaterian *Bauplan* must be interpreted to have undergone secondary simplification as well as increasing complexity. Some, but not all, species within the acoelomorphs (Fig. 1.5) exhibit the simplest nervous systems among plathelminthomorphs in that they only have a nerve plexus instead of medullary cords or lack a CNS (including a brain) entirely. These simple nervous systems resemble to a varying degree those of coelenterates. However, the acoelomorphs have two outgroups (the catenulids and the gnathostomulids) with a well-developed CNS, including a brain and longitudinal medullary cords. This strongly suggests that the simple nervous system of some acoelomorphs results from secondary simplification and loss of the bilaterian *Bauplan* (L in Fig. 1.5). Likewise, apomorphic within plathelminthomorphs is the complex brain of some polyclads (*Notoplana*, *Stylochoplana*), which is differentiated into five lobes (M in Fig. 1.5).

The Molluscan Controversy

A survey of CNS characters among the different molluscan taxa (an often used dendrogram is given in Fig. 1.6) reveals that the primitive condition for the molluscan CNS is characterized by a paired supraoesophageal ganglion (cerebral ganglion, brain) and two pairs of longitudinal medullary cords, the more dorsal pair being the pleurovisceral cords and the more ventral pair being the pedal cords (Fig. 1.1, left

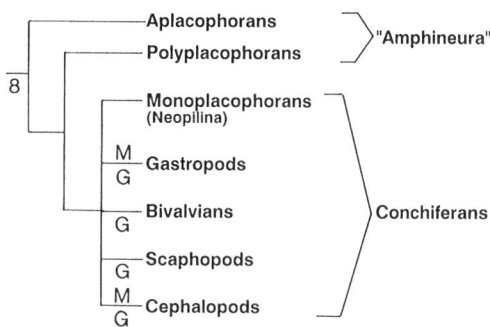

Figure 1.6. Legend on p.26.

middle panel). This is very close to the basic bilaterian *Bauplan* outlined above. A synapomorphy for molluscs, however, is the consolidation to four medullary cords (tetraneural CNS). This tetraneury is evident even in the highly derived CNS of gastropods and cephalopods.

Both aplacophorans and polyplacophorans (sometimes together called amphineurans) exhibit this simple molluscan condition, which appears to be plesiomorphic to the more complex CNS of gastropods, bivalvians, scaphopods, and cephalopods. It has alternatively been suggested, however, that molluscs and articulates share a common ancestor, which was already segmented. This would imply that a *strickleiter* nervous system is plesiomorphic for molluscs as well. An early definition of segmentation by Bateson (1894; reviewed in Jeffs and Keynes, 1990) involves that animals show a repetition of more or less identical body segments (containing most organ systems, including the coelom) along the anteroposterior axis as is seen in annelids or arthropods. Although the term *strickleiter nervous system* is used for the CNS of such overall segmented animals, the term *segmentation* today is universally used for any repetitive structures in metazoans. Do molluscs show signs of segmentation in the CNS or elsewhere?

The discovery of the monoplacophoran *Neopilina galathea* (Lemche, 1957; Lemche and Wingstrand, 1959) first fueled the theory that molluscs were ancestrally segmented. *Neopilina* shows evidence for segmental organization in a limited number of organ systems (eight pairs of muscles, six pairs of nephridia, and five pairs of gills). These organs could as well, however, have been secondarily multiplied—as is commonly assumed for the gills of polyplacophorans—and therefore would not represent remnants of a segmental organization. More importantly, in *Neopilina* there is no evidence for a segmental organization of the gonads, the coelom, and especially the nervous system. The latter conforms to the plesiomorphic molluscan *Bauplan* described above (Fig. 1.1, left middle panel): A cerebral ganglion gives off two pairs of medullary cords (i.e., neurons are distributed continuously inside the cords and are not organized into segmental ganglia as in annelids). The commissures seen in

Neopilina, which appear to have been suggestive of segmentation, also occur in plathelminths and provide no evidence of a *strickleiter* nervous system.

The distribution of central neural characters within molluscs (Fig. 1.6) strongly suggests that a cerebral ganglion with tetraneural medullary cords and commissures is the primitive condition for molluscs. This *Bauplan* is retained in monoplacophorans, and the presence of discrete ganglia instead of medullary cords in other conchiferans clearly is a derived state (Fig. 1.1, left upper panel) and may represent a synapomorphy uniting gastropods, bivalvians, scaphopods, and cephalopods, as already suggested by Hennig (1980). Furthermore, in contrast to annelids, each pair of ganglia in all derived conchiferan taxa is functionally related to a different organ system (e.g., mantle, foot, intestine; G in Fig. 1.6). Thus, there is no single mollusc exhibiting segmental ganglia associated with a segmentally organized body (i.e., a *strickleiter* nervous system). Gastropods and cephalopods in addition develop a multilobed cerebral ganglion (M in Fig. 1.6).

In contrast to Jefferies' cladogram (Fig. 1.2), the dendrograms of Conway-Morris' (1993) (Fig. 1.3) and of Halanych et al. (1995) and Aguinaldo et al. (1997) (Fig. 1.4) suggest that annelids are more closely related to molluscs than to arthropods. As demonstrated above, these dendrograms render it more parsimonious that segmentation and a *strickleiter* nervous system evolved independently in annelids and arthropods and thus offer no reason to assume that molluscs were ancestrally segmented. Again, even considering dendrograms as different as those three, the interpretation of the mollusc CNS system being very close to the basic bilaterian *Bauplan* in its plesiomorphic state and becoming more complex in derived conchiferan taxa remains the most parsimonious scenario.

The Arthropod CNS, Rather Than Being Ancestral to the Vertebrate CNS, is Equally Remote from the Basic Bilaterian *Bauplan* as the Craniate Brain

Often, annelids are viewed as the sister group of arthropods, and the two taxa would form the articulates (Ax, 1984) (Fig. 1.7). Alternatively, as has been suggested based

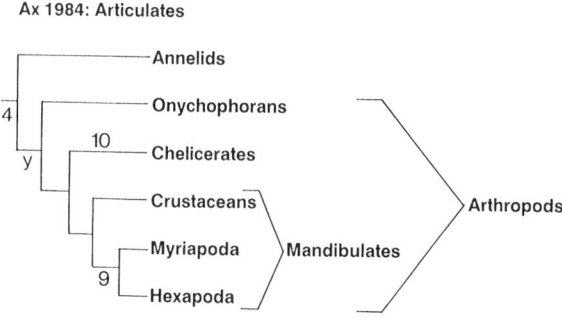

Figure 1.7. Legend on p.26.

on molecular data, annelids are only distantly related to arthropods (Conway-Morris 1993; Halanych et al., 1995; Aguinaldo et al., 1997) (Figs. 1.3 and 1.4). Contrary to the case of the origin of the plesiomorphic bilaterian and mollusc CNS condition as discussed earlier, accepting one dendrogram over the others has profound consequences for the interpretation of CNS evolution in this case.

If annelids are the sister group of arthropods (Fig. 1.7), then a *strickleiter* nervous system undoubtedly evolved only once from the basic bilaterian *Bauplan* in the last common ancestor of articulates and is ancestrally composed of a paired cerebral ganglion located in the first body part, the prostomium (Fig. 1.1, right middle panel). This cerebral ganglion is homologous to the supraoesophageal ganglion present in the basic bilaterian CNS *Bauplan* discussed earlier. The annelid supraoesophageal ganglion is connected via suboesophageal connectives to ventrally located paired cords (e.g., Telkes et al., 1996). These ventral cords (Bauchmark) are not medullary cords, however, but consist of a series of paired ganglia that are interconnected across the midline via commissures and anteroposteriorly via connectives. Ventral cord ganglia are integral parts of body segments, each of which contains a set of almost all organs including a coelomic cavity. In contrast to this plesiomorphic *Bauplan* of the *strickleiter* nervous system, the development of a trilobed cerebral ganglion through elaboration of the single prostomium ganglion (and not through fusion of several segmental ganglia; see later) in some predatory polychaetes (*Nereis, Eunice*) clearly is apomorphic within annelids. Likewise, apomorphic is the simplification of the CNS in hirudineans.

The outlined plesiomorphic condition for the *strickleiter* nervous system is altered in arthropods in many ways from the beginning. An apomorphy of arthropods is that the brain consists of fused ganglia (Fig. 1.1, right upper panel) and thus includes additional parts to the one that would appear to be homologous to the supraoesophageal ganglion located in the prostomium of annelids (which corresponds to the acron of insects). The plesiomorphic number of segmental ganglia contributing to the arthropod brain is controversial, however, because in chelicerates the minimal number is two segments (i.e., a protocerebrum containing at least the prostomium ganglion and a tritocerebrum consisting of the cheliceran ganglion), while in mandibulates (crustaceans, myriapods, and hexapods) the minimal number of brain segments is three (a protocerebrum containing at least the prostomium ganglion, a deutocerebrum consisting of the ganglion of the first antennal segment, and a tritcerebrum consisting of the ganglion belonging to the second antennal segment). The cheliceran segment is often considered to be homologous to the second antennal segment of mandibulates. Thus, the deutocerebrum with its associated segment is sometimes viewed as having been secondarily lost in chelicerates. Recently, based on homeotic gene expression patterns, it has been proposed that the deutocerebrum is present in chelicerates (Telford and Thomas, 1998). Accordingly, the cheliceran segment and the pedipalp segments would be homologous to the first antennal segment of insects/crustaceans and intercalary/second antennal segment of insects/crustaceans (i.e., to the deutocerebrum and tritocerebrum), respectively. If so, chelicerates, crustaceans, hexapods, and myriapods might share ancestrally a trisegmented brain. A recently described Cambrian arthropod with a three-segmented head supports this assumption (Chen et al., 1995). The next outgroup of chelicerates and mandibulates, the onychophorans, are ambiguous in that respect. Although the onychophoran brain is said to arise embryonically from three neuromeres, this gives no final evidence for the fusion of segmental ganglia, because the adult multiple-lobed brain of onychophorans is located in the prostomium (Schürmann, 1987). The brain of annelids as the next outgroup definitely consists of no more than the cerebral ganglion located in the prostomium.

The cladistic position of onychophorans as the outgroup of all other arthropods (except myriapods) has recently been confirmed with molecular data (Ballard et al., 1992). Surprisingly, in this molecular study, myriapods, otherwise considered to be mandibulates (Fig. 1.7) were suggested to represent the outgroup to all other arthropods, including onychophorans. This would support the assumption that the arthropod brain consists of at least three ganglia (that of the prostomium and two additional segmental ganglia) in its plesiomorphic state (y in Fig. 1.7). Also, the brain and medullary cords of onychophorans would, then, clearly be considered secondarily simplified.

In summary, while the whole brain of annelids is homologous to that of their bilaterian outgroups, in the arthropod brain two segmental ganglia—which appear to be homologous to the most anterior ventral cord ganglia of annelids—likely were added to the plesiomorphic bilaterian brain.

Increasing fusion of additional ventral cord ganglia took place independently within chelicerates, crustaceans, and hexapods (Roth and Wullimann, 1996); the most rostral of these condensations is often called *suboesophageal ganglion*. Although within chelicerates the xiphosurans and scorpionids retain many unfused ventral cord ganglia, the more derived arachnids have a single, fused suboesophageal ganglionic mass. Immediately posterior to the pedipalp segment (which might be homologous to the tritocerebral brain segment, see earlier), however, the suboesophageal cell mass always involves the ganglia of leg and of abdominal segments. A similar phylogenetic trend toward increasing fusion of ventral cord ganglia has occurred independently in crustaceans (Sandeman, 1982) and hexapods. In the latter, the suboesophageal ganglion ancestrally consists of the three ganglia belonging to the mandibular, maxillary and labial segments carrying the mouth appendages. Therefore, while at least part of the supraoesophageal ganglion (brain) has a continuous evolutionary history and may be homologous even within all bilaterians, the various manifestations of a suboesophageal ganglion definitely are homoplastic. The composition of the latter is heterogeneous in different bilaterian taxa (e.g., consisting of all ventral cord ganglia in derived arachnids and of only the most anterior three ventral cord ganglia in insects) and clearly evolved independently in annelids, chelicerates, crustaceans, and hexapods/myriapods.

If, alternatively, annelids are only distantly related to arthropods (Figs. 1.3, and 1.4), segmentation and a *strickleiter* nervous system more likely have developed twice independently from the basic bilaterian *Bauplan* (i.e., once in annelids and once in arthropods (see discussion of the molluscan controversy). Furthermore, in Conway-Morris' dendrogram (Fig. 1.3), mandibulates do not form a monophyletic group within the arthropods, and in the dendrograms by Halanych et al. (1995) and

Aguinaldo et al. (1997) not even arthropods are monophyletic. In comparison to Ax's cladogram (1984), neither dendrogram offers a more parsimonious explanation for the emergence of a multisegmented brain in arthropods or ecdysozoans, respectively. The tardigrades however, remain part of the arthropods and ecdysozoans (Figs. 1.3 and 1.4, respectively); they have a relatively simple *strickleiter* nervous system, including a brain consisting of the prostomium ganglion and very few body segments with ventral cord ganglia. Thus, there might be an independently evolved similarity of ancestral features of a *strickleiter* nervous system in the arthropod and in the annelid lineages. Strausfeld (1998), using exclusively neural characters, recently proposed a dendrogram for metazoans naturally explaining neural evolution most parsimoniously (e.g., the *strickleiter* nervous system).

Irrespective of the cladistic position of annelids, there is no good reason for assuming that segmentation and a *strickleiter* nervous system evolved before the divergence of deuterostomes and arthropods, because this would require independent losses of typical overall segmental and *strickleiter* nervous system characters in many taxa. Such an assumption is extremly unparsimonious. Furthermore, the *strickleiter* nervous system (and especially the insect brain) can in no way be considered plesiomorphic to the vertebrate CNS. Both types of CNS are equally apomorphic, and they may have arisen from the same plesiomophic condition (i.e., the bilaterian *Bauplan* as described earlier).

Deuterostome Nervous Systems

Craniates include the myxinoid fishes plus all vertebrates, and the search for the evolutionary roots of the craniate brain is of immense interest to neurobiologists. It is, however, obscured by three problems. The first problem lies in the unsatisfactorily resolved systematic position of deuterostomes, and another two problems relate to their biology.

Although deuterostomes are regarded monophyletic in all three metazoan dendrograms discussed here (Figs. 1.2–1.4), their position could not be more different in each single case. In the first case (Fig. 1.2), they are the sister group of tentaculates and range among the most derived taxa. In the second one (Fig. 1.3), they represent the sister group of all other bilaterians, with the notable exception of the plathelminths, which again form the outgroup to *all* other bilaterians. In the third dendrogram, however, deuterostomes are the outgroup of all other bilaterians, including the plathelminths. This has profound consequences for the interpretation of the phenotypic evolution of the deuterostome CNS.

At first sight, the last mentioned dendrogram allows for a provocative hypothesis. Because echinoderms are generally viewed as the outgroup to all other deuterostomes (an often used dendrogram is shown in Fig 1.8), echinoderms may have retained and altered the radial nervous system seen in their outgroup, the coelenterates. The life history and development of echinoderms, however, clearly show that they are bilaterians and acquire radial symmetry secondarily. Also, using the first and second metazoan dendrograms (Figs. 1.2 and 1.3), a hypothetical adult deuterostome

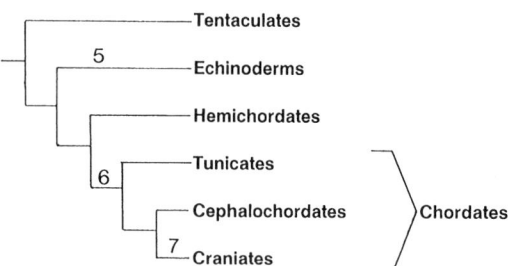

Figures 1.2–1.8. Dendrograms of diverse metazoan taxa as indicated. Numbers refer to neural characters (listed below) and, except for Figure 1.6, are plotted according to the most parsimonious explanation for their evolutionary emergence. 1, neurons; 2, cerebral ganglion; 3, longitudinal medullary cords (maximally: ventral, lateral, dorsal); 4, *strickleiter* nervous system; 5, secondary radial nervous system; 6, dorsal hollow neural tube; 7, craniate brain; 8, consolidation to four medullary cords (tetraneury); 9, ganglia of 1 and 2 antennal segment fused with cerebral ganglion; 10, ganglion of cheliceran segment fused with cerebral ganglion; L, loss of basic bilaterian *Bauplan* in some species; M, multilobed cerebral ganglion in some species; G, discrete ganglia replace medullary cords; x, alternative position for *strickleiter* nervous system (see text); y, alternative to 9 and 10, the brain consists of minimally 3 fused ganglia here.

ancestor would be concluded to exhibit the basic bilaterian CNS *Bauplan* discussed earlier. Thus, echinoderms would simply represent a special case of secondary radial symmetry and loss of the basic bilaterian CNS *Bauplan*. Two other deuterostome issues of importance here are life style (sessility vs. mobility) and life history (larval and adult nervous systems). Many deuterostomes (and tentaculates, for that matter) are characterized by sessility, and this lifestyle appears to be correlated with a certain simplification of the basic bilaterian CNS *Bauplan* as established earlier. This *Bauplan* might alternatively, however, have been simpler initially in bilaterian evolution given that deuterostomes might be the outgroup of all other bilaterians (Fig. 1.4). Clearly, more comparative studies on various critical taxa are needed to decide this question.

The most profound and related problem is that of life history of deuterostomes. Which life history stages and related nervous structures may be homologized at all? Some deuterostomes (echinoderms and hemichordates) have planktonic larvae like many other bilaterians (essentially all taxa belonging to the lophotrochozoa; see Fig. 1.4), which subsequently metamorphose into adults (Schwartz, 1973). If this biphasic sequence is ancestral for bilaterians (which would be strongly supported by the dendrogram shown in Fig. 1.4, but also by that in Fig. 1.3), it is reasonable to look in this two-step life history for how neural tissue is transformed into an adult nervous organ and to homologize nervous tissues or organs during this developmental process among bilaterians. The fact that many bilaterian taxa (the ecdysozoans, Fig. 1.4) have no planktonic larvae may be explained as a loss of that life stage (e.g., in terrestrial arthropods) and thus poses no problem for an evolutionary analysis of adult nervous structures: Although insects skipped that early stage of larval development, we may still compare their adult CNS with that of annelids because these life stages are equivalent.

Garstang (1894) has proposed such a scenario for deuterostomes: A deuterostome ancestor resembling the echinoderm auricularia-larva gave rise to the various adult recent deuterostome forms (the Auricularia hypothesis). Not all recent deuterostome taxa (Fig. 1.8), however, retain a planktonic larva. In tunicates, planktonic larvae are lost, and a more actively mobile larval type comes into existence, displaying a set of characters (i.e., a similar early embryology of the neuroectoderm leading to a hollow dorsal neural tube [neurulation] associated with a notochord and axial musculature) that is commonly recognized as the diagnostic complex of synapomorphies uniting (larval) tunicates, cephalochordates, and craniates (chordates). Garstang's additional hypothesis (1928) of secondary mobility of cephalochordates and craniates through neoteny of a tunicate ancestor is widely accepted and highly plausible (Fig. 1.8). Accordingly, the life history stage that becomes the adult mode of life in cephalochordates and craniates initially is intercalated between the planktonic and adult stages of a chordate ancestor. Thus, although it is reasonable to compare the *adult* CNS of tunicates with that of any other bilaterians, the neural tube of chordates would represent an evolutionary novelty that has no homologue in any other taxon. In fact, the whole tissues giving rise to the adult tunicate body originate from the head portion of the chordate larva; the tail containing the neural tube, chorda, and musculature is resorbed (Jeffery and Swalla, 1997). The primordial neural cells forming the adult nervous system (cerebral ganglion) of tunicates reside as an undifferentiated cell mass in the chordate stage larval head (Koyama and Kusunoki, 1993). The larval neural tube is thus not transformed into the adult tunicate CNS.

What about the collar ganglion (*Kragenmark*) of hemichordates, which, based on a neurulation like development (Schwartz, 1973) during metamorphosis of the planktonic (dipleurula) larva and adult location, has been homologized with the neural tube of chordates? For the latter to be true, one would have to accept that the adult stages of hemichordates (enteropneusts, pterobranchs) correspond to the larval (chordate) and not to the adult stage of tunicates. Although many missing developmental and adult characters (e.g., absence of a chorda and axial musculature) speak against this scenario, more detailed developmental studies are needed in hemichordates. Unfortunately, hemichordates are not treated in a recent excellent comparative embryology text of Gilbert and Raunio (1997). Alternatively, the collar ganglion of hemichordates could be interpreted as the retention of the basic bilaterian cerebral ganglion rather than being homologous to the neural tube of chordates. The existence of extensive ventral and dorsal medullary cords in enteropneusts (Knight-Jones, 1952) supports this interpretation.

Nevertheless, it is possible that a hypothetical deuterostome ancestor had a triphasic life history (i.e., a planktonic larva, a freely mobile chordate larva, and adult stage). In such a scenario, one could compare and eventually homologize the adult nervous system of echinoderms to the chordate CNS. Accordingly, we would have to assume that echinoderms alter their development during the very early chordate larval stage and become radially symmetrical, including their nervous systems. In both hemichordates and echinoderms, one would have to look during metamorphosis of the dipleurula larvae for indications of synapomorphies typical of the chordate larval stage of tunicates, such as neurulation (for echinoderms, compare Heinzeller and

Welsch, this volume, chapter 2). Neurulation clearly does not occur in nervous system development during the metamorphosis of a (trochophora-type) planktonic larva in any other bilaterian. Lacalli (1994) provides clear evidence that the development of the adult plathelminth CNS (i.e., the basic bilaterian *Bauplan*) develops differently and independently from the nervous system (i.e., the ciliary bands) of the planktonic Müller larva. This might well be the ancestral developmental pattern that is altered in deuterostomes where the ciliary bands are assumed to transform into a neural tube as part of the altered ontogeny leading to the chordate larval stage (the Auricularia hypothesis; see earlier). If this ontogenetic change occurred only at the base of the chordates (and not of the deuterostomes), however, the echinoderm and hemichordate nervous systems could be reasonably compared and homologized only with the altered ancestral basic bilaterian *Bauplan*. Because we will probably never know for sure at what stage of deuterostome evolution the triphasic life history originated, this problem may never be resolved satisfactorily. If deuterostomes turned out to be the outgroup of all other bilaterian taxa (Fig. 1.4), they might have had a different life history and consequent development from the beginning.

A rather different scenario of deuterostome evolution is given by Jefferies' (1986), who assumes that hemichordates are the outgroup of both echinoderms and chordates and that a hypothetical sessile hemichordate ancestor gave rise to both echinoderms and (secondarily) motile chordates (calcichordates, mitrates). This hypothetical ancestor is assumed to already have had a craniate-type nervous system (including major craniate brain parts and cranial nerves; compare Fig. 1.9, below). In this scenario, cephalochordates form the outgroup to a tunicata/craniate sister taxon and have a reduced nervous system, and tunicates would have become secondarily sessile again. Because this scenario is based entirely on highly controversial paleontological data, I will not further discuss it regarding CNS evolution.

Conclusion

A phylogenetic analysis at this rather general morphological level suggests that a brain (i.e., cerebral or supraoesophageal ganglion) and medullary cords originated at the base of bilaterian evolution. A cerebral ganglion and medullary cords were retained in an evolutionary continuous history in almost all evolutionary bilaterian lineages, possibly including the deuterostome lineage, and are thus homologous among them. Many alterations of the medullary cords (segmentation, fusion of ganglia) and especially of the cerebral ganglion (expansions, inclusion of other parts of the CNS) can be recognized in various bilaterian lineages independently. Besides many independent increases in complexity of the brain (insects, cephalopods, craniates), simplification must also have occurred (aceolomorph plathelminths, various times within the major arthropod groups, maybe tentaculates and early deuterostomes, salamanders among craniates). Regarding chordate CNS evolution, one must conclude that if Garstang's theory of neoteny is correct, then the craniate brain and spinal cord, as well as the cephalochordate and tunicate neural tube (but not the adult tunicate, hemichordate, and echinoderm nervous systems) are *homoplastic* to all other bilaterian CNS manifestations. If Garstang's Auricularia hypothesis is correct, at least part of the adult echinoderm and hemichordate CNS might be homologous to the craniate CNS.

EARLY GENES IN NEURAL DEVELOPMENT—DO THEY TELL A DIFFERENT STORY?

Development and *Bauplan* of the Vertebrate CNS

The morphogenetic events and molecular genetic mechanisms during early brain development are fundamental for the understanding of the craniate (vertebrate) brain *Bauplan*. In the last decade, two findings marked a considerable progress in that understanding. First, there was a rediscovery of the fact that the conventionally described five parts of the adult vertebrate brain are preceded in early development by a more fundamental segmentation (neuromery) of the brain (Puelles und Rubenstein, 1993) (Fig. 1.9A). Although segmental elements (neuromeres) in the vertebrate brain had already been described morphologically decades ago (e.g., Rendahl, 1924; Bergquist, 1932; Vaage, 1969), the reality of neuromeres was accepted only after modern methods confirmed their existence. For example, there is a spatiotemporally ordered gene expression in the early embryonic vertebrate brain, and certain neuromeres may be characterized by a selective gene expression pattern. A second important realization was that many early developmental genes also occur in invertebrates, for example, in *Drosophila*, where they are expressed in a similar fashion. In the following, I discuss these two major results of developmental biology and point out some consequences for brain evolution.

Classic embryology states that the vertebrate brain traverses a three-vesicle stage by exhibiting a most caudal rhombencephalic vesicle (rhombencephalon, including the metencephalon and myelencephalon), a middle mesencephalic vesicle (mesencephalon), and an anterior prosencephalic vesicle (prosencephalon, including the diencephalon and telencephalon). Subsequently, the brain enters the five-vesicle stage, representing the *Anlage* of the five major adult brain parts. Proponents of the neuromeric theory emphasize that slightly earlier in vertebrate development, a more fundamental compartmentalization along the longitudinal brain axis exists. According to this view, at least the rhombencephalon (hindbrain)—if not the whole brain—is subdivided into a larger number of transitory elements (neuromeres). Originally, the description of neuromeres was largely based on repetitive alternating swelling and narrowing of the rhombencephalic neural tube. These descriptions were, however, viewed as artifactual for most of the twentieth century. Nowadays, the existence of neuromeres in the rhombencephalon (i.e., rhombomeres) is widely accepted because a wealth of modern studies document specifically the segmental organization of the rhombencephalon. For example, cellular clonal restriction within a neuromere, segmental patterning of first neurons and of axonal sprouting, distribution of glia, and certain gene expression patterns respect rhombomere boundaries

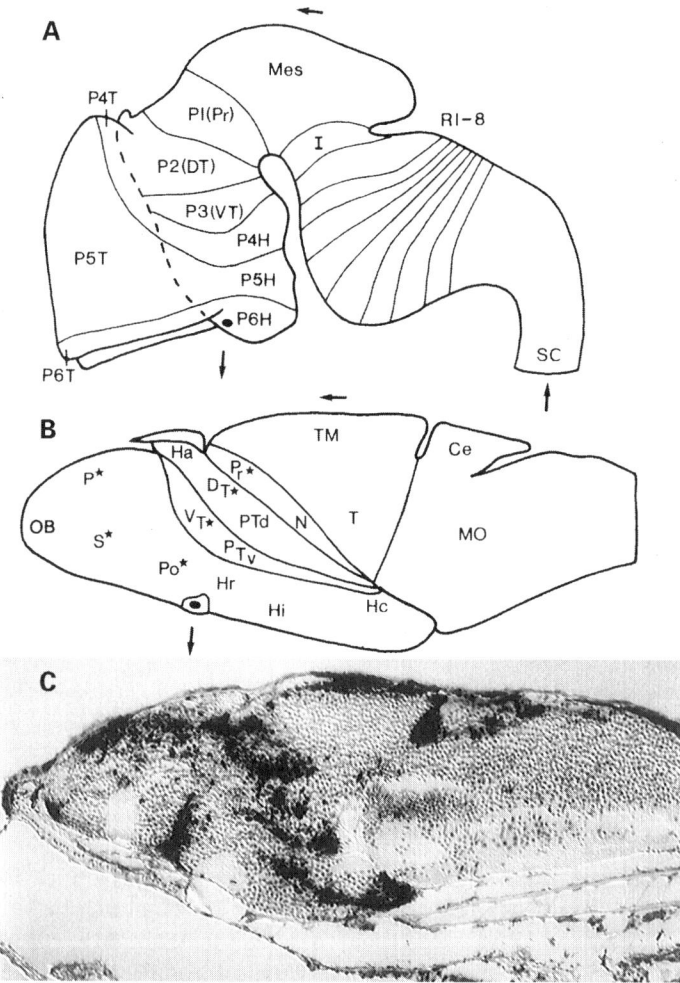

Figure 1.9. (*A*) Sagittal view of neuromeric model for the amniote brain (Puelles and Rubenstein, 1993). (*B*) Its application to the zebrafish forebrain, based on the distribution of proliferation zones (Wullimann and Puelles, 1999). (*C*) A sagittal section of the zebrafish brain immunoreacted for the proliferation marker proliferating cell nuclear antigen. In A and B, arrows designate axis of neural tube and black dot indicates the optic chiasma. The distribution of distinct proliferation centers in the mesencephalon and forebrain is consistent with the prediction of the neuromeric model that three prosomeres exist rostral to the mesencephalon, that is, the pretectal one (P1), the dorsal thalamic one (P2), and the ventral thalamic one (P3), because each of those prosomeres has separable alar plate (Pr*, DT*, VT*) and basal plate (N, PTd, PTv) proliferation zones. More rostrally (telencephalon and hypothalamus), the distribution of proliferation zones is not apparently related to the existence of three additional prosomeres in the zebrafish. Ce, corpus cerebelli; DT, dorsal thalamus; Ha, habenula; Hc, Hi, Hr, caudal, intermediate, rostral hypothalamus; I, isthmic segment; Mes, mesencephalon, MO, medulla oblongata; N, proliferation in the area of the nucleus of the medial longitudinal fascicle; OB, olfactory bulb; P*, pallial proliferation zone; Po*, preoptic proliferation zone; Pr, pretectum; PT, posterior tuberculum area; PTd, PTv, dorsal, ventral proliferation zone of PT; R1–8 rhombomeres 1–8, P4H, P5H, P6H, prosomeres 4–6 (hypothalamic portions); P4T, P5T, P6T, prosomeres 4–6 (telencephalic portions); S*, subpallial proliferation zone; SC, spinal cord; T, tegmentum, TM, tectum mesencephali; VT, ventral thalamus.

(Holland und Hogan, 1988; Lumsden, 1990; Wilkinson and Krumlauf, 1990). There is also evidence for neuromeres in the prosencephalon (forebrain, including the diencephalon and telencephalon), for example, clonal restriction of cell lines (Figdor and Stern, 1993). Also, the spatial pattern of early proliferation activity in the forebrain supports a prosomeric organization (Wullimann and Puelles, 1999), at least in the posterior forebrain (P1–P3 in Fig. 1.9B,C). The most comprehensive neuromeric model of Puelles und Rubenstein (1993) currently available integrates data from classic morphology with those mentioned from modern studies, including gene expression data.

According to this model, the vertebrate brain consists of an isthmic (0), plus seven to eight more caudally located rhombencephalic neuromeres (rhombomeres), a mesencephalic neuromere (mesomere), and six more neuromeres in the prosencephalon (prosomeres; Fig. 1.9A; note that the direction of numbering is opposite for rhombomeres and prosomeres). The essentials of the model are as follows. Early emerging neural tube flexures tilt the originally straight longitudinal axis of the brain, for example, the axis of the prosencephalon deviates almost 180° in comparison to that of the rhombencephalon. Thus, the rostral tip of the brain lies in the region of the optic chiasma (black dot located at the lower—not the left—boundary of the prosencephalon in Fig. 1.9A,B). According to this longitudinal axis, the ventral prosencephalon is directly adjacent to the ventral rhombencephalon. Furthermore, the diencephalon is not simply the caudal part of the forebrain as was assumed in some traditional models. In the neuromeric model, the diencephalon consists of three complete prosomeres plus the basal parts of three additional prosomeres. The first, most caudal prosomere (P1) includes the pretectum; the rostrally adjacent second prosomere (P2) includes the epithalamus and dorsal thalamus; and the third prosomere (P3) represents the ventral thalamus of the traditional diencephalon. The ventral portions of the final three more rostral prosomeres represent the hypothalamus (P4H–P6H in Fig. 1.9A) and complete the diencephalon. Accordingly, the hypothalamus is—with respect to the above-mentioned longitudinal axis—not considered to be the ventral part of the classic diencephalon, but is in fact the ventral part of those prosomeres giving rise to the telencephalon with their dorsal portions (P4T–P6T). The telencephalon (as well as the hypothalamus), in contrast to the remaining four classic brain parts, is not composed of complete neural tube segments, because it lacks their respective basal parts.

These differences between the neuromeric and traditional models in the allocation of brain regions based on a newly defined axis are of great importance because the ventral and dorsal aspects of the neural tube differ in many respects (e.g., origin of motor and sensory neurons from ventral basal and dorsal alar plates, respectively). In the neuromeric model, the classically recognized four longitudinal zones of the neural tube (i.e., from ventral to dorsal, the floor, basal, alar, and roof plates) do all continue up to the anterior end of the brain in the area of the optic chiasma. This newly defined longitudinal and assumed overall segmental organization of the brain of the neuromeric model is of great predictive value and is open to be tested on all levels of investigation.

Early Regulatory Genes and Neuromeres in the Vertebrate Bain

The activity of many early regulatory genes has been visualized meanwhile by in situ hybridization in various metazoans. The homeotic genes of the *Hox-B* complex are expressed (e.g., in portions of the CNS and other segmental organs; Graham et al., 1989; Hunt and Krumlauf, 1992) in an anteroposterior order that parallels their spatial order in the vertebrate genome. More specifically, the anterior ends of different *Hox-B* gene expression domains proceed successively more rostrally in a graduated manner and respect various rhombomere boundaries (Fig. 1.10). The expression domains of certain additional early regulatory genes, such as *Krox-20*, outline particular rhombomeres and thus respect anterior as well as posterior rhombomere boundaries. Such evidence is generally taken as the most convincing proof for the existence of rhombomeres. Like many other early regulatory genes, the *Hox* genes are transcription factors, (i.e., their proteins interact with the DNA and regulate the expression of various other genes). Thus, many of those regulatory genes not only act early in embryogenesis, but, by activating the transcription of other genes, they also stand at a rather high hierarchical level during development. Evidently, such genes have a much greater influence on the phenotype than structural genes, for example.

The anteroposteriorly graduated rostral expression boundaries of various *Hox-B* genes (as well as the expression of other genes) lead to a particular combination of gene activity in each rhombomere during early brain development that is thought to specify the interrhombomeric differences and, consequently, the adult hindbrain phenotype. Indeed, experimental extension of the expression domains of particular *Hox-B* genes to more anterior rhombomeres results in an altered phenotype of those rhombomeres (Krumlauf, 1993). While the homeotic genes of the *Hox* complex have no expression domains in the prosencephalon (forebrain) and mesencephalon, various other regulatory genes containing a homeobox (e.g., *Otx, Emx, Dlx, Gbx*; Simeone et al., 1992, Boncinelli et al., 1993; Bulfone et al., 1993; Millet et al., 1996) are expressed there during early development (Fig. 1.10). The caudal expression boundary of *Otx2* coincides with the midbrain–hindbrain boundary, and the rostral one extends almost to the tip of the brain in the region of the optic chiasma (see earlier discussion). Because *Otx1* as well as various *Emx* and *Dlx* genes have more restricted expression domains, a graduated expression pattern similar to that formed by the *Hox-B* genes in the rhombencephalon is observed in the midbrain and forebrain. Studies on null mutants and their phenotypes (*Otx2*: Bally-Cuif and Boncinelli, 1997; *Emx1/2*: Yoshida et al., 1997) also suggest similar functions to that of the *Hox* complex (i.e., anteroposterior patterning of the more anterior brain parts).

Early Regulatory Genes and the Insect CNS

Orthologues of many regulatoy genes now known in vertebrates were discovered much earlier in the fruit fly *D. melanogaster*. The homeotic (HOM) genes of the

Early Genes in Neural Development—Do They Tell A Different Story? 33

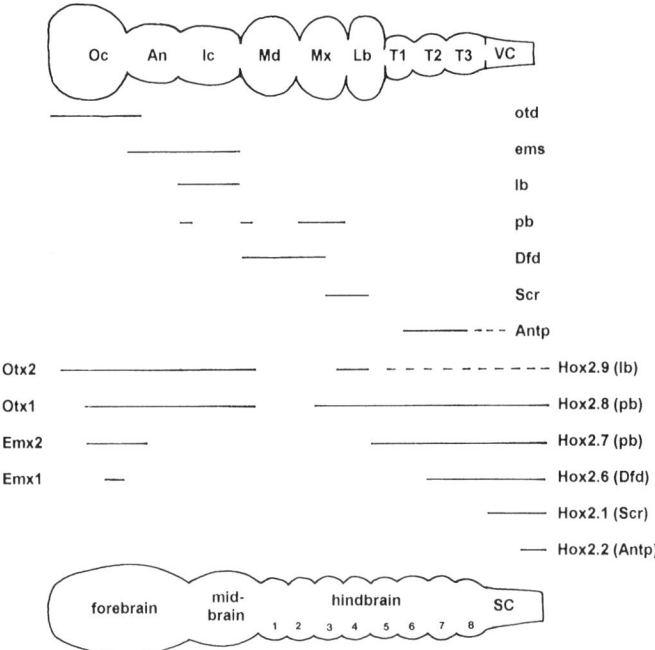

Figure 1.10. Early regulatory gene expression in insect CNS (*upper panel*) and vertebrate CNS (*lower panel*). Numbers indicate vertebrate rhombomeres. *Drosophila* genes: *Antp*, antennapedia; *Scr*, sex combs reduced; *Dfd*, deformed; *pb*, proboscipedia. Abbreviations for other genes are mentioned in the text. *Drosophila* head segments and corresponding neuromeres: Oc, ocular (protocerebrum); An, antennal (deutocerebrum); Ic, intercalary (tritocerebrum); Md, mandibular; Mx, maxillary; Lb, labium segment (last three containing together the subesophageal ganglion); T1–3, thoracal (leg) segments (and respective ganglia); VC, ventral cord ganglia. Note that whereas in vertebrates the anterior ends of expression domains of various *Hox* genes are exactly *at* the respective interrhombomeric boundaries (as summarized by Holland et al., 1992), some corresponding expression boundaries in the insect brain mark *hemisegments* (posterior boundary of *Dfd*, both boundaries of *Scr* and *Antp*; after Kaufman et al., 1990; *pb* after Telford and Thomas, 1998). The expression domains of vertebrate forebrain and midbrain genes (*Otx*, *Emx*) are not definitively assigned to neuromeric boundaries here. However, both *Otx1* and *Otx2* expressions appear to respect posteriorly the midbrain/hindbrain boundary. Although a small, most rostral telencephalic area is spared, the *Otx2* expression extends considerably more rostral than that of *Otx1*. Rostrally, the *Emx2* expression is coextensive with that of *Otx1*, and, posteriorly, it respects the P3/P2 boundary. *Emx1* has a more restricted, exclusively telencephalic expression domain (after Boncinelli et al. 1993). In insects, brain segment boundaries definitively are transgressed by the *otd*, but not the *ems*, expression pattern; in contrast to vertebrates, the two genes additionally have a more posterior CNS expression domain, that is, in the ventral cord ganglia (Reichert and Boyan, 1997).

antennapedia–ultrabithorax complex, which determine segment identity (Gehring, 1987), correspond to the *Hox-B* cluster of vertebrates. As in the latter, the corresponding homeotic genes of insects are aligned in the genome in the same order as they are phenotypically expressed in the anteroposterior axis. In particular, these orthologues in *Drosophila* of the vertebrate homeotic *Hox-B* genes have a similar spatial expression pattern in parts of the CNS when compared with vertebrates (Graham et al., 1989; Carroll, 1995). Equally striking, there are orthologues of vertebrate *Otx* and *Emx* genes in *Drosophila* (i.e., *orthodenticle* [*otd*], and *empty spiracles* [*ems*], respectively), and their expression domains are restricted to anterior head neuromeres (supraoesophageal—but not suboesophageal—ganglion), and ventral cord ganglia (Finkelstein and Perrimon, 1990; Finkelstein and Boncinelli, 1994; Reichert and Boyan, 1997; compare Fig. 1.10). For example, the *otd* gene is expressed in the protocerebrum and in the most anterior part of the deutocerebrum, and the *ems* gene is expressed in deuto and tritocerebrum (Reichert and Boyan, 1997). Accordingly, *Drosophila* that are mutant in *otd* or *ems* lack a protocerebrum or deuto- and tritocerebrum, respectively (Hirth et al., 1995). Furthermore, the vertebrate *Otx1* and insect *otd* genes can functionally replace each other in development; murine *Otx1* null mutants with an introduced *Drosophila otd* gene show a rescued brain phenotype (Acampora et al., 1998; Leuzinger et al., 1998).

Apparently, many such early regulatory genes were present in the last common ancestor of vertebrates and insects. What does this fact reveal about the brain and CNS phenotype in that ancestor? An often heard argument is that those similarities in sequence, genomic and phenotypic alignment, and developmental function of early regulatory genes support the early existence of a complex brain and its concomitant developmental plan, which were both established only once close to the origin of bilaterians (Reichert and Boyan, 1997). The similarities sometimes are further taken as evidence that segmentation (including that of the CNS) is plesiomorphic for bilaterians or even that a *strickleiter* nervous system may be plesiomorphic for the vertebrate brain and spinal cord (De Robertis, 1997). Major differences in the *Bauplan* of the vertebrate and insect CNS exist, however, and are in need of explanation. Nobody would ever mistake an insect brain for a vertebrate brain. Furthermore, comparative analyses of phenotypic CNS evolution (even on a rather general level; see earlier) are in contradiction to easily digestable generalizations such as the often heard "There is but one animal".

Phylogenetic Interpretation of Molecular Genetic and Phenotypic Data

How can these apparently contradictory conclusions drawn from neurogenetic or morphological data be reconciled? Let us consider brain subdivisions of various invertebrates. The three divisions of the insect brain (i.e., proto-, deuto-, and tritocerebrum) are phylogenetically best interpreted as having arisen through fusion of originally similar, segmentally organized ventral cord ganglia. In contrast, the trilobed brain of some polychaete annelids (*Eunice*; see earlier) most likely did *not* arise through fusion of segments, but originated through elaboration of the prostomium ganglion. Its anteroposterior specification may, however, turn out to be controlled by orthologous homeobox genes active in the insect brain. Indeed, in one leech species (which does not have a trilobed brain), the *otd*- orthologue *Lox22–Otx* is reported to be expressed mainly in the prostomium ganglion (Bruce and Shankland, 1998). The developmental program that creates a trilobed brain in polychaetes would nevertheless have a different evolutionary history in insects and annelids (i.e., the feature of having a trilobed brain could not be considered homologous in the phenotype).

Let us return to the *Hox-B* example. Craniates and, consequently, vertebrates had a rhombencephalon from the very beginning, and the said genes were undoubtedly always involved in the development of this most caudal brain part. The most rostral expression domains of the orthologous genes of the antennapedia–ultrabithorax complex of insects are in the suboesophageal ganglion, which subserves the various segmental mouth appendages, as well as in the tritocerebrum and most posterior part of the deutocerebrum, but *not* in the protocerebrum (Fig. 1.10). More specifially, only *labial* and *proboscipedia* are expressed in the brain proper (trito- and deuto- cerebrum); the other genes of the complex have more posterior expression domains in the suboesophageal ganglion. The latter is multisegmental and includes the ganglia of the mandibular, maxillary, and labium segments. Rogers and Kaufman (1996) recently confirmed the assumption of a six-segmented insect head with the *engrailed* protein pattern, although a total of seven segments (with an additional segment anterior to the ocular or protocerebral one) has also been suggested (Schmidt-Ott et al., 1994). If one accepts that the suboesophageal ganglion is the posterior part of the insect brain, then an outgroup comparison renders evidence that such a ganglion did not exist in the outgroups of insects in the primitive condition, but corresponds with several ganglia of the ventral chain that are not included in the brain. In the phenotype that represents a functional morphological unit (i.e., the brain has functions different from those of ventral cord ganglia), the expression domains of the said homeotic genes would not be included in the brain proper in the ancestral condition. Of course, the said homeotic genes can be expected to have expression domains in the corresponding ventral chain ganglia of these arthropods as well. Consistent with this, Kourakis et al. (1997) showed the anterior *Hox* gene expression boundary between ventral cord ganglia and prostomium ganglion in an annelid (i.e., leech). Although these corresponding ventral chain ganglia are homologous to the respective segmental ganglia forming the insect suboesophageal ganglion, they are not homologous when their phenotypic aspect of being a brain part is considered. These anterior ventral chain ganglia that correspond with the insect suboesophageal ganglion are not part of the brain in the plesiomorphic condition in arthropods, let alone in articulates, coleomates, or bilaterians.

Thus, the *Hox-B*/HOM cluster likely was always expressed in the posterior brain of vertebrates, but not in that of arthropods, because the latter included the suboesophageal ganglion only later into the cephalic portion of the CNS. With respect to the brain of the hypothetical ancestor of vertebrates and insects, this means that the corresponding (orthologous) genes were expressed in the CNS, but that a complex rhombencephalon or suboesophageal ganglion did not yet exist. *This shows that one cannot directly derive a particular phenotype from the mere existence and orderly expression of early regulatory genes. Molecular genetic and phenotypic data need to be jointly interpreted in a phylogenetic context.* A prediction to be made here is that plathelminths and nemertines should express orthologues of the *Hox-B* cluster in the anterior part of the medullary cords, but not in the cerebral ganglion.

The expression domains of the *Otx/otd* and *Emx/ems* genes are certainly located within the brain proper of both vertebrates and insects. A brain containing three to four neuromeres is unlikely, however, to be ancestral for all arthropods, and it certainly is not plesiomorphic for articulates or even protostomes (see earlier). Genes specific for the anterior brain would be expected to be expressed in these phenotypes within the most rostral ventral cord ganglia as well. Actually, in the leech, *labial*, which is the *Hox* gene with an expression domain extending into the trito- and deutocerebrum in *Drosophila*, is expressed up to the most rostral ventral cord ganglia, but not in the cerebral ganglion (Kourakis et al., 1997). In contrast, vertebrates had a constant anteroposterior sequence of brain parts from the very beginning, including a fore-, mid-, and hindbrain. It is therefore highly unlikely that the last common ancestor of arthropods and vertebrates had a *brain* showing a graduated gene expression pattern characterized anteriorly by *Otx/Emx* orthologues and posteriorly by *Hox* orthologues.

Current evidence suggests that the above discussed genes of the HOM/*Hox* complex and the *Otx/otd* and *Emx/ems* genes form part of the *zootype* and are plesiomorphic for metazoans (Slack et al., 1993), including those that are not segmentally organized. This suggests that homeotic genes are not strictly correlated with the phenotypic context in which they were first discovered (i.e., segment specification and *strickleiter* nervous system). Ten years ago, Akam (1989) proposed that the reason why genes of the HOM/*Hox* complex are highly conserved in bilaterian phylogeny is that they are plesiomorphically responsible for positional information, that is, for the anteroposterior specification of the bilaterian body, and that these already existing genes were used and further elaborated on by arthropods in the context of an overall segmentation (including that of the CNS) and by vertebrates in relation to segmental (metameric) organ systems independent of each other. This scenario certainly is more parsimonious than one assuming that segmentation as seen in articulates (including a *strickleiter* nervous system) was plesiomorphic for bilaterians because many phenotypic alterations leading away from an initially segmented body would then have to be invoked in all bilaterians outside the articulates.

CONCLUSION

The number of known early active genes common to invertebrates and vertebrates that share similar developmental functions is growing almost daily, and this fact is amazing in itself. There is clear evidence that genes of the HOM/*Hox* complex and eventually the *Otx/Emx* genes and their orthologues (and many other early regulatory genes) existed and were active in the developmental context of anteroposterior specification at the outset of bilaterian history. Head segmentation (including that of the CNS) of insects and neuromeres in vertebrates is a special case of this specification. The fact that these genes originated very early in bilaterian evolution does not mean that any recent phenotype (e.g., a complex insect or vertebrate brain or the *strickleiter* nervous system) may be deduced to be plesiomorphic for bilaterians or for the last common ancestor of vertebrates/insects.

Conversely, it was a misinterpretation of comparative morphology that seemingly convergent phenotypes (i.e., our example of a complex hindbrain or suboesophageal ganglion) *must* have a different genetic basis. Obviously, data from all levels of investigation have to be jointly interpreted. The stunning universality in developmental function and systematic distribution of many early regulatory genes is only half of the lesson to be learned here. The second half of the lesson is that modifications of the spatiotemporal interactions of these genes are *the* major force in creating new phenotypes on which natural selection might act in evolution. Comparative neurobiologists by definition are interested in evolutionary history and, thus, must still care about the study of phenotypic CNS evolution that complements—but cannot be replaced by—the fascinating molecular genetic work.

ACKNOWLEDGEMENTS

I am greatly indebted to the grandseigneur of comparative neurobiology, Theodore H. Bullock, for taking the time to make many illuminating remarks after reading a more immature version of the manuscript and Gerhard Roth for many clarifying discussions on metazoan brain evolution. I also thank Catherina G. Becker, Thomas Becker, Thomas Müller, Gerhard Roth, and Gerhard Schlosser for making valuable comments on the manuscript. The author's research is supported by the DFG (Wu 211/1–4).

REFERENCES

Acampora, D., V. Avantaggiato, F. Tuorto, P. Barone, H. Reichert, R. Finkelstein, and A. Simeone (1998) Murine *Otx1* and *Drosophila otd* genes share conserved genetic functions required in invertebrate and vertebrate brain development. *Development* 125:1691–1702.

Aguinaldo, A.M.A., J.M. Turbeville, L.S. Linford, M.C. Rivera, J.R. Garey, R.A. Raff, and J.A. Lake (1997) Evidence for a clade of nematodes, arthropods and other moulding animals. *Nature* 387:489–493.

Akam, M. (1989) *Hox* and HOM: homologous gene clusters in insects and vertebrates. *Cell* 57:347–349.

Ax, P. (1984) *Das phylogenetische System*. G. Fischer, Stuttgart.

Ballard, J.W.O., G.J. Olsen, D.P. Faith, W.A. Odgers, D.M. Rowell, and P.W. Atkinson (1992) Evidence from 12S ribosomal RNA sequences that onychophorans are modified arthropods. *Science* 258:1345–1348.

Bally-Cuif, L., and E. Boncinelli (1997) Transcription factors and head formation in vertebrates. *BioEssays* 19:127–135.

Bateson, W. (1894) *Materials for the Study of Variation*. Macmillan, London.

Bergquist, H. (1932) Zur Morphologie des Zwischenhirns bei niederen Wirbeltieren. *Acta Zool. (Stockh.)* 13:57–304.

Boncinelli, E., M. Gulisano, and V. Broccoli (1993) *Emx* and *Otx* homeobox genes in the developing mouse brain. *J. Neurobiol.* 24:1356–1366.

Bulfone, A., L. Puelles, M.H. Porteus, M.A. Frohmann, G.R. Martin, and J.L.R. Rubenstein (1993) Spatially restricted expression of *Dlx-1, Dlx-2 (Tes-1), Gbx-2* and *Wnt-3* in the embryonic day 12.5 mouse forebrain defines potential transverse and longitudinal segmental boundaries. *J. Neurosci.* 13:3155–3172.

Bullock, T.H., and G.A. Horridge (1965) *Structure and Function in the Nervous Systems of Invertebrates.* W.H. Freeman and Co., San Francisco.
Bruce, A.E.E., and M. Shankland (1998) Expression of the head gene *Lox22-Otx* in the leech *Helobdella* and the origin of the bilaterian body plan. *Dev. Biol.* 201:101–112.
Callaerts, P., G. Halder, and W.J. Gehring (1997) *Pax-6* in development and evolution. *Annu. Rev. Neurosci.* 20:483–532.
Carroll, S.B. (1995) Homeotic genes and the evolution of arthropods and chordates. *Nature* 376:479–485.
Chen J.-Y., G.D. Edgecombe, L. Ramsköld, and G.-Q. Zhou (1995) Head segmentation in Early Cambrian *Fuxianhuia*: implications for arthropod evolution. *Science* 268:1339–1343.
Conway-Morris, S. (1993) The fossil record and the early evolution of the metazoa. *Nature* 361:219–225
De Robertis, E.M. (1997) The ancestry of segmentation. *Nature* 387:25–26.
Ehlers, U. (1985) *Das Phylogenetische System der Plathelminthes.* G. Fischer, Stuttgart.
Figdor, M.C., and C.D. Stern (1993) Segmental organization of embryonic diencephalon. *Nature* 363:630–634.
Finkelstein, R., and E. Boncinelli (1994) From fly head to mammalian forebrain: the story of *otd* and *Otx. TIG* 10:311–315.
Finkelstein, R., and N. Perrimon (1990) The *orthodenticle* gene is regulated by *bicoid* and *torso* and specifies *Drosophila* head development. *Nature* 346:485–488.
Garstang. W. (1894) Preliminary note on a new theory of the phylogeny of the Chordata. *Zool. Anz.* 17:122–125.
Garstang, W. (1928) The morphology of the Tunicata, and its bearings on the phylogeny of the Chordata. *Q. J. Microsc. Sci.* 72:51–187.
Gehring W.J. (1987) Homeo boxes in the study of development. *Science* 236:1245–1252.
Gilbert, S.F., and A.M. Raunio (1997) *Embryology.* Sinauer, Sunderland, MA.
Graham, A., N. Papalopulu, and R. Krumlauf (1989) The murine and *Drosophila* homeobox gene complexes have common features of organization and expression. *Cell* 57:367–378.
Grimmelikhuijzen, C.J.P., I. Leviev, and K. Carstensen (1996) Peptides in the nervous system of cnidarians: structure, function and biosynthesis. *Int. Rev. Cytol.* 167:37–89.
Halanych, K.M., J.D. Bacheller, A.M.A. Aguinaldo, S.M. Liva, D.M. Hillis, and J.A. Lake, (1995) Evidence of 18S ribosomal DNA that the lophophorates are protostome animals. *Science* 267:1641–1643.
Halder, G., P. Callaerts, and W.J. Gehring (1995) Induction of ectopic eyes by targeted expression of the *eyeless* gene in *Drosophila. Science* 267:1788–1792.
Hennig, W. (1950) *Grundzüge einer Theorie der phylogenetischen Systematik.* Deutscher Zentralverlag, Berlin.
Hennig, W. (1966) *Phylogenetic Systematics.* University of Illinois Press, Urbana.
Hennig, W. (1980) *Taschenbuch der Speziellen Zoologie* (Bd. 1), Harri Deutsch, Frankfurt.
Hirth, F., S. Therianos, T. Loop, W.J. Gehring, H. Reichert, and K. Furukubo-Tokunaga (1995) Developmental defects in brain segmentation caused by mutations of the homeobox genes *orthodenticle* and *emtpy spiracles* in *Drosophila. Neuron* 15:769–778.
Holland, P.W.H., and B.L.M. Hogan (1988) Expression of homeobox genes during mouse development: a review. *Genes Dev.* 2:773–782.
Holland, P., P. Ingham, and S. Krauss (1992) Mice and flies head to head. *Nature* 358:627–628.
Hunt, P., and R. Krumlauf (1992) *Hox* codes and positional specification in vertebrate embryonic axes. *Annu. Rev. Cell. Biol.* 8:227-256.
Jefferies, R. P. S. (1986) *The Ancestry of the Vertebrates.* British Museum (Natural History), Dorset Press, Dorchester.
Jeffery, W.R., and B.J. Swalla (1997) Tunicates. In S.F. Gilbert and A.M. Raunio (eds.): *Embryology.* Sinauer, Sunderland, MA, pp. 331–364.
Jeffs, P.S., and R.J. Keynes (1990) A brief history of segmentation. *Semin. Dev. Biol.* 1:77-87.
Kaufman, T.C., M.A. Seeger, and G. Olsen (1990) Molecular and genetic organization of the *Antennapedia* gene complex of *Drosophila melanogaster. Adv. Genet.* 27:309–362.
Knight-Jones, E.W. (1952) On the nervous system of *Saccoglossus cambrensis* (Enteropneusta). *Philos. Trans. R. Soc. Lond. Biol.* 236:315–363.
Kollar, E.J., and C. Fisher (1980) Tooth induction in chick epithelium: expression of quiescent genes for enamel synthesis. *Science* 207:993–995.

References

Kourakis, M.J., V.A. Master, D.K. Lokhorst, D. Nardelli-Haefliger, C.J. Wedeen, M.Q. Martindale and M. Shankland (1997) Conserved anterior boundaries of *Hox* gene expression in the central nervous system of the leech *Helobdella*. *Dev. Biol.* 190:284–300.

Koyama, H., and T. Kusunoki (1993) Organization of the cerebral ganglion of the colonial ascidian *Polyandrocarpa misakiensis. J. Comp. Neurol.* 338:549–559.

Krumlauf, R. (1993) *Hox* genes and pattern formation in the branchial region of the vertebrate head. *Trends. Genet.* 9:106–112.

Lacalli, T.C. (1994) Apical organs, epithelial domains, and the origin of the chordate central nervous system. *Am. Zool.* 34:533–541.

Lemche, H. (1957) A new living deep-sea mollusc of the Cambro-Devonian class Monoplacophora. *Nature* 179:413–416.

Lemche, H., and K.G. Wingstrand (1959) The anatomy of *Neopilina galathea* Lemche, 1957 (Mollusca, Trybliciacea). *Galathea Rep.* 3:9–72.

Leuzinger, S., F. Hirth, D. Gerlich, D. Acampora, A. Simeone, W.J. Gehring, R. Finkelstein, K. Furukubo-Tokunaga, and H. Reichert (1998) Equivalence of the fly *orthodenticle* gene and the human *OTX* genes in embryonic brain development of *Drosophila. Development* 125:1703–1710.

Lumsden, A. (1990) The cellular basis of segmentation in the developing hindbrain. *TINS* 13:329–339.

Mackie, G.O. (1990) The elementary nervous system revisited. *Am. Zool.* 30:907–920.

McCormick, C.A. (1992) Evolution of central auditory pathways in anamniotes. In D.B. Webster, R.R. Fay and A.N. Popper (eds.): *The Evolutionary Biology of Hearing* Springer, New York, pp. 323–350.

Millet, S., E. Bloch-Gallego, A. Simeone, and R.-M. Alvarado-Mallart (1996) The caudal limit of *Otx2* gene expression as a marker of the midbrain/hindbrain boundary: a study using *in situ* hybridization and chick/quail homotopic grafts. *Development* 122:3785–3797.

Northcutt, R.G. (1984) Evolution of the vertebrate central nervous system: patterns and processes. *Am. Zool.* 24:701–716.

Northcutt, R.G. (1995) The forebrain of gnathostomes: in search of a morphotype. *Brain Behav. Evol.* 46:275–319.

Northcutt, R. G.., and C. Gans (1983) The Genesis of Neural Crest and Epidermal Placodes: a Reinterpretation of Vertebrate Origins. *Q. Rev. Biol.* 58: 1–28.

Puelles, L., and J. Rubenstein (1993) Expression patterns of homeobox and other putative regulatory genes in the embryonic mouse forebrain suggest a neuromeric organization. *TINS* 16:472–479.

Reichert, H., and G. Boyan (1997) Building a brain: developmental insights in insects. *TINS* 20:258–264.

Rendahl, H. (1924) Embryologische und morphologische Studien über das Zwischenhirn beim Huhn. *Acta Zool. (Stockh.)* 5: 241–344.

Rogers, B.T., and T.C. Kaufman (1996) Structure of the insect head as revealed by the EN protein pattern in developing embryos. *Development* 122:3419–3432.

Roth, G., K.C. Nishikawa, C. Naujoks-Manteuffel, A. Schmidt, and D.B. Wake (1993) Paedomorphosis and simplification in the nervous system of samalanders. *Brain Behav. Evol.* 42:137–170.

Roth G., and M.F. Wullimann (1996) Evolution der Nervensysteme und der Sinnesorgane. In J. Dudel, R. Menzel, R.F. Schmidt (eds.): *Neurowissenschaft: Vom Molekül zur Kognition.* Springer-Verlag, Berlin, pp. 1–31.

Sandeman, D.C. (1982) Organization of the central nervous system. In H.L. Atwood and D.C. Sandeman (eds.): *The Biology of the Crustacea*, vol. 3, Academic Press, New York, pp. 1–61.

Schmidt-Ott, U., M. González-Gaitán, H. Jäckle, and G.M. Technau (1994) Number, identity, and sequence of the *Drosophila* head segments as revelaed by neural elements and their deletion patterns in mutants. *Proc. Natl. Acad. Sci. U.S.A.* 91:8363–8367.

Schürmann, F.-H. (1987) Histology and ultrastructure of the onychophoran brain. In A.P. Gupta (ed.): *Arthropod Brain.* J. Wiley & Sons, New York, pp. 159–180.

Schwartz, V. (1973) *Vergleichende Entwicklungsgeschichte der Tiere.* G. Thieme Verlag, Stuttgart.

Simeone, A., D. Acampora, M. Gulisano, A. Stornaiuolo, and E. Boncinelli (1992) Nested expression domains of four homeobox genes in developing rostral brain. *Nature* 358:687–690.

Slack, J.M.W., P.W.H. Holland, and C.F. Graham (1993) The zootype and the phylotypic stage. *Nature* 361:490–492.

Strausfeld, N.J. (1998) Crustacean-insect relationships: the use of brain characters to derive phylogeny amongst segmented invertebrates. *Brain Behav. Evol.* 52:186–206.

Striedter, G.F. (1991) Auditory, electrosensory and mechanosensory lateral line pathways through the forebrain in channel catfishes. *J. Comp. Neurol.* 312:311–331.

Telford, M.J., and R.H. Thomas (1998) Expression of homeobox genes shows chelicerate arthropods retain their deutocerebral segment. *Proc. Natl. Acad. Sci. U.S.A.* 95:10671–10675.

Telkes, I., M. Csoknya, P. Buzás, R. Gábriel, J. Hámori, and K. Elekes (1996) GABA-immunoreactive neurons in the central and peripheral nervous system of the earthworm, *Lumbricus terrestris* (Oligochaeta, Annelida). *Cell Tissue Res.* 285:463–475.

Vaage, S. (1969) The segmentation of the primitive neural tube in chick embryos (*Gallus domesticus*). A morphological, histochemical and autoradiographical investigation. *Ergebn. Anat. Entwicklungsgesch.* 41:1–88.

Wicht, H., and R.G. Northcutt (1992) The forebrain of the Pacific hagfish: a cladistic reconstruction of the ancestral craniate forebrain. *Brain Behav. Evol.* 40:25–64.

Wiley, E.O. (1981) *Phylogenetics*. J. Wiley & Sons, New York.

Wilkinson, D.G., and R. Krumlauf (1990) Molecular approaches to the segmentation of the hindbrain. *TINS* 13:335–339.

Wullimann, M.F. (1997) The central nervous system. In D. Evans (ed): *The Physiology of Fishes.* CRC Press, Boca Raton, pp. 245–282.

Wullimann, M.F., and R.G. Northcutt (1988) Connections of the corpus cerebelli in the green sunfish and the common goldfish: a comparison of perciform and cypriniform teleosts. *Brain Behav. Evol.* 32:293–316.

Wullimann, M.F., and L. Puelles (1999) Postembryonic neural proliferation in the zebrafish forebrain and its relationship to prosomeric domains. *Anat. Embryol.* 199:329–348.

Wurmbach, H. and R. Siewing (1985) *Lehrbuch der Zoologie, vol. 2: Systematik.* G. Fischer, Stuttgart.

Yoshida, M., Y. Suda, I. Matsuo, N. Miyamoto, N. Takeda, S. Kuratani, and S. Aizawa (1997) *Emx1* and *Emx2* functions in development of dorsal telencephalon. *Development* 124:101–111.

Chapter 2

THE ECHINODERM NERVOUS SYSTEM AND ITS PHYLOGENETIC INTERPRETATION

Thomas Heinzeller and Ulrich Welsch, University of Munich, Department of Anatomy

Perhaps the most enigmatic part of any echinoderm is its nervous system. – Smiley (1994)

INTRODUCTION

One echinoderm class (crinoids = sea lilies and feather stars) includes some species that live permanently attached to the substrate. For reasons of their palmlike appearance (Fig. 2.1a), the entire class is also called *pelmatozoa*. In contrast, all remaining echinoderms move freely and thus are termed *eleutherozoa*. Four eleutherozoan classes (Fig. 2.1b–e) can be distinguished: asteroids (sea stars), ophiuroids (brittle stars), echinoids (sea urchins), and holothuroids (sea cucumbers).

Echinoderms are deuterostomians with a secondary pentaradial structure. In contrast to hemichordates and chordates, a dorsal neural tube seems to be absent in echinoderms or to be masked by the pentaradial symmetry of the body. Generally, the echinoderm nervous system consists of a circumoral nerve ring situated in the body's center and five radial cords that extend into those body parts that we usually call *arms*. This basic design apparently exists at three body levels, which is commonly (see Hyman, 1955) considered to reflect the existence of three nervous subsystems, including an ectoneural, hyponeural, and aboral nervous subsystem.

By looking somewhat closer to the different echinoderm classes, the concept of a threefold nervous supply does not satisfy in every respect. First, the three subsystems are quantitatively represented very differently in the five extant echinoderm classes (Table 2.1). Second, the term *hyponeural subsystem* summarizes structures that probably are not homologous among each other, because the hyponeural nerves of crinoids are located in the connective tissue whereas those of noncrinoids lie within coelomic epithelia. Third, important groups of neurons and fiber plexus, whose

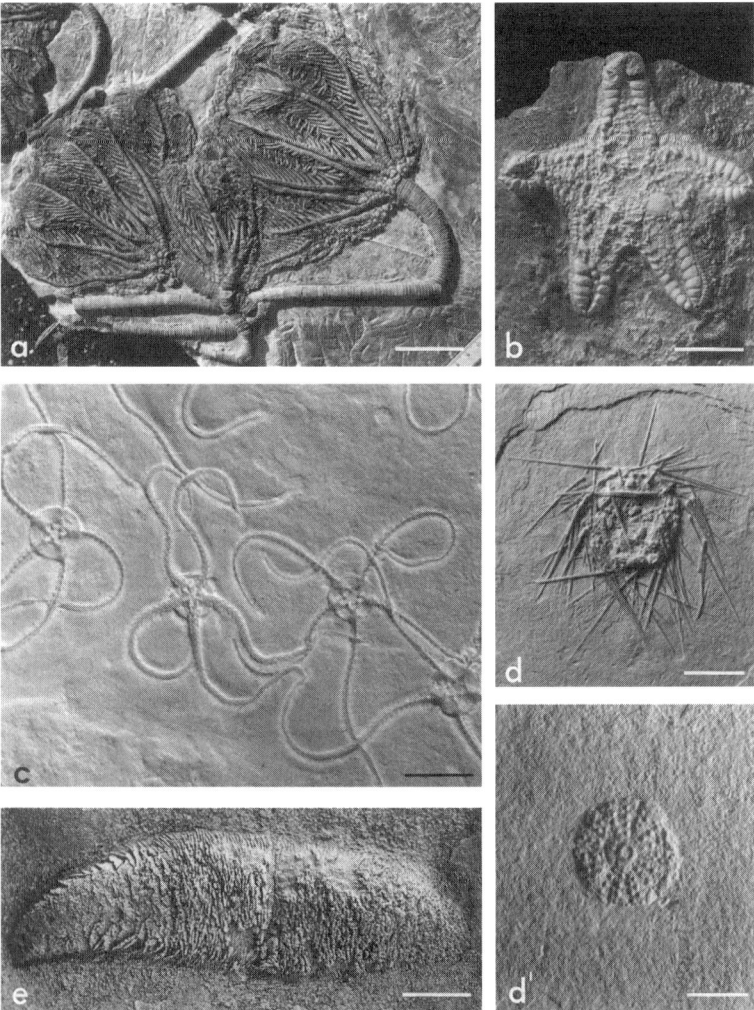

Figure. 2.1. Fossilized mesozoic echinoderm specimens already demonstrating (despite minor taphonomy-based deformations) each class-specific habitus. (a) *Traumatocrinus*, a Triassic sea "lily" (crinoid) from South China, displaying a crown with richly branched arms and a stalk composed of low cylindrical ossicles, free of cirri. (b) A Triassic asteroid, *Trichasteropsis*, showing the typical shape of a pentamerous sea "star", found close to Crailsheim, Bathe Wuerttemberg. (c) Jurassic ophiuroids of the genus *Sinosura* from Hienheim, Bavaria; note the central flat disklike body and the long crinkling arms ("serpent" stars). (d, d´) Jurassic echinoids from Brunn, Bavaria, belonging to the genus *Pseudodiadema*, fossilized with its covering spines (d, sea "urchin") or after loosing their spines (d´, aboral view with the genital plate in the center where the five rays meet). (e) Middle Triassic holothuroid *Strobilothyone* from Catalonia, Northern Spain, oral end on the right; note the cylindrical body, which led to the trivial name sea "cucumbers". Bars = 5 cm in a; 1 cm in b, d, and d´; 2´mm in c; and 4 mm in e. For these photographs, we are deeply indepted to Dr. Hans Hagdorn, Muschelkalkmuseum Hagdorn Ingelfingen (a and b); Dr. Martin Röper, Monika and Klaus Rothgänger, and Dr. Hansjörg Wunderer, Naturkundemuseum Ostbayern, Regensburg (c, d, and d´); and Dr. Andrew B. Smith, The Natural History Museum London, and Dr. Jaume Gallemí, Museu de Geologia Barcelona (e).

Table 2.1: Semiquantitative Comparison of the Conventionally Accepted Three Nervous Subsystems (Hyman, 1955) as Found in the Different Classes of Echinoderms.

		Ectoneural	Hyponeural	Aboral
Pelmatozoa	Crinoidea	+	$+^a$	$+++^a$
Eleutherozoa	Asteroidea	+++	$+^b$	$+^{b,c}$
Eleutherozoa	Ophiuroidea	+++	$++^b$	$-^{b,e,f}$
Eleutherozoa	Echinoidea	+++	$+^{b,c}$	$+^{a,c}$
Eleutherozoa	Holothuroidea	+++	$++^{b,d}$	$-^{b,e,f}$

^{a}Located in the connective tissue (i.e., subepithelial) ^{b}Located in a coelothelial epithelium ^{c}Possibly associated only with Aristotle's lantern ^{d}Possibly without circumoral ring commissure ^{e}Associated mainly with gonads ^{f}Not detectable at the light microscopical level; some neurons present at the electron microscopic level.

details escaped the classic light microscopic period, are missing in this classification (e.g., the juxtaligamental cells or the coelothelial plexus). Fourth, the intraepithelial intestinal nervous system does not fit properly into any of the three subsystems. Last, not least, the concept conceals the leading role that the ectoneural part plays in all eleutherozoan echinoderms. In the pelmatozoan crinoids, however, this subsystem quantitatively stands clearly behind the dominant aboral subsystem.

Nowadays, any classification of the echinoderm nervous system should consider the restriction of nervous tissue to two tissue compartments: basiepithelial and subepithelial. However, the well-established terms *ectoneural, hyponeural*, and *aboral* are used later, in their topographic sense—being aware that the terms *hyponeural* and *aboral* describe different neuronal populations in pelmatozoa and eleutherozoa, respectively.

The basiepithelial compartment comprises ectoneural (in the epidermis), entoneural (in the intestinal epithelium), and coelothelial (in the coelomic epithelia) neurons and fibers. The subepithelial compartment includes all neurons and their processes that are located in the connective tissue space, in particular the juxtaligamental cells (all classes; see Postmetamorphotic Nervous System: Common Features, later), the special hyponeural and aboral subsystem of crinoids, and the gonadal innervation in echinoids (Kawaguti, 1965).

It is difficult to ascribe unequivocally the traditional three subsystems to the basiepithelial or subepithelial compartment. The innervation of the intestine may demonstrate the difficulties. The traditional aboral system is told to supply the gut by a basiepithelial entoneural plexus (some authors use *entoneural* and *aboral* as synonymes) as well as the gonads by a basiepithelial coelothelial plexus (except echinoids; see earlier), but nowhere are the two plexuses interlinked, and thus they cannot be considered one common subsystem. Furthermore, the innervation of the intestinal wall may include not only the basiepithelial entoneural plexus mentioned before but also subepithelial neurons, for example, in several ophiuroids (Schechter and Lucero, 1968), and basiepithelial neurons in the coelomic lining. In this case, the latter could be appointed either to the aboral subsystem (as is usually done with the basiepithelial plexus in the coelothelial lining of gonads) or to the hyponeural subsystem located in the same somatocoelomic epithelium.

In addition, a modern evaluation of the echinoderm nervous system also should respect the prevalence of the ectoneural nerves and commissures. This is not only because of the morphological predominance of the ectoneural nerves but also because of the assessment of this system as a possible homologue of the neural plate of chordates. This view is based on the observation that orthologues of those regulatory genes that in acrania (Holland, 1996) and vertebrates control the development of the metameric trunk and its neural tube up to the third rhombomere are present also in echinoderms. Consequently, the so-called arms in echinoderms may be considered homologous with the chordate trunk, including the posterior head region: The data suggest that "pentamery may have arisen from the multiplication of an ancestral axis into five radii" (Popodi et al., 1998b; see Questions of Symmetry, later). The present study is a contribution to the question whether the nervous system of the echinoderms does indeed fit into this concept and whether the available data allow comparisons with the chordate nervous system

DESCRIPTION OF NERVOUS SYSTEMS

Larval Nervous System

Most authors agree that the nervous system of the echinoderm larva does not preform the adult nervous system, which during metamorphosis obviously develops de novo. The larval system is confined to the larval demands and is largely resorbed and replaced at metamorphosis (Chia and Burke, 1978). Therefore, it is only briefly described here.

The larval system is built up predominantly and maybe exclusively by basiepithelial neurons (Lacalli and West, 1993). These cells either aggregate to form ganglia in the anterior region, in the upper or lower lips of the mouth, and at the bases of larval arms or are found scattered throughout the epidermis and in the esophageal wall.

The most prominent part of the basiepithelial neurons, however, which has been demonstrated in all echinoderm larvae studied thus far both by electron microscopy and by histochemical methods (glyoxylic acid or anti-dopamineserum), is embedded in the ciliary bands. These basiepithelial (Burke, 1978) axon tracts, misleadingly described as underlying the ciliary bands, are formed by dopaminergic neurons and their processes (Burke et al., 1986; Bisgrove and Burke, 1987; Nakajima, 1987; Nezlin et al., 1991). In addition, serotonergic neurons have been identified in certain of the abovementioned ganglia (e.g., Chee and Byrne, 1997), as have neurons with GABA (Bisgrove and Burke, 1987) or the SALMFamide S1 (Beer and Thorndyke, 1998).

The anterior (apical) region, which presumably "is not needed for anything essential in the adult" (Lacalli, personal communication), and the ciliary nervous system with its associated ganglia will be completely replaced during metamorphosis. The formation of the adult nervous system obviously starts anew from undifferentiated tissue. Also, other important adult structures do not develop before metamorphosis (e.g. the radial hydrocoelomic channels). There is an enormous capacity of generating new structures inherent in echinoderm larvae. This is extremely expressed in asexually budding asteroid brachiolariae, as observed in a high percentage of tropical and subtropical populations (Bosch et al., 1989; Jaeckle, 1994).

Postmetamorphotic Nervous System: Common Features

Nerve cells. The perikarya of most nerve cells of echinoderms are very small, measuring a few micrometers in diameter; only certain exceptional cells reach about 20 µm in diameter (e.g., in the apical ganglion of *Leptometra phalangium*). As far as can be concluded from their shapes, the cells belong to the bipolar and multipolar types. The cytoplasm of the perikarya usually contains moderate amounts of mitochondria, groups of rough endoplasmic reticulum cisterna, and a medium-sized Golgi apparatus. Perikarya with abundant small dense-cored granules occur regularly among the ordinary neuronal perikarya.

Most nerve cell processes are extremely thin, down to 0.1 µm in diameter, but some "giant" fibers, measuring 10 or 20 µm in diameter, are described in ophiuroids (Byrne, 1994) and may occur also in other classes. Giant fibers usually contain abundant microtubules. The thin fibers form numerous varicosities, several micrometers thick, in which often different types of vesicles are colocalized (small and electron lucent; dense cored; large and electron dense). Classic synapses have been observed (*Echinus esculentus:* Peters and Campbell, 1987; *Stylometra spinifera:* Heinzeller and Welsch, 1994; *Ophiura ophiura:* Byrne, 1994), but occur very rarely, as do gap junctions, the morphological indicators of electric coupling. Thus the usual way of interneuronal transmission is that of a chemical synapse, which lacks conspicuous subsynaptic structures.

Juxtaligamental cells (Fig. 2.4c), a special kind of nerve cell, contribute to an echinoderm-specific functional system unique in the animal kingdom: the mutable connective tissue, which is characterized by the ability to rapidly change the degree of collagenous softness/stiffness (reviewed by Wilkie, 1996). The entire connective tissue of echinoderms is not of the mutable type, but many ligaments (or fibrils in the body wall of holothuroids) that support the entire animal's posture or the position of arms and spines are. The idea of the transmission of nervous impulses to juxtaligamental cells, which in turn regulate the physicochemical state of the mutable collagenous tissue, was first formulated by Wilkie (1978). Biochemical aspects of the phenomenon of mutability were recently analyzed (Erlinger et al., 1993; Thurmond et al., 1998; Trotter et al., 1996). Several types of juxtaligamental cells were described in species of all echinoderm classes. In comparison with other neurons, their somata are large and of approximately spherical shape. Juxtaligamental cells may form ganglionlike aggregates, often lined up along the border of ligaments (Fig. 2.3d). They extend one or more thick, granule-rich processes into interfibrillar spaces, where they presumably release secretory products, either de-stiffening the ligaments for changing posture or even inducing autotomy (e.g., Holland and Grimmer, 1981).

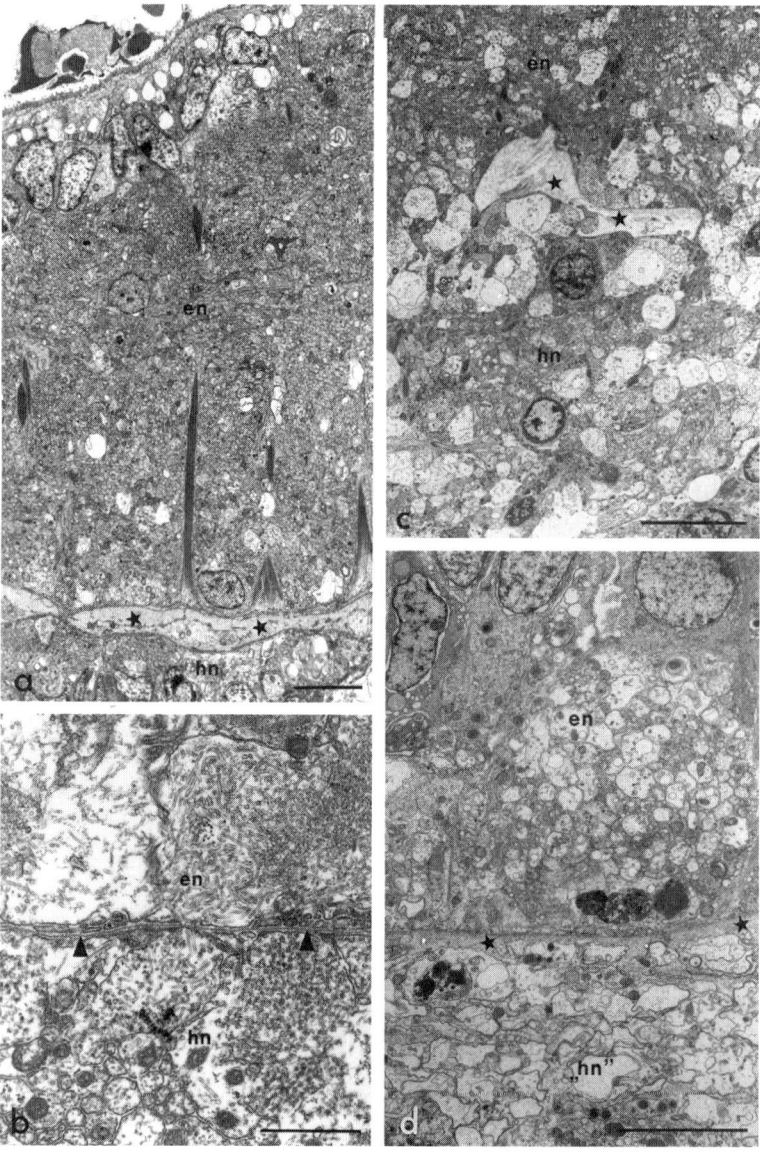

Figure 2.2. Transmission electron microscopy histology of the ectoneural (en) cord and the hyponeural (hn) plexus in the radial arm nerves of *Asterias rubens* (Asteroidea) (a), *Ophiura ophiura* (Ophiuroidea) (b), *Holothuria scabra* (Holothuroidea) (c), and *Antedon bifida* (Crinoidea) (d). (*a*) The two subsystems are separated by a connective tissue lamella (stars). (*b*) Conversely, the border is maximally reduced to a common basal lamina (arrowheads). (*c*) The situation shown here suggests that the separating connective tissue lamella (stars) is traversed freely by nerve fibers of the two plexuses. (*d*) The unique crinoid situation is shown where the basiepithelial ectoneural cord is next to the subepithelial hyponeural ("hn") nerve. The hyponeural subsystem of a, b, and c lies basiepithelially in the somatocoelomic epithelium, while the hyponeural subsystem of crinoids is directly embedded in the connective tissue (stars). Bars = 5 μm in a) and d), 10 μm in c) and 1 μm in b).

Description of Nervous System 47

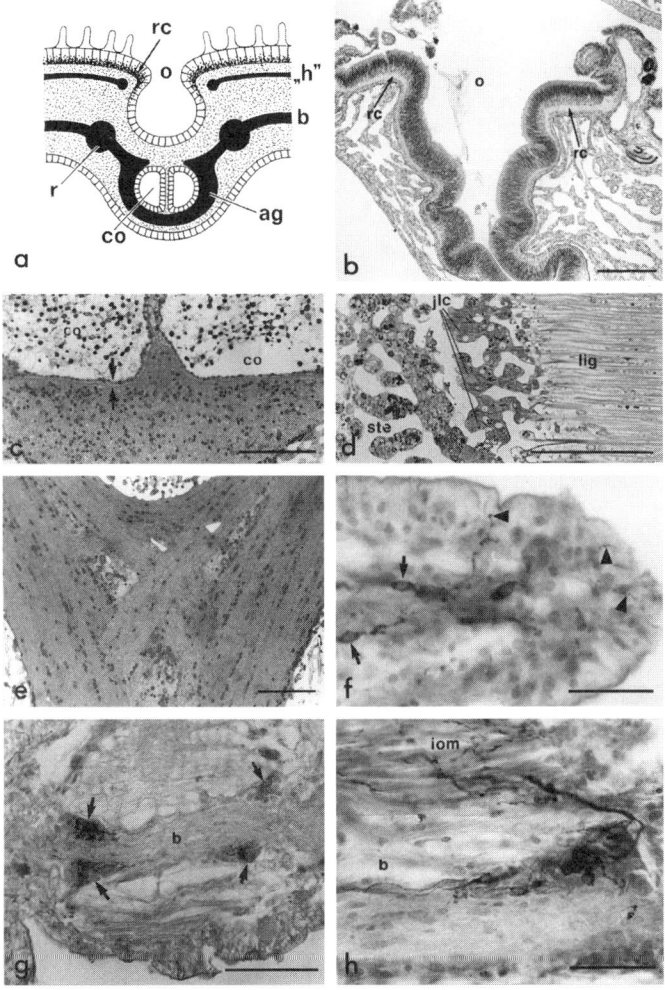

Figure 2.3. Nervous system of crinoids. (*a*) Section through the disk in the oral–aboral axis. Basiepithelial nervous tissue in the oral epidermis is stippled, and subepithelial nervous tissue is black. rc, circumoral ring commissure of the ectoneural subsystem, o, orifice, "h", = hyponeural subsystem; b, r, and ag comprise the aboral subsystem in which b = brachial nerve, r = ring commissure, and ag = apical ganglion around the chambered organ (co). (*b*) Oral–aboral section of *Leptometra phalangium*. (*c*) Oral–aboral section of the apical ganglion of *Comatella nigra* (co, somatocoelomic pouches of the chambered organ); arrows outline the somatocoelomic epithelium, which encloses the real hyponeural plexus. (*d*) Row of juxtaligamental cells (jlc) at the border of a ligament (lig), *Antedon bifida*, ste, stereom. (*e*) Crinoid aboral subsystem, dividing brachial nerve with highly ordered exchange of fiber bundles (*Comatella nigra*). (*f*) Subepithelial sensory, anti-NGF–positive cells (arrows) in the tip of a pinnula (*Antedon bifida*) with processes extending to the surface epithelium (arrowheads). (*g*) An interossicular section of the aboral brachial nerve (b) of *Antedon bifida* is shown with two ganglia each (arrows) at the border of the ossicles, many of the ganglionic neurons reacting positively with an anti-S2 serum. (*h*) In a higher magnification of one of these ganglia, fibers can be seen that supply the interossicular muscles (iom). b, brachial nerve. Bars = 200 μm in b; 100 μm in c, d, and e; 20 μm in f; 50 μm in g; and 25 μm in h, b–e stained with toluidine blue.

48   2 The Echinoderm Nervous System and its Phylogenetic Interpretation

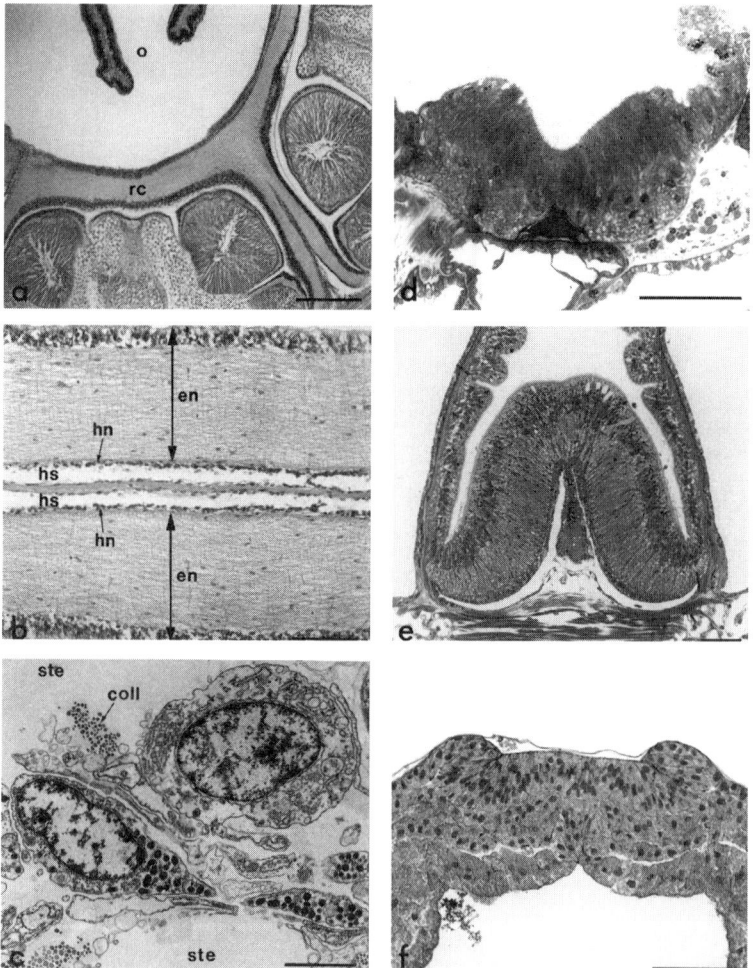

Figure 2.4. Nervous system of asteroids (a–c,e) and crinoids (d). (*a*) Horizontal section of *Echinaster sepositus* (o = orifice) with two nerve cords radiating from the ring commissure (rc). (*b*) Due to its keel-shaped form (cf. with e), the radial nerve cord of asteroids seems to be bipartitioned on horizontal sections (*Echinaster sepositus*; en, ectoneural cord; hn, hyponeural plexus; hs, hyponeural sinus). (*c*) Juxtaligamental cells, *Asterias rubens* (ste, stereom; coll, collagen fibrils). Bars = 200 µm in a and b; 2 µm in c. Ectoneural cords in the arms of crinoids (*d, Leptometra phalangium*) and asteroids (*e, Echinaster sepositus*) in comparison with the Vertebrate neural plate before neurulation (*f,* larva of *Ambystoma mexicanum*). Bars = 50 µm in d and e; 200 µm in f). Staining: hemalum/eosine (a, b, e, f), toluidine blue (d), and uranyl acetate/lead citrate (c).

Regularly, juxtaligamental cells are innervated by the same neurons, that also supply functionally correlated muscles.

Sensory cells and sensory organs. Columnar, apically monociliated cells, either singularly or in small groups, are part of the epidermis in all echinoderm classes. The filigree of their basal processes contributes to a weblike intraepidermal plexus.

Such cells are commonly agreed to be sensory, although convincing physiological evidence is poor. In echinoids, cells of this type presumably trigger the spine-convergence response and conduct it for a short distance via the basiepithelial plexus without employing the radial cords (Bullock, 1965). In crinoids, tentacles are arranged in rows aside the food grooves and serve to examine possible food particles. At the surface of the tentacles, groups of sensory cells are combined with mucous-secreting cells, forming sensory-secretory papillae (McKenzie, 1992).

In the ambulacral epithelium, sensory cells are frequent; their basal axons contribute to condensed strips of the intraepidermal plexus, which are called *ectoneural cords*. Sensory cells of the ambulacral epithelium eventually also concentrate to form small, relatively simple sensory organs such as eyespots at the distal ends of starfish ambulacra or statocysts, as recently described at the electron microscopical level in an apodous holothuroid (Ehlers, 1997).

Sensory cells are not restricted to the epidermal layer. Mainly the diffuse light sense of many echinoderms is thought to be based on subepidermal neurons (Hendler and Byrne, 1987; Byrne, 1994). In *Antedon bifida* subepidermal, spindle-shaped cells (Fig. 2.3f), (which could be visalized by their binding of an anti–nerve growth factor serum) extend one slender process straight to the epidermis and the opposite process into the aboral cords, where they compose long fiber tracts (Heinzeller et al., 1992).

Glia. Slender supporting cells, armoured with a bulk of intermediate filaments anchored at the basement membrane and traversing the entire epithelium, as demonstrated with the electron microscope (e.g., in *Asterias rubens* by Bargmann et al. [1962]), are common in ectoneural cords. In *Asterias rubens*, an antibody directed against Reissner's substance (Viehweg et al., 1998) was found to bind to such cells, an observation that lead to the interpretation of the supporting cells as glial elements. Peripheral nerve bundles of *Ophiocoma wendti* are reported to be ensheathed by gliallike cells (Byrne, 1994). Thus the traditional assessment of the echinoderm nervous tissue being devoid of glial cells may be somewhat too categorical; however, the number of candidate glia cells is very low.

Basement membrane. The term *basement membrane* plays a rather important role as a demarcation line in descriptions of the echinoderm nervous system, but it is often used differently in vertebrate histology, where it comprises three components: lamina lucida, lamina densa (together = basal lamina), and lamina fibroreticularis. In echinoderm histology, the term *basement membrane* is used either equivalently to *basal lamina* or, alternatively, indicates a thin layer of connective tissue, as described in the following.

Principally, the ectoneural ring and cords develop in close vicinity and mutual functional relationship with the ring and radial vessels of the hydrocoel (see later, Echinoderm Ectoneural Cord Versus Chordate Neural Plate; and Hydrocoel and Notochord—Are They Convergent or Homologous?) (Fig. 2.5a,c). Later, connective tissue spreads between the two structures. In addition, the somatocoelomic space (Fig. 2.5b,d) extends into that connective tissue (oral somatocoelomic tubes in asteroids and holothuroids, hyponeural sinus in ophiuroids, and "hemocoel" in echinoids). In asteroids, ophiuroids, and holothuroids (and with certain restrictions also in echinoids), the epithelium of these somatocoelomic channels houses

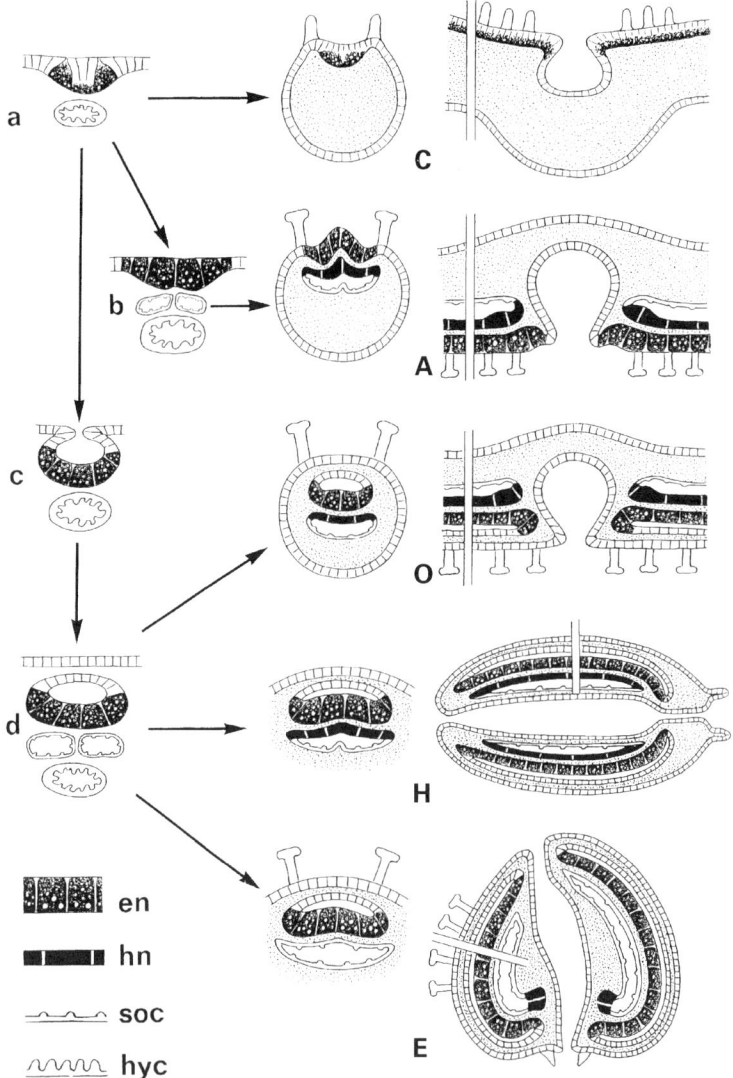

Figure 2.5. Ectoneural and hyponeural subsystem in all echinoderm classes. (a–d) Relationship with the underlying hydrocoelomic or somatocoelomic canal, respectively. In a, the initial formation of the ectoneural nerve cord is visible, which in c becomes submerged by a neurulation like process. In b and d, a section of the somatocoel has been secondarily intercalated between the ectoneural cord and the hydrocoelomic canal. en, ectoneural plexus; hn, hyponeural plexus imbedded in a section of the somatocoelomic epithelium (soc); hyc, hydrocoelomic epithelium. In all the remaining parts (C, A, O, H, E), the hydrocoel is omitted, while the somatocoel, which comes in close contact with the ectoneural cord (except in crinoids), is included as far as it generates a hyponeural subsystem of a remarkable quantity. The parts characterized by a capital (C = crinoids, A = asteroids, O = ophiuroids, H = holothuroids, E = echinoids) represent the five classes in their natural body position; the parallel-lines indicate the location of cross sections through rays that by a turn of 90° (E) or 180° (A and O) are brought to the same orientation as parts a–d, note also the direction of the podia.

hyponeural nerve cells and fibers, that are separated from the epidermis, which contains the ectoneural cords, by a sandwich of two basal laminae and a connective tissue sheet in between (Fig. 2.2a,c). Now, the connective tissue sheet is thinned out locally so far that the two basal laminae become indistinguishable from each other and persist as a common layer, a single basal lamina (Fig. 2.2b). At such sites the two closely apposed nervous plexuses communicate. Not even a thin layer of connective tissue necessarily hinders a transmitter action, as was shown physiologically for the first time by Florey and Cahill (1977, 1980) in the sea urchin tube feet.

The importance of the basal lamina for the morphological analysis of the ectoneural–hyponeural complex has been repeatedly stressed by J.L.S. Cobb (e.g., Cobb, 1985a). There are sites, however, where the continuity of the basal lamina is questionable. In ophiuroids, for instance, fibers leave the ectoneural and intrude the hyponeural compartment; whether the basal lamina is fenestrated at these sites (Stubbs and Cobb, 1981; Cobb and Stubbs, 1982) or bulges out to ensheath the ectoneural fibers is still under debate. Similar fiber transitions from the ectoneural to the hyponeural system can be observed in holothuroids (Fig. 2.2c). Even in larvae (starfish bipinnaria) the basal lamina underlying an ectodermal plexus is not continuous everywhere: Processes of mesenchymal cells, so-called subtrochal cells, "penetrate through the basement lamina and terminate adjacent to the ciliary nerve" (Lacalli, 1996).

Furthermore, it should be kept in mind that the striking ectoneural–hyponeural demarcation does not exclude a direct access of ectoneural fibers to muscle cells independently from a hyponeural mediation (e.g., spine innervation in echinoids [Peters, 1985] or retractor muscles in starfish podia [Cavey, 1998]).

Postmetamorphotic Nervous System: Group-Specific Features

Pelmatozoa: Crinoids. In terms of phylogeny, the class of crinoids is clearly separated from the remaining echinoderm classes, independently of whether paleontological criteria are applied or criteria of morphology or of molecular composition (collagen, 18S₁RNA, 28S₁RNA; reviewed by David, 1993). Also, the structures of the nervous system are exceptional and not representative for the whole phylum and therefore shall be summarized only briefly.

Basiepithelial compartment. The ectoneural subsystem is less voluminous than in other echinoderms. It is chiefly represented by ectoneural cords (Fig. 2.4d) in the basis of the ambulacral epithelia that serve for nutrition and a circumoral ring (Figs. 2.3b and 2.5C), and it probably has few or no motor functions beyond the control of ciliary movement. The connection with underlying parts of the "hyponeural" plexus (see later) is much less elaborated than in ophiuroids or asteroids. In the intestinal epithelium, neurons and their fibers are relatively sparse. In all coelomic epithelia, a well-developed nervous plexus is present, notably in the chambered organ, where it contributes to the aboral ganglion (Fig. 2.3c).

Subepithelial compartment. The so-called hyponeural subsystem of crinoids is not integrated into the somatocoelomic epithelium as in other echinoderms, but is directly embedded in the connective tissue (Fig. 2.2d), as is the aboral subsystem. Both systems are thus part of the subepithelial compartment as defined here. Together they form a crinoid-specific entity, which in the arm or pinnule, respectively, consists of two longitudinal nerves running on either side of the ambulacrum (i.e., the hyponeural nerves), and a strikingly strong unpaired nerve penetrating the brachial or pinnular ossicles (i.e., the aboral nerve). In the periphery, hyponeural and aboral nerves are frequently interconnected. In the central disk, an inconspicuous orally situated ring collects all the hyponeural nerves, while the aboral arm nerves comprise a voluminous ring commissure in the aboral half of the disk. The aboral arm nerves exchange fiber bundles at branching sites of the arms in a surprisingly geometrical order (Fig. 2.3e). In the interradial sections of the ring, additional cords (one pair per interradius) connect the ring with an enormous, cup-shaped ganglion investing the five coelomic pouches of the chambered organ. This ganglion, which lacks any equivalent in the eleutherozoan classes, extends nerves into cirri. Hyponeural and aboral cords are incompletely covered by amebocytes with specific granules.

Skeletal muscles and juxtaligamental cells are exclusively supplied by the hyponeural–aboral entity. With an antibody against the SALMFamide S2 applied to the aboral arm nerve of *Antedon bifida*, it could be demonstrated that the immunoreactive cells regularly form small ganglia where the nerve leaves or enters the ossicle (Fig. 2.3g,h); the cells extend long, profusely branching processes to the skeletal muscles and to juxtaligamental cells (Heinzeller et al., 1993). These ganglia of presumed motor neurons are interconnected intrasegmentally and intersegmentally by thin S2-positive fibers. Nevertheless, the hyponeural–aboral entity is not restricted to motor functions but obviously also receives and processes the sensory inputs from its own sensory system (cells with nerve growth factor–like immunoreactivity; see the earlier discussion of the common features of the postmetamorphotic nervous system).

Asterozoa: Asteroids. J.B. Spix (1809) first confirmed the existence of nerve cords in echinoderms by applying a galvanic setup, following a suggestion of Georges Cuvier (1769–1832). For these experiments, Spix fortunately chose the starfish *Asterias rubens*, in which the ambulacral epithelium with its ectoneural plexus is freely accessible. A detailed description of the system was not obtained, however until the improved light microscopical conditions at the end of the nineteenth century (e.g., Lange, 1876; Hamann, 1885). A contemporary review, referring also to electron microscopical observations, is given by Chia and Koss (1994).

Basiepithelial compartment. Ciliated sensory and nerve cells are integrated in the epidermis of asteroids all over the body surface. Both cell types contribute extremely thin processes to the epidermal plexus; most of these fibers contain the SALMFamide S1 (Moore and Thorndyke, 1993). Reports on moderately thick or even giant fibers are lacking. Sensory cells and neurons are grouped at the bases of podia or spines, where they form small ganglia, or in the sensory hillocks of pedicellariae, but they reach the highest concentration in the cords of the ectoneural subsystem (Figs. 2.4b,e and 2.5A). These cords are located in the thickened epidermis (100 μm and more) of the ambulacral groove, which in most asteroid species, in contrast to that of crinoids, exerts no more nutritive but almost exclusively nervous functions but contains also some mucous secreting cells. Although the circumoral ring (Fig. 2.4a) is exposed to the outside environment, as are the cords, it is less easily accessible. Ring and cords are accompanied by rows of podia on either side. In a cross-sectioned arm, the outlines of the cord resemble a "V" (Figs. 2.4e and 2.5A). Basally, ring and cords rest on a moderately thick lamella of connective tissue, which separates the ectoneural subsystem from the somatocoelomic epithelium/hyponeural plexus.

The perikarya of ectoneural sensory, neuronal, and supporting cells are arranged in two to four rows in the apical zone (Fig. 2.2A); the thick layer of neuropile below is nearly free of cell bodies. Most of the fibers run longitudinally in the cords or circularly in the ring, and some run transversely. Many of these fibers give a bright fluorescent reaction when tested for biogenic amines (v. Hehn, 1970). The majority of cells and fibers, however, bind to an antibody against the SALMFamide S1 (Moore and Thorndyke, 1993). Some cells and many fibers are GABAergic (Newman and Thorndyke, 1994). Single ectoneural cells may also synthesize nitric oxide (Martínez et al., 1994). Electron microscopical investigations (Cobb, 1970) revealed fiber varicosities containing plenty of small, clear vesicles, in particular at the ectoneural–hyponeural boundary.

Most authors agree that the ectoneural subsystem is sensory and motor in function. The assumption of a sensory function is based on the large number of ciliated cells, which are believed to be multimodal, and is most obviously exemplified by pigmented eyespots, which are regularly found on terminal tube feet (Smith, 1937). The ectoneural motor neurons have functional access across the basement membrane either to processes of muscle fibers ("muscle tails"), or to processes of hyponeural neurons.

As a flat layer, 10 to 20 µm in height, the hyponeural subsystem—occasionally also called Lange's nerve—accompanies the main ectoneural cords (Fig. 2.4b) and the ring. It is lodged in a coelomic epithelium, and myoepithelial cells are interspersed among supporting, neuronal, and neurosecretory cells (v. Hehn, 1970). Perikarya are concentrated luminally, and the basal plexus consists of fibers measuring up to 0.6 µm in diameter (Cobb, 1970). Neurons are arranged in a segmental "ganglionated fashion" (Moore and Thorndyke, 1993) with poor evidence for intersegmental connectivity. Histochemically, no indication for biogenic amines (v. Hehn, 1970) or GABA (Newman and Thorndyke, 1994) could be detected, whereas many cell bodies and axons positively react with anti-S1 (Moore and Thorndyke, 1993). Hyponeural axons supply skeletal and podial muscles.

Corresponding with the ability of starfishes to evert the stomach for external digestion, the digestive tract is equipped with a well-developed basiepithelial plexus. This plexus is rich in aminergic fibers (Cobb and Raymond, 1979). Immunohistochemistry revealed also the presence of S1 (*Asterias rubens*; Moore and Thorndyke, 1993) or cross-reactivity with several other neuropeptides (*Marthasterias glacialis:* FRMFamide, human peptide-tyrosine-tyrosine, human pancreatic polypeptide, α-melanocyte–stimulating hormone, Martínez et al., 1993; adrenomedullin, Martínez et al., 1996). Strong labeling of the plexus in the digestive epithelium was also obtained by applying antisera against GABA (Newman and Thorndyke, 1994) or nitric oxide synthase (Martínez et al., 1994).

Subepithelial Compartment. The subepithelial compartment is represented only by rows of juxtaligamental cells bordering numerous ligaments.

Cryptosyringida

If one considers the anatomical situation of the ectoneural radial cords and the circumoral ring in asteroids as being ancestral, the condition in the remaining three echinoderm classes must be concluded to be derived. Here, cords and ring are located in a "hidden" (greek *kryptos*) system of ectodermal tubes (greek *syrinx*), that is, the epineural canals (O, H, and d in Fig. 2.5; see Fig. 2.7a–c), which run inside (echinoids) or outside (ophiuroids) the axial skeleton or inside the muscular–collagenous body wall (holothuroids). Smith (1984) proposed to combine these classes into a common taxon, Cryptosyringida. The embryological processes of forming the epineural canals either may equal a neurulationlike overgrowth by lateral folds (ophiuroids and echinoids) or may not, as Smiley (1986) found in the holothuroid *Stichopus californicus*. The usually unilayered and squamous epithelial wall of the tubular epineural canal, which complements the ambulacral epithelium to form the tube, is called *epineural epithelium*. The tube resembles an early developmental state of a chordate rhombencephalon with a thick neurogenic, ciliated epithelium at the ventral side that is overlain dorsally by a non-neurogenic thin epithelium (Fig. 2.7d; for further comparative aspects, later, Are Echinoderm Arms Homologous with Bilaterian Trunks?).

Ophiuroids. In comparison with other classes, the nervous system of ophiuroids has been more intensely studied. The convenient anatomical situation (i.e., accessibility of the ectoneural cords, which can be exposed by removing the covering ventral arm plates, and the presence of "giant" axons of up to 20 µm in diameter) allowed J.L.S. Cobb and co-workers to do successful combined electrophysiological and morphological studies of the ophiuroid nervous system (Cobb, 1985a,b, 1987, 1988, 1990a,b, 1995; Cobb and Begbie, 1994; Cobb and Ghyoot, 1993; Cobb and Moore, 1986; Cobb and Stubbs, 1981; Ghyoot et al., 1994; Moore and Cobb, 1985, 1986; Pentreath and Cobb, 1972; Stubbs and Cobb, 1981, 1982).

Basiepithelial compartment. The superficial plexus consists of widespread neurons and possibly neurosecretory cells (Märkel and Röser, 1985) and their axon bundles (Cobb and Moore, 1986), which presumably innervate other epidermal cells, either secretory or ciliary (bands on the genital shields; Stubbs and Cobb, 1982). Granulated cells, which are abundantly found in the epidermis of podial tips in association with mucous-secreting cells, contain small, dense-cored vesicles. The sensory function of these cells is indicated by a single apical kinocilium; basally they give rise to axons (Ball and Jangoux, 1990).

The dominating part of the basiepithelial system are five ectoneural cords and their circumoral ring (Figs.2.6a and 2.7a), which are located in the aboral moiety of the epineural canal. In this thickened part of the epineural wall, nuclei of neurons and of supporting cells are concentrated on the luminal side. At the abluminal side, the coelothelial sheet of the hyponeural sinus is closely attached, which includes the hyponeural elements (see later discussion). The "basement membrane" (see earlier discussion) between hyponeural and ectoneural subsystems is relatively thick in the midline, where it may contain a vascular plexus, while laterally it is reduced to 40 nm in places.

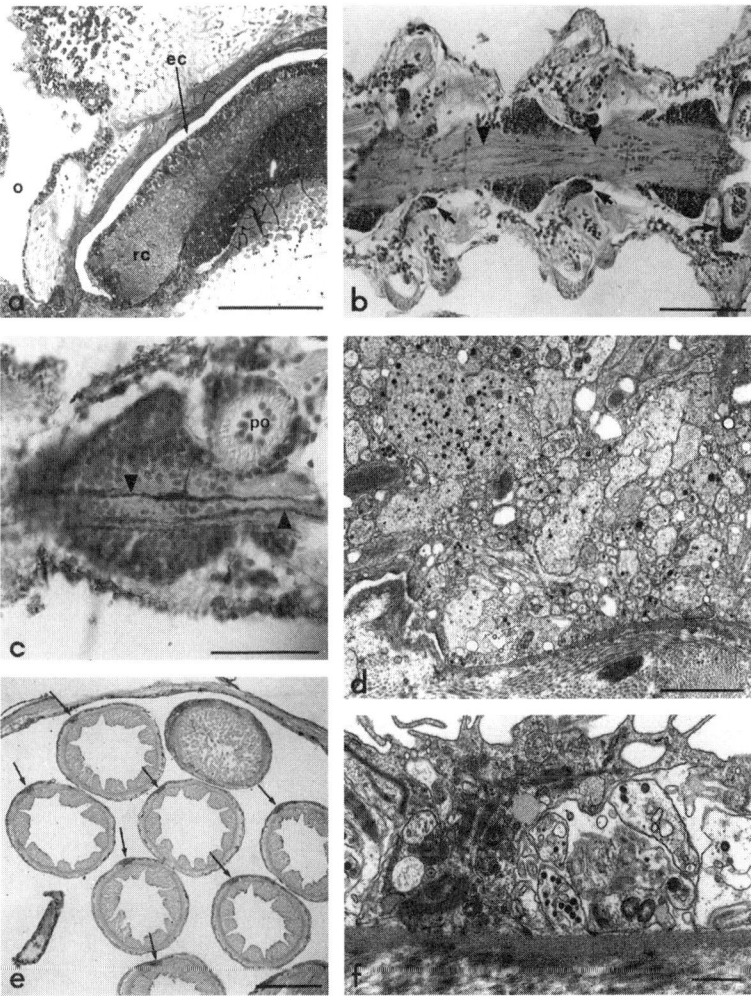

Figure 2.6. Nervous system of cryptosyringid echinoderms. (*a*) Oral aboral section of the ophiuroid *Ophioderma longicaudum* (oral side down, o, orifice, ec, epineural canal, rc, ring commissure). In b and c, horizontal sections of arms of *Ophiura ophiura* are shown. (*b*) Low-power micrograph displays three pairs of cell-rich interossicular swellings of the ectoneural cord with nearly soma-free sections in between and three pairs of podial ganglia (arrows). Delicate bundles of longitudinal fibers, marked by their reaction with a serum directed against the SALMFamide S2, are indicated by arrowheads. (*c*) Higher magnification of a segmental ganglionic swelling with through conducting S2-positive fibers (arrowheads). po, podium. (*d*) Intestinal plexus (*Echinometra*, Echinoidea). (*e*) Cross-cut podia of *Arbacia lixula* (Echinoidea) with the podial nerve (arrows) marked by its immunoreactivity against the SALMFamide S2. (*f*) Hydrocoelomic epithelium (body wall of *Paracaudina chilensis*, Holothuroidea) with basiepithelial nerve fiber profiles. Bars = 200 μm in a and e; 100 μm in b; 50 μm in c; 2 μm in d; 1 μm in f. Staining: hemalum/eosin in a; hemalum in b, c, and e; and uranyl acetate with lead citrate in d and f.

2 The Echinoderm Nervous System and its Phylogenetic Interpretation

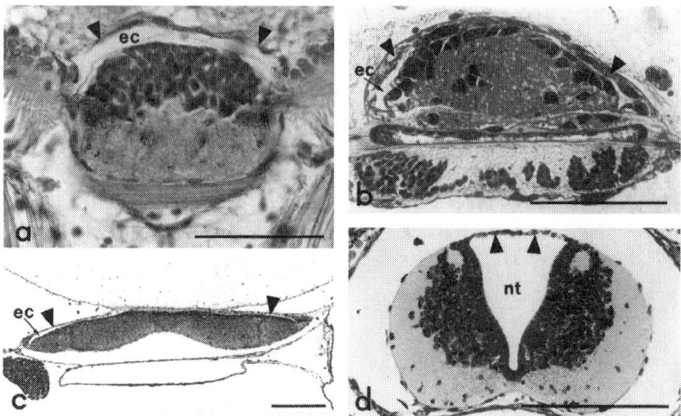

Figure 2.7. Epineural canals (ec) of cryptosyringids in comparison with the vertebrate neural tube (nt). Both epineural canals and the neural tube are closed by a thin unilayered epithelium (arrowheads). (*a*) *Ophiura ophiura*, Ophiuroidea, (*b*) Juvenile *Holothuria tubulosa*, Holothuroidea, (*c*) *Sphaerechinus granularis*, Echinoidea (courtesy of Prof. Konrad Märkel). (*d*) Tadpole of *Rana temporaria*. Bars = 50 μm in a and b; 200 μm in c and d. Staining: hemalum/eosin in a and d and toluidine blue in b and c.

Neurons in the ectoneural cords are aggregated in segmental ganglia (Fig. 2.6b), longitudinally connected by intersegmental sections, which are poor or even free of perikarya (Cobb, 1985a). Some of the long through-conducting fibers (Fig. 2.6c) were shown to be GABAergic, others serotonergic (Ghyoot and Cobb, 1994). A remarkable fraction of the perikarya and fibers are "giant" by echinoderm standards. Giant fibers are mostly oriented longitudinally, but may also connect left and right halves of the ganglion. Many of the ectoneural neurons and their intrasegmental fibers bind to an antibody against the SALMFamide S1 (DeBremaeker et al., 1997), others to the SALMFamide S2 (Fig. 2.6b,c). When carboxyfluorescein was injected into single ganglion cells (Cobb and Ghyoot, 1993), neurons were identified, usually extending over three or more segments. Among these neurons one element was highly conspicuous because of the constancy of position, shape, and axonal length: the giant through-conducting neuron. Only one of these cells was found per segment, always in a lateral position, with the axon immediately crossing contralaterally and then turning toward the disc. Such an axon runs for at least six full segments.

Lateral branches of ectoneural cords (and thus of the epineural canal) establish a connection to ring-shaped ectoneural ganglia at the podial basis, from where a podial nerve runs to the podial tip. This ectoneural nerve stays separate from the hydrocoelomic myocytes by a thin connective tissue layer. Some of the myocytes receive ectoneural innervation across the separating layer (Cavey, 1998). Other groups of podial myocytes are innervated by hyponeural fibers, which reach the podium by the same path as the ectoneural fibers and which are accompanied by an extension of the hyponeural sinus.

Corresponding with the ectoneural ganglionic swellings, two ganglia per segment are formed in the hyponeural subsystem, again located in the coelomic epithelia. The ultrastructure of these hyponeural ganglia, including that of their giant neurons and axons, was studied in detail by Stubbs and Cobb (1981). Sharply contrasting with traditional descriptions, these ganglia are not interconnected longitudinally with those in neighboring segments, at least not so in *Ophiura ophiura* (Cobb, 1985a). This new knowledge is based on the observation of more than 100 (giant) hyponeural cells, which were intracellularly injected with Lucifer yellow. Also, immunohistochemical studies, which in the ectoneural cords visualized small perikarya and tiny longitudinal fibers, failed to demonstrate any interganglionic fibers in the hyponeural system (Ghyoot and Cobb, 1994). Even for a possible left–right interganglionic fiber exchange, absolutely no hints were obtained. Consequently, hyponeural ganglia must be considered neuronal cell groups, which are isolated from each other, but are intercalated between the ectoneural plexus and skeletal muscles, to which they presumably transmit ectoneurally generated excitation. Hyponeural activity depends on excitatory (possibly S1) and inhibitory (possibly glycine) transmitters, which are released from varicosities of ectoneural axons (Cobb, 1985a) close to the basement membrane and which are thought to act across this membrane on fine dendritic endings of hyponeural cells. The hyponeural axons contact intervertebral muscles and also supply (by branching) groups of juxtaligamental cells.

In most ophiuroids, the digestive system is reduced to esophagus and stomach. Reports on its innervation are sparse but confirm the existence of two basiepithelial plexuses, one located in the digestive epithelium proper and the other integrated into the coelothelial (mesothelial) outer sheath (Byrne, 1994). In some ophiuroid species, additional neurons are described in the connective tissue layer, which separates the digestive epithelium from the coelothelium (Schechter and Lucero, 1968; Pentreath, 1969).

Subepithelial compartment. As observed in *Ophiocomina nigra* (Wilkie, 1979), juxtaligamental cells form four pairs of ganglia per segment, each associated with a ligament or another major connective tissue component. Inside the ganglia, hyponeural nerves terminate on and are tangled with processes of juxtaligamental cells. Some areas of close contact display characters of chemical synapses: thickening of the cell membrane and numerous small clear vesicles on the hyponeural side (Cobb, 1985b; Byrne, 1994).

Juxtaligamental ganglia are also reported to include another kind of modified neuron, which is responsible for luminescence (*Ophiopsila californica, Amphipholis squamata*; Brehm and Morin, 1977). These cells also depend on hyponeural innervation using a muscarinic cholinergic receptor (DeBremaeker et al., 1996).

Ophiuroids are sensitive to light, even after removal of the epidermis. Hendler and Byrne (1987) observed chromatophores in the dermis of *Ophiocoma wendti* that, depending on the illumination, covered (day) or uncovered (night) bundles of nerve fibers in clefts of the stereom. These bundles are thought to be photoreceptive; the location of the corresponding cell bodies is still unknown. Presumably the photoreceptive cells modulate the hyponeural system and its influence on the skeletal muscles, because the animals immediately freeze when shadowed. In addition, the photoreceptive cells must contact, either directly or indirectly, the ectoneural cords, because Moore and Cobb (1985) in preparations of *Ophiura ophiura* recorded responses to photic stimulation from the interganglionic region of the radial nerve cord, which is exclusively ectoneural.

Echinoids. The anatomy of the echinoid nervous system is reviewed by Cuénot (1948) and, more recently, by Cavey and Märkel (1994). Because some of the main nervous structures *grosso modo* resemble the situation as just discussed for asteroids and ophiuroids, attention is be drawn primarily to features specific for echinoids.

Basiepithelial compartment. Ciliated sensory cells are widely distributed but remarkably numerous in sensory pads inside the valves of pedicellariae (Peters and Campbell, 1987). Axons of sensory cells form tracts, which deeply intrude into the subepithelial space and directly contact valve muscles. At the base of spines, the epidermal plexus is thickened to form a ring-shaped ganglion, which, according to Peters (1985), directly contacts the spine muscles. Cobb and Begbie (1994), however, emphasize the intervention of hyponeural neurons between the epidermal ganglion and the muscles.

More than in any other eleutherozoan class, the nervous system in echinoids is dominated by the ectoneural subsystem: The five radial nerve cords entirely lack a hyponeural component (Figs. 2.5E and 2.7c). This may be related to the lack of intervertebral muscles (compare Table. 2.2). Only the spine basis and lantern muscles are supplied by hyponeural fibers. The perikarya of these fibers form hyponeural ganglia (Fig. 2.5E) attached to the ectoneural ring (10 in number in *Eucidaris tribuloides*; Birenheide, 1989). In spatangoid species, a masticatory apparatus is missing, as are hyponeural ganglia (Kaestner, 1963).

The histology and ultrastructure of the ectoneural cord has been studied in several species (*Echinus esculentus, Psammechinus miliaris, Heliocidaris erythrogramma, Patiriella calcar*, Cobb, 1970; *Mespilia globulus*, Märkel and Röser, 1991).

Table 2.2. Highly Generalized Scheme of the Muscle Groups that Enable the Animals to Their Usual Kind of Locomotion

	Intervertebral or Comparable Arm Muscles	Hydrocoelomic Musculature of Podia and Tentacles	Spine Muscles	Body Wall Musculature
Rays forming free arms: Crinoidea	++	–	–	–
Rays forming free arms: Asteroidea	+	++	+	+
Rays forming free arms: Ophiuroidea	++	–	+	–
Rays integrated into body wall: Echinoidea	–	+	++	–
Rays integrated into body wall: Holothuroidea	–	++	–	++

Commonly the cord includes numerous sensory cells, which—among other functions—probably accounts for the cord's immediate photosensitivity (Yoshida et al., 1984). In echinoids, the epineural canal opens by many small pores: Close to a podial base, the epineural canal gives off a fine lateral branch canal, which traverses the test and opens at the animal's surface. The thickened wall of such a branch canal is in continuity with that thickened wall of the epineural canal that includes the ectoneural cord. Thus, the lateral branch canal includes a so-called lateral nerve. The oral part of this lateral nerve passes to the epidermal plexus, while the aboral part forms the podial nerve (Märkel and Röser, 1991) (Fig. 2.6e), the varicosities of which are presynaptic to muscle tails of ampullar myoepithelial cells across a thin lamella of connective tissue (Cobb, 1987).

In the intestinal wall of echinoids, an entoneural, basiepithelial plexus is well developed, most conspicuously in the pharyngeal and esophageal sections (DeRidder and Jangoux, 1982), and, in addition, there is a basiepithelial plexus in the accompanying coelothelium. In the irregular echinoid *Echinocardium cordatum*, strands of nerve fibers run in the connective tissue along the esophagus that emerge from the entoneural plexus and again enter the entoneural plexus of certain intestinal glands. Thus, these nerves are part of the basiepithelial subsystem, although they are observed in the connective tissue (DeRidder and Jangoux, 1993).

Subepithelial compartment. Echinoids possess only few ligaments in their shell-like skeleton. Nevertheless, examples of juxtaligamental cells have been described, that control the tensility of (1) the conical cylinder of collagenous fibers, which attach a spine to the test (Cobb and Begbie, 1994); (2) the collagenous tooth support, with its "dense vesicle cells" (Birenheide, 1990); (3) certain ligaments of Aristotle's lantern (*Paracentrotus lividus*; Wilkie et al., 1992); and (4) the peristomial membrane (e.g., Wilkie et al., 1994).

Holothuroids. A fundamental description of the nervous system of holothuroids is given by Semon (1883). The moderate progress in our knowledge about this topic (Smiley, 1994) is only briefly summarized here.

Basiepithelial compartment. The dominating part of the nervous system of sea cucumbers is again the ectoneural subsystem, which consists of a circumoral ring, five cords descending aborally, and at least 10 nerves that ascend from the ring into buccal tentacles and distally merge with the superficial epidermal plexus (Bouland et al., 1982). During early develotment, the entire ectoneural subsystem sinks below the surface so that it is paralleled everywhere by epineural canals (Figs. 2.5H and 2.7b) or clefts; the latter have been described in the locomotory podia (Flammang and Jangoux, 1992). In the descending ectoneural cords, the metameric organization is restricted to the supply of ambulacral podia or even absent in apodid species. Sensory organs such as photoreceptive cell patches at the base of buccal tentacles (Yamamoto and Yoshida, 1978) or statocysts are specializations of the ectoneural cords.

Only descending cords (and not the oral nerves) are combined with a hyponeural layer, which is integrated in the wall of a somatocoelomic tube. No hyponeural ring can be observed (Haanen, 1914), and no hyponeural nerves extend into the buccal tentacles (McKenzie, 1987, 1988). Where present, the hyponeural plexus is assumed to innervate the muscle cells of the body wall. Many of the neurons and processes of both the ectoneural and the hyponeural layer were shown to bind specifically to antisera raised against a holothuroid peptide, GFSKLYFamide (Díaz-Miranda et al., 1995).

In the digestive tract of holothuroids, the entoneural plexus is reported to be missing (Jangoux, 1982; Feral and Massin, 1982), while the coelothelial one is well developed in all perivisceral coelothelia (Smiley, 1994).

Subepithelial compartment. The connective tissue of the dermis has plenty of juxtaligamental cells (Matsuno and Motokawa, 1992). It is one of the classic objects for studying the mutable characteristics of echinoderm collagenous fibers (Lindemann, 1900; Trotter et al., 1996).

Interclass Comparison of Sensory Versus Motor Function

As elucidated in the preceding descriptions, J.L.S. Cobb's hypothesis, according to which the hyponeural subsystem is exclusively motor, has been repeatedly confirmed. This should not, however, be interpreted in the sense that locomotion depends exclusively on the hyponeural subsystem. Table 2.2 lists the muscle groups that are used mainly for locomotion in the different classes. The relative predominance of nervous subsystems in the different classes shows no clear correlation to the presence or absence of certain muscle groups (compare Table 2.1). Only one conclusion can be drawn with some certainty, namely, that the two groups (Echinoidea, Holothuroidea) with the rays integrated into the body wall (and, thus, trivially lacking intervertebral arm muscles) both reduce the hyponeural nerve cords to those regions where musculature is present and use the ectoneural compartment as a main innervation system.

In contrast, the ectoneural subsystem is sometimes considered exclusively sensory. Although sensory abilities must be ascribed to many ectoneural cells, there exist examples for a sensorimotor co-function within a certain subsystem. For instance, in crinoids the subepidermal sensory neurons extend their processes into the aboral cords, which clearly contain motor neurons (Heinzeller and Welsch, 1994). The ectoneural cord of echinoids serves as a second example: The nerve cells that, across a basement membrane, supply the ampullar myocytes lie next to primary sensory cells contacting the lumen of the epineural canal (Cavey and Märkel, 1994).

QUESTIONS OF SYMMETRY

Central Part of the Body

With regard to the oral–aboral axis, some of the organs included in the central disk, that is, the central part of the body of adult echinoderms, are asymmetrical or have an eccentric position (e.g., the stone canal in echinoids or the spongy organ of crinoids). Other organs of the disk, such as the pyloric diverticula of asteroids, the gonads of asteroids and echinoids, the chambered organ of crinoids, or the adult organization of the hydrocoel (all classes) display a faultless pentaradial symmetry. During metamorphosis, such rotatory symmetry develops starting from a bilateral organization. The very first indicator of this process is the crescent-like outgrowth of the left hydrocoel, gradually transforming into a complete circular ring, which then develops five radial tubes. The hydrocoelomic ring and its five radial extensions dominate the morphogenesis of echinoderms.

The radial symmetrical disk defines the oral–aboral axis, which might be founded by the gradient of a morphogen already existing in the eight–cell blastula (*Asterina pectinifera*;Tosuji, 1998). When the oral–aboral axis becomes visible in the early free-living larva, it is not necessarily identical with the larva's anteroposterior axis. The two axes are aligned more or less in the same direction in holothuroids and crinoids, whereas they are nearly perpendicular to each other in echinoids, asteroids, and ophiuroids (Smiley, 1986). Consequently, the oral–aboral axis of echinoderms is neither constant in all echinoderm classes nor should it parallel the body axis of bilaterians.

Bilateral Symmetry and Segmentation of the Arms

Each arm is bilaterally organized with segmentlike repetitive units. In ophiuroids this can be seen directly in the arrangement of ossicles, muscles, and paired podia and in the nervous system displaying a pronounced pair of ectoneural ganglia and a pair of hyponeural ganglia per segment (Fig. 2.6b).

In other classes, bilateral symmetry is somewhat hidden by podia that serially alternate on the left and right sides. This does not necessarily, however, reflect the original branching pattern of the radial hydrocoelomic channel, which is symmetrical, because at least the developmentally earliest lateral evaginations arise in pairs from the radial channel (asteroids: Gemill, 1914; Hörstadius, 1939; Popodi et al., 1998a; comatulid crinoids: e.g., Seeliger, 1892; isocrinid crinoids: Heinzeller et al., 1997). During further outgrowth, the branches of the hydrocoelomic main channel favor the right or left side in alternating fashion. In echinoids, this accords with the alternate formation of covering ossicles (ocular plate rule; Mooi et al., 1994). In crinoids, the lateral branches alternatively turn to left or right pinnules and, thus, give the arms their characteristic zigzag pattern. Nevertheless, these arms also include segments of evident bilateral symmetry, the so-called axials. Similar to proximal axials in crinoids, also in asteroids and ophiuroids symmetrical points of dichotomous branching close to the disk generate the 10 arms, which is a common number in many species of these three classes. Thus the arms should be considered primarily bilateral symmetrical with a tendency to somewhat mask this primary situation during outgrowth.

Today the questions related to symmetry and metamery no longer depend on merely morphological considerations, but increasingly become supported by molecular data.

In *Drosophila*, in *Amphioxus* (Holland et al., 1997), and in vertebrates, the *engrailed* gene acts as one of the segment polarity genes that demarcate segmental borders. Similarly, *engrailed* is expressed in a segment-like fashion along the arms in early postmetamorphic stages of sea urchins (*Heliocidaris erythrogramma*, Popodi et al., 1998b; *Psammechinus miliaris*, Beer and Thorndyke, 1998) and of the ophiuroid *Amphipholis squamata* (Lowe and Wray, 1997).

Are Echinoderm Arms Homologous with Bilaterian Trunks?

If genes coding for bilaterian segmentation can be demonstrated in the arms of echinoderms, this might indicate that their arms represent modules possibly homologous to bilaterian trunks, provided that the genes maintained their developmental task also in echinoderms (cf. Phylogenetic Aspects, below).

Assessment of homology, however, depends on the data accessible. Therefore, a structural homology must be hypothesized by careful comparison of detailed morphological data. The criteria for recognizing homology are, according to Remane (1952), the position in a set of structures, the specific qualities, and the certain phylogenetic continuity. The first criterion may be neglected in the case of multiple body axes. The other two criteria evidently become fulfilled by the increasing molecular genetic evidence.

Homeotic genes in bilaterian development define the identity of certain segments and were demonstrated in echinoderms during metamorphosis, although data on their temporospatial expression are scarce. These genes include orthologues of the *Hox* genes of all three groups (anterior, central, and posterior; Popodi et al.,1996) and display high-grade similarity with those of the mouse (*Tripneustes gratilla:* Dolecki et al., 1988; *Paracentrotus lividus:* DiBernardo et al., 1994; *Heliocidaris erythrogramma:* Popodi et al., 1998a; *Holopneustes purpurescens*: Morris et al., 1998; *Stomopneustes variolaris* and *Tripneustes gratilla:* Wu et al., 1998; *Asterina minor:* Mito, 1998). Even the most anterior cognate groups of *Hox* genes, which in chordates are expressed in the developing rhombencephalon, were reported in echinoderms (first report of a group 1 cognate: Mito, 1998; first report of a group 2 cognate: Wu et al., 1998). These findings refute the former assumption of a gene loss at the 3' end of the cluster in echinoderms.

Echinoderm Ectoneural Cord Versus Chordate Neural Plate

Some of the regulatory genes that organize the chordate neural plate are also expressed in the echinoderm ectoneural cord, for example, *Wingless* and (again) *engrailed* (Joyner, 1996; Lowe and Wray, 1997; Popodi et al., 1998b). Furthermore, there is a series of morphological parallelisms, which are briefly discussed.
1. Although composed of segmental units, both the ectoneural cord and the neural plate show neurons whose axons transgress the segment borderline. In the spinal cord (derived from the neural plate) of chordates this is profusely so, but also in echinoderms the giant fibers at least of the brittlestar radial nerve span several segments (Cobb, 1988; Ghyoot and Cobb, 1994; Fig. 2.6c).

2. In the ectoneural cord, the fiber plexus is located basally, as it is in the epithelium of the developing vertebrate neural tube (compare, e.g., Fig. 2.7a with Fig. 2.7d).

3. Both chordates and (cryptosyringid) echinoderms have an ectodermal tube consisting of a voluminous part on one side (ventrolateral in chordates; aboral in cryptosyringid echinoderms) as well as the thin closing part on the other side of the tube, which is of low or no neurogenic potency (roof plate of the spinal cord and ventricle coverings of the brain) (Figs. 2.7a–c and 2.8d).

4. After being submerged under the body surface, both chordate and echinoderm tubes stay separate from the surrounding connective tissue, demarcated by a basement membrane.

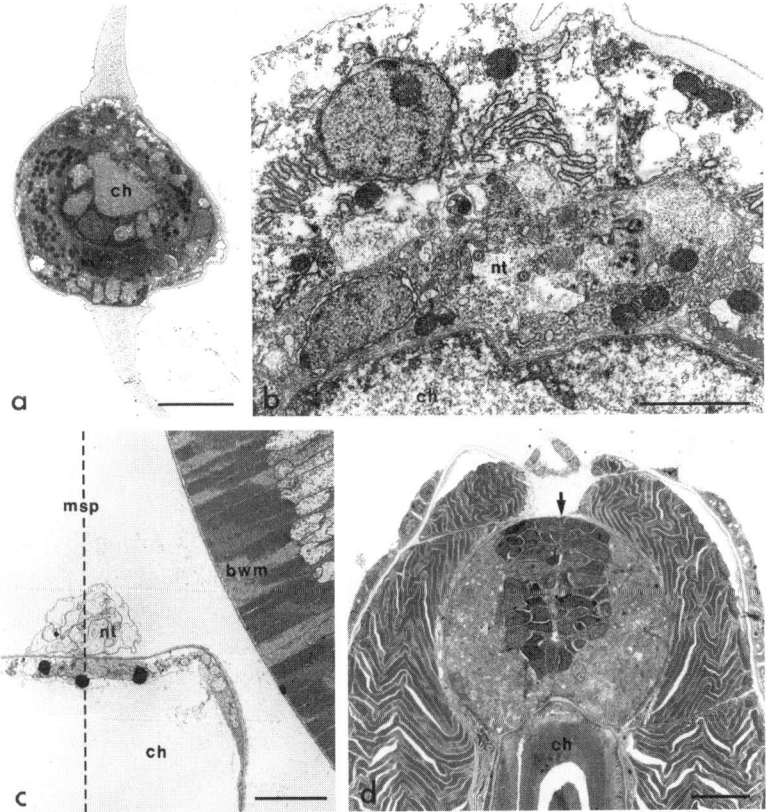

Figure 2.8. Tubular notochord (ch) and neural tube (nt) in nonvertebrate chordates. (*a*) Larva of *Ciona intestinalis* (Tunicata), cross section of the tail. The lumen of the notochord includes masses of a flocculent material, as do vacuoles of the notochord cells. (*b*) Higher magnification, the lumen of the neural tube includes two kinocilia. (*c*) *Oikopleura dioica* (Copelata), cross section of the tail (msp, medial sagittal plane; bwm, body wall muscle). The neural tube is already degenerating, and the voluminous notochord consists of a jelly-filled tube that is formed by a single layer of squamous epithelial cells. (*d*) Larva of *Branchiostoma floridae* (Acrania), the neural tube is closed dorsally by a thin roof plate (arrow). Bars = 10 µm in a and d; 2 µm in b, 5 µm in c.

5. In both systems, this basiepithelial nervous system is supported by a second neuronal population, which in contrast to the tube neurons is located in the connective tissue space (i.e., neural crest and/or placodes in chordates and the subepithelial compartment in echinoderms). It seems unlikely, however, that these additional groups of neurons are homologous: Gans and Northcutt (1983) claim the neural crest a craniate autapomorphy, and Jefferies et al. (1996) attribute vestiges of spinal ganglia already to calcichordates but argue the echinoderm lineage to branch off before.

In addition, as is the case in the chordate spinal cord, the echinoderm ectoneural cord covers important functional fields:

1. Reflectory control of movements.

2. The ability of coordinate reaction to external stimuli. Attractive stimuli in echinoderms are, for instance, the immediate contact with food particles. Such stimulation is answered by local secretory and motor reactions of podia, tentacles, or the stomach wall. The smell of distant food is answered by target-oriented locomotion. Adverse stimuli (e.g., being touched or hurt) are locally answered by retracting or enrolling arms, by stiffening the body wall, or by directed and coordinated flight of the animal.

3. Flight can also be observed when an echinoderm is likely to become attacked. Shadowing may be a sufficient stimulus, as is an approaching predator: It has been repeatedly observed that an approaching *Marthasterias* causes an ophiuroid to escape from its expected route (P. Lambert, personal communication). Sea urchins (*Tetrapygus niger*) reduce motility when a predator is present (Rodriguez et al., 1998). Such examples illustrate that the echinoderm nervous system may also guide more complex behavioral patterns. Furthermore, there are reports of starfish that behave successfully in the Y maze (*Asterias forbesi*, Lepper and Moore, 1998).

In this last respect, the echinoderm ectoneural cord even exceeds the abilities of the vertebrate spinal cord, which has no special sensory organs associated with it and is controlled largely by the brain and by sensory inputs originating from peripheral (neural crest–derived) ganglia (spinal ganglia). *Amphioxus* has primary sensory cells in its neural cord and lacks spinal ganglia in the dorsal roots.

Additional Body Axes

Because several nonchordate and chordate deuterostomians form colonies (e.g., *Rhabdopleura* or many members of the Ascidians and Thaliacea), some authors—beginning with Duvernoy (1848)—thought that the rays of echinoderms might represent body axes, and thus an individual echinoderm constitutes a centrally cohering colony. Recent molecular genetic data furnish increasing evidence: "Comparison of these expression patterns to chordates suggests that each radial nerve may correspond to an ancestral anterior-posterior axis" (Popodi et al., 1998b).

Also, the process of how a body axis forms has been elucidated to some extent in recent years. In contrast to insects, where the distribution of maternal mRNA (e.g., *bicoid*) defines the body axis, the longitudinal axis of chordates is not necessarily identical with that of the egg cell. In birds, for instance, these two axes are roughly perpendicular to each other. The prospective body axis is established somewhat later by cells of the embryo itself (i.e., by the organizer at the dorsal lip of the blastoporus). In *Xenopus* these cells were shown to express a gene (*goosecoid*) whose product is responsible for the formation of the notochord (Niehrs et al., 1994). Injections of *goosecoid* mRNA into early *Xenopus* embryos induce formation of additional body axes with not only a notochord but also a neural tube (Cho et al., 1991).

The notochord, once established, presumably hinders the rise of another body axis. It may be speculated that a restriction of such an inhibitory process marks the embryological origin of an echinoderm. This may also be reflected in the phylogenetic stem lineage of the phylum. Jefferies et al. (1996) have detailed a series of transformations, starting from a unirayed condition (Raff, 1996), that are characterized by duplication, triplication, and at last quintuplication of the ambulacra (trunk axes in our terms). Although speciation by multiplication of body parts is only one possibility among a variety of others (Hotchkiss, 1998; Raff, 1996), all the opinions are based on a similar molecular process, by which new axes are generated.

Hydrocoel and Notochord—Are They Convergent or Homologous?

Because the echinoderm ectoneural cord may be homologous to the chordate neural plate (see earlier discussion of echinoderm ectoneural chord versus chordate neural plate), a similar relationship between the echinoderm hydrocoel and the chordate notochord must be examined more closely.

Orthologues of genes that in vertebrates and in *Amphioxus* (Holland et al., 1995; Zhang et al., 1997) take part in the formation of the notochord (*Brachyury* and *HNF-3β*) were demonstrated in early sea urchin embryos. These genes were intensely expressed first in cells around the blastoporus, in a later stage in the entire archenteron, and finally in the tip of the archenteron and the founder cells of the secondary mesenchyme (Harada et al., 1996). From these cells, all coelomic sacs are derived, including the left hydrocoel, which plays an eminent role in the formation of rays during metamorphosis, as does the notochord with respect to the body axis of chordates.

Furthermore, both notochord and hydrocoel induce neurons to differentiate in the overlying ectoderm. This has been definitely demonstrated in the chordate neural tube and is also very likely to happen in the echinoderm ectoneural cord (Kaestner, 1963; David and Mooi, 1996). Consequently, both structures immediately underlie the neural tube or ectoneural cord, respectively.

Furthermore, notochord and hydrocoel share two morphological features: Both are hollow tubes and both are surrounded by a specific thickening of the extracellular matrix. As is the case with the hydrocoelomic channel, the notochord of many chordates is hollow, at least transiently in early embryogenesis, as can be seen immediately in mammals and several birds and reptiles, where it originates by invagination. In the urochordates *Oikopleura* and free-swimming Ascidian larvae, the chorda dorsalis is a jelly-filled tube (Fig.2.8a,c) bordered by a squamous epithelium throughout life (Olsson, 1965; Burighel and Cloney, 1997). The specific surrounding matrix has been interpreted as "the most consistent unifying morphological characteristic of chordate notochords" (Balser and Ruppert, 1990). Such a fibrous layer was observed also in the enteropneust stomochord (Welsch and Storch, 1970; Balser and Ruppert, 1990) and around the notochord of several nonvertebrate chordates. Also, the echinoderm hydrocoelomic channels, in particular their peripheral parts, often are ensheathed by a thickened basement membrane and/or a layer of specific fibrillar connective tissue. Particularly interesting also is that some enteropneusts share a basiepithelial nervous plexus in their stomochord epithelium (Welsch and Storch, 1970) with that in echinoderm hydrocoelomic tubes (i.e., hyponeural system). Thus, there is accumulating evidence allowing us to consider the hydrocoelomic channel and the notochord as homologues.

LOCOMOTION OF ECHINODERMS

Echinoderms are principally composed of five modules resembling chordate trunks, including an ectoneural cord each, that are fused by a ring in the center. Individual arms are normally not able to survive. There are only few but well-known exceptions (e.g., species of the sea star genus *Linckia*, which regenerate complete five-rayed animals from a single arm). Even these regenerates always complete a disk and further rays, indicating that not a solitary ray but the cooperation of circularily arranged rays is the model "approved" by evolution.

On the one hand, this points to the limited efficiency of a single ectoneural cord which is improved by cooperation. According to Hotchkiss (1998), Raff (1996) pointed out that Cambrian nonpentameral, asymmetrical, and nearly bilaterally symmetrical echinoderm classes became extinct, and only pentameral echinoderms survive to the present.

On the other hand, the coordinating ring structure in the disk is not comparable with the brain of chordates or the cerebral ganglion of protostomians in many respects (e.g., great independence of the rays). Refraining from forming a distinct cerebral superior control unit might have been a main condition for the successful echinoderm model. The echinoderm model thus combines the advantage of relatively independent units (i.e., arms) with that of a coordinating structure (i.e., the disk).

The highest degree of independence is seen in the segments of the ectoneural cords in ophiuroids and asteroids or of the aboral cords in crinoids (see earlier discussion). In echinoids and holothuroids, where arms are integrated into the body wall, the radial nerves lack a morphologically demonstrable metamery; however, the existence of locally restricted, segment-like subunits must be assumed on the basis of locally restricted reflectory responses (e.g., foot retraction following upon gentle contact, *Echinus esculentus*, Anton, 1927, or *Holothuria surinamensis*, Crozier, 1915).

Comparable with the link of a chain, the segment contributes to various movements of the entire arm. These movements include all kinds of bending and stiffening, enrolling, and waving, which enables echinoderms with free arms to swim, crawl, stand on the five tips, or sweep the substrate. In different behavioral patterns, the single arms act simultaneously or alternately, or thus transiently provide the entire animal with a target-oriented anterior pole. In most ophiuroids and asteroids, for instance, two kinds of directed movement were observed: Either two arms walk on each side of the animal with the fifth ray being dragged behind, or one ray leads with two walking on each side, a form of ambulation that has also been observed in crinoids (Langeloh, 1937). Behavioral observation suggests that it is always the arm that receives the most intense sensory input, either of light (*Asterias rubens*, Just, 1927) or of a chemoattractant (*Asterias forbesi*, Dale, 1998), that assumes leading function. *Pycnopodia helianthoides*, an asteroid with 20 arms, in which a particular arm is reported always to lead (Cuénot, 1948), is an exceptional example, not representing the phylum. Echinoids and holothuroids also display a wide spectrum of coordinated movements (e.g., unilinear walking on spicules or directed swimming in the open waters). Echinoids mostly move perpendicular to the oral–aboral axis, holothuroids mostly with the oral pole leading.

The contribution of an arm to the coordinated patterns of movements is altered or disappears entirely when the ectoneural cord or the connecting ring structures in the disk are injured. Pronounced reactions of this kind were observed in sea stars and brittle stars and also in crinoids (although referring in the latter animals to injury of the aboral nerves and their central aboral ring and the ganglion around the chambered organ), while in echinoids and holothuroids the central ring seems to play a less important role. According to Smith (1965), isolated arms of *Asterias rubens* walk in opposite directions depending on whether a sector of the central ring is still present or not. In an animal with a ring transsected twice, the podia of different arms lose their common direction of step. Isolated arms of the brittle star *Ophioglypha* sp. remain much longer active when containing a part of the ring (Mangold, 1909). In echinoids, tube feet and spines move independently on the two sides of a transsected radial nerve (Kinosita, 1941). In crinoids (several species of *Antedon*), removal of the central ring and the chambered organ made the arms rigidly stretched out (Carpenter, 1876), while an isolated sector with two arms continues to strike similarly as in normal swimming (Moore, 1924). Normal swimming by the entire feather star requires the central parts to be unsevered (Langeloh, 1937).

On the basis of the behavioral observations described above, integration tuners must be postulated, that harmonize the actions of the arms in changing situations. In crinoids, such integrative tuners may be located in the ring commissure and chambered organ of the aboral system (Langeloh, 1937). In the other four classes, the integrative tuners are localized in the radial cords themselves and may also be in the rings (Smith, 1965), which possess many neuronal perikarya of various sizes, arranged mostly in a clear geometric order. It remains unresolved to date whether these tuners should be assessed as central nervous systems or even a brain. Some coordinating functions of these tuners are certainly comparable, however, with functions of the central nervous system of other metazoans.

PHYLOGENETIC ASPECTS

Consistency Versus Flexibility of Regulatory Genes

It is widely accepted that homeobox genes were conserved for hundreds of millions of years. Nevertheless, this genetic stability did not block evolution either at the DNA level or at the level of the gene product. One possibility for adopting new developmental roles is gene duplication (Holland, 1990; Sharman and Holland, 1996). As far as we know, this possibility is not true for echinoderms, because in this class homeobox genes are present as single copies only. Therefore, the presence of orthologous genes in echinoderms is difficult to interpret in terms of function, in particular when the structures that these genes code in chordates—in particular in vertebrates—apparently are missing in echinoderms.

There are two possible ways of handling this problem, namely, either to state that there is a gene but the structure depending on it not yet known or to look for the missing structure. Harada et al. (1996), who demonstrated the expression of the notochord-bound gene *forkhead* in the sea urchin embryo, point out that "Echinoderms lack a notochord or any structures obviously homologous with it." Lowe and Wray (1997), who substantiated the expression of *engrailed* in brittle star larvae, state that "the superficial similarity between brittle stars and bilateral animals is probably convergent," but also concede that "it is possible that a neurogenic role for *engrailed* is widely conserved among triploblastic animals." Thus, the question about the detailed functions that these genes (*engrailed*, or the anterior group of homeotic genes) take over in echinoderms have to remain open at the moment. However, as discussed in Question of Symmetry, above, echinoderms do possess structures that may be homologous with a notochord or a neural plate, respectively, and that, therefore, could be the result of the same genetic regulation. There are also, however, genetic parallels without morphological equivalents: *Orthodenticle*, which in vertebrate embryos is expressed in the anlage of the prosencephalon (Brand and Wurst, 1997), is found activated in the ectoderm at the tips of the arms of ophiuroid larvae (Lowe and Wray, 1997), which would be at the "wrong end" of the ectoneural tube.

Garstang's hypothesis

In 1894, Garstang postulated a common ancestor for echinoderms, enteropneusta, and chordates, a bilateral ancestor looking like a young auricularia larva. As described earlier in Larval Nervous System, the nervous tissue of such a larva is related to densely ciliated epidermal regions (i.e., with the apical tuft and with the ciliary bands). Reevaluating Garstang's hypothesis on the background of modern embryological knowledge, Lacalli (1994) presumes that the neural plate of the hypothetical ancestor is derived from the aboral ectoderm, which is *Hox* positive. This aboral ectodermal field is bordered on both sides by ciliary bands and their ciliary nerve plexus, which in the dorsal midline closely approach each other. The resulting double band markedly resembles a chordate neural plate and an ambulacral groove of adult echinoderms. The latter may be located superficially and be engaged in food acquisition (crinoids), superficially and be exclusively neuronal in function (asteroids), or hidden and be exclusively neuronal (remaining classes).

Systematics of Echinoderms

Textbooks often allot a somewhat peripheral place to echinoderms within deuterostomians as an ancient, highly derived group with secondary rotatory symmetry and a low differentiation level of the nervous system. The auricularia (dipleurula) hypothesis of Garstang or Lacalli, respectively, brings echinoderms much closer to the chordates. Moreover, the entry into the club of true notoneuralians (i.e., deuterostomians with a dorsal neural tube) would be facilitated if the traditional view of the echinoderm body axis (represented either by the rotatory oral–aboral axis or by a line through one, "leading", ray and its opposite interray), is given up in favor of the concept of trunklike modules that hitherto were looked at as arms and, furthermore, if the ectoneural cord that dominates the nervous system of all classes except crinoids becomes substantiated as homologous to the chordate neural plate.

Missing Brain

Neurulation is a necessary condition for the formation of a chordate central nervous system. When submerged into the deeper parts of the body wall, the (cryptosyringid) echinoderm ectoneural cord reflects in every respect the result of a neurulationlike process. Outbulging of the neural tube at its anterior end characterizes the developing chordate brain. In no echinoderm has a comparable process been observed hitherto, probably because a persistent anterior end is lacking. In chordates the evolution of prosencephalic structures is correlated with increasing cognitive abilities. As echinoderms lack a brain and thus also a forebrain, it can be assumed that they lack the substrate of advanced cognition. Nevertheless, echinoderms can be dated back into the Cambrium. They have survived all geological periods of crisis (e.g., at the end of Permian), and the efficiency and adaptive capability of their nervous system might have been involved in this successful history.

REFERENCES

Anton, H. (1927) Die Koordination der Saugfüsschenreflexe der regulären Echiniden. Ein Beitrag zur Zentrumsfrage. *Z. Vergl. Physiol.* 5:801–816.

Ball, B.J., and M. Jangoux (1990) Ultrastructure of the tube foot sensory–secretory complex in *Ophiocomina nigra* (Echinodermata, Ophiuroidea). *Zoomorphology* 109:201–209

Balser, E., and E.E. Ruppert (1990) Structure, ultrastructure, and function of the preoral heart–kidney in *Saccoglossus kowalevskii* (Hemichordata, Enteropneusta) including new data on the stomochord. *Acta zool.* 71(4):235–249.

Bargmann, W., M.V. Harnack, and K. Jacob (1962) Über den Feinbau des Nervensystems des Seesternes (*Asterias rubens* L.). I. Ein Beitrag zur vergleichenden Morphologie der Glia. *Z. Zellforsch.* 56:573–594.
Beer, A.-J., and M.C. Thorndyke (1998) Studies on the developing nervous system of *Psammechinus miliaris*. In R. Mooi and M. Telford (eds.): *Echinoderms*. Rotterdam, Balkema, PP.567–570.
Birenheide, R. (1989) Ultrastrukturelle und experimentelle Untersuchungen am Kauapparat und am Darmkanal des Seeigels. Doctoral Thesis, Ruhr, Universität Bochum.
Birenheide, R. (1990) Functional analysis of the tooth support in echinoids. In DeRidder et al. (eds.):*Echinoderm Research*, Balkema, Rotterdam, pp. 203–206.
Bisgrove, B.W., and R.D. Burke (1987) Development of the nervous system of the pluteus larva of *Strongylocentrotus droebachiensis*. *Cell Tissue Res.* 248:335–343
Bosch, I., R.B. Rivkin and S.P. Alexander (1989) Asexual reproduction by oceanic planktotrophic echinoderm larvae. *Nature*, 337:169–170.
Bouland, C., C. Massin, and M. Jangoux (1982) The fine structure of the buccal tentacles of *Holothuria forskali* (Echinodermata, Holothuroidea). Zoomorphology 101:133–149.
Brand, M., and W. Wurst (1997) Regionale determination in der Neuralplatte der Wirbeltiere: Entstehung und Organization der Mittel-Hinterhirn-Region. *Neuroforum* 1.97:8–14.
Brehm, P., and J.G. Morin (1977) Localization and characterization of luminescent cells in *Ophiopsila californica* and *Amphipholis squamata* (Echinodermata: Ophiuroidea). *Biol. Bull.* 152:12–25.
Bullock, T.H. (1965) Comparative aspects of superficial conduction systems in echinoids and asteroids. *Am. Zool.* 5:545–562.
Burighel, P., and R.A. Cloney (1997) Urochordata: Ascidiacea. In F.W. Harrison and E.E. Ruppert (eds.): *Microscopic Anatomy of Invertebrates, vol. 15, Hemichordata, Chaetognatha, and the Invertebrate Chordates*. Wiley-Liss, New York, pp. 221–347.
Burke, R.D. (1978) The structure of the nervous system of the pluteus larva of *Strongylocentrotus purpuratus*. *Cell Tissue. Res.* 191:233–247.
Burke, R.D., D.G. Brand, and B.W. Bisgrove (1986) Structure of the nervous system of the auricularia larva of *Parastichopus californicus*. *Biol. Bull.* 170:450–460.
Byrne, M. (1994) Ophiuroidea. In F.W. Harrison and F.S. Chia (eds.): *Microscopic Anatomy of Invertebrates, vol. 14, Echinodermata*. Wiley-Liss, New York, pp. 247–344.
Carpenter, P.H. (1876) Remarks on the anatomy of the arms of the crinoids. *J. Anat. Lond.* 10:571–585.
Cavey, M.J. (1998) Neuromyoepithelial relationships in the starfish ambulacrum and excitation–contraction coupling among the podial retractor cells. In R. Mooi and M. Telford (eds.): *Echinoderms*. Balkema, Rotterdam, pp. 215–219.
Cavey, M.J., and K. Märkel (1994) Echinoidea. In F.W. Harrison and F.S. Chia (eds.): *Microscopic Anatomy of Invertebrates, vol. 14, Echinodermata*. Wiley-Liss, New York, pp. 345–400.
Chee, F., and M. Byrne (1997) Visualization of the developing serotonergic nervous system in the larvae of the sea star, *Patiriella regularis* using confocal microscopy and copmputer generated 3-D reconstructions. *Inverteb. Reprod. Dev.* 31:151–158.
Chia, F.S., and R.D. Burke (1978) Echinoderm metamorphosis: fate of larval structures. In F.S. Chia and M.E. Rice (eds.): *Settlement and Metamorphosis of Marine Invertebrate Larvae*. Elsevier, New York, pp. 219–234.
Chia, F.S., and R. Koss (1994) Asteroidea. In F.W. Harrison and F.S. Chia (eds.): *Microscopic Anatomy of Invertebrates, vol. 14, Echinodermata*. Wiley-Liss, New York, pp. 169–246.
Cho, K.W.Y., B. Blumberg, H. Steinbeisser, and E.M. DeRobertis (1991) Molecular nature of Spemann's organizer: the role of the *Xenopus* homeobox gene *goosecoid*. *Cell* 67:1111–1120.
Cobb, J.L.S. (1970) The significance of the radial nerve cords in Asteroids and Echinoids. *Z. Zellforsch.* 108:457–474.
Cobb, J.L.S. (1985a) The neurobiology of the ectoneural/hyponeural synaptic connection in an echinoderm. *Biol. Bull.* 168:432–446.
Cobb, J.L.S. (1985b) The motor innervation of the oral plate ligament in the brittle star *Ophiura ophiura* (L.). *Cell Tissue Res.* 242:685–688.
Cobb, J.L.S. (1987) The neurobiology of the echinodermata. In M.A. Ali (ed.): *Invertebrate Nervous Systems*, Nato ASI Ser. A. Plenum Press, New York, pp. 483–525.
Cobb, J.L.S. (1988) A preliminary hypothesis to account for the neural basis of behavior in echinoderms. In R.D. Burke (ed.): *Echinoderm Biology*. Rotterdam, Balkema, pp. 565–573.

Cobb, J.L.S. (1990a) The significance of a non-centralized nervous system to general studies on echinoderm biology. In C. De Ridder, P. Dubois, M.C. Lahaye, and M. Jangoux (eds.): *Echinoderm Research.* Balkema, Rotterdam, pp. 3–7.

Cobb, J.L.S. (1990b) A physiological study of the correlation between motor output in hyponeural nerves and arm movements in the brittlestar *Ophiura ophiura. Mar. Behav. Physiol.* 17:147–157.

Cobb, J.L.S. (1995) The nervous systems of Echinodermata: recent results and new approaches. In O. Breidbach and W. Kutsch (eds.): *The Nervous Systems of Invertebrates: An Evolutionary and Comparative Approach* Birkhäuser, Basel, pp. 407–424

Cobb, J.L.S., and K.M. Begbie (1994) Aspects of the hyponeural nervous system. In B. David et al. (eds): *Echinoderms Through Time*, Balkema, Rotterdam, pp. 25–29.

Cobb, J.L.S., and M. Ghyoot (1993) The giant through conducting neuron of the brittlestar *Ophiura ophiura*—a key neuron? *Comp. Biochem. Physiol.* 105A: 697–703.

Cobb, J.L.S., and A. Moore (1986) Comparative studies on the receptor structure in the brittlestar *Ophiura ophiura. J. Neurocytol.* 15:97–108.

Cobb, J.L.S., and A.M. Raymond (1979) The basiepithelial nerve plexus of the viscera and coelom of Eleutherozoan Echinodermata. *Cell Tissue Res.* 202:155–163.

Cobb, J.L.S., and T.R. Stubbs (1981) The giant neurone system in Ophiuroids. I. The general morphology of the radial nerve cords and circumoral ring. *Cell Tissue Res.* 219:197–207.

Cobb, J.L.S., and T.R. Stubbs (1982) The giant neuron system in ophiurois. III. The detailed connections of the circumoral nerve ring. *Cell Tissue Res.* 226:675–687.

Crozier, W.J. (1915) The sensory reactions of *Holothuria surinamensis* Ludwig. *Zool. Jb. (All. Zool.)* 35:233–297.

Cuénot, L. (1948) Anatomie, éthologie et systématique des Échinodermes. In P.P. Grassé (ed.): *Traité de Zoologie*, 11. Masson, Paris, pp. 3–363.

Dale, J.H. (1998) Coordination of chemosensory orientation in the starfish *Asterias forbesi*. In R. Mooi and M. Telford (eds.): *Echinoderms*. Balkema, Rotterdam, p. 233

David, B. (1993) How to study evolution in echinoderm? In M. Jangoux and J.M. Lawrence (eds.): *Echinoderm Studies* vol 4. Balkema, Rotterdam, pp. 1–80.

David, B., and R. Mooi (1996) Embryology supports a new theory of skeletal homologies for the phylum Echinodermata. *C.R. Acad. Sci. Paris*, 319:577–584.

DeBremaeker, N., D. Deheyn, M.C. Thorndyke, F. Baguet, and J. Mallefet (1997) Localization of S1- and S2-like immunoreactivity in the nervous system of the brittle star *Amphipholis squamata* (Delle Chiaje 1828). *Proc. R. Soc. Lond. Biol.* 264:667–674.

DeBremaeker, N., J. Mallefet, and F. Baguet (1996) Luminescence control in the brittlestar *Amphipholis squamata*: effect of cholinergic drugs. *Comp. Biochem. Physiol.* 115C:75–82.

DeRidder, C., and M. Jangoux (1982) Digestive systems: Echinoidea. In M.Jangoux and J.M. Lawrence (eds.): *Echinoderm Nutrition* Balkema, Rotterdam, pp. 213–234

DeRidder, C., and M. Jangoux (1993) The digestive tract of the spatangoid echinoid *Echinocardium cordatum* (Echinodermata): morphofunctional study. *Acta Zool. (Stockh.)* 74:337–351

Díaz-Miranda, L., R.E. Blanco, and J.E. García-Arrarás (1995) Localization of the heptapeptide GFSKLYFamide in the sea cucumber *Holothuria glaberrima* (Echinodermata): a light and electron microscopic study. *J. Comp. Neurol.* 352:626–640.

DiBernardo, M., R. Russo, P. Oliveri, R. Melfi, and G. Spinelli (1994) Expression of homeobox-containing genes in the sea urchin (*Paracentrotus lividus*) embryo. *Genetica* 94:141–150.

Dolecki, G.J., G. Wang, and T. Humphreys (1988) Stage- and tissue-specific expression of two homeobox genes in sea urchin embryos and adults. *Nucleic Acids Res.* 16:11543–11558.

Duvernoy, G.L. (1848) Sur les analogies de composition et sur quelques points de l'organization des échinodermes. *C. R. Acad. Sci. Paris* 26:76–83, 266–271, 290–294.

Ehlers, U. (1997) Ultrastructure of the statocysts in the apodous sea cucumber *Leptosynapta inhaerens* (Holothuroidea, Echinodermata). *Acta Zool.* 78:61–68.

Erlinger, R., U. Welsch, and J.E. Scott (1993) Ultrastructure and biochemical observations on proteoglycans and collagen in the mutable connective tissue of the feather star *Antedon bifida* (Echinodermata, Crinoidea). *J. Anat.* 183:1–11.

Feral, J.P., and C. Massin (1982) Digestive sytems: Holothuroidea. In M.Jangoux and J.M. Lawrence (eds.): *Echinoderm Nutrition.* Balkema, Rotterdam, pp. 191–212.

Flammang, P., and M. Jangoux (1992) Functional morphology of the locomotory podia of *Holothuria forskali*. Zoomorphology 111:167–178.
Florey, E., and M.A. Cahill (1977) Ultrastructure of sea urchin tube feet. Evidence for connective tissue involvement in motor control. *Cell Tissue Res.* 177:195–214.
Florey, E., and M.A. Cahill (1980) Cholinergic motor control of the sea urchin tube feet: evidence for chemical transmission without synapses. *J. Exp. Biol.* 88:281–292.
Gans,C., and R.G. Northcutt (1983) Neural crest and the origin of vertebrates: a new head. *Science* 220:268–274.
Garstang, W. (1894) Preliminary note on a new theory of the phylogeny of the Chordata. *Zool. Anz.* 17:122–125.
Gemill, J.F. (1914) The development and certain points in the adult structure of the starfish *Asterias rubens*. *Philos. Trans. R. Soc. Lond. Biol.* 205:213–294.
Ghyoot, M., and J.L.S. Cobb (1994) Immunocytochemical investigations on the radial nerve cord of *Ophiura ophiura*. In B. David et al. (eds.): *Echinoderms through Time*, Balkema, Rotterdam, pp. 429–434.
Ghyoot, M., J.L.S. Cobb, and M.C. Thorndyke (1994) Localization of neuropeptides in the nervous system of the brittle star *Ophiura ophiura*. *Philos. Trans. R. Soc. Lond. Biol.* 346:433–444.
Haanen, W. (1914) Anatomische und histologische Studien an *Mesothuria intestinalis* (Ascanius und Rathke). Engelmann, Leipzig, pp. 1–255.
Hamann, O. (1885) Beiträge zur Histologie der Echinodermen. Heft 2. Die Asteriden. Fischer, Jena, 1–126.
Harada, Y., K. Akasaka, H. Shimada, K.J. Peterson, E.H. Davidson, and N. Satoh (1996) Spatial expression of a forkhead homologue in the sea urchin embryo. *Mech. Dev.* 60(2):163–174.
Heinzeller, T., J.L.S. Cobb, A. Lange, and U. Welsch (1993) SALMFamid-immunoreaktive Neurone im aboralen Subsystem von *Antedon bifida*. *Verh. Dtsch. Zool. Ges.* 86:160.
Heinzeller, T., H. Fechter, N. Améziane-Cominardi, and U. Welsch (1997) Development of *Cyathidium foresti* (Echinodermata: Crinoidea, Cyrtocrinida) from early attached larvae to adult-like juveniles. *J. Zool. Syst. Evol. Res.* 35:11–21.
Heinzeller, T., and U. Welsch (1994) Crinoidea. In F.W. Harrison and F.S. Chia (eds.): *Microscopic Anatomy of Invertebrates, Vol. 14, Echinodermata*. Wiley-Liss, New York, pp. 9–148.
Heinzeller, T., U. Welsch, A. Lange, and J.L.S. Cobb (1992) Anti-NGF-positive Nervenzellen und -fasern bei *Antedon bifida*, ein sensibles Subsystem? *Verh. Dtsch. Zool. Ges.* 85:225.
Hendler, G., and M. Byrne (1987) Fine structure of the dorsal arm plate of *Ophiocoma wendti*: evidence for a photoreceptor system (Echinodermata, Ophiuroidea). *Zoomorphology* 107:261–272.
Hörstadius, S. (1939) Über die Entwicklung von *Astropecten aranciacus* L. *Publ. Della Stat. Zool. Napoli* 17:221–312.
Holland, L.Z., M. Kene, N.A. Williams, and N.D. Holland (1997) Sequence and embryonic expression of the amphioxus *engrailed (AmphiEn)*: the metameric pattern of transcription resembles that of its segment-polarity homolog in *Drosophila*. *Development* 124:1723–1732.
Holland, N.D., and J.C. Grimmer (1981) The fine structure of the cirri and a possible mechanism for their motility in stalkless crinoids (Echinodermata). *Cell Tissue Res.* 214:207–217.
Holland, P.W.H. (1990) Homeobox genes and segmentation: co-option, co-evolution, and convergence. *Sem.in.Dev.Biol.* 1:135–145.
Holland, P.W.H. (1996) Molecular biology of lancelets: insights into development and evolution. *Israel J. Zool.* 42:S247–S272.
Holland, B., P.W.H., L.Z. Koschorz, Holland, and B.G. Hermann (1995) Conservation of *Brachyury (T)* genes in amphioxus and vertebrates—developmental and evolutionary implications. *Development* 121:4283–4291.
Hotchkiss, F.H.C. (1998) Diskussion on pentamerism: the five-part pattern of *Stomatocystites*, Asterozoa and Echinozoa. In R. Mooi and M. Telford (eds.): *Echinoderms*. Balkema, Rotterdam, pp. 37–42.
Hyman, L.H. (1955) *The Invertebrates, vol. 4: Echinodermata. The Coelomate Bilateria.* McGraw-Hill, New York.
Jaeckle, W.B. (1994) Multiple modes of asexual reproduction by tropical and subtropical sea star larvae: an unusual adaptation for genetic dispersal and survival. *Biol. Bull.* 186:62–71.
Jangoux, M. (1982) *Digestive systems: general considerations.* In M.Jangoux and J.M. Lawrence (eds.): Echinoderm Nutrition. Balkema, Rotterdam, pp. 185–186.
Jefferies, R.P.S., N.A. Brown, and P.E.J. Daley (1996) The early phylogeny of chordates and echinoderms and the origin of chordate left-right asymmetry and bilateral symmetry. *Acta Zool.* 77 (2):101–122

References 73

Joyner, A.L. (1996) *Engrailed, Wnt* and *Pax* genes regulate midbrain–hindbrain development. *Trends Genet.* 12:15–19

Just, G. (1927) Untersuchungen über Ortsbewegungsreaktionen. I. Das Wesen der phototaktischen Reaktionen von *Asterias rubens. Z. Vergl. Physiol.* 5:247–282.

Kaestner, A. (1963) *Lehrbuch der Speziellen Zoologie.* Fischer, Jena.

Kawaguti, S. (1965) Electron microscopy on the ovarian wall of the echinoid with special references to its muscles and nerve plexus. *Biol. J. Okayama Univ.* 11:66–74.

Kinosita, H.J. (1941) Conduction of impulse in superficial nervous system of sea urchin. *Jpn. J. Zool.* 9:221–232.

Lacalli, T.C. (1994) Apical organs, epithelial domains, and the origin of the chordate central nervous system. *Am. Zool.* 34:533–541.

Lacalli, T.C. (1996) Mesodermal pattern and patern repeats in the starfish bipinnaria larva, and related patterns in other deuterostome larvae and chordates. *Philos. Trans. R. Soc. Lond. Biol.* 351:1737–1758.

Lacalli, T.C., and J.E. West (1993) A distinctive nerve cell type common to diverse deuterostome larvae: comparative data from echinoderms, hemichordates and Amphioxus. *Acta Zool. (Stockh.)* 74 (1):1–8.

Lange, W. (1876) Beitrag zur Anatomie und Histologie der Asteriden und Ophiuren. *Morphol. Jb.* 2:241–286.

Langeloh, H.-P. (1937) Über die Bewegung von *Antedon rosaceus* und ihre nervöse Regulierung. *Zool. Jb.* 57: 236–279.

Lepper, D.M.E., and P.A. Moore (1998) The role of chemical signals in the foraging behavior of the sea star *Asterias forbesi.* In R. Mooi and M. Telford (eds.): *Echinoderms.* Balkema, Rotterdam, p. 266.

Lindemann, W. (1900) Über einige Eigenschaften der Holothurienhaut. *Z. Biol.* 39: 18–36.

Lowe, C.J., and G.A. Wray (1997) Radical alterations in the roles of homeobox genes during echinoderm evolution. *Nature* 389(6652):718–721.

Märkel, K., and U. Röser (1985) Comparative morphology of echinoderm calcified tissues: histology and ultrastructure of ophiurid scales (Echinodermata, Ophiuroidea). *Zoomorphology* 105:197–207.

Märkel, K., and U. Röser (1991) Ultrastructure and organization of the epineural canal and the nerve cord in sea urchins (Echinodermata, Echinoidea). *Zoomorphology* 110:267–279.

Mangold, E. (1909) Studien zur Physiologie des Nervensystems der Echinodermen. III. Über die Armbewegungen der Schlangensterne und v. Uexkülls Fundamentalgesetz für den Erregungsverlauf. *Pflügers. Arch. Ges. Physiol.* 126: 371–406.

Martínez, A., J. López, L.M. Montuenga, and P. Sesma (1993) Regulatory peptides in gut endocrine cells and nerves in the starfish *Marthasterias glacialis. Cell Tissue Res.* 271:375–380.

Martínez, A., V. Riveros-Moreno, J.M. Polak, S. Moncada, and P. Sesma (1994) Nitric oxide (NO) synthase immunoreactivity in the starfish *Marthasterias glacialis. Cell Tissue Res.* 275:599–603.

Martínez, A., E.J. Unsworth, and F. Cuttitta (1996) Adrenomedullin-like immunoreactivity in the nervous system of the starfish *Marthasterias glacialis. Cell Tissue Res.* 283:169–172.

Matsuno, A., and T. Motokawa (1992) Evidence for calcium translocation in catch connective tissue of the sea cucumber *Stichopus chloronotus. Cell Tissue Res.* 267:307–312.

McKenzie, J.D. (1987) The ultrastructure of the tentacles of eleven species of dendrochirote holothurians studied with special reference to the surface coats and papillae. *Cell Tissue Res.* 248:187–199.

McKenzie, J.D. (1988) Ultrastructure of the tentacles of the apodous holothurian *Leptosynapta* spp., with special reference to the epidermis and surface coats. *Cell Tissue Res.* 251:387–397.

McKenzie, J.D. (1992) Comparative morphology of crinoid tube feet. In L. Scalera-Liaci and C. Canicatti (eds.): *Echinoderm Research 1991.* Balkema, Rotterdam, pp. 73–79.

Mito, T. (1998) A PCR survey of Hom/Hox-class homeobox genes in the sea star, *Asterina minor.* In R. Mooi and M. Telford (eds.): *Echinoderms.* Balkema, Rotterdam, p. 285.

Mooi, R., B. David, and D. Marchand (1994) Echinoderm skeleton homologies: classical morphology meets modern phylogenesis. In B. David et al., (eds.): *Echinoderms Through Time.* Balkema, Rotterdam, pp. 87–95.

Moore, A.R. (1924) The nervous mechanism of coordination in the crinoid *Antedon rosaceus. J. Gen. Physiol.* 6:281–288.

Moore, A., and J.L.S. Cobb (1985) Neurophysiological studies on photic responses in *Ophiura ophiura. Comp. Biochem. Physiol.* 80A:11–16.

Moore, A., and J.L.S. Cobb (1986) Neurophysiological studies on the detection of mechanical stimuli by *Ophiura ophiura* (L.). *J. Exp. Mar. Biol. Ecol.* 104:125–141

Moore, S.J., and M.C. Thorndyke (1993) Immunocytochemical mapping of the novel echinoderm neuropeptide SALMFamide 1 (S1) in the starfish *Asterias rubens*. *Cell Tissue Res.* 274:605–618.

Morris, V.B., J. Brammall, M. Frommer, and M. Byrne (1998) Homeobox gene sequences identified in the sea urchin *Holopneustes purpurescens*. In R. Mooi and M. Telford (eds.): *Echinoderms*. Balkema, Rotterdam, pp. 759–760.

Nakajima, Y. (1987) Localization of catecholaminergic nerves in larval echinoderms. *Zool. Sci.* 4:293–299.

Newman, S.J., and M.C. Thorndyke (1994) Localisation of gamma aminobutyric acid (GABA)-like immunoreactivity in the echinoderm *Asterias rubens*. *Cell Tissue Res.* 278:177–185.

Nezlin, L.P., I.M. Prudnikov, and P.V. Davydov (1991) Catecholaminergic neurons in the larval nervous system of starfishes during metamorphosis. *J. Evol. Biochem. Physiol.* 27:19–27.

Niehrs, C., H. Steinbeisser, and E.M. DeRobertis (1994) Mesodermal patterning by a gradient of the vertebrate homeobox gene *goosecoid*. *Science* 263:817–820.

Olsson, R. (1965) Comparative morphology and physiology of the *Oikopleura* notochord. *Isr. J. Zool.* 14:213–220.

Pentreath, R.J. (1969) The morphology of the gut and a qualitative review of digestive enzymes in some New Zealand ophiuroids. *J. Zool. Lond.* 159:413–423.

Pentreath, V.W., and J.L.S. Cobb (1972) Neurobiology of Echinodermata. *Biol. Rev.* 47:363–392.

Peters, B.H. (1985) The innervation of spines in the sea-urchin *Echinus esculentus* L. An electron-microscopic study. *Cell Tissue Res.* 239:219–228.

Peters, B.H., and A.C. Campbell (1987) Morphology of the nervous and muscular systems in the heads of pedicellariae from the sea urchin *Echinus esculentus* L. *J. Morphol.* 193:35–51.

Popodi, E., J.A. Bolker, M.J. Ferkowicz, M.E. Andrews, and R.A. Raff (1998a) Development of the sea urchin central nervous system in *Heliocidaris erythrogramma*. In R. Mooi and M. Telford (eds.): *Echinoderms:* Balkema, Rotterdam, p. 791.

Popodi, E., M.J. Ferkowicz, M.E. Andrews, and R.A. Raff (1998b) Expression of *engrailed* and *wnt5* in the developing sea urchin nervous system. In R. Mooi and M. Telford (eds.): *Echinoderms*. Balkema, Rotterdam, p. 792.

Popodi, E., J.C. Kissinger, M.E. Andrews, and R.A. Raff (1996) Sea urchin *Hox* genes: insights into the ancestral hox cluster. *Mol. Biol. Evol.* 13(8):1078–1086.

Raff, R.A. (1996) The shape of life: genes, development, and the evolution of animal form. University of Chicago Press, Urbana, pp. 417–423.

Remane, A. (1952) *Die Grundlagen des natürlichen Systems, der vergleichenden Anatomie und der Phylogenetik*. Akademische Verlagsgesellschaft, Leipzig.

Rodriguez, S.R., J.M. Farina, and F.P. Ojeda (1998) Behavior and spatial distribution patterns of the sea urchin *Tetrapygus niger* (Echinodermata: Echinoidea) in presence of predators, food, and topography. In R. Mooi and M. Telford (eds.): *Echinoderms*. Balkema, Rotterdam, p. 804.

Schechter, J., and J., Lucero (1968) A light and electron microscopic investigation of the digestive system of the ophiuroid *Ophiuroiderma panamensis* (brittle star). *J. Morphol.* 124:451–482.

Seeliger, O. (1892) Studien zur Entwicklungsgeschichte der Crinoiden. *Zool. Jb. Abt. Anat. Ontogenie* 6:161–444.

Semon, R. (1883) Das Nervensystem der Holothurien. *Jen. Z. Nat. Wiss.* 16:578–600.

Sharman, A.C., and P.W.H. Holland (1996) Conservation, duplication, and divergence of developmental genes during chordate evolution. *Neth. J. Zool.* 46:47–67.

Smiley, S. (1986) Metamorphosis of *Stichopus californicus* (Echinodermata: Holothuroidea) and its phylogenetic implications. *Biol. Bull.* 171:611–631.

Smiley, S. (1994) Holothuroidea. In F.W. Harrison and F.S. Chia (eds.): *Microscopic Anatomy of Invertebrates, Vol. 14, Echinodermata*. Wiley-Liss, New York, pp. 401–472.

Smith, A.B. (1984) Classification of the Echinodermata. *Paleontology*, 27(3): 431–459.

Smith, J.E. (1937) On the nervous system of the starfish *Marthasterias glacialis* (L.). *Philos. Trans. R. Soc. Lond.* 227:111–173.

Smith, J.E. (1965) Echinodermata. In T.H. Bullock and G.A. Horridge (eds.): *Structure and Function in the Nervous System of Invertebrates*. Freeman & Co., San Francisco, pp. 1520–1558.

Spix, J.B.V. (1809) Mémoire pour servir a l'histoire de l'Asterie Rouge. *Ann. Mus. Hist. Nat. Paris* 13:438–459.

Stubbs, T.R., and J.L.S. Cobb (1981) The giant neuron system in Ophiuroids. II. The hyponeural motor tracts. *Cell Tissue Res.* 220:373–385.

Stubbs, T.R., and J.L.S. Cobb (1982) A new ciliary feeding structure in an ophiuroid echinoderm. *Tissue Cell* 14:573–583.

Thurmond, F.A., J.A. Trotter, T.J. Koob, and J.M. Bowness (1998) Microfibrils from sea cucumber dermis belong to the fibrillin family, and their long-range elasticity is a crucial component of mutable collagenous tissues. In R. Mooi and M. Telford (eds.): *Echinoderms*. Balkema, Rotterdam, p. 528.

Tosuji, H. (1998) Determination of oral-aboral axis in larvae of the starfish, *Asterina pectinifera*. In R. Mooi and M. Telford (eds.): *Echinoderms*. Balkema, Rotterdam, p. 311.

Trotter, J.A., G. Lyons-Levy, D. Luna, T.J. Koob, D.R. Keene, and M.A.L. Atkinson (1996) Stiparin: a glycoprotein from sea cucumber dermis that aggregates collagen fibrils. *Matrix Biol.* 15:99–110.

v. Hehn, G. (1970) Über den Feinbau des hyponeuralen Nervensystems des Seesternes (*Asterias rubens* L.). *Z. Zellforsch.* 105:137–154.

Viehweg, J., W.W. Naumann, and R. Olsson (1998) Secretory radial glia cells in the ectoneural system of the sea star *Asterias rubens* (Echinodermata). *Acta Zool.* 79:119–131.

Welsch, U., and V. Storch (1970) The fine structure of the stomochord of the Enteropneusts *Harrimannia kupfferi* and *Ptychodera flava*. *Z. Zellforsch.* 107:234–239.

Wilkie, I.C. (1978) Nervously mediated change in the mechanical properties of brittlestar ligament. *Mar. Behav. Physiol.* 5:289–306.

Wilkie, I.C. (1979) The juxtaligamental cells of *Ophiocoma nigra* (Abilgaard) (Echinodermata: Ophiuroidea) and their possible role in mechano-effector function of collagenous tissue. *Cell Tissue Res.* 197:515–530.

Wilkie, I.C. (1996) Mutable collagenous tissues: extracellular matrix as mechano-effector. In M. Jangoux and J.M. Lawrence (eds.): *Echinoderm Stud.* 5:61–102.

Wilkie, I.C., M.D. Candia Carnevali, and F. Andrietti (1994) Microarchitecture and mechanics of the sea-urchin peristomial membrane. *Boll. Zool.* 61:39–51.

Wilkie, I.C, M.D. Candia Carnevali, and F. Bonasoro (1992) The compass depressors of *Paracentrotus lividus* (Lamarck) (Echinodermata: Echinoidea): ultrastructural and mechanical aspects of their variable tensility and contractility. *Zoomorphology* 112:143–153.

Wu, J.-Y., C.-P. Chen, C.-F. Hui, S.P.L. Hwang, and D.J. Miller (1998) Preliminary studies on Hox type homeoboxes in the echinoids *Stomopneustes variolaris* and *Tripneustes gratilla*. In R. Mooi and M. Telford (eds.): *Echinoderms*. Balkema, Rotterdam, p. 893.

Yoshida, M., N. Takasu, and S. Tomatsu (1984) Photoreception in echinoderms. In M.A. Ali (ed.): Photoreception and vision in invertebrates. New York, Plenum, pp. 743–771.

Yamamoto, M., and M. Yoshida (1978) Fine structure of the ocelli of a synaptid holothurian, *Opheodesoma spectabilis*, and the effects of light and darkness. *Zoomorphologie* 90:1–17.

Zhang, S., N.D. Holland, and L.Z. Holland (1997) Topographic changes in nascent and early mesoderm in amphioxus embryos studied by DiI labeling and in situ hybridization for a *Brachyury* gene. *Dev. Genes Evol.* 206:532–535.

Chapter 3

EVOLUTION OF VERTEBRATE MOTOR SYSTEMS

Hans J. ten Donkelaar, Departments of Anatomy/Embryology and Neurology, University of Nijmegen

INTRODUCTION

During the evolution of vertebrates, various locomotor patterns such as swimming, crawling, walking, running, jumping, brachiation, flying, and burrowing were developed (Fig. 3.1). Each of these diverse locomotor modes is derived from the fundamental swimming pattern (i.e., lateral undulation) present in most aquatic chordates (see Romer and Parsons, 1977; Young, 1981). Paired fins did not evolve until later. When the land vertebrates arose, most probably from the crossopterygian rhipidistians (Carroll, 1988), the lateral paired fins were converted into organs of locomotion on the ground or in the air. The basic pattern of terrestrial locomotion consists of a combination of lateral undulation of the trunk with protraction and retraction of the limbs in a sprawling way (Edwards, 1977; Rewcastle, 1981). Secondarily, limbs were lost in caecilians (apodans), snakes, and limbless lizards, and aquatic adaptations appeared in various extinct reptiles (e.g., mesosaurs, ichthyosaurs, and mosasaurs), cetaceans, and pinnipeds. Most birds use their modified forelimbs for flight. In birds, the beak functions in reaching, grasping, and manipulation of food. In mammals, particularly in primates, modifications of the distal parts of the extremities (usually the forelimbs) allowed the manipulation of the environment.

Neural control of locomotion results from an interplay of three major elements (Wetzel and Stuart, 1976, 1977; Grillner, 1981; Rossignol, 1996): (1) central pattern generators within the spinal cord capable of generating stereotypical, cyclic patterns, (2) peripheral input, and (3) descending supraspinal control (Fig. 3.2). The cerebellum plays an important role in the coordination of rhythmical movements such as locomotion (Arshavsky et al., 1986). The manipulation of the environment involves specialized forms of supraspinal control. The descending pathways from the forebrain and brain stem to the spinal cord represent the instruments by which the central nervous system (CNS) steers movements of the trunk, the tail, and the extremities. All vertebrates have a certain repertoire of descending brain stem pathways in common (ten Donkelaar, 1982). Reticulospinal neurons constitute the

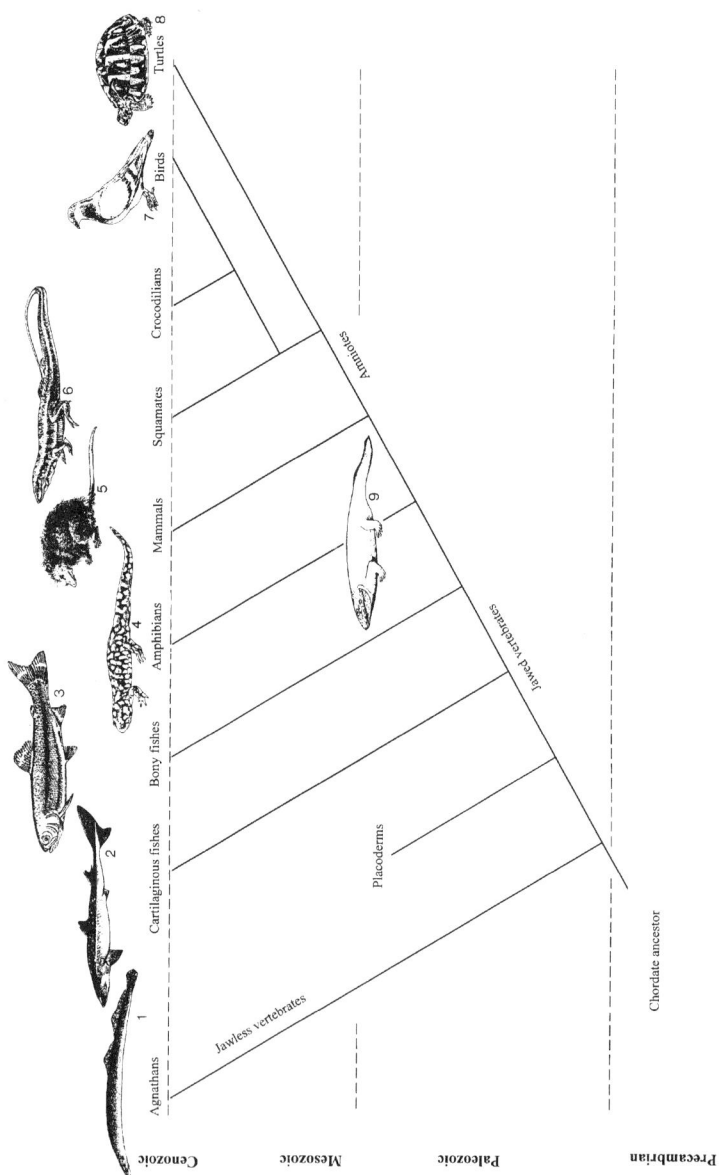

Figure 3.1. Evolution of the chordates (after a diagram from, Carroll, 1988). The living vertebrates illustrated are 1, the lamprey, *Lampetra fluviatilis*; 2, the spiny dogfish *Squalus acanthias*; 3, the rainbow trout *Salmo gairdneri*; 4, the tiger salamander *Ambystoma tigrinum*; 5, the North American opossum *Didelphis virginiana*; 6, the tegu lizard *Tupinambis teguixin*; 7, the pigeon *Columba livia*, and 8, the tortoise *Testudo hermanni*. (From Nieuwenhuys et al., 1998, by permission of Springer, Berlin). The oldest tetrapod known, *Ichthyostega* (9), from the late Devonian of East Greenland, is also shown (after Jarvik, 1955).

Introduction

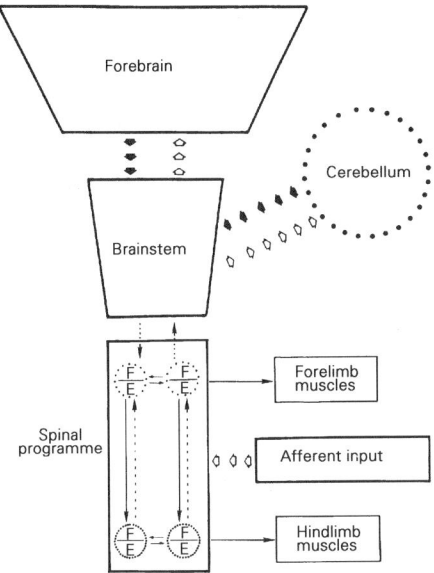

Figure 3.2. The neural control system for quadrupedal locomotion. F, E, flexor and extensor pool motoneurons. (After Wetzel and Stuart, 1977.)

most ancestral descending motor system by which the vertebrate brain exerts control over movements in all classes from cyclostomes to mammals (Shapovalov, 1972, 1975; Rovainen, 1979). With the appearance of extremities, the development of an adequate neural control system for the steering of limb movements became apparent. It is likely that the rubrospinal tract plays an important role in this mechanism (ten Donkelaar, 1988).

The most notable difference between the motor circuitry of nonmammalian vertebrates and mammals is the apparent absence of somatomotor cortical areas giving rise to long descending projections to the spinal cord in nonmammalian vertebrates. The corticospinal tract is unique to mammals, and its development appears to be associated with the acquisition of dexterous motor skills (Kuypers, 1981; Heffner and Masterton, 1983; Nudo and Masterton, 1990a,b). In birds, a unique sensorimotor circuit is present that is related to handling ("mandibulation") of food (Wild et al., 1985). Its anatomical organization is analogous to that of the sensorimotor pathways controlling the forelimbs of mammals.

In the present survey, after some introductory notes on the various types of locomotion found in vertebrates and on prehensile extremities, aspects of the spinal and supraspinal networks for locomotion and the neural circuitry for the manipulation of the environment are discussed. The examples presented show the basic features in motor control found in vertebrates, but, moreover, various ways in which the CNS has adapted to the specific requirements posed by the major structural and physiological changes in the history of vertebrates.

BASICS OF VERTEBRATE LOCOMOTION

The ancestral vertebrate evolved in an aquatic environment and, presumably, swam using its axial musculature (Romer and Parsons, 1977). Studies in the cephalochordate *Branchiostoma lanceolatum* (Webb, 1973), larval lampreys, salamander larvae, and adult eels (Blight, 1977) showed that Amphioxus, cyclostomes, and various fishes as well as amphibian larvae move by means of an undulatory wave, which is transmitted along the body from head to tail (Fig. 3.3). All fish and the larval stages of most amphibians are *primary swimmers* and show a great diversity of locomotor adaptations (Gray, 1968; Webb, 1982; Webb and Blake, 1985). Fish with paired fins use these for postural stability and steering control, but also to maneuver and propel the body at low speed. For ordinary steady or rapid swimming most species depend on body propulsion. *Secondary swimmers* include aquatic and semiaquatic reptiles, birds, and mammals, which have returned to the water from terrestrial habitats. Throughout early tetrapod evolution, there is a tendency to return

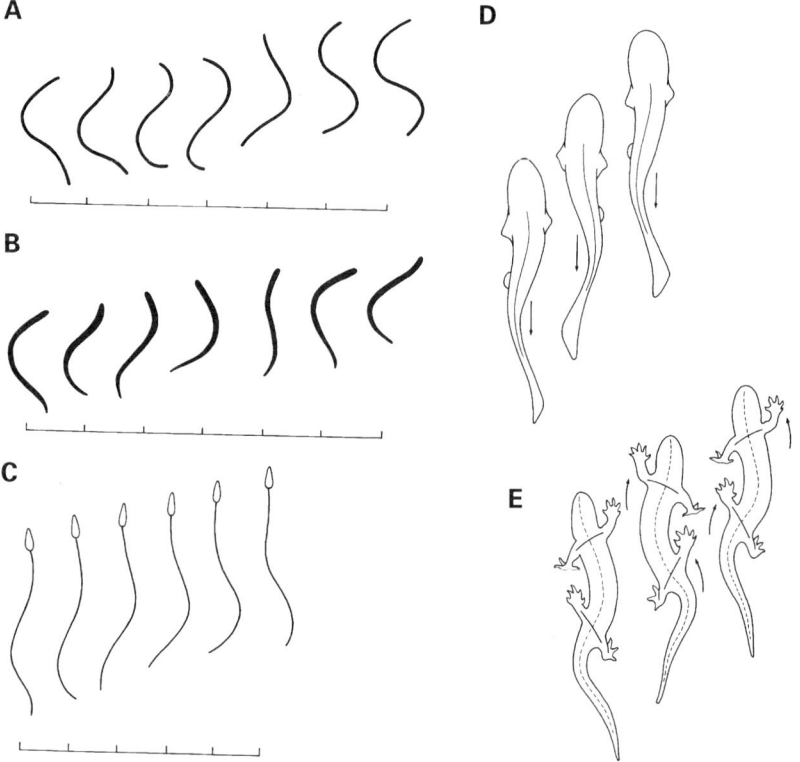

Figure 3.3. (*A–C*), Swimming movements traced from ciné film (after Blight, 1977) of A, the midline positions of a 45 mm adult Amphioxus (based on data by Webb, 1973); B, a 7 mm stage 17 *Petromyzon marinus* larva; C, an adult eel. (*D,E*) The evolution of terrestrial locomotion (after Romer and Parsons, 1977).

to the water, particularly among reptiles. Basically, all swimmers use one of two types of propulsion (Webb and Blake, 1985): axial undulatory propulsion or appendage propulsion (undulatory or oscillatory). In undulatory movements, waves are passed along the body or fin propulsors. Oscillatory propulsors are usually paired ppendages such as the large pectoral flippers of sea turtles.

During the conquest of the land, the lateral paired fins were converted into pentadactyl limbs. The earliest amphibians, the Upper Devonian ichthyostegids found in late Devonian sediments from East Greenland (Jarvik, 1955), were ponderous and clumsy-looking animals (see Fig. 3.1), over a meter long with large skulls, short trunks, and stocky limbs. Their skeletal pattern is basic to all terrestrial vertebrates, while the proximal limb bones, girdles, vertebrae, and dermal bones of the skull are all directly comparable with those of osteolepiform rhipidistians (Carroll, 1988). Changes in the skeleton between the rhipidistian fish and early amphibians are related to the requirements of support, feeding, and locomotion on land. The ancestral tetrapod pattern was most probably a quadrupedal gait in which the limbs became of major importance in providing propulsive thrust. Early tetrapods possessed the sprawling limb posture and, presumably, a traveling wave lateral undulation system (Fig. 3.3E) as an inheritance (Edwards, 1977; Rewcastle, 1981).

Terrestrial locomotion requires the movements of elongated appendages in regularly repeated cycles. The neural activation of limb muscles must also by cyclic. Such cycles result in specific patterns of footfalls or gaits (see Sukhanov, 1974; Hildebrand, 1976; Alexander, 1977). A quadruped can only be stable when it has three or four feet on the ground. Locomotion involving lateral undulation may have favored retention of the sprawling limb posture (Edwards, 1977), but there was a shift to increased limb dependence. The upright or erect posture arose independently in both the sauropsid (reptiles and birds) and mammalian lineages. The Archosauria ("ruling reptiles"), including dinosaurs and crocodilians, reduce or eliminate the lateral flexure of the vertebral column and bring the limbs more directly under the body (Romer, 1966).

Adaptations for terrestrial locomotion include various advanced types such as running adaptations, bipedal walking and running, limbless locomotion, climbing, and locomotion among trees (arm swinging of brachiation), in soil (digging), and in air (parachuting, gliding, and flying).

Several lineages of tetrapods, including caecilians, plethodontid salamanders, snakes, skinks, and amphisbaenians (worm lizards) have reduced their limbs or lost them entirely. Such reduction or loss of limbs is always associated with elongation of the body (Gans, 1974, 1975, 1985). Except for snakes, almost all limbless terrestrial forms are shelterers or burrowers. *Limbless locomotion* can be quite efficient. Snakes crawling on a treadmill have a cost of transport only about half of that of comparably sized limbed reptiles (Chodrow and Taylor, 1973). Limbless locomotion can be divided into various types of undulatory movements, including lateral undulation—the most common mode of limbless locomotion—concertina locomotion, and sidewinding (Fig. 3.4A–C). These modes are powered by waves of contraction that travel from rostral to caudal along the axial musculature of alternating sides of the trunk (Gans, 1974, 1975, 1985; Edwards, 1985). Rectilinear locomotion is common in

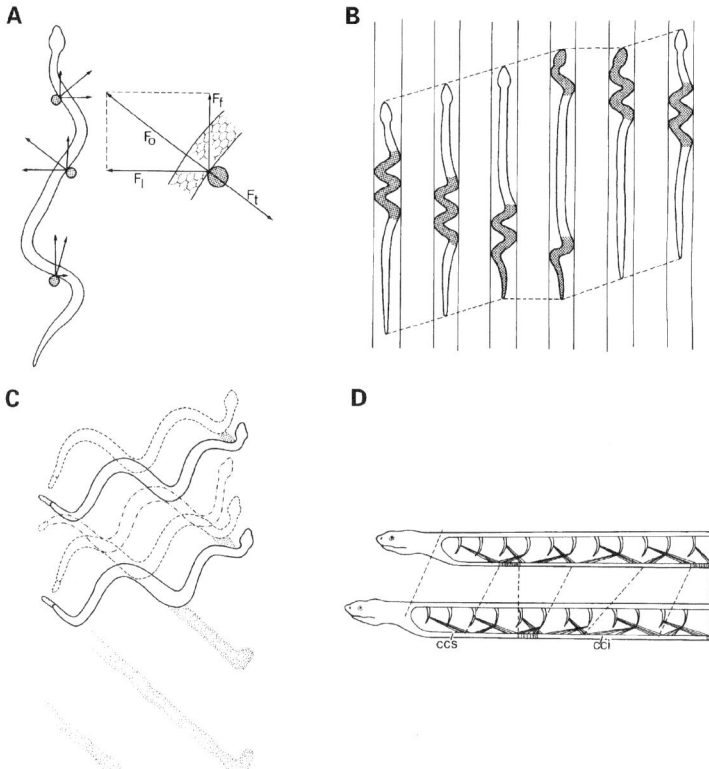

Figure 3.4. Limbless locomotion. (*A*) Lateral undulation, (*B*) Concertina locomotion, (*C*) Sidewinding, (*D*) Rectilinear locomotion. During lateral undulation, the thrust of the snake (F_t) against an object (e.g., a plant stem) is opposed by an equal and opposite force (F_o) exerted by the object against the body. This force has a forward component (F_f) in the direction that the snake is moving and a lateral component (F_l). cci, inferior costocutaneous muscles; ccs, superior costocutaneous muscles. (A–C, after Gans, 1974; D, after Lissmann, 1950; from ten Donkelaar, 1998 by permission of Springer, Berlin).

amphisbaenians and in stout-bodied snakes such as many boids and some vipers. In rectilinear locomotion, the body is held in a more or less straight line, and waves of contraction pass down the costocutaneous musculature of both sides of the body simultaneously (Fig. 3.4D). The costocutaneous muscles rapidly pull a segment of ventral skin forward into temporarily immobile contact with the ground, while the body moves uniformly over that segment. Rectilinear locomotion requires obvious structural modifications. Connective tissue attachments are reduced between skin and axial musculature, and costocutaneous muscles produce rectilinear movement (Lissmann, 1950): The large inferior costocutaneous muscles provide the propulsive action for the majority of the body, whereas the slender superior muscles are only required to lift and transport the scutes. By means of rectilinear locomotion, snakes can only move forward. In their underground tunnels, amphisbaenians, however, use this mode of locomotion both forward and backward. Amphisbaenians possess another set of costocutaneous muscles connecting the dorsal portion of each rib to the skin anterior to the rib. It is apparently this third set of costocutaneous muscles, coupled with the loose (to reduce friction), annulate skin, that allows posterior rectilinear locomotion in amphisbaenians (Gans, 1974).

Jumping has evolved independently among vertebrates at least six times (Emerson, 1985). It is dependent on great enlargement of the hindlimbs. Schmalhausen (1968) suggested that jumping was developed as a special technique for escaping from predators in small animals inhabiting the banks of ponds and rivers. Jumping vertebrates are characterized by a diversity of body forms and saltatory behaviors: Frogs usually make only one or a few jumps at a time, whereas kangaroos and springhares use jumping for sustained locomotion (hopping). Jumping results from the synchronized *(in-phase coordination)* extension of the two hindlimbs.

Most *climbing vertebrates* live in the branches of trees. The ability to climb evolved from the more common terrestrial modes of locomotion. The greatest problem with climbing is gravity, which results in a hazardous tendency to fall. Therefore, tree-living animals require special means of maintaining themselves in their precarious habitat. Several solutions were developed in arboreal vertebrates (Cartmill, 1985). Some use sharp claws for the purpose, others adhesion (arboreal frogs and salamanders, geckos) or suction (plethodontid salamanders and tropical bats) mechanisms, whereas primates have evolved prehensile hands and feet. In all primates, the limbs have a greater branch-grasping ability than is found in other placental mammals. Associated with *grasping* are the replacement of claws by flattened nails and the expansion of the plantar pads, which become covered with roughened skin. The skin pad pattern of the tree shrew likely is the retention of the ancestral mammalian pattern. In tree shrews, the palms and soles bear a number of separate and well-defined elevated pads, 11 pads per extremity (see Fig. 3.5, below). In many tree-climbing primates, but also in sloths and koalas, the volar pads are fused into a broad, soft contact surface like those of human hands. The epidermis covering the volar pads is commonly reorganized into a system of dermatoglyphic friction ridges or "fingerprints". Such ridges are found in all primates and are variably developed in arboreal marsupials, carnivores, and insectivores.

Grasping specializations on the hindfeet allow a firm grip on the support. A broadly divergent, grasping first toe is characteristic of all primates except humans (Cartmill, 1985). Specialized grasping hindfeet with divergent marginal digits are also found in chameleons, bamboo-climbing rodents, and certain tree frogs. The development of a grasping tail greatly enhanced the prehensility of the trailing end of the body in chameleons, some arboreal snakes and salamanders, and a variety of arboreal mammals. Extraordinarily specialized tails are found among spider monkeys and other atelines, which end in a fingertip-like apical pad covered with dermatoglyphics. These monkeys are capable of fine manipulation with their tail (Cartmill, 1985; Lemelin, 1995). *Brachiation* is an extension of climbing that allows relatively free movement among the branches of trees. The hands of brachiators such as gibbons are highly specialized.

Digging is used by caecilians, amphisbaenians, and many quadrupeds. Most fossorial vertebrates are highly modified for their mode of life (Hildebrand, 1985). Digging tools can be teeth, claws, feet, and even the head (e.g., in amphisbaenians).

An unusual way of digging is used by moles. They rotate the humerus around its long axis. Moles are highly fossorial, spending their entire life under ground in a system of tunnels. The most obvious adaptations to this environment are the powerful shovel-like forelimbs that are positioned laterally for digging (Yalden, 1966). Their senses are also specialized for the fossorial lifestyle. Moles seem to depend almost exclusively on their sense of touch to navigate in tunnels and locate food. There are many small sensory vibrissae on the snout and forelimbs but, moreover, a touch-sensitive patch of glabrous tissue at the end of the snout (Catania, 1995).

PREHENSILE EXTREMITIES

The intelligent use of the hand as a sensorimotor organ for exploring the visible world and to locate, identify, and appropriately use objects within reach has been an important factor in the biological success of primates (Darian-Smith et al., 1996). Apart from some specialized nonprimate mammals such as the raccoon, the sensorimotor capacities of the hand develop best in primates (Napier, 1980). In Figure 3.5, hands of the tree shrew (*Tupaia glis*), and of some primates, illustrating stages in functional organization, are presented. Modern tupaiids appear to represent the retention of an ancestral stage in the evolution of eutherians, and their general appearance may differ little from that of their Upper Cretaceous ancestors (Carroll, 1988). Moreover, the tree shrews are closely related to the primates (Novacek, 1992). A number of characteristics have been found that indicate an early separation in the phylogeny of tree shrews and primates. The primates include the prosimians (lemurs and tarsiers), monkeys, apes, and humans.

The clawed hand of the tree shrew resembles the forepaw in a number of nonprimate mammals. On a scale of digital dexterity (Table 3.1), it represents the simplest form of a hand. Specializations for locomotion such as fused or restrained digits have developed in ungulates, and nonconvergent digits are found in most carnivores. The tree shrew does not grasp small objects with one hand, but instead picks them up and manipulates them using both hands. Tree shrews show the ancestral arrangement of volar pads. Prosimians have hands with terminal fingerpads backed by nails and a clear-cut differentiation of a thumb, and they use their hands in a stereotypical prehensile pattern. The digits all extend together as the hand approaches its target and together close over it. There is no independent movement of individual fingers and no opposition of the thumb (Bishop, 1964). The hand still acts as a single functional unit. Prosimians do not explore surfaces with their fingerpads.

In the Anthropoidea, precision and power grips are added. Napier (1956) differentiated the "power grip" of the whole hand from the "precision grip" of the thumb and index finger. New World monkeys have pseudo-opposable thumbs and are not much better equipped than prosimians. They can, however, use their fingerpads to explore the surfaces and shapes of objects. The acrobatic spider monkeys (*Ateles*) and woolly monkeys (*Lagothrix*) have no external thumbs, but they can pick up small objects with the glabrous-skinned tips of their prehensile tails. The tail of these monkeys is

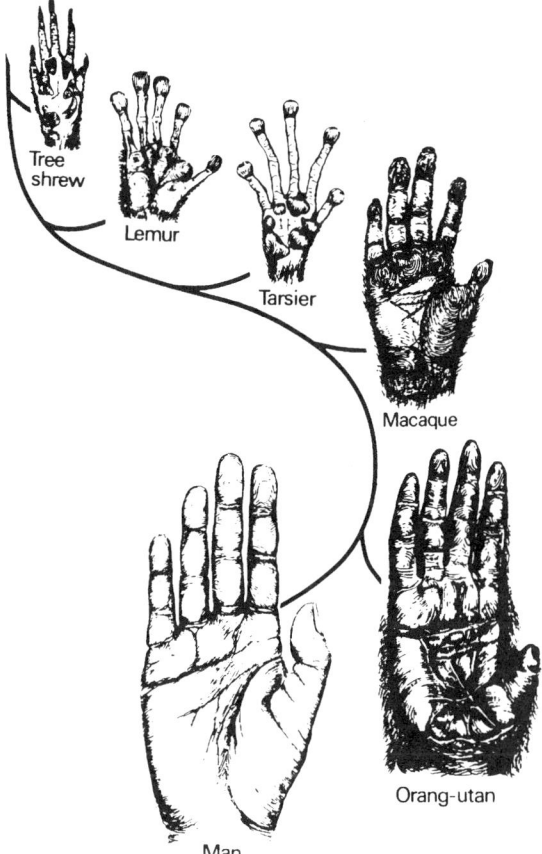

Figure 3.5. Hands of the tree shrew and some primates. (From Darian-Smith, 1984 by permission of American Physiological Society, Bethesda.)

both a power and a precision organ (Napier, 1980). It can be used to suspend the body from an overhead branch (power grip) or to delicately pick up such small items as a shelled peanut (precision grip). In the Old World monkeys, apes, and humans, the thumb is rotated through 90° in embryonic life and is truly opposable. Moreover, the tactile role of the fingerpads has developed much further, and the thumb and index fingers become independently controlled. Further development of the sensorimotor function of the hand of the apes and humans depends essentially on increasingly independent control of the movements of the remaining fingers (Darian-Smith, 1984).

FEATURES OF THE ANCESTRAL VERTEBRATE MOTOR SYSTEM

The musculature of early vertebrates was almost certainly myomeric axial musculature (see Carroll, 1988; Fetcho, 1992). Myomeric musculature is also present in living chordates such as Amphioxus and in most anamniotes (Nursall, 1956; Bone,

Table 3.1. Index of Dexterity in Different Mammals (After Heffner and Masterton (1983); based on Napier (1961) and Bishop (1964).

Function	Dexterity Index	Digit Type	Species
Specialization for locomotion	1	Fused or restrained digits	Ungulates
	2	Separate digits that do not converge when flexed	Hedgehogs, most carnivores
Simple hand	3	Convergent but not prehensile (not capable of holding an object in one hand)	Opossums, tree shrews
Specialization for manipulation	4	Prehensile digits, non opposable thumb	Tarsiers
	5	Prehensile digits, pseudo-opposable thumb	Lemurs
	6	Opposable thumb, capable of power and limited precision grips	Old World monkeys, apes
	7	Opposable thumb, capable of precision grip in opposition to each finger	Humans

1978; Fetcho, 1987). It is seen in agnathans, cartilaginous and bony fishes (Fig. 3.6), urodeles, and anuran tadpoles. A segmental origin of the musculature is also evident during the development of amniotes but greatly transformed in adults. Bone (1978) emphasized a plain phylogenetic increase in complexity of shape of the myotomes, from the simple "V" shape in Amphioxus via the shallow "W" shape of agnathans, to the deep "W" shape of gnathostomes (see Fig. 3.6).

The myomeric musculature in Amphioxus and in most anamniotes can be divided into two major muscle fiber types or muscle units (Bone, 1978; Fetcho, 1987): a slow fiber type, relatively slow-contracting and long-lasting; and a fast type, contracting and relaxing quickly. Typically, the slow fibers form only a small part of all muscle fibers and occupy a superficial position. In *Branchiostoma lanceolatum*, the muscle fibers are flattened sheets or lamellae (Fig. 3.6E) the slow components of which extend only a short distance medially from the lateral surface. The fast fibers span the whole mediolateral extent of the myomeres (Flood, 1968). The muscle fibers send processes medially to contact the spinal cord. These processes (the "ventral roots") contact a specialized region of the ventral part of the spinal cord that can be divided into a dorsal and a ventral compartment (Flood, 1968). The processes of the two different types of muscle fibers contact these compartments: The superficial lamellae send long thin processes to the dorsal compartment, whereas the deep lamellae send relatively large processes to the ventral compartment. Although Bone (1978) distinguished at least two types of motoneurons, it remains to be established which neurons contact the two compartments. In agnathans, the myomeres are formed by subunits containing groups of fast fibers, surrounded by slow ones (Rovainen, 1979; Fetcho, 1987). In lampreys, motoneurons supplying the dorsal and ventral parts of the

Features of the Ancestral Vertebrate Motor System   87

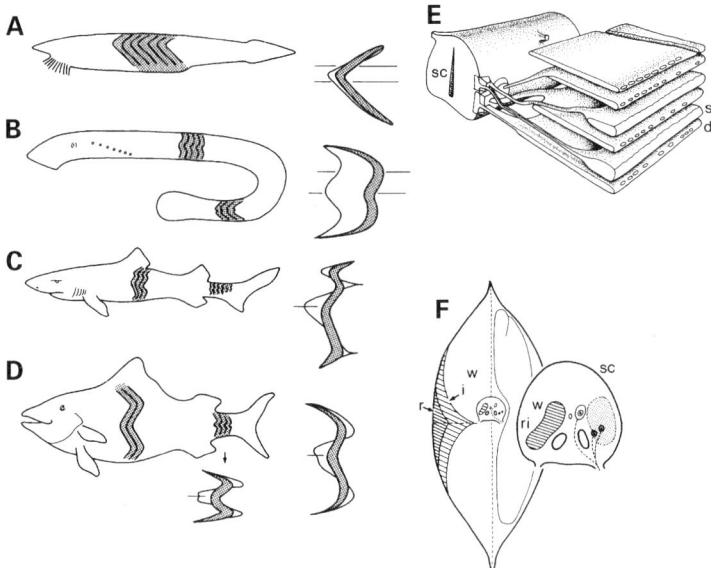

Figure 3.6. (*A–D*) The myomere pattern of fishlike chordates (after Nursall, 1956). Lateral views of the chordates in question are shown as well as horizontal sections through a myomere. A, Amphioxus; B, a lamprey (*Petromyzon*); C, a cartilaginous fish (*Squalus*); D, a teleost (*Perca*). (*E*) Various muscle types of Amphioxus (after Flood, 1968). In Amphioxus, the ventral roots consist of medial projections from the myotomal muscle cells synapsing directly at the ventral part of the spinal cord. (*F*) Various muscle types and corresponding motoneurons of zebrafish (after van Asselt et al., 1990). d, s, deep and superficial muscle lamellae in Amphioxus; r, i, w, red, intermediate, and white muscle fibers as well as the localization of their motoneurons in zebrafish; sc, spinal cord.

myotomes have different morphological characteristics (Wallén et al., 1985). In both cartilaginous and bony fishes, the slow fibers form a red band of muscle along the superficial surface of the myomere just beneath the skin (Bone, 1978; Fetcho, 1987) (Fig. 3.6F). The red muscle fibers are responsible for slow cruising movements. The fast fibers are recruited if the speed of swimming has to be increased. Thus, throughout anamniotes, two major classes of motoneurons are present, suggesting that they were present in early vertebrates (Fetcho, 1992).

The spinal motoneurons are controlled by spinal and supraspinal networks. In the living anamniotes and likely in ancestral vertebrates (see Fetcho, 1992), the major movement produced by the central circuits is lateral bending of the body. Such swimming can be initiated in lampreys, cartilaginous and bony fishes, frog embryos, and turtles. It is produced by a *central pattern generator* (CPG) within the spinal segments that can produce the basic swimming pattern independent of sensory feedback and input from the brain (see Grillner et al., 1988). A CPG can be defined as a network of interconnected neurons that produces rhythmic output with neither rhythmic input nor reflexes (Cohen, 1988; Arshavsky et al., 1993). The spinal circuitry underlying locomotion has been extensively studied in lampreys, particularly because in vitro preparations of the isolated spinal cord or brain stem-spinal cord have proved

3 Evolution of Vertebrate Motor Systems

to be excellent models for such studies (see Brodin and Grillner, 1990). The *Xenopus* embryo model has also been analyzed extensively (Roberts, 1989, 1990).

In Figure 3.7A, the spinal network of premotor interneurons in the lamprey spinal cord is shown. The segmental locomotor interneurons include one excitatory (EIN) and two inhibitory (CCIN, LIN) types, and their synaptic interactions have been demonstrated with electrophysiological techniques (Rovainen, 1979; Grillner et al., 1988). EINs excite all ipsilateral neurons, CCINs inhibit all contralateral neurons, whereas LINs discharge only at the peak of the depolarization and inhibit CCINs, therefore disinhibiting the contralateral side. Provided that the background excitation is sufficient, the neurons on the contralateral side will start discharging, thereby

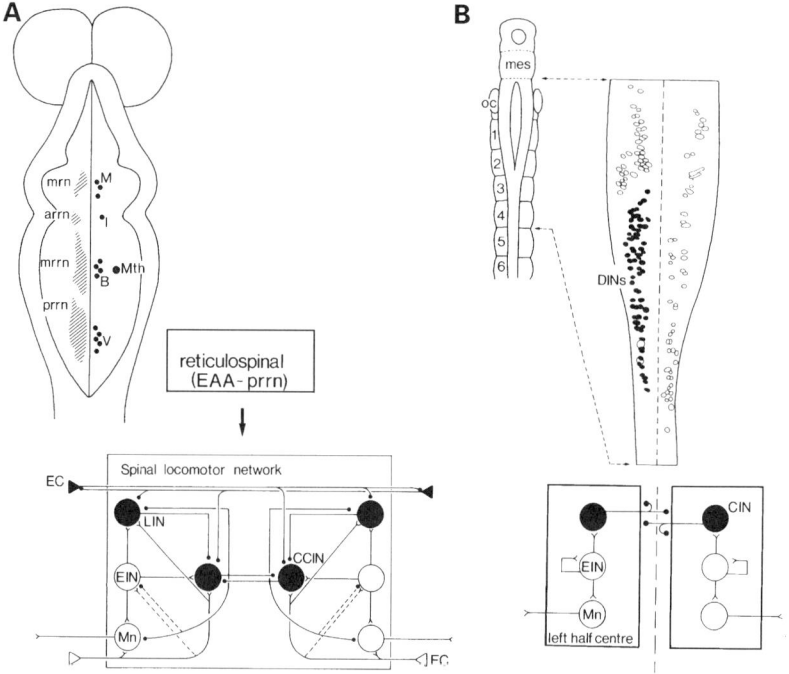

Figure 3.7. (*A*) Schematic drawings of the lamprey brain from a dorsal view. The reticular formation (left side) consists of posterior (prrn), middle (mrrn), and anterior (arrn) rhombencephalic and mesencephalic (mrn) reticular nuclei and the mesencephalic (M), isthmic (I), bulbar (B), and vagal (V) Müller cells. These structures as well as the Mauthner (Mth) cell form the supraspinal centers innervating the segmental network of premotor interneurons shown below (after Brodin and Grillner, 1990). This segmental network is composed of one excitatory interneuron (EIN), two inhibitory type neurons (CCIN, a crossed caudal interneuron; LIN, a lateral interneuron), and a motoneuron (Mn). Edge cells (EC) feed back information to this network. (*B*) A dorsal view of the brain and rostral spinal cord (the first six postotic myotomes [1–6] are shown) of a stage 37/38 *Xenopus laevis* embryo (after Roberts and Alford, 1986). The enlarged part shows the labeled neurons after horseradish peroxidase application at the left half of the fourth spinal segment. The dark cells indicate the "descending interneurons" (DINs) in the rhombencephalic reticular formation. These cells drive the half centers present in the spinal cord (after Arshavsky et al., 1993). CIN, commissural (inhibitory) interneuron; EAA, excitatory amino acid–mediated transmission; EIN, excitatory interneuron; mes, mesencephalon; Mn, motoneuron; oc, otic capsule.

inhibiting neurons on the initially active side. Therefore, *reciprocal inhibition* between groups of interneurons that control the motoneurons for antagonistic pairs of muscles, primarily active in alternation, forms the basis for CPG organization (Grillner and Matsushima, 1991; Arshavsky et al., 1993). Brown (1911) called such groups "half-centres". Data in frog embryos are summarized in Figure 3.7B. Great similarities exist in terms of overall CPG organization, cellular components, and transmitters involved between lamprey and anuran embryos.

Movement feedback interacts with the central network underlying locomotion in all species studied. Under normal conditions, the spinal network will generate the motor patterns, whereas the sensory input will feed back information about the instantaneous movements that actually occur. In lampreys, the lateral undulation of the body activates sensory stretch receptors (edge cells), which are located in the lateral margin of the spinal cord itself. The edge cells are of two types (Fig. 3.7A): an excitatory type, which via excitatory amino acid–mediated transmission excites ipsilateral motoneurons and interneurons of the locomotor network; and an inhibitory, glycinergic type, which inhibits the contralateral inhibitory interneurons and contralateral stretch receptors as well (Grillner et al., 1995). This type of stretch receptor appears to be present in several classes of vertebrates with lateral undulatory movement, including urodeles (Schroeder and Egar, 1990) and reptiles (Schroeder and Richardson, 1985).

Locomotor activity can be initiated by stimulation of reticulospinal pathways, by sensory stimuli, and, in isolated preparations of the CNS, by application of excitatory amino acid agonists (Brodin et al., 1989; McClellan, 1988; Grillner and Matsushima, 1991). Throughout vertebrates, reticulospinal neurons are large. Their coarse axons conduct rapidly and make direct connections with spinal motoneurons and interneurons (Shapovalov, 1972, 1975). Tracing studies (see Figs. 3.10, and 3.12, below). show that throughout vertebrates a basic pattern in the organization of descending pathways is present with a dominant role for reticulospinal projections. In anamniotes, a pair of giant reticulospinal neurons, called the *Mauthner cells*, plays a crucial role in escape behavior.

In lampreys, the posterior rhombencephalic reticular nucleus is the major descending drive of the spinal locomotor circuitry (McClellan, 1988; Ohta and Grillner, 1989) (see Fig. 3.7A). The reticulospinal neurons can be activated by rostral brain stem structures and by a variety of sensory stimuli. The *brain stem locomotor region* extends from the mesencephalon (the "mesencephalic locomotor region", a structure first identified in decerebrated cats by Shik et al., 1966) to the lower brain stem (McClellan, 1986). After the initial activation, most reticulospinal neurons become modulated in phase with the ipsilateral locomotor activity in rostral spinal segments (Kasicki et al., 1989). This modulation results from ascending information from the spinal locomotor circuits, which provide supplementary alternating phasic and inhibitory synaptic drives (Grillner et al., 1995). Part of this ascending projection has a relay in a dorsal column nucleus (Dubuc et al., 1993).

The neural control system for locomotion is basically similar in all classes of vertebrates (Grillner, 1981; Grillner and Matsushima, 1991) despite the fact that the mode of locomotion differs enormously among vertebrates. Essentially, locomotion is initiated from brain stem locomotor areas, and reticulospinal neurons activate spinal networks, which produce the motor pattern, activating the various muscle groups in the order necessary to produce locomotor movements. Sensory information from the ongoing movements is fed back to the spinal networks and adapts the network activity to the external conditions.

The extensive studies of the spinal and supraspinal motor networks of anamniotes, outlined above for the lamprey, likely indicate some of the features of the motor system of early vertebrates (Fetcho, 1992) (Table 3.2). Most probably, the ancestral motor system consisted of myomeric axial musculature composed of at least two types of muscle fibers: nonspiking slow muscle fibers and spiking fast muscle fibers, which are innervated by small and large motoneurons, respectively. Early vertebrates used their axial muscles to bend the body and their various types of motor units to produce slow swimming movements as well as rapid bending associated with fast swimming or escape reactions. The spinal network producing lateral undulation was most probably a circuit composed of at least two types of interneurons: an *excitatory interneuron* that produces excitation of ipsilateral motoneurons and other interneurons and an *inhibitory commissural interneuron* that blocks contralateral activity. Two major descending supraspinal systems can activate the spinal networks:

Table 3.2. Evolutionary Changes in the Ancestral Motor System

Features of the ancestral motor system

> Myomeric axial musculature
>
> Two types of muscle fibers: nonspiking slow muscle fibers and spiking fast muscle fibers
>
> Two types of motoneurons: small and large motoneurons innervating the slow and fast muscle fibers, respectively
>
> A spinal network composed of at least two types of interneurons: an excitatory interneuron and an inhibitory commissural interneuron
>
> Two major descending supraspinal systems to activate the spinal networks: reticulospinal neurons and, for rapid escape movements, Mauthner cells

Evolutionary changes in the motor apparatus

> Substantial differentiation of the ancestral myomeric musculature into many individual axial muscles
>
> Development of paired appendages and their associated musculature
>
> Loss of segregation of muscle fiber types in many muscles
>
> Development of a topographic map of the motor column onto the embryonic myotome
>
> Development of muscle spindles and, in mammals, a separate gamma motor innervation of muscle spindles
>
> Development of an adequate neural control system for the steering of limb movements
>
> Development of the corticospinal tract in mammals

After Fetcho (1992).

Reticulospinal neurons are important for the initiation of rhythmic swimming and the production of turning movements, whereas the Mauthner cells activate rapid escape or startle movements.

These features of the early motor system can be interpreted to have been retained in living anamniotes (Table 3.2). Major changes occur among amniotes, including the breakup of the myomeres into a large number of discrete axial muscles, the development of paired fins and limbs with the associated musculature, the loss of segregation of muscle fiber types in many muscles, the development of a topographic map of the motor column onto the embryonic myotome, and changes in the activation of axial musculature (Fetcho, 1992).

NEURAL CONTROL OF QUADRUPEDAL LOCOMOTION

The likely ancestors of the land vertebrates, the lobe-finned rhipidistian crossopterygians (Fig. 3.8A), presumably used their paired fins to "walk" on the bottom as the related modern lungfish do (Hinchliffe and Johnson, 1980). The only living crossopterygian, the coelacanth, *Latimeria chalumnae*, found near the islands of the Comores in the Indian Ocean at a depth of about 200 m, uses alternating coordination of the paired fins during low swimming movements in a pattern common to tetrapods and lungfish (Fricke et al., 1987). Fin muscles are derived from part of the myomeric musculature. Dorsal and ventral muscle masses, above and below the fins, respectively, raise and lower or abduct and adduct the fins (Fig. 3.8B). In land vertebrates, the dorsal and ventral muscle masses are split up into discrete muscles (Fig. 3.8C,D).

For locomotion on land an increased efficiency of the limbs was necessary. Salamanders are sprawlers and use walking gaits characterized by a standing wave mode of axial undulation in which points on the vertebral column having no lateral movement ("nodes") alternate with regions of large lateral movements (Edwards, 1977). Salamanders use traveling wave undulation when trotting. Edwards (1977) suggested that the first terrestrial gait was a trot that employed a traveling wave of axial undulation, because this is the type of wave used by fish and amphibian larvae. Frolich and Biewener (1992), however, showed that the motor control system to produce a standing wave is present in amphibian embryos and larvae. Moreover, many fish that use traveling waves during constant-velocity swimming probably have the capability to use standing waves for fast starts and escape responses (Webb and Blake, 1985). Thus, traveling waves may not be ancestral for terrestrial vertebrates. Based on extensive studies on salamander embryos, Brändle and Székely (1973) suggested that traveling waves are mediated by reticulospinal pathways to spinal motoneurons. The limbs are more or less passively carried along by the traveling waves, resulting in a trot. The walking gait is associated with a standing wave generated by *limb-moving generators*, one for each limb. The limb-moving spinal cord segments alone are incapable of controlling the alternating coordination of pairs of limbs. For this function a critical length of the medulla or, for the lumbar cord innervating the hindlimbs, that of the thoracic spinal cord must be in contact with the limb

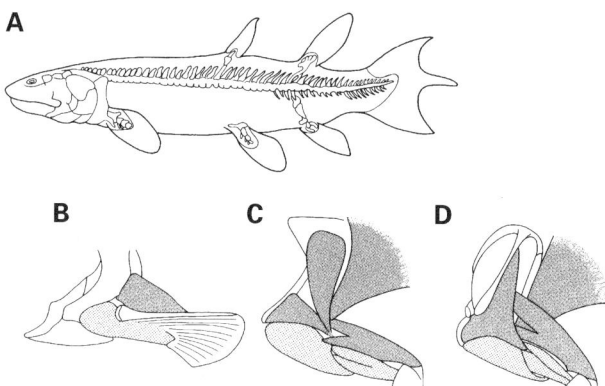

Figure 3.8. (*A*) *Eusthenopteron*, a lobe-finned rhipidistian crossopterygian representing a possible ancestor of the land vertebrates (after Hinchliffe and Johnston, 1980). (*B–D*) Dorsal (dark gray) and ventral (light gray) muscle masses and their derivatives in B, the pectoral fin of a teleost; C, the forelimb of a lizard; and D, the forelimb of an opossum (after Hinchliffe and Johnston, 1980). The pectoral fin of a teleost is abducted and adducted by dorsal and ventral muscle masses, respectively. In the lizard and opossum, the dorsal and ventral muscle masses are split into discrete muscles.

segments. It seems likely that the control of alternating limb movements is associated with the control of sinusoid movements during locomotion (Székely and Czéh, 1976).

The limb movements of salamanders are rather complicated. In the freely moving newt, *Triturus cristatus*, Székely and co-workers (1969) recorded the activity pattern of eight forelimb muscles electromyographically. Antagonistic muscle pairs co-contract extensively at both protraction and retraction (Fig. 3.9). Co-contraction of antagonistic muscle pairs is an important factor in the stabilization of the joints and in grading the movement. Similar co-contractions were recorded in the varanid lizard *Varanus exanthematicus* and in the North American opossum *Didelphis virginiana* (Jenkins and Goslow, 1983). A number of shoulder muscles in *Varanus exanthematicus* and in *Didelphis virginiana* are similar in attachment, in activity pattern with respect to phases of the step cycle, and in apparent actions. These similarities can be interpreted as a pattern inherited from the ancestors of amniote tetrapods (Jenkins and Goslow, 1983).

For locomotion, turtles depend on the use of their extremities. In the red-eared turtle, *Pseudemys scripta elegans*, electrical stimulation of the dorsolateral funiculus of intact as well as spinal turtles can elicit rhythmic limb movements similar to those observed during swimming (Lennard and Stein, 1977; Stein, 1978). These data suggest that spinalization interrupts descending pathways utilized by the intact turtle to activate CPGs for locomotion largely resident in the spinal cord. Studies in other turtle species showed that electrical stimulation of the brain stem in decerebrated turtles may evoke cyclic coordinated movements of the limbs (Kazennikov et al., 1980). As in other vertebrates, the brain stem locomotor region forms a rostrocaudally oriented strip extending from the caudal part of the mesencephalon to the caudal part of the medulla oblongata. Reticulospinal neurons serve as a final common supraspinal pathway for locomotion.

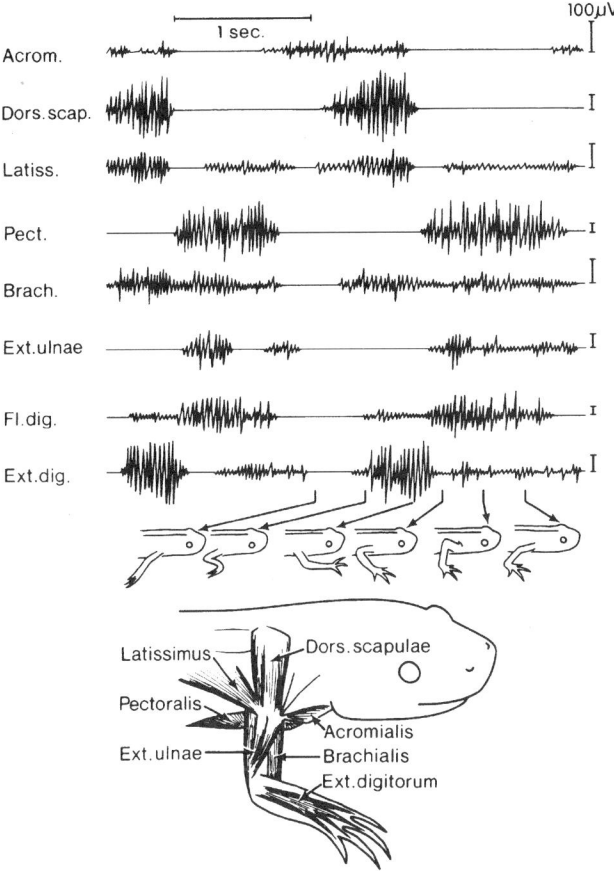

Figure 3.9. Activity pattern of eight forelimb muscles recorded electromyographically in the freely moving newt. The position of the limb is shown in different phases of the step, corresponding with the electromyographic data from muscles. (From Székely et al., 1969 by permission of Elsevier, Amsterdam.)

SUPRASPINAL CONTROL

Descending control systems from the motor cortex and the brain stem function generally in the visuomotor coordination of motor behavior. Vestibulospinal pathways are involved in equilibrium and postural activities. The cerebellum is intimately involved in the sensory to motor transformation, as will be exemplified for the cerebellorubrospinal limb control system.

Descending Supraspinal Pathways

A number of invariant motor centers and pathways are found throughout vertebrates. This is particularly evident for the descending supraspinal pathways from the brain stem (Table 3.3). In Figure 3.10, the cells of origin of descending supraspinal

Table 3.3. Major Sources of Descending Supraspinal Pathways in Vertebrates

Class	Reticular Formation	Vestibular Nuclear Complex	Interstitial Nucleus of flm	Red Nucleus	Cerebellar Nuclei	Dorsal column nuclei	Raphe Complex	Locus Coeruleus	Hypothalamus	Sub pallium	Pallium
Agnatha	+	+	+	−	−	−	+	+	?	−	−
Chondrichthyes	+	+	+	±	−	+	+	+	+	−	?
Osteichthyes	+	+	+	±	−	−	+	+	+	−	−
Amphibia	+	+	+	±	+	+	+	+	+	+	−
Reptilia	+	+	+	+	+	+	+	+	+	+	−
Mammalia	+	+	+	+	+	+	+	+	+	±	+
Aves	+	+	+	+	+	+	+	+	+	?	±

+, Present; −, absent; ±, present in certain species, absent in others; ?, questionable.

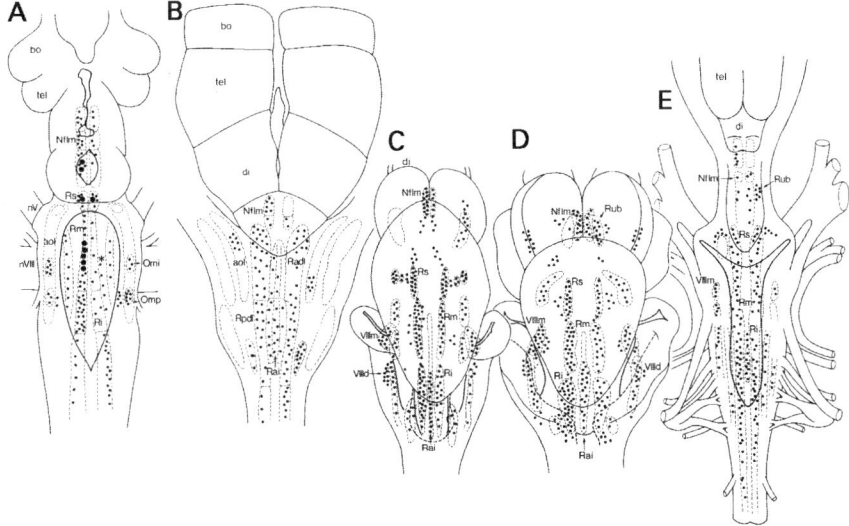

Figure 3.10. The distribution of retrogradely labeled cells in the brain stem after horseradish peroxidase injections into the left side of the spinal cord in (*A*) the silver lamprey *Ichthyomyzon unicuspis*; (*B*) the Pacific hagfish *Eptatretus stouti*; (*C*) the spotted dogfish *Scyliorhinus canicula*; (*D*) the ray *Raja clavata*; and (*E*), the African lungfish *Protopterus amphibians*. In A, the large dots indicate Müller (large reticulospinal) cells, and the asterisk indicates the Mauthner cell (A,B, after Ronan, 1989; C,D, after Smeets and Timerick, 1981; E, after Ronan and Northcutt, 1985). aol, area octavolateralis; bo, bulbus olfactorius; di, diencephalon; Nflm, nucleus of the fasciculus lengitudinalis medialis; nV, nervus trigeminus nVIII, nervus octavus; Omi, Omp, intermediate and posterior octavomotor nuclei; Radl, dorsolateral part of nucleus reticularis anterior; Rai, nucleus raphes inferior; Ri, Rm, Rs, nucleus reticularis inferior, medius, and superior; Rpdl, dorsolateral part of nucleus reticularis posterior; Rub, nucleus ruber; tel, telencephalon; VIIId, VIIIm, descending and magnocellular vestibular nuclei.

projections are shown for agnathans, cartilaginous fishes, and a lungfish. It is evident that a basic pattern is found in this series of anamniotes. Medial (reticulospinal) and lateral (octavomotor or vestibulospinal) columns are found in the brain stem. These two columns give rise to the bulk of the descending motor pathways in anamniotes. Reticulospinal projections arise from the mesencephalon (the nucleus of the fasciculus longitudinalis medialis) and throughout the rhombencephalic reticular formation. Moreover, serotonergic raphespinal and noradrenergic coerulospinal projections are common to all vertebrates (see Table 3.3) and complement the "vertebrate common plan" of descending spinal pathways (Nudo and Masterton, 1988). Spinal projections from the red nucleus, cerebellar nuclei, and the dorsal column nucleus are apparently absent in agnathans and in many cartilaginous and bony fishes. Spinal projections from the cerebellar nuclei and the dorsal column nucleus can be viewed as a *tetrapod augmentation* (Nudo and Masterton, 1988).

In anamniotes, a *red nucleus* is indistinct or cannot be identified cytoarchitectonically. Possibly, in gnathostomes, a small, unspecialized red nucleus may have originated with paired appendages. Apparently, some of its connections were lost in some fish species again. Criteria used to identify a structure as a (primordial) red nucleus are, apart from its relative position, the mesencephalic site of termination of the

3 Evolution of Vertebrate Motor Systems

brachium conjunctivum and its contralateral spinal projection (ten Donkelaar, 1988). Based on such criteria, a crossed rubrospinal tract could be unequivocally identified in the thornback ray, *Raja clavata* (Fig. 3.11B), in the common goldfish, *Carassius auratus* (Prasada Rao et al., 1987), in the African lungfish, *Protopterus amphibians* (Fig. 3.11C), in a salamander, *Salamandra salamandra* (Naujoks-Manteuffel et al., 1988), and in anurans (the clawed toad, *Xenopus laevis*: Fig. 3.11D; ranid frogs: Tóth et al., 1985; Larson-Prior and Cruce, 1992). No rubrospinal tract could be identified in a shark (Fig. 3.11A) or in a limbless amphibian, the apodan *Ichthyophis kohtaoensis* (Naujoks-Manteuffel et al., 1988). These data suggest that the presence of a rubrospinal tract is related to the presence of paired appendages. The thornback ray (*Raja clavata*) uses its enlarged pectoral fins for locomotion. In teleosts, paired fins are used for postural stability and steering control but also to maneuver and propel the body at low speed (see Webb, 1982). In this respect, it would be of great interest to know whether a well-developed rubrospinal tract is present in the mudskipper (*Periophthalmus koelreuteri*), which habitually emerges from the water, spends considerable periods of time on land, and uses its pectoral fins as struts (Harris, 1960). Snakes presumably have lost their rubrospinal tract secondarily because in boid snakes no rubrospinal tract could be demonstrated (ten Donkelaar and Bangma, 1983). On the other hand, they retain a nucleus ruber with a distinct rubro-bulbar projection, presumably involved in the neural control of mastication.

Unfortunately, in most anamniotes the site of termination in the spinal cord of descending motor pathways is hardly known. Tract-tracing data from amphibians (Fig. 3.12A), reptiles (Fig. 3.12B–D), birds (see Cabot et al., 1982), and mammals (Fig. 3.12E,F) show that throughout terrestrial vertebrates *medial* and *lateral* systems

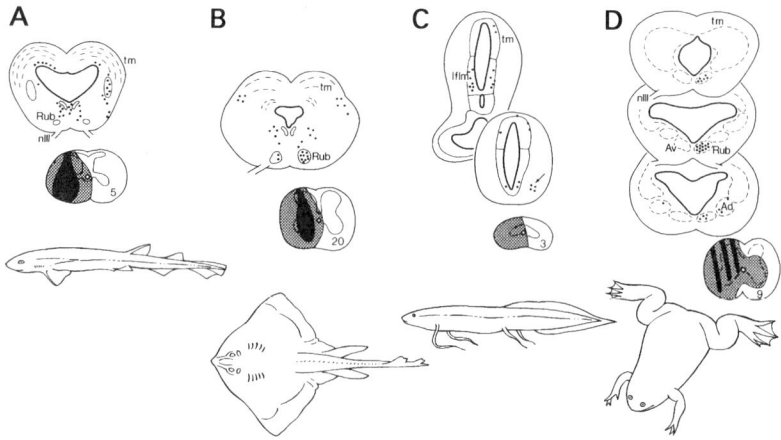

Figure 3.11. The distribution of retrogradely labeled neurons in the mesencephalon (at the level of the oculomotor nerve) after horseradish peroxidase injections into the spinal cord in (*A*) a shark, the spotted dogfish *Scyliorhinus canicula*; (*B*) the thornback ray *Raja clavata*; (*C*) the African lungfish *Protopterus amphibians*; and (*D*) the clawed toad *Xenopus laevis* (A,B, after Smeets and Timerick, 1981; C, after Ronan and Northcutt, 1985; D, after ten Donkelaar et al., 1981; from ten Donkelaar, 1988.) Ad, Av, anterodorsal and anteroventral tegmental nuclei; Iflm, interstitial nucleus of the fasciculus longitudinalis medialis; nIII, oculomotor nerve; Rub, nucleus ruber; tm, tectum mesencephali. Numbers refer to spinal segments

of descending brain stem pathways as advocated by Kuypers (1981) can be distinguished. Interstitiospinal, reticulospinal, and vestibulospinal pathways pass via the ventral funiculus and ventral part of the lateral funiculus and terminate in the mediodorsal parts of the ventral horn and the adjacent parts of the intermediate zone. This *medial* system is functionally related to postural activities and progression and constitutes a basic system by which the brain exerts control over movements. The *lateral* system consists of fibers occupying a lateral position in the lower brain stem and descending into the lateral funiculus of the spinal cord. This system is mainly composed of rubrospinal fibers. The rubrospinal tract terminates in lateral and dorsal parts of the intermediate zone. In mammals, the rubrospinal pathway has been found to influence distal joint muscles with direct motoneuronal connections to the cervical enlargement, at least in cats (Holstege, 1987; McCurdy et al., 1987) and some primates (Houk et al., 1988; Cheney et al., 1991). Moreover, in mammals, a direct corticospinal tract gradually supersedes the descending projections from the brain stem.

The *corticospinal tract* arises invariably from layer V pyramidal cells, particularly from rostral, frontal parts of the cerebral cortex (Fig. 3.13). Both motor and somatosensory cortices give rise to corticospinal projections (see Kuypers, 1981; Nudo and Masterton, 1990a,b). In opossums, the motor and somatosensory cortices overlap. The somatosensory cortex innervates the dorsal horn of the spinal cord and the dorsal column nuclei. The corticospinal projection is predominantly contralateral, but in many insectivores (e.g., moles) largely ipsilateral. Moles have dense corticospinal projections from the forelimb representation of the somatosensory and motor cortices that may reflect sensorimotor specializations related to digging (Catania and Kaas, 1997). The sensorimotor cortex of the Eastern mole has the densest concentration of corticospinal neurons per unit brain weight of any mammal yet investigated (Nudo et al., 1995).

With regard to the terminal distribution of corticospinal fibers, the various mammals tend to fall into four groups (Table 3.4) that show an increasingly wider distribution area of cortical fibers in the spinal gray (Kuypers, 1981). By ranking the motor skill of the hands of 69 different mammals from 1 to 7 (see Table 3.1), Heffner and Masterton (1983) came to the conclusion that the extent and the site of termination of the corticospinal tract most closely correspond with dexterity. Direct *corticomotoneuronal* connections to motoneurons innervating hand and finger muscles are only found in primates (see Kuypers, 1981) and a few carnivores such as raccoons and kinkajous (Petras, 1969; Wirth et al., 1974). This suggests that the presence of direct corticomotoneuronal connections is a derived characteristic that has evolved independently, along with manual dexterity, in both primates and carnivores (Heffner and Masterton, 1983). Direct corticomotoneuronal projections are not restricted to forelimb motoneurons, however. In many monkeys, the motor cortex also projects to hindlimb motoneurons, and, in spider, (*Ateles*) and woolly (*Lagothrix*) monkeys, moreover, to motoneurons innervating the muscles of the prehensile tail (Petras, 1968).

Telencephalic projections to the spinal cord are not restricted to mammals. Minor telencephalospinal projections were found in the nurse shark *Ginglymostoma cirratum* (Ebbesson and Schroeder, 1971) and in birds. Moreover, the avian Wulst innervates the dorsal column nuclei and the spinal cord. The avian "corticobulbar" projections, (i.e., the septomesencephalic and occipitomesencephalic tracts) are discussed later.

98   3 Evolution of Vertebrate Motor Systems

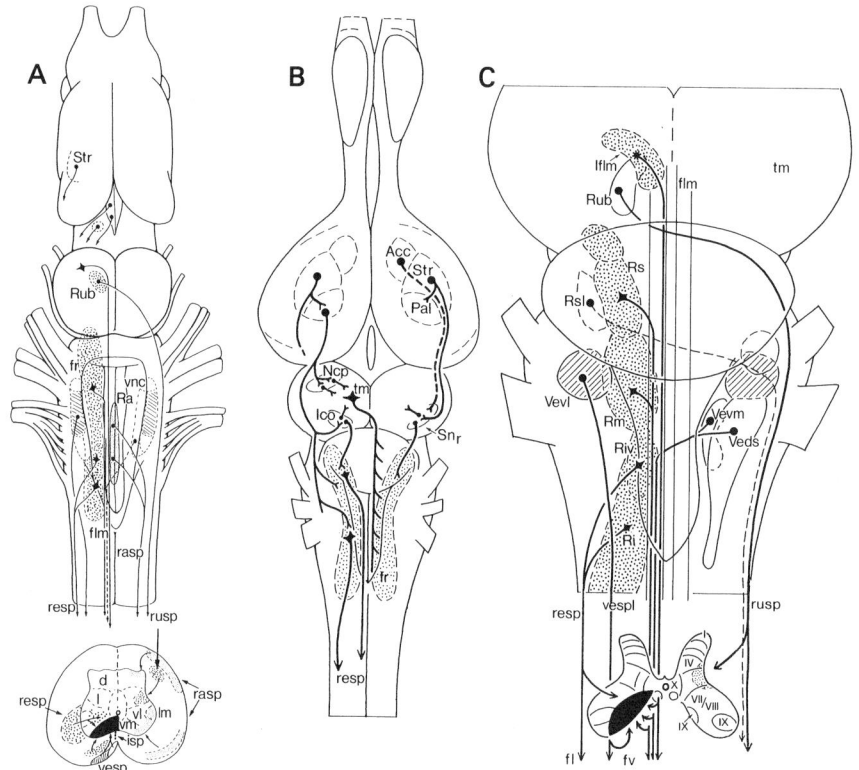

Figure 3.12. Diagrams summarizing experimental data in anurans (*A*), lizards (*C,D*) and the North American opossum *Didelphis virginiana* (*E,F*) on origin, course, and site of termination of descending brain stem projections (after ten Donkelaar, 1982, 1992; ten Donkelaar et al., 1987; opossum data based on Martin et al., 1975, 1982). In (*B*), the basal ganglia projections to the reticular formation (directly or via the tectum mesencephali) in *Varanus exanthematicus* are indicated (from ten Donkelaar et al., 1987, by permission of Springer, Berlin). *Continued on opposite page*

The Cerebellorubrospinal Limb Control System

Goal-directed limb movements are controlled mainly by the rubrospinal tract, in mammals by the corticospinal tract as well. The red nucleus, cerebellum, and their extensive interconnections form a premotor network for controlling limb movements (Keifer and Houk, 1994). Major differences are present in this circuitry among terrestrial vertebrates (Fig. 3.14). In amphibians, the cerebellar cortex innervates a single cerebellar nucleus that gives rise to both an ascending projection (the brachium conjunctivum) to the contralateral red nucleus and a descending projection to the vestibular nuclear complex (González et al., 1984; Larson-Prior and Cruce, 1992). Between the red nucleus and the cerebellar nucleus reciprocal connections exist. In amniotes, two or more separate cerebellar nuclei can be distinguished, each of which is innervated by a particular longitudinal strip of Purkinje cells (see ten Donkelaar

Supraspinal Control 99

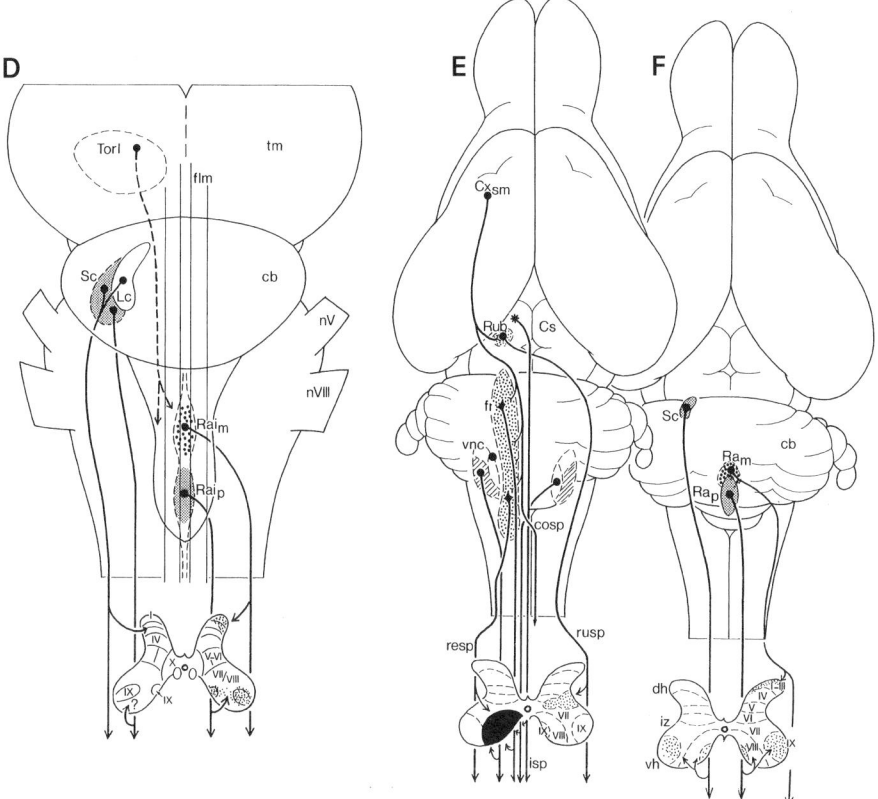

Figure 3.12. contd.
Acc, nucleus accumbens; cb, cerebellum; cosp, corticospinal tract; C_s, colliculus superior; Cx_{sm}, somatomotor cortex; d, l, lm, vl, vm, dorsal, lateral, lateral motor, ventrolateral, and ventromedial fields of spinal gray; dh, dorsal horn; fl, fv, lateral and ventral funiculi; flm, fasciculus longitudinalis medialis; fr, fasciculus retroflexus; Ico, nucleus intercollicularis; Iflm, nucleus interstitialis of the flm; isp, interstitiospinal tract; iz, intermediate zone; Lc, locus coeruleus; Ncp, nucleus of the commissura posterior; nV, nervus trigeminus; nVIII, nervus vestibulocochlearis; Pal, pallidum; Ra, nucleus raphes; Ra_m, Ra_p, nucleus raphes magnus, and pallidus; Raim, Raip, nucleus raphes inferior, magnocellular part, and pallidal part; rasp, raphe spinal projections; resp, reticulospinal projections; Ri, Riv, nucleus reticularis inferior, and pars ventralis; Rm, nucleus reticularis medius; Rs, Rsl, nucleus reticularis superior, and pars lateralis; Rub, nucleus ruber; rusp, rubrospinal tract; Sc, subcoeruleus area; Sn_r, substantia nigra pars reticulata; Str, striatum; tm, tectum mesencephali; Torl, torus semicircularis, nucleus laminaris; Veds, Vevl, Vevm, descending, ventrolateral, and ventromedial vestibular nuclei; vesp, vestibulospinal projections; vespl, lateral vestibulospinal tract; vh, ventral horn; vnc, vestibular nuclear complex; I–X, laminar subdivision of the spinal gray.

and Bangma, 1992). In reptiles, the medial cerebellar nucleus mainly influences the vestibular nuclear complex, whereas the lateral cerebellar nucleus gives rise to a well-developed brachium conjunctivum. This ascending projection extensively innervates the contralateral red nucleus and more sparsely the diencephalon (Bangma et al., 1984; Belekhova and Gaidaenko, 1985; Künzle, 1985b; Sarrafizadeh and Houk,

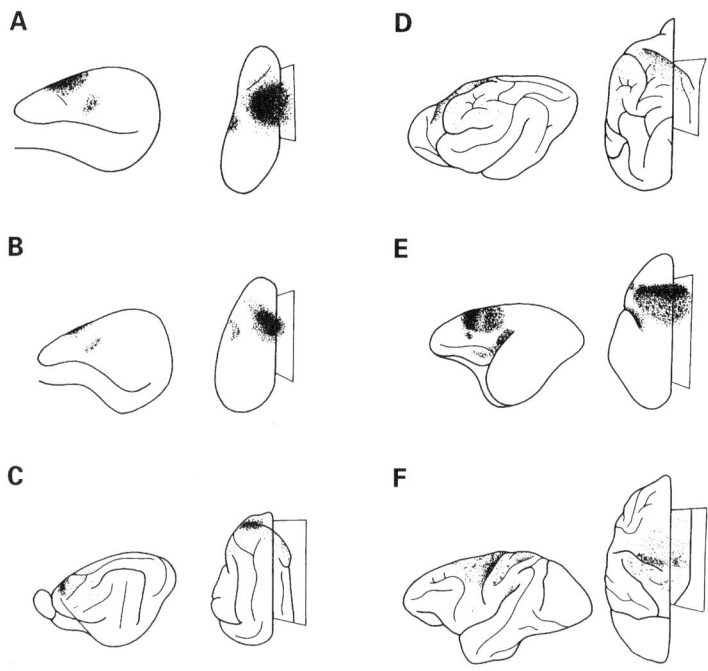

Figure 3.13. The distribution of the cells of origin of the corticospinal tract shown in lateral (left drawing of each panel) and dorsal (right drawing of each panel) views of (*A*) the North American opossum *Didelphis virginiana*; (*B*) the tree shrew *Tupaia glis*; (*C*) the domestic cat *Felis catus*; (*D*) the raccoon *Procyon lotor*; (*E*) the lesser bushbaby *Galago senegalensis*, and (*F*) the rhesus monkey *Macaca mulatta* (after Nudo and Masterton, 1990a). The mirrors in the dorsal views show the medial extent of corticospinal neurons on the medial side of the hemisphere.

1994). The red nucleus gives rise to a distinct crossed rubrospinal and rubrobulbar tract, but also to a small ipsilateral rubro-olivary tract to the inferior olive (ten Donkelaar and de Boer-van Huizen, 1981). The inferior olive innervates the contralateral cerebellum (Bangma and ten Donkelaar, 1982; Künzle, 1985a). It is unclear whether any telencephalic projections reach the red nucleus. In birds, a comparable cerebellorubral circuit is found (Arends and Zeigler, 1991a,b). Moreover, a telencephalic projection from the hyperstriatum accessorium of the anterior Wulst innervates the red nucleus (Wild, 1992; Wild and Williams, 2000).

In mammals, three cerebellar nuclei are found of which the interposed and lateral cerebellar (or dentate) nuclei innervate the red nucleus and the ventrolateral thalamic complex (e.g., Martin et al., 1974b). The ventrolateral thalamic complex projects to the motor cortex. In the North American opossum (Fig. 3.14C), the red nucleus can roughly be divided into large-celled parts which project contralaterally to the brain stem and spinal cord, and a rostromedial part that innervates the inferior olive ipsilaterally (King et al., 1972; Martin et al., 1974a). In primates, a further spatial segregation of rubral projection neurons is found. Rubrospinal neurons are found only in the

Table 3.4. The Corticospinal Tract: Patterns of Spinal Termination

Group 1
  Mammals with corticospinal fibers extending *only* to cervical or midthoracic segments and terminating in the *dorsal horn* (opossums, tree shrews, rabbits)

Group 2
  Mammals with corticospinal fibers extending *throughout* the spinal cord and terminating in the *dorsal horn* and *intermediate zone* (rat, most carnivores)

Group 3
  Mammals with corticospinal fibers extending *throughout* the spinal cord and terminating in the *dorsal horn, intermediate zone,* and *dorsolateral* parts of the *lateral* motoneuronal cell groups (raccoon, primates including *Saimiri, Galago,* and rhesus monkeys)

Group 4
  Mammals with corticospinal fibers extending throughout the spinal cord and terminating in the *dorsal horn, intermediate zone,* and both *dorsolateral* and *ventromedial* parts of the *lateral* motoneuronal cell groups (*Cebus*, apes such as chimpanzee, humans)

After Kuypers (1981).

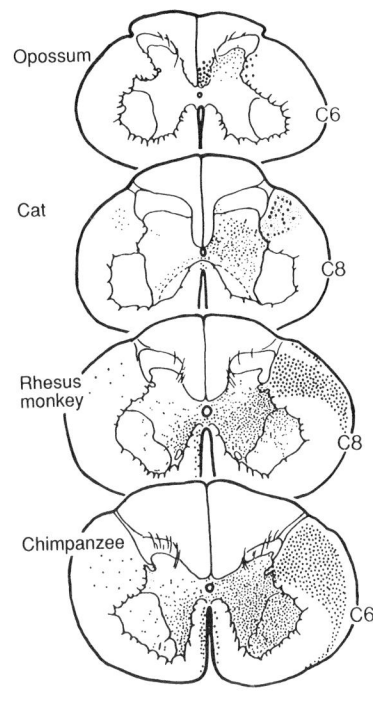

caudal magnocellular part of the red nucleus, whereas the rostral parvocellular part gives rise to the ipsilateral rubro-olivary pathway (see Kuypers, 1981). The magnocellular part of the red nucleus receives its input mainly from the interposed nucleus, whereas the parvocellular part is innervated by the dentate nucleus (Kennedy et al., 1986) and extensively by corticorubral projections (Kuypers and Lawrence, 1967; Humphrey et al., 1984). Only a minority of cortical fibers innervates the magnocellular part of the red nucleus. In monkeys, neurons of the magnocellular red nucleus are preferentially related to movements of the hand and fingers (see Cheney et al., 1991). Particularly in anthropoid primates such as the gibbon, the magnocellular part is much reduced (Padel et al., 1981). In humans, the rubrospinal tract is very small. Only a few fibers reach the spinal cord and usually do not extend beyond the upper cervical segments (Nathan and Smith, 1982).

The functional role of the cerebellorubrospinal circuit has been analyzed nicely in freshwater turtles (Keifer and Houk, 1994; Sarrafizadeh and Houk, 1994). The turtle brain has an unusual resistance to anoxia (Hounsgaard and Nicholson, 1990). Therefore, in vitro preparations of isolated parts of the CNS offer excellent

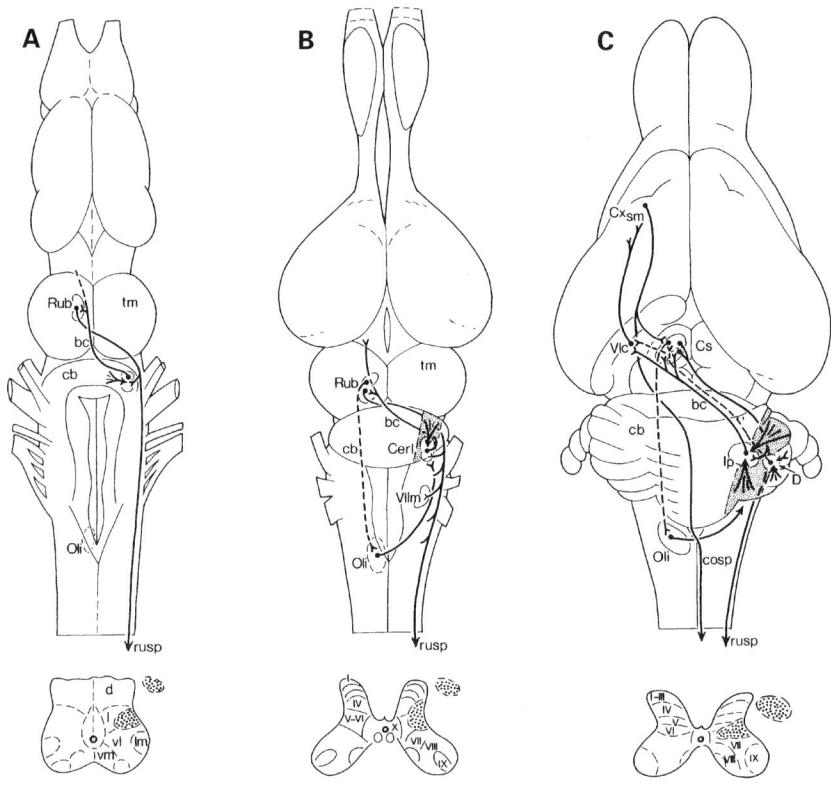

Figure 3.14. Cerebellorubrospinal circuitry in (*A*) the clawed toad *Xenopus laevis*; (*B*) the savannah monitor lizard *Varanus exanthematicus*, and (*C*) the North American opossum *Didelphis virginiana*. bc, brachium conjunctivum; cb, cerebellum; Cerl, nucleus cerebellaris lateralis; cosp, corticospinal tract; Cs, colliculus superior; Cx_{sm}, somatomotor cortex; D, dentate (lateral) nucleus; d, l, lm, vl, vm, dorsal, lateral, lateral motor, ventrolateral and ventromedial fields of the spinal gray; Ip, interposed nucleus; Oli, oliva inferior; Rub, nucleus ruber; rusp, rubrospinal tract; tm, tectum mesencephali; Vlc, ventrolateral (thalamic) nuclear complex; VIIm, facial motor nucleus; I–X, laminar subdivision of the spinal gray. (From ten Donkelaar et al., 1987 by permission of Springer, Berlin.)

opportunities for combined tracing and electrophysiological studies as well as for pharmacological manipulations of the turtle brain. In freshwater pond turtles (*Chrysemys picta*), Sarrafizadeh and Houk (1994) found that the chelonian red nucleus receives a dense input from the contralateral lateral cerebellar nucleus, projects back to that nucleus sparsely, and innervates more heavily the lateral reticular nucleus (Fig. 3.15). Lateral reticular axons heavily innervate the lateral cerebellar nucleus before terminating in the lateral part of the cerebellum.

These prominent recurrent loops between the lateral cerebellar nucleus, red nucleus, and lateral reticular nucleus constitute the rubrocerebellar limb premotor network in turtles. Sensory input to the red nucleus originates in the contralateral dorsal column nucleus, the principal trigeminal sensory nucleus and the spinal cord.

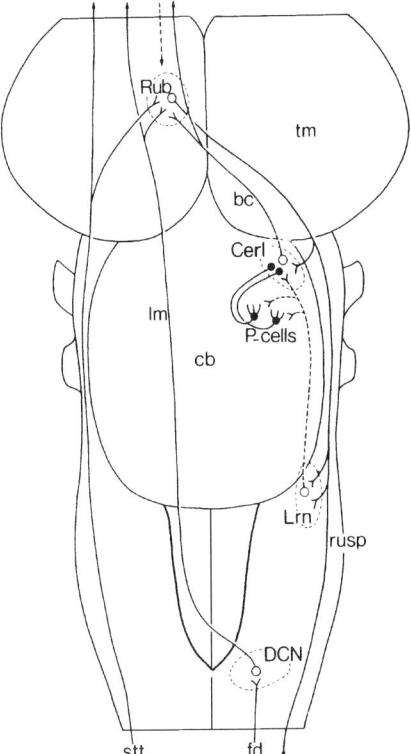

Figure 3.15. The limb rubrocerebellar premotor network in freshwater turtles (based on data by Sarrafizadeh and Houk [1994] and earlier data reviewed by ten Donkelaar and Bangma [1992]). bc, brachium conjunctivum; cb, cerebellum; Cerl, lateral cerebellar nucleus; DCN, dorsal column nuclei; fd, funiculus dorsalis (primary spinal afferent fibers); lm, lemniscus medialis; Lrn, lateral reticular nucleus; P-cells, Purkinje cells; Rub, nucleus ruber; rusp, rubrospinal tract; stt, spinothalamic tract; tm, tectum mesencephali.

Sensory input may be used to preselect motor programs, to trigger their initiation, to influence when they terminate, and to evaluate the success or failure of the patterns in controlling a motor behavior (Houk et al., 1993; Keifer and Houk, 1994). Sensory input is thought to be used by the cerebellar cortex to preselect motor programs before their execution. This preselection may take the form of an organized reduction in Purkinje cell inhibition of a select group of lateral cerebellar nucleus neurons, thereby allowing specific rubrocerebellar loops to become activated upon presentation of a trigger stimulus. Sensory inputs to the red nucleus are thought to be of special importance in the triggering of rubral descending commands. Once initiated, these motor commands could be sustained by positive feedback activity between brain stem, cerebellum, and red nucleus. The cerebellar cortex could terminate motor programs by using proprioceptive and efference copy information to turn Purkinje cells back on, thereby restraining premotor network activity (Houk et al., 1993; Keifer and Houk, 1994).

104   3   Evolution of Vertebrate Motor Systems

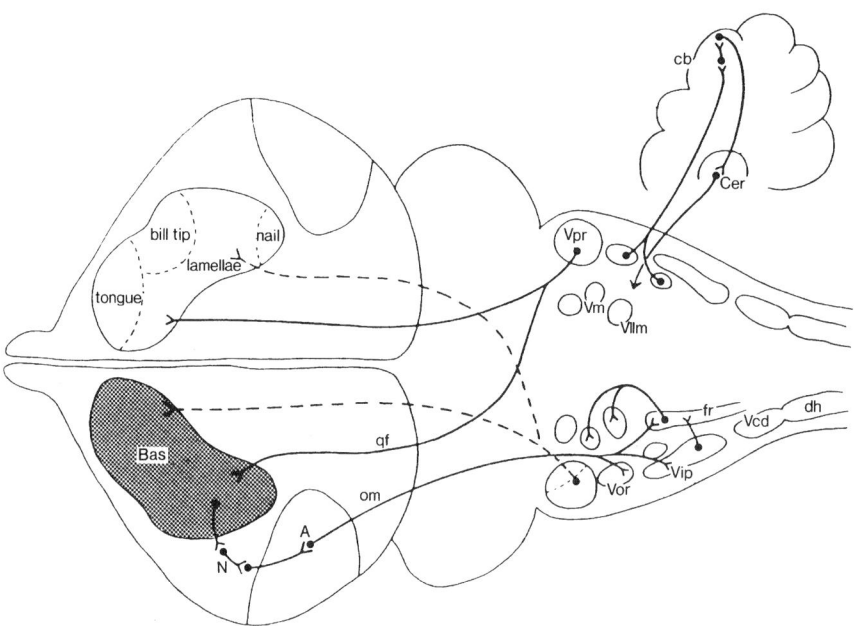

Figure 3.16. Diagram showing the "trigeminal feeding system" in birds, exemplified for the mallard. A, archistriatum; Bas, nucleus basalis; cb, cerebellum; Cer, cerebellar nucleus; dh, dorsal horn; fr, formatio reticularis; N, neostriatum; om, occipitomesencephalic tract; qf, quintofrontal tract; Vm, trigeminal motor nucleus; Vcd, Vip, Vor, caudal, interpolar, and oral subnuclei of the nucleus of the descending trigeminal tract; Vpr, principal trigeminal sensory nucleus; VIIm, facial motor nucleus. (After Dubbeldam, 1984.)

The Special Case for Birds

A quite different solution for the manipulation of the environment than in mammals is found in birds. The beak of birds functions in reaching, grasping, and manipulation analogously with the forelimb of mammals and the primate hand (Wild et al., 1985). In primates, the manipulation of the environment involves sensorimotor mechanisms controlling the steering of the hand. This sensorimotor circuit includes cortical control of spinal motoneurons and sensory feedback via the dorsal column–medial lemniscal system. In birds, the tactile sense is very important in the various types of feeding behavior and other beak functions. Tactile information from mechanoreceptors in the beak, tongue, and palatum is relayed to sensory nuclei of the trigeminal system, the principal trigeminal sensory nucleus in particular (Dubbeldam, 1984). Via the quintofrontal tract the latter nucleus innervates the nucleus basalis in the telencephalon (Fig. 3.16) *without* a thalamic relay as usual for sensory information to the telencephalon.

The nucleus basalis forms part of the dorsal ventricular ridge (DVR). The DVR, a large intraventricular protrusion (see Ulinski, 1983), and the Wulst, a swelling present on the dorsal surface of the avian telencephalon, contain cell groups that are assumed

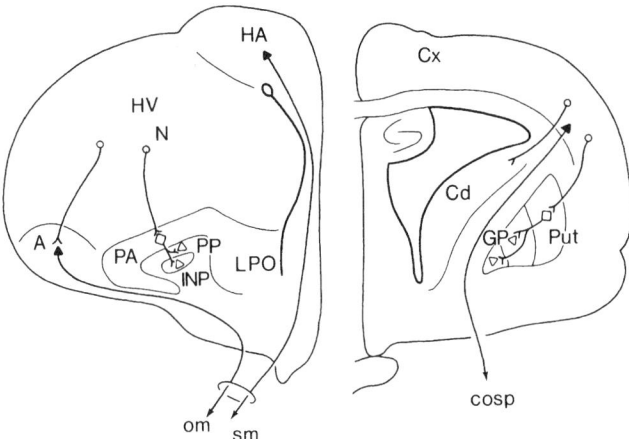

Figure 3.17. Origins of somatomotor projections in birds (left) and mammals (right). A, archistriatum (rostral part); Cd, caudate nucleus; cosp, corticospinal tract; Cx, cerebral cortex; GP, globus pallidus; HA, hyperstriatum accessorium (part of Wulst); HV, hyperstriatum ventrale (part of dorsal ventricular ridge); INP, intrapeduncular nucleus; LPO, lobus parolfactorius; N, neostriatum; om, occipitomesencephalic tract; PA, PP, paleostriatum augmentatum and -primitivum; Put, putamen; sm, septomesencephalic tract. (After Karten and Dubbeldam, 1973.)

to be homologous to those in the mammalian isocortex (Nauta and Karten, 1970). Both pallial structures comprise end stations of ascending systems, telencephalic "motor" output areas and large areas with predominantly intratelencephalic connections (see Dubbeldam, 1991; Rehkämper and Zilles, 1991). Via a relay in the frontal neostriatum or hyperstriatum ventrale, the nucleus basalis innervates the rostral part of the archistriatum (Fig. 3.16). In this part of the DVR a major pallial efferent pathway originates—the *occipitomesencephalic tract*—which projects to various brain stem nuclei including premotor groups in the reticular formation innervating the motor nucleus of the jaw muscles (Wild et al., 1985; Dubbeldam and Visser, 1987; Dubbeldam et al., 1997). In the pigeon and the mallard, the occipitomesencephalic tract extends into the rostral part of the spinal cord (Zeier and Karten, 1971; Dubbeldam et al., 1997). The occipitomesencephalic tract represents the *telencephalic output channel* for the trigeminal "feeding circuit" (Dubbeldam, 1984, 1991) as well as for the "vocalization circuit" found in songbirds (Nottebohm et al., 1982) and resembles the corticobulbar tract found in mammals.

In birds, another corticobulbar projection—the *septomesencephalic tract*—arises from the Wulst (Fig. 3.17). The caudal, visual part of the Wulst plays a role in modulating the activity of tectal projections to premotor structures in the brain stem reticular formation. The rostral, somatosensory part of the Wulst projects to the red nucleus (Wild, 1992), pontine nuclei, dorsal column nuclei, and to the contralateral spinal cord (Karten, 1971; Wild and Williams, 2000). This system may be related specifically to motor control of the talons in birds of prey (Ulinski and Margoliash, 1990). In parrots, which possess brains with the most highly developed telencephala among birds (see Rehkämper et al., 1991), the basal branch of the septo-mesencephalic tract reportedly reaches the cervical cord (Zecha, 1962). Moreover, parrots appear to be particularly dexterous in manipulating objects with their feet. Prehension is facilitated by a tendon arrangement that allows simultaneous flexion and extension of the paired opposing toes (Raikow, 1985). In zebra and green finches, rather extensive projections to the cervical spinal cord were found (Wild and Williams, 2000). The evidence for an avian "pyramidal tract" descending into the spinal cord, however, is not very convincing as a general feature. In prehensile birds (a cockatoo, *Cacatua galerita*, and a rosella, *Platycerus eximius*), Webster et al. (1990) failed to find evidence for telencephalospinal projections with retrograde tracing techniques. Moreover, parrots have no greater development of the rubrospinal tract than nonprehensile birds. Therefore, in birds there is no general direct palliospinal control of refined motor skills of the extremities beyond the examples listed above.

SUMMARY

The present survey discusses the basic features in motor control found in vertebrates and various ways in which the brain has adapted to the specific requirements posed by the major structural and physiological changes in the history of vertebrates. The neural control system for locomotion is basically similar in all classes of vertebrates. Essentially, locomotion is initiated from brain stem locomotor areas, and reticulospinal neurons activate spinal networks. Vestibulospinal pathways are involved in equilibrium and postural activities. With the appearance of extremities, the development of an adequate neural control system for the steering of limb movements became apparent. It is likely that the rubrospinal tract plays an important role in this mechanism. Goal-directed limb movements are controlled mainly by the rubrospinal tract and in mammals also by the corticospinal tract.

Although minor telencephalospinal projections are found in some sharks and birds, a corticospinal tract is a derived feature of mammals. Its emergence appears to be associated with the acquisition of dexterous motor skills. For prehensile extremities and tails, corticospinal projections are essential. The sensorimotor capacities of the hand for exploring the visible world develop best in primates. Direct corticomotoneuronal connections from the sensorimotor cortex to motoneurons innervating hand, finger, foot, or tail muscles are found only in primates and a few specialized carnivores such as the raccoon, which are capable of some form of precision grip. Birds have found a quite different solution for the manipulation of the environment. In birds, the beak functions in reaching, grasping, and manipulation of food. A unique trigeminal feeding circuit forms the neural substrate for these behaviors. Its anatomical organization is analogous to that of the sensorimotor pathways controlling the forelimbs of mammals.

ACKNOWLEDGMENTS

It is a pleasure to acknowledge the help of Marlu de Leeuw with the drawings and of Inge Eijkhout for secretarial assistance. This research was supported by a NATO Collaborative Research Grant (No. 930542).

REFERENCES

Alexander, R. M. (1977) Terrestrial locomotion. In R.M. Alexander and G. Goldspink (eds.): *Mechanisms and Energetics of Animal Locomotion*. Chapman and Hall, London, pp. 168–203.
Arends, J.J.A., and H.P. Zeigler (1991a) Organization of the cerebellum in the pigeon (*Columba livia*). I. Corticonuclear and corticovestibular connections. *J. Comp. Neurol.* 306:221–244.
Arends J.J.A., and H.P. Zeigler (1991b) Organization of the cerebellum in the pigeon (Columbia livia). II. Projections of the cerebellar nuclei. *J. Comp. Neurol.* 306:245–272.
Arshavsky, Y.I., I.M. Gelfand, and G.N. Orlovsky (1986) *Cerebellum and Rhythmical Movements. Studies of Brain Function*, vol.13. Springer Verlag, Berlin.
Arshavsky, Y.I. G.N. Orlovsky, Y.V. Panchin, A. Roberts, and S.R. Soffe (1993) Neuronal control of swimming locomotion: analysis of the pteropod mollusc *Clione* and embryos of the amphibian *Xenopus. Trends Neurosci.* 16:227–233.
Bangma, G.C., and H.J. ten Donkelaar, (1982) Afferent connections of the cerebellum in various types of reptiles. *J. Comp. Neurol.* 207:255–273.
Bangma, G.C., ten H.J. Donkelaar, P.J.W. Dederen, and R. de Boer-van Huizen (1984) Cerebellar efferents in the lizard *Varanus exanthematicus*. II. Projections of the cerebellar nuclei. J. Comp. Neurol. 230:218–230.
Belekhova, M.G., and G.V. Gaidaenko (1985) A study of cerebellar connections in turtles by means of horseradish peroxidase axonal transport [in Russian]. *Neurophysiology (Kiev)* 17:786–794.
Bishop, A. (1964) Use of the hand in lower primates. In J. Buettner-Janusch (ed.): *Evolutionary and Genetic Biology of Primates*, vol.2. Academic Press, New York, pp. 133–225
Blight, A.R. (1977) The muscular control of vertebrate swimming movements. *Biol. Rev.* 52:181–218.
Bone, Q. (1978) Locomotor muscle. In W.S. Hoar and D.J. Randall (eds.): *Fish Physiology, vol VII: Locomotion*. Academic Press, New York, pp. 361–424.
Brändle, K. and G. Székely (1973) The control of alternating coordination of limb pairs in the newt (*Triturus vulgaris*). *Behav. Brain Evol.* 8:366–385.
Brodin, L., and S. Grillner (1990) The lamprey CNS in vitro, an experimentally amenable model for synaptic transmission and integrative functions. In H. Jahnsen (ed.): *Preparations of Vertebrate Central Nervous System In Vitro*. Wiley, New York, pp. 103–153.
Brodin, L., Y. Ohta T. Hökfelt, and S. Grillner (1989) Further evidence for excitatory amino acid transmission in lamprey reticulospinal neurons: selective retrograde labeling with (3H)D-aspartate. *J. Comp. Neurol.* 281:225–233.
Brown, T.G. (1911) The intrinsic factor in the act of progression in the mammal. *Proc. R. Soc. (Lond.) Biol.* 84:308–319.
Cabot, J.B., A. Reiner, and N. Gogan (1982) Avian bulbospinal pathways: anterograde and retrograde studies of cells of origin, funicular trajectories and laminar termination. *Prog. Brain. Res.* 57:79–108.
Carroll, R.L. (1988) *Vertebrate Paleontology and Evolution*. Freeman, New York.
Cartmill, M. (1985) Climbing. In M. Hildebrand, D.M. Bramble, K.F. Liem, and D.B. Wake (eds.): functional vertebrate morphology. Harvard University Press, Cambridge, pp. 73–88.
Catania, K.C. (1995) The structure and innervation of the sensory organs on the snout of the star-nosed mole. *J. Comp. Neurol.* 351:549–567.
Catania, K.C. and J.H. Kaas (1997) Organization of somatosensory cortex and distribution of corticospinal neurons in the Eastern mole (*Scapolus aquaticus*). *J. Comp. Neurol.* 378:337–353.
Cheney, P.D., E.E. Fetz, and K. Mewes (1991) Neural mechanisms underlying corticospinal and rubrospinal control of limb movements. *Prog. Brain. Res.* 87:213–252.
Chodrow, R.E., and C.R. Taylor (1973) Energetic cost of limbless locomotion in snakes. *Fed. Proc.* 32:422.

Cohen, A.H. (1988) Evolution of the vertebrate central pattern generator for locomotion. In A.H. Cohen, S. Rossignol, and S. Grillner (eds.): *Neural Control of Rhythmic Movements in Vertebrates.* Wiley, New York, pp. 129–166.
Darian-Smith, I. (1984) The sense of touch: performance and peripheral neural processes. In I. Darian-Smith (ed.): *Handbook of Physiology—The Nervous System, vol.III: Sensory Processes.* American Physiology Society, Bethesda, pp. 739–788.
Darian-Smith, I., M.P. Galea, C. Darian-Smith, M. Sugitani, A. Tan, and K. Burman (1996) The anatomy of manual dexterity: the new connectivity of the primate sensorimotor thalamus and cerebral cortex. *Adv. Anat. Embryol. Cell Biol.* Vol 133, pp. 1–142.
Dubbeldam, J.L. (1984) Brainstem mechanisms for feeding in birds: interaction or plasticity. A functional–anatomical consideration of the pathways. *Brain Behav. Evol.* 25:85–98.
Dubbeldam, J.L. (1991) The avian and mammalian forebrain: correspondences and differences. In Andrew, R.J. (ed.): *Neural and Behavioural Plasticity. The Use of the Domestic Chick as a Model.* Oxford University Press, New York, pp. 65–91.
Dubbeldam, J.L., A.M. den Boer-Visser, and R.G. Bout (1997) Organization and efferent connections of the archistriatum of the mallard, *Anas platyrhynchos* L.: an anterograde and retrograde tracing study. *J. Comp. Neurol.* 388:632–657.
Dubbeldam, J.L., and A.M. Visser (1987) The organization of the nucleus basalis–neostriatum complex of the mallard (*Anas platyrhynchos* L) and its connections with the archistriatum and the paleostriatum complex. *Neuroscience* 21:487–517.
Dubuc, R., F. Bongianni, Y. Ohta, and S. Grillner (1993) Anatomical and physiological study of brainstem nuclei relaying dorsal column inputs in lampreys. *J. Comp. Neurol.* 327:260–270.
Ebbesson, S.O.E., and D.M. Schroeder (1971) Connections of the nurse shark's telencephalon. *Science* 173:254–256.
Edwards, J.L. (1977) The evolution of terrestrial locomotion. In M.K. Hecht, P.C. Goody, and B.M. Hecht (eds.): *Major Patterns in Vertebrate Evolution.* Plenum Press, New York, pp. 553–577.
Edwards, J.L. (1985) Terrestrial locomotion without appendages. In M. Hildebrand D.M. Bramble K.F. Liem, and D.B. Wake (eds.): *Functional Vertebrate Morphology.* Harvard University Press, Cambridge, pp. 159–172.
Emerson, S.B. (1985) Jumping and leaping. In M. Hildebrand, D.M. Bramble, K.F. Liem, D.B. Wake (eds.): *Functional Vertebrate Morphology.* Harvard University Press, Cambridge, pp. 58–72.
Fetcho, J.R. (1987) A review of the organization and evolution of motoneurons innervating the axial musculature of vertebrates. *Brain. Res. Rev.* 12:243–280.
Fetcho, J.R. (1992) The spinal motor system in early vertebrates and some of its evolutionary changes. *Brain. Behav. Evol.* 40:82–97.
Flood, P.R. (1968) Structure of the segmental trunk muscle in *Amphioxus. Z. Zellforsch. Mikrosk. Anat.* 84:389–416.
Fricke, H. O. Reinicke, H. Hofer, and W. Nachtigall (1987) Locomotion of the coelacanth *Latimeria chalumnae* in its natural environment. *Nature* 329:331–333.
Frolich, L.M., and A.A. Biewener (1992) Kinematic and electromyographic analysis of the functional role of the body axis during terrestrial and aquatic locomotion in the salamander *Ambystoma tigrinum. J. Exp. Biol.* 162:107–130.
Gans, C. (1974) *Biomechanics: An Approach to Vertebrate Biology.* J.B. Lippincott, Philadelphia.
Gans, C. (1975) Tetrapod limblessness: evolution and functional corollaries. *Am. Zool.* 15:455–467.
Gans, C. (1985) Limbless locomotion—a current overview. *Fortschr Zool.* 30:13–22.
González, A., H.J. ten Donkelaar, and R. de Boer-van Huizen (1984) Cerebellar connections in *Xenopus laevis.* An HRP study. *Anat. Embryol.* 169:167–176.
Gray, J. (1968) *Animal Locomotion.* Wiedenfeld and Nicholson, London.
Grillner, S. (1981) Control of locomotion in bipeds, tetrapods and fish. In V.B. Brooks (ed.): *Handbook of Physiology—The Nervous System, vol.II: Motor Control.* American Physiology Society, Bethesda, pp. 1179–1236.
Grillner, S., J.T. Buchanan, P. Wallén, and L. Brodin (1988) Neural control of locomotion in lower vertebrates—From behavior to ionic mechanisms. In A.H. Cohen, S. Rossignol, and S. Grillner (eds.): *Neural Control of Rhythmic Movements in Vertebrates.* Wiley, New York, pp. 1–40.
Grillner, S. T. Deliagina, Ö. Ekeberg, A. El Manira, R.H. Hill, A. Lansner, G.N. Orlovsky, and P. Wallén (1995) Neural networks that co-ordinate locomotion and body orientation in lamprey. *Trends Neurosci.* 18:270–279.

Grillner, S., and T. Matsushima (1991) The neural network underlying locomotion in lamprey—Synaptic and cellular mechanisms. *Neuron* 7:1–15.
Harris, V.A. (1960) On the locomotion of the mudskipper *Periophthalmus koelreuteri*. *Proc. Zool. Soc. (Lond.)* 134:107–135.
Heffner, R., and R.B. Masterton (1983) The role of the corticospinal tract in the evolution of human digital dexterity. *Brain. Behav. Evol.* 23:165–183.
Hildebrand, M. (1976) Analysis of tetrapod gaits: general considerations and asymmetrical gaits. *Adv. Behav. Biol.* 18:203–236.
Hildebrand, M. (1985) Digging of quadrupeds. In M. Hildebrand, D.M. Bramble, K.F. Liem, and D.B. Wake (eds.): *Functional vertebrate morphology*. Harvard University Press, Cambridge, pp. 89–109
Hinchliffe, J.R., and D.R. Johnson (1980) *The Development of the Vertebrate Limb. An Approach Through Experiment, Genetics and Evolution*. Clarendon Press, Oxford.
Holstege, G. (1987) Anatomical evidence for an ipsilateral rubrospinal pathway and for direct rubrospinal projections to motoneurons in the cat. *Neurosci. Lett.* 74:269–274.
Houk, J.C., A.R. Gibson, C.F. Harvey, P.R. Kennedy, and P.L.E. van Kan (1988) Activity of primate magnocellular red nucleus related to hand and finger movements. *Behav. Brain. Res.* 28:201–206.
Houk, J.C., J. Keifer, and A.G. Barto (1993) Distributed motor commands in the limb premotor network. *Trends Neurosci* 16:27–33.
Hounsgaard, J., and C. Nicholson (1990) The isolated turtle brain and the physiology of neuronal circuits. In H. Jahnsen (ed.): *Preparations of Vertebrate Central Nervous System In Vitro*. Wiley, Chichester, pp. 279–294.
Humphrey, D.R., R. Gold, and D.J. Reed (1984) Sizes, laminar and topographic origins of cortical projections to the major divisions of the red nucleus in the monkey. *J. Comp. Neurol.* 255:75–94.
Jarvik, E. (1955) The oldest tetrapods and their forerunners. *Sci. Monthly* 80:141–154.
Jenkins, F.A., and G.E. Goslow (1983) The functional anatomy of the shoulder of the savannah monitor lizard *(Varanus exanthematicus)*. *J. Morphol.* 174:195–216.
Karten, H.J. (1971) Efferent projections of the Wulst of the owl. *Anat. Rec.* 169:353
Karten, H.J., and J.L. Dubbeldam (1973) The organization and projections of the paleostriatal complex in the pigeon *(Columba livia)*. *J. Comp. Neurol.* 148:61–90.
Kasicki, S., S. Grillner, Y. Ohta, R. Dubuc, and L. Brodin (1989) Phasic modulation of reticulospinal neurons during dictive locomotion and other types of motor activity in lamprey. *Brain Res.* 484:203–216.
Kazennikov, O.V., V.A. Selionov, M.L. Shik, and G.V. Yakovleva (1980) The rhombencephalic "locomotor" region in turtles *Neurophysiology (Kiev)* 12:251–258.
Keifer, J., and J.C. Houk (1994) Motor function of the cerebellorubrospinal system. *Physiol. Rev.* 74:509–542.
Kennedy, P.R., A.R. Gibson, and J.C. Houk (1986) Functional and anatomic differentiation between parvicellular and magnocellular regions of the red nucleus in the monkey. *Brain. Res.* 364:124–136.
King, J.S., G.F. Martin, and J.B. Conner (1972) A light and electron microscopic study of corticorubral projections in the opossum, *Didelphis marsupialis virginiana*. *Brain Res.* 38:251–265.
Künzle, H. (1985a) Climbing fiber projection to the turtle cerebellum: longitudinally oriented terminal zones within the basal third of the molecular layer. *Neuroscience* 14:159–168.
Künzle, H. (1985b) The cerebellar and vestibular nuclear complexes in the turtle. I. Projections to mesencephalon, rhombencephalon and spinal cord. *J. Comp. Neurol.* 242:102–121.
Kuypers, H.G.J.M. (1981) Anatomy of the descending pathways. In J.M. Brookhart, V.B. Mountcastle (eds.): *Handbook of Physiology—The Nervous System, vol.II: Motor Control*. American Physiology Society, Bethesda, pp. 597–666.
Kuypers, H.G.J.M., and D.G. Lawrence (1967) Cortical projections to the red nucleus and the brainstem in the rhesus monkey. *Brain Res.* 4:151–188.
Larson-Prior, L.J., and W.L.R. Cruce (1992) The red nucleus and mesencephalic tegmentum in a ranid amphibian: a cytoarchitectonic and HRP connectional study. *Brain Behav. Evol.* 40:273–286.
Lemelin, P. (1995) Comparative and functional myology of the prehensile tail in New World monkeys. *J. Morphol.* 224:351–368.
Lennard, P.R., and P.S.G. Stein (1977) Swimming movements elicited by electrical stimulation of turtle spinal cord. I. Low-spinal and intact preparations. *J. Neurophysiol.* 40:768–778.
Lissmann, H.W. (1950) Rectilinear locomotion in a snake *(Boa occidentalis)*. *J. Exp. Biol.* 26:368–379.

Martin, G.F., M.S. Beattie, J.C. Bresnahan, C.K. Henkel, and H.C. Hughes (1975) Cortical and brain stem projections to the spinal cord of the American opossum (*Didelphis marsupialis virginiana*). *Brain. Behav. Biol.* 12:270–310.

Martin, G.F., T. Cabana, F.J. DiTirro R.H.Ho, and A.O. Humbertson (1982) Reticular and raphe projections to the spinal cord of the North American opossum. Evidence for connectional heterogeneity. *Prog. Brain. Res.* 57:109–129.

Martin, G.F., R. Dom, S. Katz J.S. King (1974a) The organization of projections neurons in the opossum red nucleus. *Brain Res.* 78:17–34.

Martin, G.F., J.S. King, and R. Dom (1974b) The projections of the deep cerebellar nuclei of the opossum. *J. Hirnforsch.* 15:545–573.

McClellan, A.D. (1986) Command systems for initiating locomotion in fish and amphibians: parallels to initiation systems in mammals. In S. Grillner, et al. (eds.): *Neurobiology of Vertebrate Locomotion*. MacMillan Press, Houndmills, pp. 3–20.

McClellan, A.D. (1988) Brainstem command systems for locomotion in the lamprey: localization of descending pathways to the spinal cord. *Brain Res.* 457:338–349.

McCurdy, M.L., D.I. Hansma, J.C. Houk, and A.R. Gibson (1987) Selective projections from the cat red nucleus to digit motor neurons. *J. Comp. Neurol.* 265:367–379.

Napier, J.R. (1956) The prehensile movements of the human hand. *J. Bone. Joint Surg.* 38B:902–913.

Napier, J.R. (1961) Prehensibility and opposability in the hands of primates. *Symp. Zool. Soc. Lond.* 5:115–132.

Napier, J.R. (1980) *Hands*. Allen and Unwin, London.

Nathan, P.W., and M.C. Smith (1982) The rubrospinal and central tegmental tracts in man. *Brain* 105:223–269.

Naujoks-Manteuffel, C., G. Manteuffel, and W. Himstedt (1988) On the presence of a nucleus ruber in the urodele *Salamandra salamandra* and the caecilian *Ichthyophis kohtaoensis*. *Behav. Brain Res.* 28:29–32.

Nauta, W.J.H., and H.J. Karten (1970) A general profile of the vertebrate brain, with sidelights on the ancestry of cerebral cortex. In F.O. Schmitt (ed.): *The Neurosciences: Second Study Program*. Rockefeller University Press, New York, pp. 7–26.

Nieuwenhuys, R., H.J. ten Donkelaar, and C. Nicholson (1998) *The Central Nervous System of Vertebrates*. Springer Verlag, Berlin.

Nottebohm, F., D.B. Kelley, and J.A. Paton (1982) Connections of vocal control nuclei in the canary telencephalon. *J. Comp. Neurol.* 207:344–357.

Novacek, M.J. (1992) Mammalian phylogeny: shaking the tree. *Nature* 356:121–125.

Nudo, R.J., and R.B. Masterton (1988) Descending pathways to the spinal cord: an HRP study in 22 mammals. *J. Comp. Neurol.* 277:53–79.

Nudo, R.J., and R.B. Masterton (1990a) Descending pathways to the spinal cord. III. Sites of origin of the corticospinal tract. *J. Comp. Neurol.* 296:559–583.

Nudo, R.J., and R.B. Masterton (1990b) Descending pathways to the spinal cord. IV. Some factors related to the amount of cortex devoted to the corticospinal tract. *J. Comp. Neurol.* 296:584–597.

Nudo, R.J., D.P. Sutherland, and R.B. Masterton (1995) Variation and evolution of mammalian corticospinal somata with special reference to primates. *J. Comp. Neurol.* 358:181–205.

Nursall, J.R. (1956) The lateral musculature and the swimming of fish. *Proc. Zool. Soc. (Lond)* 126:127–143.

Ohta, Y., and S. Grillner (1989) Monosynaptic excitatory amino acid transmission from the posterior rhombencephalic reticular nucleus to spinal neurons involved in the control of locomotion in lamprey. *J. Neurophysiol.* 62:1079–1089.

Padel, Y., P. Angaut. J. Massion, and R. Sedan (1981) Comparative study of the posterior red nucleus in baboons and gibbons. *J. Comp. Neurol.* 202:421–438.

Petras, J.M. (1968) Corticospinal fibers in New World and Old World simians. *Brain Res.* 8:206–208.

Petras, J.M. (1969) Some efferent connections of the motor and somatosensory cortex of simian primates and felid, canid and procyonid carnivores. *Ann. N.Y. Acad. Sci.* 167:469–505.

Prasada Rao, P.D., A.G. Jadhao, and J.C. Sharma (1987) Descending projection neurons to the spinal cord of the goldfish, *Carassius auratus*. *J. Comp. Neurol.* 265:96–108.

Raikow, R.J. (1985) Locomotor system. In A.S. King, and J. McClelland (eds.): *Form and Function in Birds*, vol.3. Academic Press, London, pp. 57–158.

References

Rehkämper, G., H.D. Frahm, and K. Zilles (1991) Quantitative development of brain and brain structures in birds (Galliformes and Passeriformes) compared to that in mammals (Insectivores and Primates). *Brain Behav. Evol.* 37:125–143.

Rehkämper, G., and K. Zilles (1991) Parallel evolution in mammalian and avian tissues: Comparative cytoarchitectonic and cytochemical analysis. *Cell Tissue Res.* 263:3–28.

Rewcastle, S.C. (1981) Stance and gait in tetrapods: an evolutionary scenario. *Symp. Zool. Soc. (Lond)* 48:239–267.

Roberts, A. (1989) The neurons that control axial movements in a frog embryo. *Am. Zool.* 29:53–63.

Roberts, A. (1990) How does a nervous system produce behaviour? A case study in neurobiology. *Sci. Prog. (Oxf.)* 74:31–51.

Roberts A., and S.T. Alford (1986) Descending projections and excitation during fictive swimming in *Xenopus* embryos: neuroanatomy and lesion experiments. *J. Comp. Neurol.* 250:253–261.

Romer, A.S. (1966) *Vertebrate Paleontology*, 3rd ed. University of Chicago Press, Chicago.

Romer, A.S., and T.S. Parsons (1977) *The Vertebrate Body*. 5th ed. W.B. Saunders, Philadelphia.

Ronan, M. (1989) Origins of the descending spinal projections in petromyzontid and myxinoid agnathans. *J. Comp. Neurol.* 281:54–68.

Ronan, M., and R.G. Northcutt (1985) The origins of descending spinal projections in lepidosirenid lungfishes. *J. Comp. Neurol.* 241:435–444.

Rossignol, S. (1996) Neural control of stereotypic limb movements. In L.B. Rowell, and J.T. Sheperd (eds.): *Handbook of Physiology—Exercise: Regulation and Integration of Multiple Systems*. American Physiology Society Bethesda, pp. 173–216.

Rovainen, C.M. (1979) Neurobiology of lampreys. *Physiol Rev.* 59:1007–1077.

Sarrafizadeh, R., and J.C. Houk (1994) Anatomical organization of the limb premotor network in the turtle (*Chrysemys picta*) revealed by in vitro transport of biocytin and neurobiotin. *J. Comp. Neurol.* 344:137–159.

Schmalhausen, I.I. (1968) *The Origin of Terrestrial Vertebrates*. Academic Press, New York.

Schroeder, D.M., and M.W. Egar (1990) Marginal neurons in the urodele spinal cord and the associated denticulate ligaments. *J. Comp. Neurol.* 301:93–103.

Schroeder, D.M., and S.C. Richardson (1985) Is the intimate relationship between ligaments and marginal specialized cells in the snake's spinal cord indicative of a CNS mechanoreceptor? *Brain Res.* 328:145–149.

Shapovalov, A.I. (1972) Evolution of neuronal systems of suprasegmental motor control. *Neurophysiology (Kiev)* 4:346–359.

Shapovalov, A.I. (1975) Neuronal organization and synaptic mechanisms of supraspinal motor control in vertebrates. *Rev. Physiol. Biochem. Pharmacol.* 72:1–54.

Shik, M.L., E.V. Severin, and G.N. Orlovsky (1966) Control of walking and running by means of electrical stimulation of the midbrain. *Biophysics* 11:756–765.

Smeets, W.J.A.J., and S.J.B. Timerick (1981) Cells of origin of pathways descending to the spinal cord in two chondrichthyans, the shark *Scyliorhinus canicula* and the ray *Raja clavata*. *J. Comp. Neurol.* 202:473–491.

Stein, P.S.G. (1978) Swimming movements elicited by electrical stimulation of the turtle spinal cord: the high spinal preparation. *J. Comp. Physiol.* 124:203–210.

Sukhanov, V.B. (1974) General System of Symmetrical Locomotion of Terrestrial Vertebrates and Some Features of Movement of Lower Tetrapods [original edition, in Russian: 1968, Nauka, Leningrad] Amerind Publishing, New Delhi.

Székely, G., and G. Czéh (1976) Organization of locomotion. In R. Llinás, and W. Precht (eds.): *Frog Neurobiology*. Springer Verlag, Berlin, pp. 765–792.

Székely, G., and G. Czéh, and G. Vörös (1969) The activity pattern of limb muscles in freely moving normal and deafferented newts. *Brain Res.* 9:53–62.

ten Donkelaar, H.J. (1982) Organization of descending pathways to the spinal cord in amphibians and reptiles. *Prog. Brain. Res.* 57:25–67.

ten Donkelaar, H.J. (1988) Evolution of the red nucleus and rubrospinal tract. *Behav. Brain. Res.* 28:9–20

ten Donkelaar, H.J. (1992) Development of motor systems: a comparative approach. *Eur. J. Morphol.* 30:9–22.

ten Donkelaar, H.J. (1994) Some notes on the organization of spinal and supraspinal premotor networks for locomotion. *Eur. J. Morphol.* 32:156–167.

ten Donkelaar, H.J. (1998) Reptiles. In R. Nieuwenhuys ten H.J. Donkelaar, and C. Nicholson (eds.): The Central Nervous System of Vertebrates. Springer Verlag, Berlin, pp. 1315–1524.

ten Donkelaar, H.J., and G.C. Bangma (1983) A crossed rubrobulbar projection in the snake *Python regius*. *Brain Res.* 279:229–232.

ten Donkelaar, H.J., and G.C. Bangma (1992) The cerebellum. In C. Gans, and P.S. Ulinski (eds.): *Biology of the Reptilia, vol 17:Neurology C—Sensorimotor Integration*. University of Chicago Press, Chicago, pp. 496–586.

ten Donkelaar, H.J., G.C. Bangma, H.A. Barbas-Henry R. de Boer-van Huizen, and J.G. Wolters (1987) The brain stem in a lizard, *Varanus Exanthematicus*. *Adv. Anat. Embryol. Cell Biol.* 107: 1–168.

ten Donkelaar, H.J., and R. de Boer-van Huizen (1981) Basal ganglia projections to the brain stem in the lizard *Varanus exanthematicus* as demonstrated by retrograde transport of horseradish peroxidase. *Neuroscience* 6:1567–1590.

ten Donkelaar, H.J., R. de Boer-van Huizen F.T.M. Schouten, and S.J.H. Eggen (1981) Cells of origin of descending pathways to the spinal cord in the clawed toad *(Xenopus laevis)*. *Neuroscience* 6:2297–2312.

Tóth, P., Gyorgi Csank, and Gyorgi Lázár (1985) Morphology of the cells of origin of descending pathways to the spinal cord in *Rana esculenta*. A tracing study using cobaltic-lysine complex. *J. Hirnforsch.* 26:365–383.

Ulinski, P.S. (1983) *Dorsal Ventricular Ridge: A Treatise on Forebrain Organization in Reptiles and Birds*. Wiley, New York

Ulinski, P.S., and D. Margoliash (1990) Neurobiology of the reptile bird transition. In E.G. Jones, and Peters A. (eds.): *Cerebral Cortex*, vol.8A. Plenum Press, New York, pp. 217–265.

van Asselt, E., W. van Raamsdonk, F. de Graaf, M.J. Smit-Onel, P.C. Diegenbach, and B. Heuts (1990) Enzyme histochemical profiles of fish spinal motoneurons after cordotomy and axotomy of motor nerves. *Brain Res.* 531:25–35.

Wallén, P., S. Grillner J.C. Feldman, and S. Bergelt (1985) Dorsal and ventral myotome motoneurons and their input during fictive locomotion in lamprey. *J. Neurosci.* 5:654–661.

Webb, J.E. (1973) The role of notochord in forward and reversed swimming and burrowing in the amphioxus *Branchiostoma lanceolatum*. *J. Zool. (Lond.)* 170:325–338.

Webb, P.W. (1982) Locomotor patterns in the evolution of actinopterygian fishes. *Am. Zool.* 22:329–342.

Webb, P.W., and R.W. Blake (1985) Swimming. In M. Hildebrand, D.M. Bramble, K.F. Liem, and D.B. Wake (eds.): *Functional Vertebrate Morphology*. Harvard University Press, Cambridge, pp. 110–128.

Webster, D.M.S., L.J. Rogers J.D. Pettigrew, and J.D. Steeves (1990) Origins of descending spinal pathways in prehensile birds: do parrots have a homologue to the corticospinal tract of mammals? *Brain Behav. Evol.* 36:216–226.

Wetzel, M.C., and D.G. Stuart (1976) Ensemble characteristics of cat locomotion and its neural control. *Prog. Neurobiol.* 7:1–98.

Wetzel, M.C., and D.G. Stuart (1977) Activation and co-ordination of vertebrate locomotion. In R.M. Alexander, and G. Goldspink (eds.): *Mechanics and Energetics of Animal Locomotion*. Chapman and Hall, London, pp. 115–152.

Wild, J.M. (1992) Direct and indirect "cortico"-rubral and rubrocerebellar cortical projections in the pigeon. *J. Comp. Neurol.* 326:623–636.

Wild J.M., J.J.A. Arends, and H.P. Zeigler (1985) Telencephalic connections of the trigeminal system in the pigeon (*Columba livia*): a trigeminal sensorimotor circuit. *J. Comp. Neurol.* 234:441–464.

Wild, J.M., and M.N. Williams (2000) Rostral Wulst in passerine birds. I. Origins, course, and terminations of an avian pyramidal tract. *J. Comp. Neurol.* 416: 429–450.

Wirth, F.P., J.L. O'Leary, J.M. Smith, and J.M. Jenny (1974) Monosynaptic corticospinal-motoneuron path in the raccoon. *Brain Res.* 77:344–348.

Yalden, D.W. (1966) The anatomy of mole locomotion. *J. Zool. (Lond.)* 149:55–64.

Young, J.Z. (1981) *The Life of Vertebrates*. 3rd ed. Oxford University Press, London.

Zecha, A. (1962) The "pyramidal tract" and other telencephalic efferents in birds. *Acta Morphol. Neerl. Scand.* 5:194–195.

Zeier, H., and H.J. Karten (1971) The archistriatum of the pigeon: organization of afferent and efferent connections. *Brain Res.* 31:313–326.

Chapter 4

SENSORY SYSTEM EVOLUTION IN VERTEBRATES

William Hodos and Ann B. Butler, Krasnow, Department of Psychology, University of Maryland (W.H.) Institute for Advanced Study and Department of Psychology, George Mason University (A.B.B.)

Sensory receptors and their anatomical and physiological representations in the central nervous system are major factors in the evolution of vertebrates. Because they are vital for the exploration and manipulation of the environment, the senses provide the way for vertebrates to enter new adaptive zones and to exploit effectively the opportunities for evolution that they encounter. Sensory evolution progresses by increasing the animals' sensitivity to already detectable stimuli and by the development of entirely new sensory modalities. If these new dimensions are effective in increasing reproduction and survival of offspring, they establish a trend for evolutionary changes both in the sensory periphery and the central cell groups and pathways that constitute sensory systems. For example, the animals with the best color vision are birds and primates, especially Old World primates. This high degree of specialized ability may well have evolved in both groups as an adaptation to enhance the visibility of objects from their background, such as food objects and predators. It may further have aided them to distinguish between ripe and unripe fruit, to discriminate toxic from nontoxic insects and plants, to discriminate between males and females, to ascertain sexual receptiveness, and to detect or discriminate other aspects of the visual environment that could enhance survival (Jacobs, 1981).

HOW MANY SENSES?

Sensory systems are the means by which animals detect and respond to certain physical properties of the external and internal environments. These physical properties of the environment are known as stimuli. We traditionally speak of five human senses: taste and smell (chemical senses), touch and hearing (mechanical senses), and vision (electromagnetic radiation sense). This is, of course, a gross underestimate. Humans have a vestibular sensory system for the detection of gravity and acceleration, plus an elaborate system of mechanoreceptors for muscle stretch and the position of joints, as well as a number of chemical interoreceptors for glucose, oxygen, pH, osmotic pressure, blood pressure, and other physical properties. We must, however, add to this list the stimuli and their corresponding senses that our fellow vertebrates can detect, such as infrared and ultraviolet radiation and both electrical and magnetic fields (Shepherd, 1988; Butler and Hodos, 1996). Table 4.1 summarizes the classes of stimuli and the senses that detect them. The list is not exhaustive, and experts in almost any sensory system surely would insist on further subdivision and refinement to fully explicate the subtleties of which that sense is capable.

In addition to a greater qualitative range of physical stimuli that impinge on living organisms, nonhuman animals have evolved, in many instances, greater sensitivity than humans to the senses that both possess. Detection of various segments of the electromagnetic spectrum are excellent examples of this phenomenon (Butler and Hodos, 1996). Many birds and insects can detect light in the ultraviolet range, which humans cannot detect, and crotalid and some boid snakes can detect infrared radiation, which humans also cannot detect (Hartline, 1974). Many ray-finned fishes and sharks can detect electric fields (Bullock et al., 1982, 1983) and probably magnetic fields as well. Among the chemical senses, humans are able to detect only relatively strong concentrations in comparison with many other vertebrates as well as a narrower range of chemical compounds (Finger, 1991). In addition, animals with good chemical sensitivity also appear able to detect the spatial properties of the chemical world, an aspect of the gustatory and olfactory worlds of which humans make little use.

Table 4.1. Vertebrate Sensory Modalities

Physical Stimuli	Sensory Modality	Receptor Location
Chemical	General chemical	Skin and visceral surfaces
	Olfactory	Nasal and vomeronasal organs
	Gustatory	Skin and oral surfaces
	Oxygen tension	Arteries
	Glucose	Hypothalamus
	pH	Medulla
	Toxins	Gut
	Osmotic	Hypothalamus
Mechanical	Touch	Skin
	Pressure	Skin, muscles, visceral surfaces
	Stretch	Skin, muscles, visceral surfaces, swim bladder
	Joint position	Joints
	Gravity	Vestibular labyrinth
	Acceleration	Vestibular labyrinth
	Pressure waves in water	Lateral line canals or skin pores
	Audition	Lagena, cochlea
Electromagnetic	Photoreception	Retina, epiphysis
	Infrared	Body surface (nerve terminals), face region (pit organs)
	Electroreception	Lateral line canals or skin pores
	Magnetoreception	Lateral line canals or skin pores, retina (?)

HOW MANY CRANIAL NERVES?

How many cranial nerves are required to process the information presented by the multiplicity of senses? Those who have studied neuroanatomy have dutifully memorized the names and numbers of the traditional 12 cranial nerves. Unfortunately for the student of comparative neuroanatomy and brain evolution, the list is considerably longer. The left column of Table 4.2 lists the traditional 12 cranial nerves with their familiar Roman numeralization. The right column presents the 26 cranial nerves currently recognized by comparative neuroanatomists (Butler and Hodos, 1996). Here, too, experts on any of these nerves almost certainly would insist on further subdivision. The shaded cells in the left column indicate where there is no counterpart among the traditional 12.

Table 4.2. The Cranial Nerves

The Original Human XII	The Current Vertebrate XXVI
	Terminal (T)
Olfactory (I)	Olfactory (I)
	Vomeronasal (VN)
Optic (II)	Optic (II)
	Epiphyseal (E)
Oculomotor (III)	Oculomotor (III)
Trochlear (IV)	Trochlear (IV)
Trigeminal (V)	Profundus (P)
	Trigeminal (V)
Abducens (VI)	Abducens (VI)
Facial (VII)	Dorsal facial (VII_D)
	Ventrolateral facial (VII_{VL})
Vestibulocochlear (VIII)	Vestibular (VIII_V)
	Cochlear (VIII_C)
	Anteroventral lateral line (AVLL)
	Anterodorsal lateral line (ADLL)
	Otic lateral line (OLL)
	Middle lateral line (MLL)
	Supratemporal lateral line (STLL)
	Posterior lateral line (PLL)
Glossopharyngeal (IX)	Dorsal Glossophyaryngeal (IX_D)
	Ventrolateral glossopharyngeal (IX_{VL})
Vagus (X)	Dorsal vagus (X_D)
	Ventrolateral vagus (X_{VL})
Spinal accessory (XI)	Spinal accessory (XI)
Hypoglossal (XII)	Hypoglossal (XII)

116   4 Sensory System Evolution in Vertebrates

Moreover, cranial nerve experts have recognized that a number of the traditional 12 actually comprise two or more separate nerves, such as the cochlear and vestibular divisions of cranial nerve VIII. Similarly, the gustatory components of cranial nerves VII, IX, and X long have been recognized by virtue of their separate terminations in the central nervous system and their diverse embryological origins to be quite separate from the general viscerosensory components of these same nerves. These distinctions are recognized in the right column by assigning separate names to these diverse nerves and nerve components. Furthermore, the lateral line nerves are separate nerves in their own right but are not included in the traditional 12.

TRENDS IN SENSORY SYSTEM EVOLUTION

A study of the comparative anatomy and embryology of the central nervous system reveals certain trends in the evolution of sensory systems. These trends consist of patterns of both conservatism and innovation. For example, the portion of the somatosensory system associated with the spinal cord and caudal brain stem as well as the vestibular and lateral line mechanosensory systems of the hindbrain are remarkably consistent in their overall organization across vertebrate classes. Other senses, such as electroreception, infrared reception, and color vision appear to have independently evolved multiple times.

Table 4.3 (Hodos and Butler, 1997) recapitulates the sensory systems according to two characteristics: their presumed age among the vertebrate lineages and their relative breadth of distribution across the vertebrate lineages. This table is derived from extensive data produced by many workers and reviewed by Butler and Hodos (1996). It indicates that, with the exception of infrared reception, and possibly audition and magnetoreception, all of the remaining senses can be traced to the earliest vertebrates. This suggests that these senses, or at least some of them, may represent a heritage from our invertebrate ancestors. Table 4.3 also summarizes the distribution of the senses across the vertebrate lineages. Thus, some senses, such as photoreception, vestibular sense, somesthesis, and olfaction, are widely distributed across lineages. This stands in sharp contrast to those senses, such as vomeronasal, the lateral line senses, or infrared reception, that are restricted to a narrower range of taxonomic groups.

Despite the great diversity of both lineages and adaptive zones, a relatively stable pattern of sensory system organization nevertheless seems to have endured. Even though certain senses appear to have waxed and waned with increasing and decreasing specialization, consistent patterns nevertheless have persisted. Sensory system evolution thus appears to have been relatively conservative in its course. This is quite a different perspective from that of neuroanatomists of 40 or 50 years ago, when the prevailing view was that the evolution of mammals brought with it sweeping changes in sensory system organization (Butler and Hodos, 1996).

What are some of these conservative features? Shepherd (1988) has observed that despite the range of stimuli that animals can detect and the variety of receptors that

Table 4.3. Evolutionary Characteristics of Sensory Systems, from : Hodos and Butler (1997) by permission of Karger, Basel

Sense	Age		Distribution Across Lineages	
	Ancient	Relatively Recent	Wide	Narrow
Photoreception, retinal	✓		✓	
Photoreception, epiphyseal	✓		✓	
Vestibular (vestibulospinal and vestibulocerebellar)	✓		✓	
Olfactory	✓		✓	
Somatosensory	✓		✓	
Viscerosensory	✓		✓	
Mechanosensory Lateral Line	✓			✓
Gustatory	✓		✓	
Electroreceptive	✓			✓
Auditory	✓(?)		✓	
Vomeronasal		✓		✓
Infrared		✓		✓
Magnetoreceptive		✓(?)		✓

detect them, a striking similarity exists both among the sensory neurons and receptors themselves and in the overall organization of the central sensory systems that process their output. Sensory receptors are either discrete, specialized neurons, such as those of the visual and octavolateralis systems, or they are bipolar neurons that have specialized receptor endings. All of the discrete, specialized, sensory receptor cells terminate on bipolar neurons. The term *bipolar neuron* is used here to encompass pseudounipolar ganglion cells, as found in the dorsal root ganglia of the spinal cord and in the hindbrain cranial nerve ganglia, as well as the bipolar neurons of the forebrain sensory systems. Whatever their type, all bipolar sensory neurons terminate on comparable populations of cells that we refer to as *first-order multipolar neurons* (Butler, 2000) (Fig. 4.1). These first-order multipolar neurons include, for example, the mitral cells of the olfactory system, the retinal ganglion cells, the principal and descending trigeminal nuclei, the cochlear, vestibular, and lateral line nuclei, the gustatory nucleus, the dorsal column nuclei, and the dorsal horn spinothalamic neurons.

As shown in Figure 4.2, Shepherd (1988) noted this type of commonality in the visual and olfactory systems. Both senses display parallel pathways that connect their receptors and/or bipolar neurons to the first-order multipolar neurons—the retinal ganglion cells and the olfactory mitral cells, respectively. An additional similarity is that both the retina and olfactory bulb contain specialized interneurons that modulate the straight-through processing of the sensory information by the

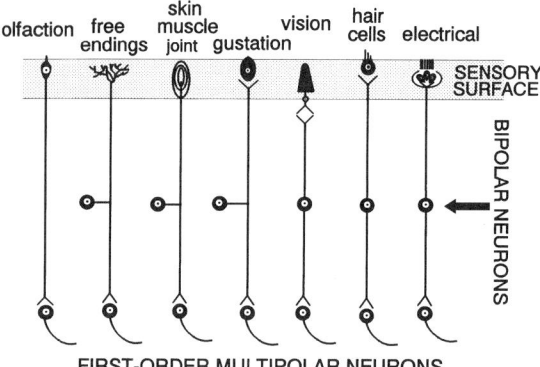

Figure 4.1. A comparison of different types of sensory neurons to show the overall similarity of their relationships to the central nervous system. Bipolar (or pseudo-unipolar) neurons are either primary receptors or are in synaptic contact with specialized receptor cells. The bipolars, in turn, terminate on first-order multipolar neurons that conduct the sensory information into the central nervous system.

first-order multipolar neurons. The interneurons are present both at the sensory receptor–bipolar interface and at the bipolar–first-order multipolar interface.

These similarities in organization could be viewed as mere coincidences. One should consider, however, that vision and olfaction are the only forebrain senses and both involve complex (albeit different) biochemical transduction mechanisms. Even though the proximal stimulus for a retinal photoreceptor is a photon of light, what occurs thereafter is a complex biochemical process, as are the events that occur in a chemosensory olfactory receptor.

Other parallels in the organization of diverse sensory-processing systems can be seen in the work of Mugnaini and his colleagues (Mugnaini et al., 1980; Mugnaini and Morgan, 1987) and Ryugo and his colleagues (Wright and Ryugo, 1996). These investigators report that the nucleus cuneatus, which is one of the dorsal column nuclei of the

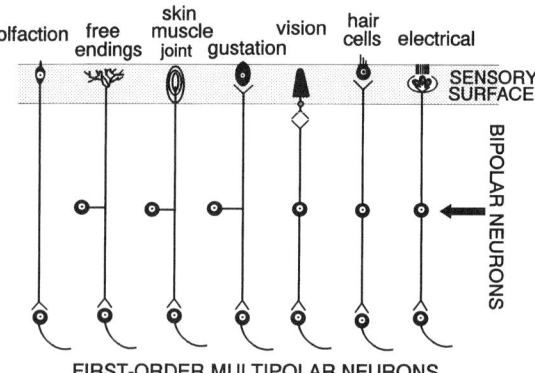

Figure 4.2. A comparison of the basic neuronal architecture of the retina and the olfactory bulb to show the similarity in their organization. (Adapted from Shepherd, 1988.)

somatosensory system, supplies mossy fibers, similar to those of the cerebellum, to the dorsal cochlear nucleus. The dorsal cochlear nucleus, in turn, has an internal organization that is quite similar to that of the cerebellar cortex, including granule cells, the axons of which form parallel fibers, inhibitory interneurons, and efferent neurons that send their dendrites into the layer of parallel fibers. To extend the comparison, both the cerebellum and the dorsal cochlear nucleus combine somatosensory inputs and inputs from the vestibular and lateral line systems (in those anamniote vertebrates that possess a lateral line system). Wright and Ryugo (1996) suggest that the dorsal cochlear nucleus may be an acoustic "cerebellum" specialized for stabilization of the head and ear pinnae in relation to a sound source. Other parallel organizational schemes may be seen between the electrosensory lateral line lobe of weakly electric gymnotiform fishes and the cerebellar cortex (Maler and Mugnaini, 1994).

ASCENDING SENSORY PATHWAYS

Most ascending sensory pathways that originate in the first-order mulitpolar neurons tend to have one or both components of a basic pattern as shown in Figure 4.3 and as fully represented in the somatosensory and visual systems. This pattern consists of each sense sending ascending axons to the dorsal thalamus and then to the telencephalon via two separate routes, one direct and one indirect. The direct routes comprise the so-called lemniscal pathways or lemnothalamic pathways (Butler, 1994a,b) in which the first-order multipolar neurons project directly to the lemnothalamus. Given the diverse afferent sources that contribute to this set of inputs, Butler (1994a) used the prefix "lemno-" in the broad sense of Nauta and Karten (1970), referring "somewhat loosely to fiber systems originating from secondary sensory cell groups and ascending toward . . . the thalamus." The indirect routes to the dorsal thalamus originate from first-order multipolar neurons that terminate on neurons located in the midbrain tectum, or colliculi. Collothalamic pathways (Butler, 1994a) comprise the sets of tectal neurons and their axons that project to the collothalamus. The lemnothalamic and collothalamic neurons of the dorsal thalamus form separate sets of nuclei. Their efferent pathways ascend to the telencephalon and terminate in separate but interconnected telencephalic areas.

Among the exceptions to this general plan are some of the olfactory, octavolateralis, and gustatory pathways. The olfactory system differs from all the other senses in that it enters directly into the telencephalon without a primary pathway via the dorsal thalamus. Although not shown in Figure 4.3, there is, however, an additional olfactory pathway, at least in amniotes, from olfactory cortex to the dorsal thalamus and back to the telencephalon (see Butler and Hodos, 1996). The olfactory system thus also has two routes to the telencephalon, but neither is via the midbrain tectum. A different variation occurs in the auditory part of the octavolateralis system, which has a collothalamic pathway but appears to lack a lemnothalamic component altogether. The vestibular system complements the latter arrangement with its direct lemnothalamic pathway (Jones, 1985) and an apparent lack of a collothalamic component. On the other hand, independently evolved, caudal diencephalic nuclei present in ray-finned

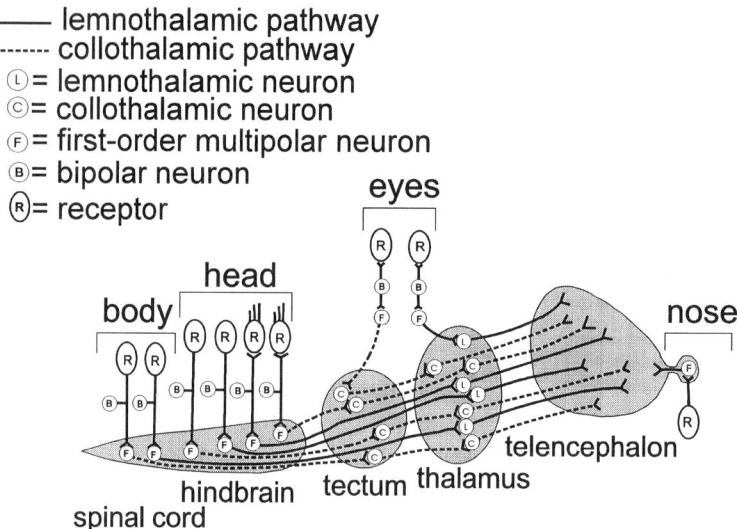

Figure 4.3. A schematic representation of vertebrate sensory pathways to the telencephalon. The pathways shown are for (left to right) the somatosensory (body and head), vestibular, auditory, visual, and olfactory systems. Similar systems exist for gustatory and other senses, but these have not been shown in the interest of clarity. Each of the receptors shown in the body region terminates on a first-order multipolar neuron located in the spinal cord or hind brain; head receptors terminate on first-order multipolar neurons in the hind brain. The first-order multipolar neurons of the visual system are the retinal ganglion cells, the somata of which are located within the retina. Both the visual and somatosensory first-order multipolar neurons have connections with the midbrain tectum and the dorsal thalamus, which respectively give rise to the ascending collothalamic and lemnothalamic pathways to the telencephalon. Vestibular and auditory first-order multipolar neurons give rise to lemnothalamic and collothalamic pathways, respectively. Olfactory receptors terminate on first-order multipolar neurons in the olfactory bulb at the rostral end of the telencephalon. Olfactory first-order multipolar neurons are unique in that they terminate directly in the telencephalon.

and cartilaginous fishes relay lateral line and gustatory information to the telencephalon and thus mimic lemnothalamic pathways (Butler, 1994a). Finally, although gustation and olfaction are both chemical senses, their sensory pathways suggest that they have quite different evolutionary histories. Gustation follows the typical route of the somatosensory system, which suggests an evolutionary relationship between gustatory receptors and cutaneous receptors (see Finger, 1997). This arrangement stands in sharp contrast to the direct telencephalic entry of the first-order multipolar olfactory neurons, which is unique among sensory systems.

NEUROEMBRYOLOGY AND THE EVOLUTION OF SENSORY SYSTEMS

How do the central components of the sensory systems become remodeled in response to the appearance of new receptors? Wilczynski (1984) pointed out that both genetic and epigenetic mechanisms are involved in the process of sensory and motor reorganization in response to adaptive pressures in the periphery. He observed that changes in the periphery are able to induce extensive and wide-ranging reorganization of central pathways by interacting with ontogenetic processes and inducing compensatory reactions. The rapid progress of the past decade in understanding the molecular and genetic bases of these phenomena has led to a rethinking of the possible mechanisms that result in sensory system evolution. For example, Raff (1996) recently summarized and interpreted the literature on the relationships between genes, embryology, and the evolution of animal form. He stressed the theme that selection affects variation in the phenotype as a result of events that occur in the developing embryo. Embryos are basically modular in organization, with the modules forming the body segments and organs, such as limbs or vertebral segments, and also components of the central nervous system. Certain internal evolutionary processes, which act on the modules, result in phenotypic changes that can be acted on by external selection pressures. Among these internal evolutionary processes are

- *Dissociation:* Heterochrony, which is the dissociation of the timing of ontogenetic events, is an example of a dissociative process.

- *Co-option*: An existing module is altered to have a new structure and/or function.

- *Duplication and divergence*: A module is duplicated one or more times. The duplicate is then moved to a new location where it can come under the influence of dissociation or co-option. Because a new module and the original module cannot occupy the same space, changes in size, location, and interaction among modules occur.

New modules often are modifications of existing modules; hence any changes in their number, their size, their location, or interactions between or among them will increase the likelihood that a new module will become co-opted for a new function. In addition, selective pressures that have the effect of increasing the time required for neurogenesis can result in larger neuronal populations (Finlay and Darlington, 1995), which themselves offer important adaptive advantages (Jerison 1973).

The mechanism by which developmental processes are related to the evolution of morphological entities, such as sensory systems, is via structural genes and regulatory genes. Structural genes are those that build the modules; regulatory genes determine how the modules function during various stages of development. Thus, the interaction between embryonic events and external selection offers insights into the mechanisms by which evolution shapes sensory systems. Gans and Northcutt (1983), Noden (1991), Puelles and Rubenstein (1993), Northcutt (1996), and others have used both genetic and ontogenetic data to explain the major events in the evolution of the craniate head, the organization of the forebrain and hindbrain, and the cranial nerves. These new approaches and the data that they have yielded offer the possibility for new answers to some perplexing questions about sensory system evolution, such as

- How do new sensory receptors evolve?

- How do new primary, secondary, and higher order sensory nuclei develop in response to novel peripheral detectors?

- How does an animal become a sensory specialist, and does it do so at the expense of other senses?
- How do sensory system axons accurately arrive at their appropriate target populations?
- How do new nuclear groups arise within a sensory system as specialization increases?
- How does the sensory world become mapped in the central nervous system?
- When peripheral sensory mechanisms are lost, what is the fate of their central neuronal populations?
- What are the mechanisms for organization and reorganization of sensory systems?

Evolution of New Sensory Receptors

One mechanism that led to the appearance of new types of sensory receptors may have been the modification of existing receptors that permitted them to detect a different range of stimuli within the same modality. A reasonable line of speculation could be that the earliest receptor types were mechanoreceptors and chemoreceptors, with all other sensory receptors being derived from them. When a receptor type became sufficiently extreme, so as to allow detection of a different stimulus or different category of stimulus, that extreme type effectively became a new class of sensory receptor. For example, the infrared detectors of the pit organs of crotalid snakes are derived from trigeminal thermal detectors (Bullock and Fox, 1957; Hartline, 1974; Molenaar, 1991). Electroreceptors, which evolved in ancestral vertebrates but occur sporadically in ray-finned fishes (Bullock et al., 1982, 1983) and which evolved independently in monotremes (Scheich et al., 1986), may have been derived from other cutaneous receptors. For example, the electroreceptors found on the snouts of platypuses are derived from receptors that innervate a mucous-secreting gland and are quite different from those of bony fishes or sharks.

Moreover, platypus electroreceptors are innervated by a branch of the trigeminal nerve rather than by branches of the lateral line nerves (Gregory et al., 1988). Similarly, color vision appears to have evolved independently several times in vertebrates (Jacobs, 1981). All of these changes could have been accomplished by relatively minor genetic mutations followed by the operation of selection on the phenotype of the new population to produce these new classes of receptors.

Evolution of New Primary, Secondary, and Higher Order Sensory Nuclei

The appearance of novel central nuclei often occurs in conjunction with the appearance of novel sensory systems, such as electroreception or infrared detection. Examples of this may be seen in the lateral trigeminal nucleus, which is the primary sensory nucleus of the infrared detectors and is found only in infrared-detecting snakes (Schroeder and Loop, 1976; Molenaar, 1978), and the nucleus electrosensorius, which is present in the pretectum only in electroreceptive ostariophysine teleosts (Bullock and Heiligenberg, 1986; Striedter, 1992). What is the mechanism by which these nuclear groups evolve? Morphological duplication and relocation of the embryonic modules that make up the central neuronal populations of the sensory systems from which the new receptor was derived would appear to be likely mechanisms, followed by co-option to a new function. Thus, the infrared sensory system is associated not with the visual system, to which it is functionally analogous as an electromagnetic-spectrum detector, but rather with the trigeminal system, to which it is morphologically related as a cutaneous sensory system. Likewise, monotreme electroreception is associated with the trigeminal system rather than the lateral line system as it is in anamniotes.

The Evolution of Sensory Specialists

A sensory specialist is an animal that has developed a particular sense to such an extent that it can detect exceptionally weak stimuli, or it can detect an exceptionally broad range of stimuli, and/or it can make exceptionally fine distinctions between different sensory qualities. Among the best examples of sensory specialization are the macrosmatic mammals, such as bloodhounds and other canids, which have very large olfactory bulbs. Another example of sensory specialists are the silurid and cyprinid fishes, in which gustation is highly developed and which possess enormous and highly differentiated brain regions for processing gustatory information (Finger, 1997). Likewise, audition in bats, spatial vision in primates, and both spatial and color vision in birds are further examples of sensory specialization.

Some evidence exists that suggests that sensory specializations may occur at the expense of other senses. For example, while color vision enhances the discriminability of the size and shape of objects, it appears to reduce the ability to see fine details of the colored objects (Jacobs, 1981). Hodos (1993) reports that although birds have excellent ability to see both color and fine details compared with many mammals, their ability to detect subtle variations in contrast is considerably less than that of mammals, even those with inferior spatial resolution. Similarly, among bats, their extraordinary specialization for audition may have come at the expense of their vision. Bats that are specialized for echolocation, as estimated from relative length of the ear pinnae, tend to have relatively small eyes, whereas many of the bat species with large eyes tend to have relatively small ear pinnae (Richardz and Lumbrunner, 1993).

Some recent studies by Kelley et al. (1994, 1995) on the development of photoreceptors may offer some clues to the mechanisms by which these specializations develop. These workers applied retinoic acid to cultures of retinal cells from rat embryonic day 18 fetuses and found that they could affect the fate of uncommitted progenitor cells so that they subsequently developed into rod photoreceptors. Likewise, when they administered T_3 thyroxin to the same type of culture, they changed the fate of the progenitor cells to become cone photoreceptors. They suggested that variations in the proportions of T_3 and retinoic acid can affect the progenitor cells to determine the relative proportions of rods, cones, and amacrine cells in the developing retina. Thus, a relatively minor change in regulatory gene expression, such has the *Hox* or *Pax* genes, which affect the production of retinoic acid, easily could affect the proportions of the different retinal cell types. Similar minor genetic changes could have resulted in the variations in the spectral sensitivities of cone photopigments that are the basis of color vision. Kelley et al. (1994) also describe similar effects in the auditory system in the development of the proportions of hair cells and supporting cells. A similar mechanism also could have resulted in the differentiation of the various types of hair cell mechanoreceptors that are present in octavolateralis system.

Evolution of Central Sensory Pathways

The different classes of cell adhesion molecules are important in the neural development of sensory pathways. These molecules attach to cell surfaces or to part of the extracellular matrix. They play important roles, not only in directing the growth of axons toward or away from certain cell populations, but also in determining the branching of axons, the formation of synapses, and the growth or inhibition of growth of the developing axons. Goodman (1996) described the varieties of cell surface guidance and adhesion molecules and has classified them into four functional categories:

- Short-range, contact-mediated attraction molecules
- Short-range, contact-mediated repulsion or inhibition molecules
- Long-range attraction molecules
- Long-range repulsion molecules

Goodman (1996) notes that the classification into long-range and short-range types is for convenience; in fact, the long-range and short-range molecules form a continuum. Included among the guidance and cell adhesion molecules are the superfamily of immunoglobulins, the netrins, and the semaphorins. These molecules have many effects on developing neurons, among which are the transient and/or permanent cessation of axonal growth and the transformation of an axon terminal into a presynaptic terminal arbor. Many of these cell adhesion molecules are of dual function; that is, they can either attract or repel growing axons according to the molecular properties of the growing axon's growth cone. Thus, guidance toward one cell population or guidance away from another population, whether the axon sends a collateral into a cell population, and whether it forms connections are determined by a complex of chemical signals from that cell population and neighboring ones, as well as the chemical properties of the growth cone itself. The axonal guidance system contains many relevant molecules so that removal of a single component might not be very disruptive to the pattern of connections being formed. If, however, that component were moved to a novel location, it could have a dramatic effect on the total signal pattern. In other words, small variations in the patterns of guidance molecules are not likely to offer a basis for selection to operate to evolve a new sensory pathway. In contrast, a mutation that changes the location of a major chemical signal or that disrupts the pattern of signals could have a major impact on the direction and extent of axonal growth.

The Evolution of New Central Sensory Nuclei

Among the cell adhesion molecules are a group known as the cadherins. These molecules appear to play a major role in the aggregation of neuroblasts into brain nuclei. They also may contribute in an important way to the differentiation of nuclei into distinct subdivisions as described by Redies et al. (1992, 1993) and Gänzler and Redies (1995). Cadherins are glycoproteins that promote cell adhesion. Cells that express the same cadherin aggregate together. Thus, a single population that is composed of cells that express different cadherins will segregate themselves into separate groups, each expressing the same cadherin. More than a dozen cadherins have been reported in the developing central nervous systems of a variety of vertebrates. In addition to the strong binding between cadherins, a weaker bond occurs between different types of cadherins and other types of cell adhesion molecules.

Two cadherins that are of particular interest in this regard are N-cadherin and R-cadherin. N-cadherin is expressed in the chicken embryo in two stages: (1) early in embryogenesis, during which time this molecule is very widely distributed; and (2) at embryonic days 5 to 8 and continuing until embryonic day 15, during which time its expression is confined to a restricted group of nuclei and axon pathways. R-cadherin also is expressed in a restricted group of cell groups and pathways during embryonic days 6 to 11.

An example of the specificity of N- and R-cadherins to particular sensory cell groups may be seen in the efferents of the optic tectum, especially those that terminate in the nucleus rotundus of the thalamus and in the pretectum (Redies et al., 1993). Figure 4.4 is a schematic representation of N-cadherin and R-cadherin expression at approximately emgryonic days 8 to 11 in the embryonic brain of a chicken. It shows the optic tectum and several of its efferent pathways: the tectorotundal pathway from the tectum to nucleus rotundus; the tectopretectal pathway from tectum to n. pretectalis, n. subpretectalis, and n. interstitio-pretecto-subpretectalis; and the tectoisthmal pathway from the tectum to the magnocellular and parvocellular nuclei isthmi and the n. semilunaris. Figure 4.4 shows that N-cadherin is expressed only in the axons and cells in the tectorotundal and tectopretectal pathways, whereas R-cadherin is expressed only in the tectoisthmal pathway. Moreover, no other tectal efferent pathway expresses either R-cadherin or N-cadherin.

Redies and co-workers (1992) also report that cadherins are expressed in other regions of the developing chick brain. The data strongly imply that cadherins and other cell adhesion molecules play an important role in determining the number and

126   4   Sensory System Evolution in Vertebrates

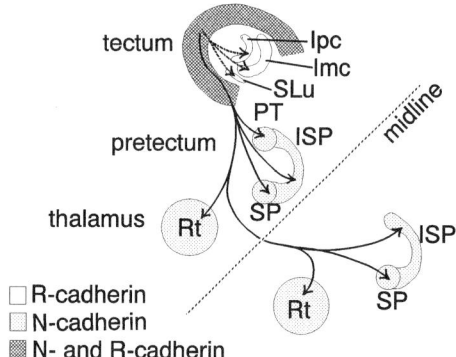

Figure 4.4. Expression of two cadherins in the optic tecum, pretectum, and dorsal thalamus of a chicken embryo during embryonic days 8 to 11. N-cadherin is expressed in the tectum, in several pretectal nuclei (PT, SP, and ISP), and in the thalamus (Rt). R-cadherin is expressed in the tectum and the nuclei isthmi (Ipc, Imc, and SLu). Imc, nucleus isthmi, pars magnocellularis; Ipc, nucleus isthmi, pars parvocellularis; ISP, nucleus interstitio-pretecto-subpretectalis; PT, nucleus pretectalis; Rt, nucleus rotundus; SLu, nucleus semilunaris; SP, nucleus subpretectalis. (Adapted from Redies et al., 1993, from : Hodos and Butler 1997, by permission of Karger, Basel.)

the location of neuronal populations in a sensory system as well as the axonal links between them. Moreover, cadherins and other cell adhesion molecules may play important roles in the formation of new components of sensory systems as sensory specialization develops.

The Evolution of Sensory Maps

A sensory specialist often is characterized by the presence of a precisely organized, highly detailed topographical map of the sensory surface or the sensory space around the animal. The high degree of precision in the organization of these topographical maps also may be a consequence of interactions between chemical guidance molecules on the growth cones of developing axons and the dendrites of neurons in topographically organized neuronal fields. Indeed, the presence of a set of common markers at different levels of the central nervous system could be the basis for maintaining the topography throughout the entire sensory pathway. One of the most dramatic aspects of these topographical maps is the registration of the representations of diverse senses within a single structure. Thus, in the optic tectum, visual, auditory, and somatosensory maps are arranged in a closely overlapping fashion (Stein and Meredith, 1993). Likewise, the tectal visual and infrared maps of rattlesnakes are in register in the tectum (Hartline et al., 1978). A specific point in space or on the body surface could be represented by a combination of chemical markers common to several sensory layers, which could account for the high degree of precision in alignment of tectal maps (Walter et al., 1987; Roskies and O'Leary, 1994; see also Goodman, 1996, for a detailed review).

Perhaps the most extreme example of detailed topographical mapping of a sensory surface occurs when the central representation of a sensory surface, such as the skin or the retina, forms such a precise representation of the peripheral organization that it takes on the actual appearance of the peripheral organ. Such precise mapping of a sensory surface onto the central nervous system has been termed an *isomorphic representation* (Hodos and Butler, 1997). The best known isomorphic representations of the periphery are the precise mappings of the retina and the cochlea onto their respective higher order cell populations in the visual and auditory systems. Four dramatic examples of isomorphic representations are shown in Figure 4.5.

The first example is the well-known distribution of the vibrissae barrel fields of the somatosensory cortex of rodents, in which the layout of the vibrissae fields is isomorphic with the spatial arrangement of vibrissae on the animal's snout (Woolsey and van der Loos, 1970; Johnson, 1990). The location of each vibrissa on the animal's snout is mirrored by a corresponding barrel field on the snout region of the somatosensory cortex. Similarly, the central representation of the palm pads and digits in a rodent (Welker and Seidenstein, 1959; Johnson, 1990) bears a striking similarity to the palmar surface of the animal's paw. Less well known, perhaps, but no less dramatic, is the isomorphism between the central organization of the barbels of a sea catfish, each studded with thousands of taste buds, and the central representation of each barbel in the animal's facial lobe (Kiyohara and Caprio, 1996). Another impressive topographic organization is the isomorphism between the peripheral distribution of the fleshy nasal rays that form the snout of the star-nose mole and their central representation (Catania and Kaas, 1996). Because the specialized peripheral structures and central isomorphisms of both the catfish and the star-nose mole represent increases in the number of elements, the two adaptations would appear to be good examples of duplication and relocation producing an extreme effect.

The occurrence of occasional extreme effects in evolution, such as highly isomorphic topographical representations, has led Gans (1993) to comment that "excessive phenotypes," as he calls them, have a significance for understanding evolutionary trends. He observes that any population that contains sizeable variability inevitably will produce a certain number of individuals with phenotypes that far exceed the demands of the environment. If these excessive variants occupy a new adaptive zone, or if the demands of their formerly comfortable environment change, what was previously excessive could then become only "adequate." Being only adequate in a challenging environment can be the basis for further selection and the development of a new phenotypic trend.

Loss of Sensory Receptors and Central Pathways

A number of recent investigations have described the invasion of one sensory system by another as a naturally occurring phenomenon or as a consequence of experimental manipulation of the embryo (for review, see Pallas, 1991). The large literature on the effects of embryonic manipulation indicates that retinal axons are capable of forming

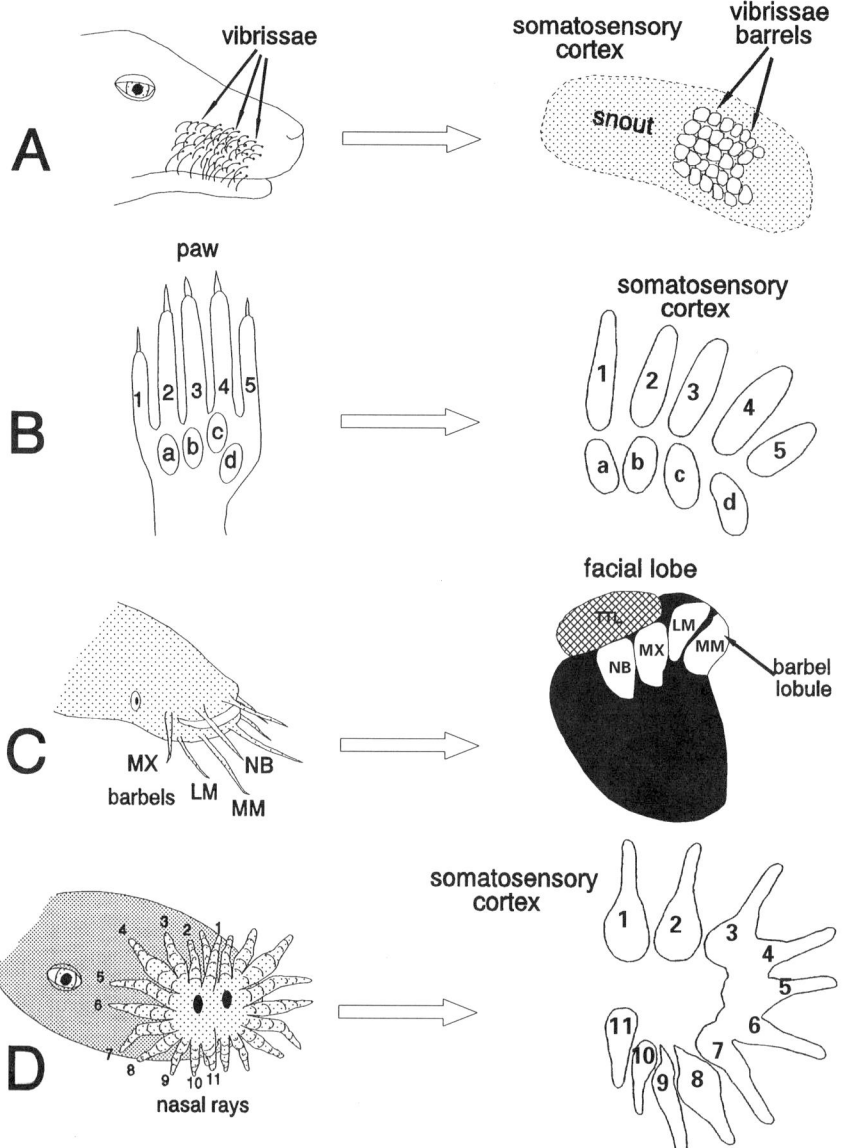

Figure 4.5. Isomorphic representations in the central nervous system of peripheral sensory structures. (*A*) Distribution of each vibrissa in the snout region of the somatosensory cortex of a mammal. (Adapted from Butler and Hodos, 1996.) (*B*) Each digit (numerals) and each palm pad (letters) is represented in the hand area of the somatosensory cortex of a mammal. (Adapted from Butler and Hodos 1996.) (*C*) Each barbel is represented in the facial lobe of a catfish. LM, lateral mandibular barbel; MM, medial mandibular barbel; MX, maxillary barbel; NB, nasal barbel; TTL, central projection of the trunk and tail taste buds. (Adapted from Kiyohara and Caprio, 1996.) (*D*) Each of the 11 fleshy nasal rays of the snout of a star-nose mole is represented in the animal's somatosensory cortex. (Adapted from Catania and Kaas, 1996.) from : Hodos and Butler (1997) by permission of Karger, Basel.

a variety of other connections. For example, when retinal axons are induced to invade the normally auditory medial geniculate nucleus in ferrets (Pallas, 1991), the retinal axons impose a two-dimensional retinotopic map on the normally one-dimensional tonotopic organization of the medial geniculate nucleus. This finding illustrates the ability of an ingrowing sensory pathway to affect the organization of its target population.

A further observation was made by Roe et al. (1993), who report that the experimentally rerouted axons of neonatal ferrets were a subset of the retinal ganglion cell type known as W-cells, which are the principal source of afferents to the optic tectum in cats (Berson and Stein, 1990) and hence part of the collothalamic visual pathway. The lateral geniculate is the thalamic target of the lemnothalamic visual pathway, whereas the medial geniculate is the thalamic target of the collothalamic auditory pathway. What is most intriguing about these results is that when a lemnothalamic visual target was not available, and a collothalamic nucleus was the new target, collothalamic visual axons were the ones to redirect themselves to it.

An illustration of this phenomenon that occurs naturally may be seen in blind mole rats (*Spalax ehrenbergi*). These animals live their entire lives in lightless, underground tunnels and communicate by using vocalization and audition, as well as by seismic signaling (i.e., vibrations of the tunnels). They are born with eyes, but these virtually degenerate as they become covered with skin and fur during postnatal maturation. As the mole rats develop, axons of the auditory system invade the visual system at both the cortical and the thalamic levels. Both 2-deoxyglucose and single-unit recordings indicate that neurons of the visual system in these animals are strongly responsive to auditory stimulation (Heil et al., 1991). Another natural occurrence of sensory invasion was reported by Voneida and Fish (1984) in the blind cavefish *Astyanax hubbsi*. These fishes, like blind mole rats, also have become adapted to a world of total darkness. In blind cavefishes, however, the reorganization occurs in the tectum such that somatosensory system fibers invade the optic layers. These findings suggest that, at least in some sensory systems, invasion of sensory nuclei that are little used because of loss of peripheral receptors may be invaded by other sensory systems. This phenomenon may account for some part of the reorganization of the target sensory system and could result in increased specialization and elaboration.

The mechanosensory lateral line system is a major sensory system in vertebrates except for amniotes (reptiles, mammals, and birds). In amphibians, it typically is present in the larval phase, but in many terrestrial species it disappears during metamorphosis. In amniotes, did some remnants of the lateral line system remain after the anamniote–amniote transition to be invaded or co-opted for a new function? The electrosensory system has been lost and reappeared sporadically among ray-finned fish taxa. How might this have come about? Perhaps the modules that direct expression of these neuronal populations were not removed from the genotype when the cell populations themselves disappeared from the phenotype, thus allowing these populations to reappear at a later time. This issue has been addressed by Butler and Saidel (2000), and they have termed this phenomenon *syngeny*, which refers to the "same genesis" for a given character regardless of its phylogenetic distribution at the phenotypic level. This is in contrast to *allogeny*, which refers to "different genesis" for different phenotypic characters with superficial similarity that occur in cases of genetically independent convergence.

The relationship of the lateral line, vestibular, and electrosensory systems to the evolutionary history of the auditory system has been the subject of considerable analysis and speculation (Fritzsch, 1992; McCormick, 1992). McCormick (1992) noted that while the auditory system appears to have had its inception in the earliest vertebrates, it has undergone independent development in different lineages. Moreover, a variety of peripheral receptors are known to supply afferents to the auditory system. McCormick asked "If different vertebrates utilize different acoustic receptors, has hearing evolved independently several times?" A possible answer to this question might be that the basic octaval pathway is a conservative system of modules, some of which can be co-opted for a variety of functions to serve the class of receptors that are hair cells or their derivatives. Interchangeability among hair cell receptors and their derivatives could be the basis of a variety of sensory organizations and reorganizations. Such a hypothesis has its own difficulties, of course, and almost certainly would require further refinement. For example, it does not explain the intermodal compensation that occurs in blind mole rats with auditory invasion of the visual system.

Mechanisms of Sensory System Evolution

Pallas (1991) suggested three possible mechanisms that could account for both organization and reorganization in sensory systems. Although her discussion was oriented toward cortical sensory areas, her conclusions have been generalized here and have been somewhat enlarged in their focus to include entire sensory systems:

- Sensory systems are essentially the same in their intrinsic organization and processing, as may be seen in the strikingly similar bipolar and first-order multipolar cell populations present in all sensory systems. The differences that are observed among them occur as a result of differences imposed by the physical properties of their stimuli and the transduction processes of their receptors.

- Specific patterns of organization from a lower level of a sensory system are capable of inducing an organization on a higher level, as seen in central isomorphic representations of peripheral structures.

- Some regions of a sensory system can develop unique patterns of organization that are independent of afferentation from lower levels. For example, lateral geniculate lamination and some aspects of thalamocortical projections may not be completely dependent for their development on information from peripheral receptors.

The differences in the chemical specifications of sensory systems most likely account for the differences in their development and functional organization, as well as their reorganization and restructuring. All sensory receptors may have evolved from a relatively few, primitive types of cells, not necessarily sensory cells. The similarities of the organization of central sensory pathways suggest strongly that a common genetic patterning mechanism underlies all of them. A better understanding of these genetic mechanisms and their interactions with developmental processes may lead us to a general understanding of the principles that guide the evolution of sensory systems in vertebrates.

ACKNOWLEDGMENTS

The authors thank Catherine Carr and Jaikun Song for their valuable comments and suggestions on an earlier version of this paper. This work was partly supported by NSF grant IBN-9728155 to ABB.

REFERENCES

Berson, D.M., and J.J. Stein (1990) Topographic variation in W-cell input to cat superior colliculus. *Exp. Brain Res.* 79:459–466.
Bullock, T.H., D.A. Bodznick, and R.G. Northcutt (1983) The phylogenetic distribution of electroreception: evidence for convergent evolution of a primitive vertebrate sense modality. *Brain Res. Rev.* 6: 25–46.
Bullock, T.H., and W. Fox (1957) The anatomy of the infrared sense organ in the facial pit of pit vipers. *Q. J. Microsc. Sci.* 98:219–234.
Bullock, T.H., and W. Heiligenberg (eds.) (1986) *Electroreception.* John Wiley and Sons, New York.
Bullock, T.H., R.G. Northcutt, and D.A. Bodznick (1982) Evolution of electroreception. *Trends Neurosci.* 5:50–53.
Butler, A.B. (1994a) The evolution of the dorsal thalamus of jawed vertebrates, including mammals: cladistic analysis and a new hypothesis. *Brain Res.Rev.* 19:29–65.
Butler, A.B. (1994b) The evolution of the dorsal pallium in the telencephalon of amniotes: cladistic analysis and a new hypothesis. *Brain Res. Rev.* 19:66–101.
Butler, A.B. (2000) Chordate evolution and the origin of craniates: an old brain in a new head. *Anat. Rec. (New Anat.)* 261:111–125.
Butler, A.B., and W. Hodos, (1996) *Comparative Vertebrate Neuroanatomy.* Wiley-Liss, New York.
Butler, A.B., and W.M. Saidel (2000) Defining sameness: historical, biological and generative homology. *BioEssays* 22, in press.
Catania, K.C., and J.H. Kaas (1996) The unusual nose and brain of the star-nosed mole. *BioScience* 46:578–586.
Finger, T.E. (1991) Gustatory nuclei and pathways in the central nervous system. In T.E. Finger and W.L. Silver (eds.): *Neurobiology of Taste and Smell.* Krieger Publishing Co., Malabar, FL, pp. 331–353.
Finger, T.E. (1997) Evolution of taste and solitary chemoreceptor cell systems. *Brain Behav. Evol.* 50:234–243.
Finlay, B.L., and R.B. Darlington (1995) Linked regularities in the development and evolution of mammalian brains. *Science* 268:1578–1584.
Fritzsch, B. (1992) The water-to-land transitional evolution of the tetrapod basilar papilla, middle ear, and auditory nuclei. In D.B. Webster, R.R. Fay, and A.N. Popper (eds.): *The Evolutionary Biology of Hearing.* Springer Verlag, New York, pp. 351–375.
Gans, C. (1993) On the merits of adequacy. *Am. J. Sci.* 293A:391–406.
Gans, C., and R.G. Northcutt (1983) Neural crest and the origin of vertebrates: a new head. *Science* 220:268–274.

Gänzler, S.I.I., and C. Reddies (1995) R-cadherin expression during nucleus formation in chicken forebrain neuromeres. *J. Neurosci.* 15:4157–4172.
Goodman, C.S. (1996) Mechanisms and molecules that control growth cone guidance. *Ann. Rev. Neurosci.* 19:341–377.
Gregory, J.E., A. Iggo, A.K. McIntyre, and U. Proske (1988) Receptors in the bill of the platypus. *J. Physiol. (Lond.)* 400:349–366.
Hartline, P. (1974) Thermoreception in snakes. In A. Fessard (eds.): *Electroreceptors and Other Specialized Receptors, Handbook of Sensory Physiology*, vol. III/3. Springer Verlag, Berlin, pp. 297–312.
Hartline, P.H., L. Kass, and M.S. Loop (1978) Merging of modalities in the optic tectum: infrared and visual integration in rattlesnakes. *Science* 199:1225–1228.
Heil, P., G. Bronchti, Z. Wollberg, and H. Scheich (1991) Invasion of visual cortex by the auditory system in the naturally blind mole rat. *Neuroreport* 2:735–738.
Hodos, W. (1993) The visual capabilities of birds. In H.P. Zeigler and H.-J. Bischof (eds.): *Vision, Brain, and Behavior in Birds.* MIT Press, Cambridge, MA, pp. 63–74.
Hodos, W., and A.B. Butler, (1997) Evolution of sensory systems in vertebrates. *Brain, Behav. Evol.* 50:189–197.
Jacobs, G.H. (1981) *Comparative Color Vision.* Academic Press, New York.
Jerison, H.J. (1973) *Evolution of Brain and Intelligence.* Academic Press, New York.
Johnson, J.I. (1990) Comparative development of somatic sensory cortex. In E.G. Jones and A. Peters (eds.): *Cerebral Cortex, vol. 8B, Comparative Structure and Evolution of Cerebral Cortex, Part II.* Plenum Press, New York, pp. 335–449.
Jones, E.G. (1985) *The Thalamus.* Plenum Press, New York.
Kelley, M.W., J.K. Turner, and T.A. Reh (1994) Retinoic acid promotes differentiation of photoreceptors in vitro. *Development.* 120:2091–2102.
Kelley, M.W., J.K. Turner, and T.A. Reh (1995) Ligands of steroid/thyroid receptors induce cone photoreceptors in vertebrate retina. *Development.* 121:3777–3785.
Kiyohara, S., and J. Caprio (1996) Somatotropic organization of the facial lobe of the sea catfish *Arius felis* studied by transganglionic transport of horseradish peroxidase. *J. Comp. Neurol.* 368:121–135.
Maler, L., and E. Mugnaini (1994) Correlating gamma-aminobutyric acidergic circuits and sensory function in the electrosensory lateral line lobe of a gymnotiform fish. *J. Comp. Neurol.* 345:224–252.
McCormick, C.A. (1992) Evolution of central auditory pathways in anamniotes. In D.B. Webster, R.R. Fay, and A.N. Popper (eds.): *The Evolutionary Biology of Hearing* Springer Verlag, New York, pp. 323–351.
Molenaar, G.J. (1978) The sensory trigeminal system of a snake in possession of infrared receptors. I. The sensory trigeminal nuclei. *J. Comp. Neurol.* 179:123–136.
Molenaar, G.J. (1991) Anatomy and physiology of infrared sensitivity in snakes. In C. Gans and P.S. Ulinski (eds.): *Biology of the Reptilia, vol. 17, Neurology C, Sensorimotor Integration.* University of Chicago Press, Chicago, pp. 367–453.
Mugnaini, E., and J.I. Morgan (1987) The neuropeptide cerebellin is a marker for two similar neuronal circuits in rat brain. *Proc. Natl. Acad. Sci. U.S.A.* 84:8692–8696.
Mugnaini, E., K.K. Olsen, A.-L. Dahl, V.L. Freidrich, and G. Korte (1980) Fine structure of granule cells and related interneurons (termed Golgi cells) in the cochlear complex of cat, rat, and mouse. *J. Neurocytol.* 9:537–570.
Nauta, W.J.H., and H.J. Karten (1970) A general profile of the vertebrate brain, with sidelights on the ancestry of cerebral cortex. In F. O. Schmitt (eds.): *The Neurosciences: Second Study Program.* The Rockefeller University Press, New York; pp. 7–26.
Noden, D.M (1991) Vertebrate craniofacial development: the relation between ontogenetic process and morphological outcome. *Brain Behav. Evol.* 38: 190–225.
Northcutt, R.G. (1996) The origin of craniates: neural crest, neurogenic placodes and homeobox genes. *Isr. J. Zool.* 42:S273–S313.
Pallas, S.L. (1991) Cross-modal plasticity in sensory cortex. In B.L. Finlay, G. Innocenti, and H. Scheick (eds.): *The Neocortex.* Plenum Press, New York, pp. 205–218.
Puelles, L., and J.L.R. Rubenstein (1993) Expression patterns of homeobox and other putative regulatory genes in the embryonic mouse forebrain suggest a neuromeric organization. *Trends Neurosci.* 16:472–479.

Raff, R.A. (1996) *The Shape of Life: Genes, Development, and the Evolution of Animal Form*. University of Chicago Press, Chicago.

Redies, C., K. Engelhart, and M. Takeichi (1993) Differential expression of N- and R-cadherin in functional neuronal systems and other structures of the developing chicken brain. *J. Comp. Neurol.* 333:398–416.

Redies, C., H. Inuzuka, and M. Takeichi (1992) Restricted expression of N- and R-cadherin on neurites of the developing chicken CNS. *J. Neurosi.* 12:3525–3534.

Richardz, K., and A. Lumbrunner (1993) *The World Book of Bats*. T.H. F. Publications, New York.

Roe, A.W., P.E. Garraghty, M. Esguerra, and M. Sur (1993) Experimentally induced visual projections to the auditory thalamus in ferrets: evidence for a W cell pathway. *J. Comp. Neurol.* 334;263–280.

Roskies, A.L., and D.D. O'Leary (1994) Control of topographic retinal axonal branching in inhibitory membrane-bound molecules. *Science* 265;799–803.

Scheich, H., G. Langner, C. Tidemann, R.B. Coles, and A. Guppy (1986) Electroreception and electrolocation in the platypus. *Nature* 319:401–402.

Schroeder, D.M., and M.S. Loop (1976) Trigeminal projections in snakes possessing infrared sensitivity. *J. Comp. Neurol.* 169:1–14.

Shepherd, G.M. (1988) *Neurobiology*. Oxford University. Press, New York.

Stein, B.E., and M.A. Meredith (1993) *The Merging of the Senses*. The MIT Press, Cambridge, MA.

Striedter, G.F. (1992) Phylogenetic changes in the connections of the lateral preglomerular nucleus in ostariophysan teleosts: a pluralistic view of brain evolution. *Brain Behav. Evol.* 39:329–357.

Voneida, T.J., and S.E. Fish (1984) Central nervous system changes related to the reduction of visual input in a naturally blind fish (*Astyanax hubbsi*). Am. Zool. 24:775–782.

Walter, J., R. Kern-Veits, J. Huf, B. Stolze, and F. Bonhoefer (1987) Recognition of position-specific properties of tectal cell membranes by retinal axons in vitro. *Development* 101:685–696.

Welker, W.I., and S. Seidenstein (1959) Somatosensory representations in the cerebral cortex of the raccoon (*Procyon lotor*). 111:469–501.

Wilczynski, W. (1984) Central neural systems subserving a homoplasous periphery. *Am. Zool.* 24:755–763.

Woolsey, T.A., and H. van der Loos (1970) The structural organization of layer IV in the somato-sensory region (S1) of mouse cerebral cortex. The description of a cortical field composed of discrete cytoarchitectonic units. *Brain Res.* 17:205–242.

Wright, D. D., and D. Ryugo (1996) Mossy fiber projections from the cuneate nucleus to the cochlear nucleus in the rat. *J. Comp. Neurol.* 365:159–172.

Chapter 5

EVOLUTION OF THE FOREBRAIN IN TETRAPODS

Toru Shimizu, Department of Psychology, University of South Florida

While there can be no doubt that evolution has resulted in some dramatic improvements in the design of brains and bodies, one should not necessarily assume that ancient, ancestral forms were "primitive" in the sense of being crude and poorly adapted versions of modern animals. Animals generally are well adapted to their environments at whatever geological age they may have existed, and many of the adaptations of ancestral forms were quite sophisticated and efficient for the environments in which they lived. Indeed, we should only speak of "primitive" characteristics, not "primitive" species. (—Butler and Hodos) (1996, p. 71)

INTRODUCTION

The tissue of the nervous system does not fossilize. There is no fossil record to study the internal brain organization of animals that have already become extinct. To reconstruct the evolutionary history of the vertebrate brain, one must essentially rely on logical inference by comparing the brains of living taxa. Consequently, only a comparative approach allows us to formulate hypotheses concerning the brains of ancestral animals that we cannot examine directly.

Since the late nineteenth century, studies in comparative neurobiology have made significant contributions to understanding the evolution of the vertebrate brain. Early interpretations about brain evolution, however, were markedly different from more recent views. The early school of comparative neurobiology assumed that the vertebrate brain evolved through a steady linear progression from a simple neural tube to a more differentiated complex brain (e.g., Ariëns Kappers et al., 1967). The underlying assumption was the Aristotelian concept of phylogenetic scale, *scala naturae*, which holds that living animals can be ranked in a continuous ascending order from "lower," "primitive" species to "higher," "more advanced" animals, with humans at the pinnacle (Hodos and Campbell, 1969).

Today, the *scala naturae* views are completely rejected based on analyses of fossil records and phyletic comparative studies (e.g., Carroll, 1988). These data lead to the

5 Evolution of the Forebrain in Tetrapods

conclusion that, instead of a linear progression, distinct radiations occurred at least four times throughout the evolutionary history of vertebrates (Northcutt, 1981). Separated from a common ancestral stock for at least 400 million years, the four radiations evolved independently and concurrently, and each produced a group of living representatives. These four radiations are agnathans (jawless vertebrates), chondrichthyes (cartilaginous fishes), osteichthyes (ray-finned fishes), and tetrapods (amphibians, reptiles, birds, and mammals). Enlargement and elaboration of the brain—the forebrain in particular—became more or less manifest independently in the four radiations (Northcutt, 1981).

The main objective of this chapter is to provide a brief overview of forebrain evolution. The scope here is limited to one particular radiation of vertebrates, the tetrapods. The geological time scale and an outline of tetrapod phylogeny are shown in Figure 5.1. Of all vertebrates, the tetrapod forebrain and its function have been most extensively studied, as demonstrated in other chapters of this book. Such studies are important in that they provide critical data for phyletic analysis to investigate the origin of the human brain and intelligence. At the same time, these studies are also significant for adaptation analysis in order to understand how animals and their forebrains adapted to altering environmental conditions.

The forebrain organization of extant tetrapods can be grouped roughly into three distinct patterns: amphibian, sauropsid (reptiles and birds), and mammalian patterns (Butler and Hodos, 1996; Northcutt and Kaas, 1995). In this chapter, the three patterns are compared by discussing the following four issues: (1) when the three groups diverged in vertebrate evolution; (2) how the three patterns are different in forebrain organization; (3) how the three patterns evolved from the common ancestor; and (4) why the three patterns became differentiated throughout evolution. The discussion of the first issue will clarify the phyletic relationships of the three groups of tetrapods. This perspective will thus provide information about the evolutionary histories of amphibians, sauropsids, and mammals. The second section provides a neuroanatomical view, explicating the differences and similarities of the three patterns of forebrain organization. The third section presents recent hypotheses of forebrain evolution from the ancestral tetrapods to the three patterns. The discussion

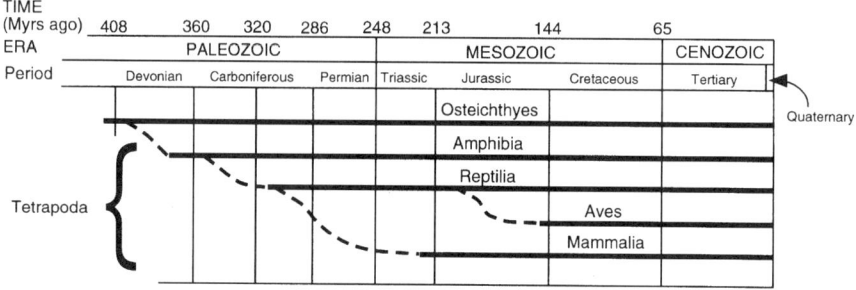

Figure 5.1. Temporal distribution of the four tetrapod classes (amphibians, reptiles, birds, and mammals) and their probable relationships. (Adapted from Harland et al., 1982.)

in the final section provides a link between the three issues by postulating what external and internal changes were involved in the differentiation of forebrain organization.

Because there are many extensive reviews of studies on vertebrate forebrain evolution (Butler and Hodos, 1996; Butler, 1994a,b; Ebbesson, 1980; Jerison, 1973; Jones and Peters, 1990; Macphail, 1982; Northcutt, 1981; Parent, 1986; Sarnat and Netsky, 1981; Striedter, 1997; Smeets and Reiner, 1994; Ulinski, 1983, 1990a), the references cited here are limited to those directly relevant to the selected topics. In particular, the first section on tetrapod paleontology relies heavily on the work of Romer (1966) and Carroll (1988), and its intention is to provide readers with the generally accepted views of the taxonomy and phylogeny of tetrapods.

EVOLUTION OF TETRAPODS

Early Tetrapods—Ancestral Amphibians

The phylogenetic relationships of the extant groups of tetrapods are shown in Figure 5.2. The first tetrapods to appear on earth were amphibians. Fossil records show that the earliest amphibians, ichthyostegids (which belong to the subclass labyrinthodonts), were most likely descended from crossopterygian fishes. They appeared over 360 million years ago in the Late Devonian period of the Paleozoic era. The emergence of amphibians is one of the most significant episodes in vertebrate evolution for at least two reasons. First, the ancestral amphibians moved from water to land and became basically the first terrestrial animals. Although many amphibians lay their eggs in water and have aquatic embryonic and larval stages, they spend the majority of their adult life on land. Adaptation from aquatic to terrestrial

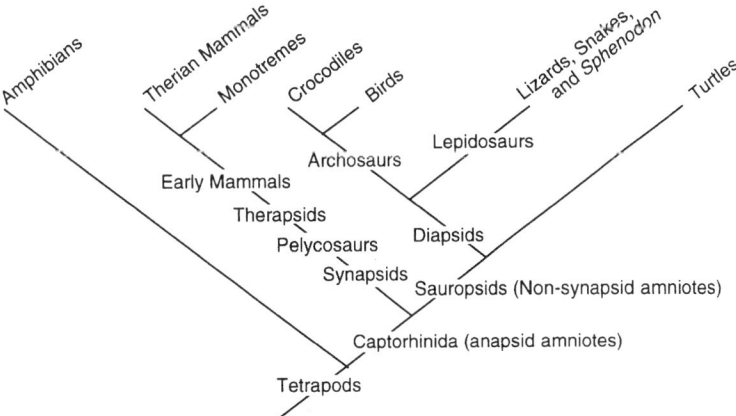

Figure 5.2. Phylogenetic relationships of the extant groups of tetrapods. (Adapted from Butler, 1994a,b.)

environments required significant changes and reorganizations in many structures and behaviors, such as respiration, feeding, reproduction, and sensory systems. Most of all, the early amphibians were distinguished from their fish ancestors by the possession of well-developed, large limbs, thereby enabling locomotion on land (Fig. 5.3A). They also had a large body—some were 1.5m in length—and a large head with sharp teeth, suggesting that they were carnivorous.

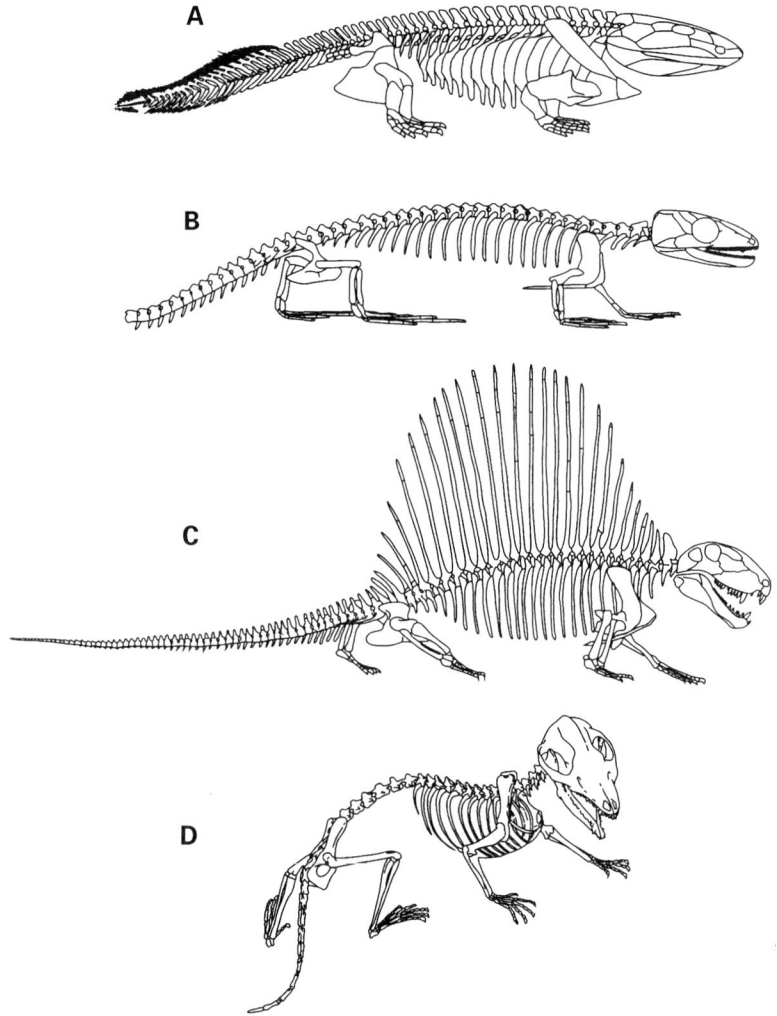

Figure 5.3. Reconstruction of the skeletons of a Paleozoic amphibian (*A*; *Ichthyyostega*, from the Upper Devonian, about 1 m long; adapted from Jarvik, 1955), an early amniote (*B*; *Hylonomus lyelli* from the early Pennsylvanian, about 10 cm long; adapted from Carroll and Baird, 1972), a carnivorous pelycosaur. (*C*; *Dimetrodon* from the Lower Permian, about 3 m long; adapted from Romer, 1966), and one of the oldest mammals (*D*; *Marganucodon* from the early Jurassic, about 10 cm long; adapted from Jenkins and Parrington, 1976).

The second point of significance in the emergence of amphibians is that they gave rise to all modern amphibians and other terrestrial vertebrates (reptiles, birds, and mammals). The Paleozoic amphibians had a major radiation during the Carboniferous period (360 to 286 million years ago), and consequently two major groups appeared: labyrinthodonts and lepospondyls. Labyrinthodonts are further divided into temnospondyls, from which frogs (anurans) evolved, and anthracosaurs, from which reptiles arose. Lepospondyls consisted of a heterogeneous assemblage of distinct groups, most of which had small bodies. Salamanders (urodeles) and caecilians (gymnophionans) probably evolved from the lepospondyls.

In light of this issue, one important fact is that all living amphibians evolved from the Mesozoic and Cenozoic ancestors after most Paleozoic amphibians became extinct between the Early Permian and Jurassic periods (286 to 213 million years ago). Living amphibians include three orders: Anura, Urodela, and Gymnophiona. The Anura includes approximately 2600 species of frogs and toads, with which most neuroanatomical studies of the amphibian brain are conducted. A possible ancestor of frogs, *Triadobatrachus,* emerged in the Early Triassic, and other frogs have been known only since the Jurassic. The Urodela includes about 300 species of newts and salamanders, which are also traced back only to the Late Jurassic. The Gymnophiona consist of about 150 species of caecilians (burrowing or aquatic limbless animals with a reduced visual system), the earliest of which are found in the Late Cretaceous and Early Tertiary periods. Collectively, lineages of living amphibians and other terrestrial vertebrates diverged from the common ancestral stock over 300 million years ago, and both evolved separately and independently. The Paleozoic amphibians were thus very heterogeneous, and it is likely that different groups included the ancestors of frogs, caecilians/salamanders, and amniotes (See below). All of the extant representatives of tetrapods have diverged dramatically from their ancestors. Consequently, the brains of modern amphibians cannot simply be assumed to represent an ancestral state of living tetrapods. This issue is eloquently argued by Ann Butler and William Hodos (1996, quoted at the beginning of this chapter). As they point out, the nervous systems of animals that existed at any point of vertebrate evolution, including those of the Paleozoic and modern amphibians, were shaped by the process of natural selection. What the brains of modern amphibians provide is the information about how the neural systems have adapted to their unique internal and external environments.

Early Amniotes—Ancestral Reptiles

Reptiles, birds, and mammals are collectively designated as *amniotes*. All animals in these three classes have extraembryonic membranes (allantois, chorion, and amnion; Fig. 5.4) that protect and relay essential nutrients and gases to embryos during the early stages of development. Due to the extraembryonic membranes, amniotes are independent of the aquatic environment during embryonic stages, and thus they do not undergo metamorphosis from an aquatic larval stage to a terrestrial adult stage. With this significant change in the development of eggs, amniotes became truly terrestrial vertebrates.

140   5   Evolution of the Forebrain in Tetrapods

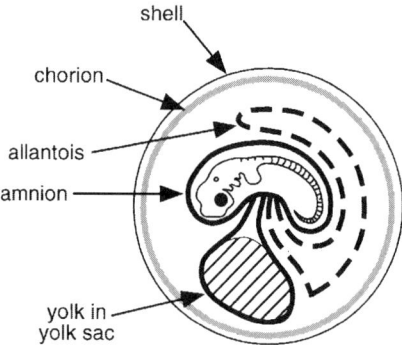

Figure 5.4. Generalized diagram of the embryonic membranes of amniotes. (Adapted from Romer, 1959.)

The earliest amniotes are included in the order Captorhinida, and they were probably derived from the anthracosaurs, a group of Paleozoic amphibians, in the Early Carboniferous period (360 million years ago). In contrast to anthracosaur amphibians, the early amniotes had a smaller body size (about 10 cm) and smaller skull, similar to living lizards. Their dental and mandible characteristics suggest an insectivorous diet. They probably moved swiftly with their slender limbs (Fig. 5.3B).

By the end of the Carboniferous period (286 million years ago), the amniotes diversified greatly, as seen with different body sizes, diets, and environments where they lived. There were three major amniote lineages, which can be broadly categorized based on cranial anatomy. The early amniotes had a solidly roofed skull behind the orbits, and this pattern is termed *anapsid* (Fig. 5.5A). The turtles, which also have no opening, are usually included in this group. Synapsids, or mammal-like reptiles, were the first lineage to separate from the common ancestral amniote stock. They had one temporal opening and became the ancestors of mammals (Fig. 5.5B). Diapsids were the second group to diverge from the ancestral stock, and they had two openings in the skull on the low cheeks (Fig. 5.5C). They became the ancestors of birds and all reptiles except turtles. Although the specific origin of turtles has not been established, they may have diverged from the early Captorhinida later than the synapsids or the diapsids. All reptiles and birds are thus collectively referred to as *sauropsids* or *nonsynapsid amniotes*.

Synapsids–Mammals

These mammal-like reptiles comprise two successive orders: Pelycosaurs and Therapsids. Pelycosaurs first appeared in the Late Carboniferous (290 million years ago), and they were similar to large lizards with their large body and skull (e.g., iguanids; Fig. 5.3C). They had a major radiation during the later Permian, during which they became the most successful amniotes (70% of the amniote genera). They became extinct, however, before the first dinosaur emerged in the Triassic. The

Evolution of Tetrapods   141

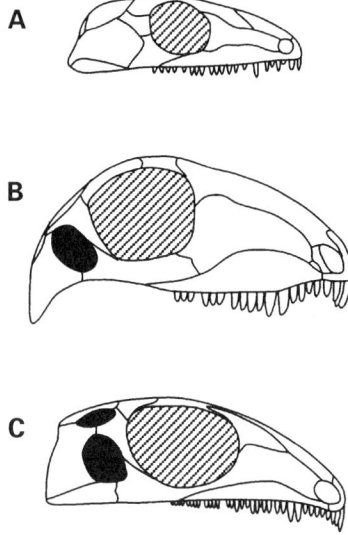

Figure 5.5. Skulls of early amniotes showing different patterns of temporal openings (black) behind the orbits (shaded). The anapsid (*A*), synapsid (*B*), and diapsid (*C*) conditions are exemplified by the *Paleothyri*, *Haptodus*, and *Petrolacosaurus*, respectively. (Adapted from Carroll, 1988.)

therapsids were derived from pelycosaurs during the middle Permian and diversified in the Early Triassic. Therapsids are further divided into the carnivorous theriodonts and the herbivorous anomodonts. In contrast to pelycosaurs, which had many skeletal similarities with early reptiles, advanced therapsids showed anatomical features of both reptiles and mammals. Based on many skeletal features, one of the major differences between early amniotes and advanced therapsids likely was the higher metabolic rate in the latter.

The earliest mammals probably evolved from the theriodonts in the Late Triassic and Early Jurassic period (over 200 million years ago). These mammals had three distinct characteristics in addition to the advanced therapsids. First, early mammals were very small, about 10 cm long, and weighed 20 grams (Fig. 5.3D). Their size, overall morphology, and dentition suggest that they were similar to living shrews. Second, they had improved sensory systems. At this time, the land was occupied by the diurnal dinosaurs. Similar to some living mammals today, the early mammals were probably nocturnal in order to avoid their predators (i.e., carnivorous reptiles). The visual abilities of the first mammals were probably severely limited, and they depended on olfactory and auditory senses. The earliest mammals likely had hair for insulation and sensory function, as seen in vibrissae of modern carnivores and rodents. Third, early mammals had an increased brain size. According to the cranial cavity size, the brain of the early mammals was about three to four times larger than that of the therapsids of overall corresponding size (Jerison, 1973).

Extant mammals include over 4500 species and are divided into two subclasses: the Prototheria and the Theria. The Prototheria is now represented only by the monotremes in Australia. The monotremes are unique mammals in that they lay eggs. Other than the reproductive system, however, many features of their anatomy and physiology (including milk producing glands) indicate that they nevertheless belong to the Mammalia. Although the origin of the monotremes is still controversial, what seems likely is that the ancestors of monotremes were isolated in Australia during the Early Jurassic.

All living mammals except the monotremes are categorized as the Therian mammals. Modern therians include two infraclasses: (1) Metatheria (i.e., the marsupials) and (2) Eutheria (i.e., the placentals). Although both groups of mammals evolved almost simultaneously from a common stock in the Early Cretaceous, they (especially the placentals) had a major radiation in the Cenozoic era after the ruling reptiles died. A likely scenario is that, with the disappearance of dangerous predators, these mammals became diurnal, and the improved visual sense was integrated in the nervous system with the already developed olfactory, somatosensory, and auditory senses.

The reproduction patterns of the marsupials and placentals are fundamentally different even though both are viviparous. Without a true placenta, the marsupials have a shorter gestation period, lay their young at a very immature stage of development, and nurture them in a pouch. In contrast, the placentals have a long gestation period, during which embryos develop within a placenta. The placentals have become the most successful mammals since the end of the Mesozoic for 65 million years. Primates appeared early, at the end of the Cretaceous period.

Sauropsids—Reptiles

The earliest diapsids, the *Petrolacosaurs*, appeared in the Late Carboniferous (Fig. 5.6A). They were about 20 cm in body size with long limbs and many marginal teeth, suggesting that they were insectivorous, like the early amniotes. Although no information is available about the evolution of diapsids during the Permian, there were many lineages by the end of the Permian. Based on locomotion patterns, these advanced diapsids can be further categorized into two groups: (1) the Lepidosauromorpha and (2) the Archosauromorpha. Similar to the early tetrapods, the lepidosauromorphs probably had sinusoidal trunk movements. They acquired a large sternum, however, which increased the force of their forelimbs. Within this large assemblage of lepidosauromorphs, the Lepidosauria today consists of about 6000 species of lizards, snakes, and *Sphenodon*. Lizards first emerged by the end of the Permian, and most living infraorders evolved by the end of the Jurassic. The oldest snake emerged in the Late Cretaceous, much later than lizards and sphenodontids. Although their ancestors had already appeared in the Late Triassic, only one species of sphenodontids still exists.

Archosauromorphs can be distinguished from lepidosauromorphs by several skeletal features, such as an elongated neck (Fig. 5.6B). Within the archosauromorphs, the archosaurs include the Thecodontia, the Crocodylia, two orders of dinosaurs (the Saurischia and Ornithischia), and the Pterosaurs (flying reptiles). Many of them had a characteristic of skeletal arrangement allowing for a

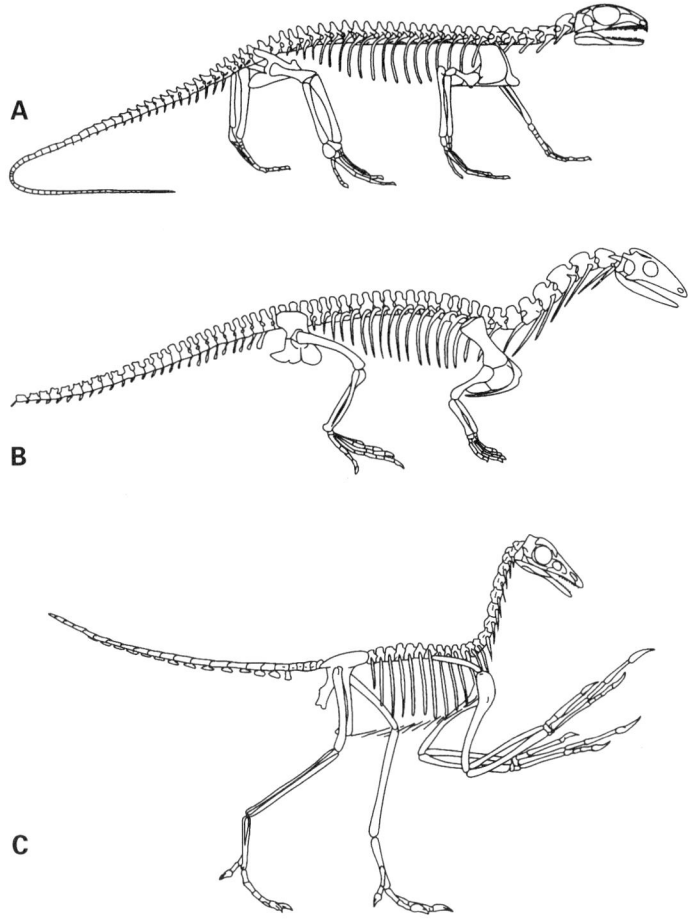

Figure 5.6. Reconstruction of the skeletons of an early diapsid (*A*) *Petrolacosaurus* from the Upper Carboniferous, about 20 cm long without including the tail; (adapted from Reisz, 1981); an early archosauromorph (*B*) *Protorosaurus* from the Upper Permian, about 1 to 2 m long; (adapted from Seeley, 1888); and a Mesozoic bird (*C*) *Archaeopteryx* from the Upper Jurassic, about 30 cm long; (adapted from Ostrom, 1976).

more upright posture compared with lepidosauromorphs. Most Triassic archosaurs belong to the Thecodontia, a large assemblage, from which crocodiles, pterosaurs, and dinosaurs ultimately arose. Thecondonts left an extensive fossil record of four heterogeneous suborders, which exhibited different body sizes, diets (carnivores, herbivores), as well as locomotive patterns (bipedal, quadrupedal). Crocodiles probably arose from the thecodont radiation during the Late Triassic and Early Jurassic, and the modern families were traced back to the Late Cretaceous.

Of all the reptiles, dinosaurs were clearly the most successful vertebrates for 150 million years from the Late Triassic to the end of the Cretaceous. They are differentiated from most thecodonts by posture and locomotion. Thecondonts had their limbs under the body. In contrast, the anatomy of limbs and records of footprints suggest that the early dinosaurs had an upright posture, and many of them were bipedal. This indicates that dinosaurs lived in a more three-dimensional environment with the additon of a vertical element. Dinosaurs continued to diversify throughout the Mesozoic (248 to 65 million years ago), and they have been categorized into the saurischians and the ornithischians based on the pelvic structure. The saurichians are further subdivided into carnivorous theropods (e.g., Tyrannosaurids) and herbivorous sauropodomorphs (e.g., Brachiosauridae), whereas the ornithischians are all herbivorous (e.g., Stegosaurs). At the end of the Mesozoic, during which dinosaurs dominated the terrestrial environment, they abruptly became extinct.

Pterosaurs diverged from the thecodont stock in the Late Triassic. They had a long tail, a large skull, and membranous wings. Pterosaurs were probably capable of active, powered flight based on their skeletal characteristics (e.g., broad sternum and anteriorly directed cristospine for the flight muscle). Furthermore, cranial endocasts show remarkable similarities between the brains of pterosaurs and living birds, such as a large optic tectum and a well-developed flocculus (vestibular cerebellum) (Fig. 5.7, also see Fig. 5.8C). Pterosaurs, however, became extinct at the end of the Cretacious. Meanwhile birds, which appeared in the Late Jurassic, survived somehow in this catastrophic period.

The earliest turtles with shells appeared in the Late Triassic. The structure of the shells was already remarkably similar to modern turtles. Modern reptiles today include four orders: Squamata (lizards and snakes); Rhynchocephalia (only one species, the tuatara *Sphenodon punctatus*); Crocodilia (crocodiles and alligators); and Chelonia (turtles and tortoises).

Sauropsids—Birds

Although the origin of birds is currently a hotly debated topic in paleontology (Feduccia, 1996; Ji et al., 1998), many paleontologists assert that ancestral birds probably originated from the saurischian dinosaurs in the Late Jurassic (Carroll, 1988). One of the convincing pieces of evidence supporting their argument for the

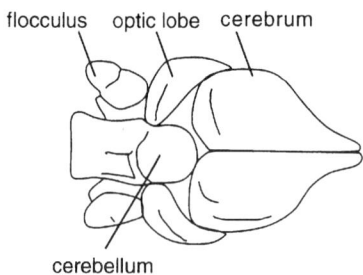

Figure 5.7. Reconstruction of an endocast of the pterosaur *Parapsicephalus*. (Adapted from Wellnhofer, 1978.)

dinosaur to bird transition is the fossil record of *Archaeopteryx*. The skeletal features of this pigeon-sized animal show that they had a dinosaurlike body with a long bony tail, three well-developed, unfused forelimb digits, and teeth, but no trace of a sternum (Fig. 5.6C). These features are very similar to the small coelurosaurian dinosaurs, but are distinctly absent in modern birds. Nevertheless, *Archaeopteryx* is considered to belong to birds because of their unique feature common to all birds—feathers. Major radiations of birds occurred by the Early Cenozoic, but all extant species appear to have evolved within the last 1 million years.

Modern birds consist of at least 28 orders and 8700 species. They include, among others, Passeriformes (perching birds), that are the largest group (5000 species); Apodiformes (swifts and hummingbirds); Falconformes (eagles, hawks, and vultures); Galliformes (chickens); Charadriiformes (shorebirds and gulls); Colombiformes (pigeons and doves); Psittaciformes (parrots); and Strigiformes (owls). Most studies of the central nervous system have been conducted in only a limited number of species, such as pigeons, chickens, owls, and finches.

Conclusion

To establish a comparative view of forebrain organization, the evolutionary history of tetrapods encourages us to be aware of two important points. First, tetrapods experienced two major divergences during their evolution, resulting in three large assemblages: amphibians, sauropsids, and synapsids. Over 300 million years ago, the tetrapod lineages of anamniotes (amphibians) and amniotes diverged from the common ancestral tetrapod stock. Soon after, diapsids–reptiles/birds and synapsids–mammals were derived from the ancestral amniotes. These three groups are today represented by modern amphibians, diapsid reptiles/birds, and mammals, all of which show unique and distinct patterns of forebrain organization. The second important point is the fact that the three groups evolved independently and separately for over 280 million years. The brains of extant amphibians thus are not ancestral versions of modern reptilian brains. Similarly, no reptilian, let alone avian, brain is less modern than that of living mammals.

FOREBRAIN ORGANIZATION OF LIVING TETRAPODS

In all vertebrates, the forebrain consists of two parts: the diencephalon and the telencephalon. The diencephalon is divided into four subdivisions: epithalamus, dorsal thalamus, ventral thalamus, and hypothalamus. The telencephalon can be further divided into two subdivisions: pallium and subpallium. The diencephalon and telencephalon are extensively interconnected, and their functional significance cannot be characterized separately. Comparative studies have also indicated that enlargement and elaboration of the telencephalon would have never been attained without the corresponding development of the diencephalon and vice versa (Butler, 1994a,b).

This section presents a comparative overview of the three major patterns of forebrain organization. Although more detailed reviews for the amphibian, avian/reptilian, and mammalian brains are covered by other authors in this book, a special focus is placed here on the ascending sensory and related pathways from the dorsal thalamus to the telencephalon—the pallium in particular. This asymmetrical approach was selected for three reasons. First, in all tetrapods, the dorsal thalamus plays a major role in processing information from the external world and sends a major projection to the telencephalon (Hodos and Butler, this volume, Chapter 4). An increase in forebrain size and in the degree of its cytoarchitectonic elaboration appears to be correlated with the hypertrophy of the thalamopallial pathways in tetrapods (Northcutt, 1981). Not surprisingly, the sensory pathways connecting the dorsal thalamus with the telencephalon have been one of the most extensively studied subjects in comparative neurobiology. Second, the subpallium—the basal ganglia in particular—is generally considered to be, in comparison with the pallium, conservative among all tetrapods in terms of connections, chemistry, and physiology (Marín et al., 1997–; Parent, 1986; Reiner et al., 1984). This is also more or less true concerning the thalamic structures other than the dorsal thalamus. Finally, the origin and evolution of the pallium has been one of the most controversial topics in comparative studies (Bruce and Neary, 1995c; Butler 1994b; Díaz et al., 1990; Karten, 1969, 1991, 1997; Karten and Shimizu, 1989; Lohman and Smeets, 1991; MacLean, 1990; Northcutt, 1981; Northcutt and Kaas, 1995; Reiner, 1991, 1993; Striedter, 1997; Ulinski, 1983, 1990a). This is a fascinating topic already from a neuroanatomical perspective. It is even more intriguing, however, to conjecture about the evolution of intelligence, which has often been associated with the enlargement and differentiation of the pallium (Jerison and Jerison, 1988).

Amphibian Pattern

Overview. Among tetrapods, amphibians are unique in that they are the only terrestrial anamniotes. The majority of studies of amphibian brains have used anurans as subjects. All three orders of living amphibians, however—anurans, urodeles, and gymnophionans—have generally similar forebrains. They are small and cylindrical with proportionally large olfactory bulbs (Northcutt and Kicliter, 1980) (Fig 5.8A). The ratio of the forebrain and body weights of amphibians is comparable with that of bony fishes (Northcutt, 1981).

The dorsal thalamus of all tetrapods consists of a group of nuclei sending sensory and related projections to the telencephalon. Butler (1994a) proposes two subdivisions in all tetrapod dorsal thalami: rostrally located lemnothalamic and caudally situated collothalamic nuclear groups (L and C in Fig. 5.9). The lemnothalamus receives lemniscal pathways that are not relayed through the mesencephalon. The collothalamus receives sensory and related input from the roof of the midbrain, which is the tectum mesencephali, consisting of optic tectum and torus semiciruluris in nonmammalian tetrapods, or the superior and inferior colliculus in mammals.

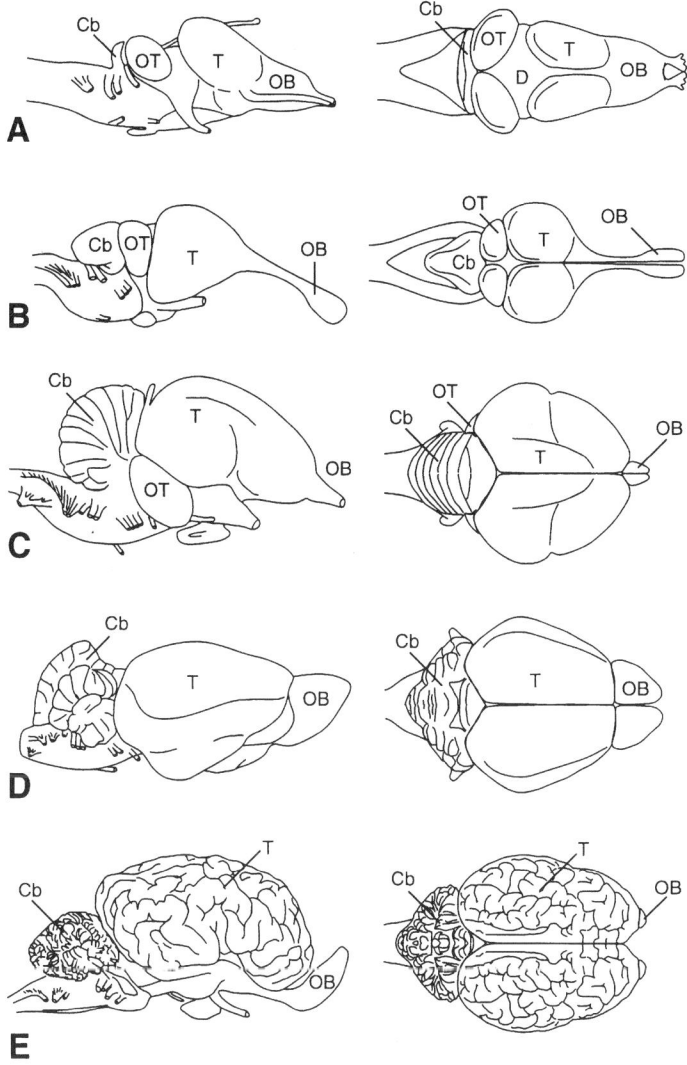

Figure 5.8. The side and top views of brains of an extant amphibian (*A*; frog), reptile (*B*; alligator), bird (*C*; goose), and mammals (*D*; tree shrew; *E*; horse). Cb; cerebellum; D; diencephalon; OB; olfactory bulb; OT; optic tectum; T; telencephalon. (Adapted from Romer, 1970.)

All tetrapods have a main olfactory bulb, an extension of the rostral telencephalon, which receives information from the olfactory receptors (Northcutt and Kicliter, 1980). In addition, some tetrapods (e.g., frogs, snakes, and lizards) possess an accessory olfactory bulb, which receives information from the vomeronasal organ (Jacobson's organ), which detects pheromones secreted by other animals for social communication.

148   5   Evolution of the Forebrain in Tetrapods

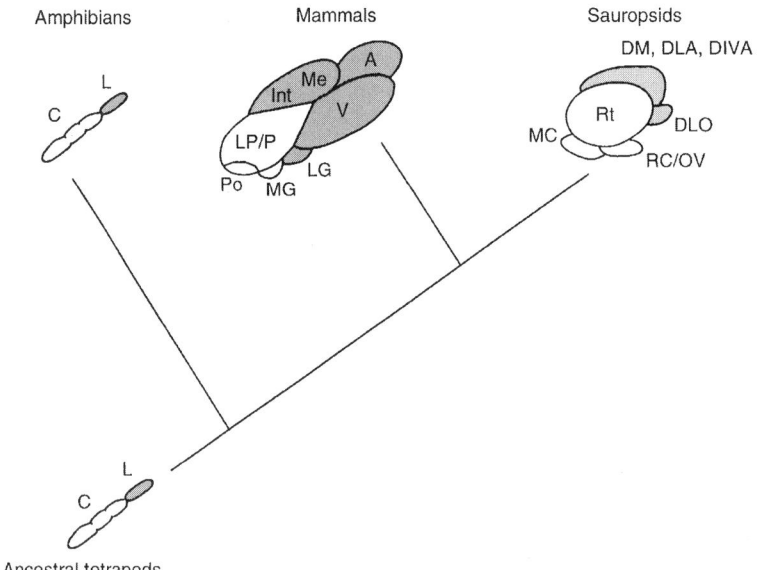

Figure 5.9. Schematic Figure illustrating the two subdivisions of the dorsal thalamus in three tetrapod patterns (amphibians, sauropsids, and mammals) (Butler, 1994a). A; anterior nuclear group; C; collothalamus; DIVA; nucleus dorsalis intermedius ventralis anterior (birds); DLA; nucleus dorsalis anterior; DLO; dorsal lateral optic nucleus; DM; nucleus dorsomedialis; Int; intralaminar nuclear group; L; lemnothalamus; LG; lateral geniculate; LP/P; lateral posterior/pulvinar complex; MC; medialis complex; Me; medial nuclear group; MG; medial geniculate; Po; posterior nuclear group; RC/OV; nucleus reuniens pars compacta (reptiles)/nucleus ovoidalis (birds); Rt; nucleus rotundus; V; ventral nuclear group. (Adapted from Butler and Hodos, 1996.)

As in other tetrapods, the pallium of amphibians is located in the dorsal roof of the cerebral hemispheres and divided into at least three parts: medial, lateral, and dorsal regions (Butler, 1994b; Northcutt and Kicliter, 1980) (MP, LP, and DP in Fig. 5.10, respectively). In frogs, the medial pallium is a very well-developed structure and at least twice as thick as the lateral and dorsal pallia (Northcutt and Kicliter, 1980; Northcutt and Ronan, 1992). The main constituent of the medial pallium is the hippocampal complex, located dorsal to the septum and amygdalar area. The lateral pallium is referred to as the *olfactory pallium* or *piriform*, which receives a projection from the main olfactory bulb (Northcutt and Kicliter, 1980; Northcutt and Royce, 1975; Scalia et al., 1968, 1991). The dorsal pallium is located between the medial and lateral pallia and is found in all tetrapods, although its evolutionary origin remains subject to controversy (Bruce and Neary, 1995c; Northcutt, 1981).

Lemnothalamo-telencephalic pathways. The amphibian lemnothalamus, as in other anamniotes, consists of a single nucleus, which is called the *nucleus anterior*. The nucleus predominantly receives retinal input (Gruberg, 1972; Scalia and Gregory, 1970). In addition, the nucleus in frogs is known to receive projections from diverse brain stem sources, including optic tectum (visual), torus semicircularis (auditory), dorsal column (somatosensory), and hypothalamus (Rubinson, 1968;

Forebrain Organization of Living Tetrapods   149

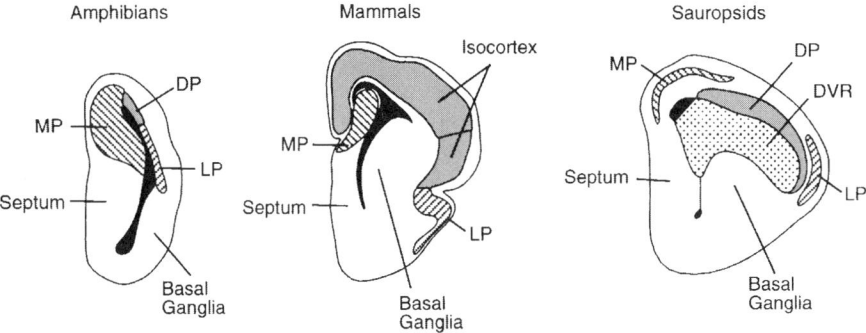

Figure 5.10. Schematic transverse telencephalic sections illustrating the basic organization of three tetrapod patterns (amphibians, sauropsids, and mammals). Black areas, ventricle; DP; dorsal pallium; DVR; dorsal ventricular ridge; LP; lateral pallium; MP; medial pallium. (Adapted from Butler [1994b] and Northcutt and Kaas [1995].)

Neary and Wilczynski, 1977; Neary, 1990). From the telencephalon, the medial pallium sends a projection to this nucleus (Northcutt and Ronan, 1992). The nucleus anterior in turn sends bilateral projections to the medial pallium and the medial part of the dorsal pallium via the medial forebrain bundle (Neary, 1984; Northcutt and Ronan, 1992) (Fig. 5.11). Furthermore, the optic tectum, posterior dorsal thalamus, and hypothalamus receive input from the anterior thalamic nucleus (Neary, 1990). The pattern of these connections suggests that the nucleus anterior sends multisensory information to the pallial region (Neary, 1990).

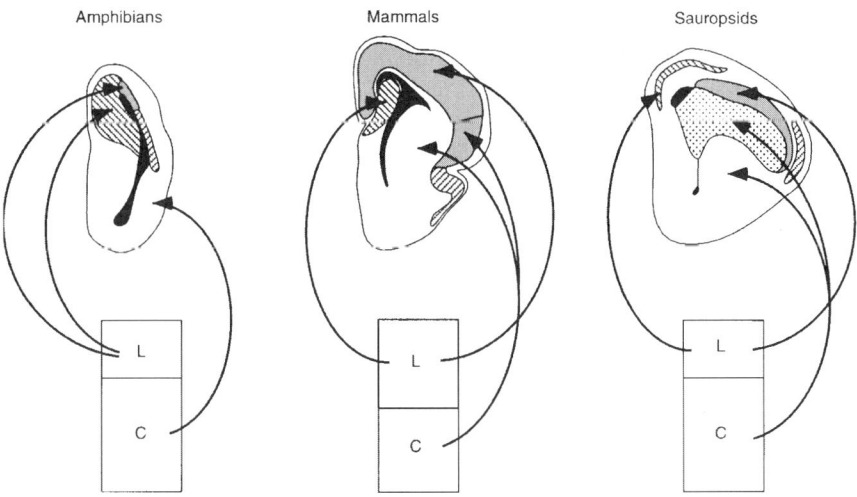

Figure 5.11. Schematic figures showing the basic pattern of major projections from the lemnothalamus (L) and collothalamus (C) to the telencephalon in the three tetrapod patterns.

Collothalamo-telencephalic pathways. The collothalamus of frogs consists of at least three nuclei: central nucleus, anterior lateral nucleus, and posterior lateral nucleus. The central nucleus receives auditory input from the medial part of the torus semicircularis (Neary, 1974, 1990; Hall and Feng, 1987). The anterior lateral and posterior lateral nuclei receive visual input from the optic tectum (Rubinson, 1968; Montgomery and Fite, 1991). The central and anterior lateral nuclei send ipsilateral projections to the basal ganglia (the striatum in particular) via the lateral forebrain bundle (Fig. 5.11), whereas no projections have been found from the posterior lateral nucleus to the telencephalon (Gruberg and Ambros, 1974; Hall and Feng, 1987; Kicliter, 1979; Neary, 1990; Wilczyniski and Northcutt, 1983a; Marín et al., 1997a). The same pattern of circuitry has been found in urodeles as well (Wicht and Himstedt, 1988).

Medial pallium. In addition to the anterior thalamic input, the thickened medial pallium of anurans receives massive afferents from the ipsilateral telencephalon (e.g., dorsal and lateral pallia, lateral and medial septal nuclei, pars medialis of the amygdala, bed nucleus of the pallial commissure, and olfactory tubercle) and the contralateral medial pallium via the pallial commissure (Neary, 1990; Northcutt, 1981; Northcutt and Ronan, 1992). Most of these telencephalic nuclei and areas are directly or indirectly involved in processing olfactory information (Northcutt and Ronan, 1992). In addition, the raphe system in the medulla sends serotonergic input to the medial pallium (Neary, 1990; Northcutt and Ronan, 1992). The medial pallium then gives rise to extensive projections to (1) various telencephalic structures (e.g., dorsal and lateral pallia, olfactory bulb, both septal nuclei, bed nucleus of the pallial commissure, and pars lateralis and medialis of the amygdala); and (2) multiple extratelencephalic structures mainly via the medial forebrain bundle; (e.g., nucleus anterior, preoptic area, and infundibular hypothalamus) (Neary, 1990; Northcutt and Ronan, 1992). Based on these connections, the medial pallium is considered to be involved in the integration of olfactory and other ascending sensory signals (Neary, 1990; Northcutt and Ronan, 1992). The olfactory information is sent to the medial pallium from many olfactory-related nuclei in the ipsilateral telencephalon, while visual, auditory, and somatosensory signals are conveyed via the nucleus anterior.

Dorsal pallium. In contrast to the medial pallium, the dorsal and lateral pallia have more limited connections. The dorsal pallium receives bilateral fibers from the olfactory bulb and the nucleus anterior and ipsilateral input from the medial, and probably lateral, pallia (Neary, 1984, 1990; Northcutt, 1981; Northcutt and Ronan, 1992; Northcutt and Royce, 1975; Scalia et al., 1968, 1991). The dorsal pallium sends ipsilateral projections to the lateral and medial pallia, whereas no projections to the basal ganglia or extratelencephalic regions have been found (Neary, 1990; Northcutt, 1981; Wilczyniski and Northcutt, 1983a). The dorsal pallium, like the medial pallium, is also suggested to be involved in the integration of olfactory and other sensory information based on these data, although it has much more limited connections with the thalamic structures than the medial pallium (Neary, 1990).

Lateral pallium. The lateral pallium is primarily involved in processing olfactory information because the lateral pallium is the major target of input from the main olfactory bulb via the lateral olfactory tract (Northcutt and Royce, 1975; Scalia et al.,

1968, 1991). In addition, the lateral pallium receives projections from the ipsilateral medial (and possibly dorsal) pallium and the dorsal thalamus (Neary, 1990; Northcutt, 1981; Northcutt and Ronan, 1992). The lateral pallium sends projections almost exclusively to structures within the ipsilateral telencephalon, such as the olfactory bulb, septum, dorsal pallium, and medial pallium (Northcutt, 1981; Northcutt and Ronan, 1992).

Basal ganglia. The amphibian basal ganglia can be divided into a striatum (caudate-putamen) and a nucleus accumbens (Marín et al., 1997a, b, c). Although some researchers (Marín et al., 1997b) have proposed that a cell group in the caudal basal telencephalon in amphibians may be homologous to the globus pallidus of amniotes, they also emphasize the necessity of further chemoarchitectonic analysis of the area. In addition to its strongest input from the collothalamic nuclei, the anuran striatum receives a heavy bilateral projection from the anterior entopeduncular nucleus, which is a caudal cell group in the striatal region (Marín et al., 1997a; Wilczyniski and Northcutt, 1983a). Other inputs to the striatum are present from many subcortical structures, including the preoptic area, torus semicircularis, and tegmental nuclei (Marín et al., 1997a; Wilczyniski and Northcutt, 1983a). Part of these tegmental cell groups is considered to be equivalent to the substantia nigra of amniotes (Marín et al., 1997a,b). There are also telencephalic projections from the ipsilateral lateral amygdala, olfactory bulb, striatopallial transition area, and medial pallium (Marín et al., 1997a). The striatum in turn gives rise to major descending projections to the cell groups in the tegmentum, as in other tetrapods (Marín et al., 1997b; Wilczyniski and Northcutt, 1983b). The anterior entopeduncular nucleus, pretectal nuclei, and midbrain roof (optic tectum and torus semicircularis) also receive input from the striatum.

These data suggest significant striatal influences on the midbrain roof directly and indirectly through the anterior entopeduncular nucleus, pretectal nuclei, and the tegmental structures, all of which send projections to the optic tectum and/or torus semicircularis (Marín et al., 1997c; Wilczyniski, 1981; Wilczyniski and Northcutt, 1977). Thus, descending striatal efferents affect motor behaviors through (1) the tegmental motor centers, which receive a direct striatal projection and send projections to the spinal cord (ten Donkelaar et al., 1981); and (2) the midbrain roof, which receives direct and indirect striatal projections and also has descending projections (Rubinson, 1968; ten Donkelaar et al., 1981).

Amygdala. The amygdala of amphibians can be divided into two subdivisions: a pallial pars lateralis and a subpallial pars medialis (Northcutt, 1981). The lateral division receives a major projection from the ipsilateral accessory olfactory bulb (Northcutt and Royce, 1975; Scalia, 1972; Scalia et al., 1991), as well as bilateral input from the medial pallium (Northcutt and Ronan, 1992). The targets of the efferents include the hypothalamus and dorsal/ventral thalamus (Halpern, 1972; Neary, 1990, 1995). The lateral amygdala and/or its surrounding region has also been suggested as a possible source of a long descending projection to the medulla and cervical spinal cord (Kokoros and Northcutt, 1977; Northcutt, 1981). The medial amygdala has reciprocal connections with the ipsilateral septum (Kicliter, 1979) and bilateral medial pallium (Northcutt and Ronan, 1992).

Mammalian Pattern

Overview. In amniotes, there are many highly differentiated discrete nuclei in the dorsal thalamus in comparison with amphibians (Fig. 5.9). These nuclei, however, are also divided into the lemnothalamic and collothalamic groups based on the source of their input (Butler, 1994a). In mammals in particular, both the lemnothalamic and collothalamic groups of the dorsal thalamus are even much more differentiated and enlarged than in nonmammals.

The mammalian pallium—the cerebral cortex—is a highly developed laminated structure, which is unique to the mammalian telencephalon. The dorsal pallium of mammals is called the *isocortex* and is characterized by hypertrophy and a six-layered organization (Butler and Hodos, 1996; Zilles and Wree, 1995) (Fig. 5.10). Layer 4 is called the *granular layer*, in which neurons receive primary ascending sensory projections. Neurons in layers 2 and 3 send projections to the deeper cortical layers and other cortical regions, whereas layers 5 and 6 contain cells that give rise to projections to the striatum and subcortical structures (e.g., the dorsal thalamus, superior colliculus, and spinal cord).

The medial and lateral pallia form three-layered cortices called the *limbic* and *olfactory* cortex, respectively, and are together designated the *allocortex* (Butler and Hodos, 1996; Zilles and Wree, 1995). As in other tetrapods, the limbic cortex includes the hippocampal formation, which is greatly expanded in placentals in contrast to monotremes, marsupials, and nonmammals. The mammalian hippocampus plays a critical role in the learning and memory systems. The olfactory cortex consists of the anterior olfactory nucleus, olfactory tubercle, piriform cortex, and corticomedial amygdala, all of which receive direct input from the olfactory bulb. The area between these allocortices and isocortices is called the *transitional cortex* and includes the subicular cortices and entorhinal cortex (Butler and Hodos, 1996).

Extensive research in this area has revealed tremendous variability between different mammalian species with regard to the extent of the cerebral cortex (Fig. 5.8D,E). I will thus concentrate on the general organization of the cerebral cortex in the therian mammals. More detailed information is available in published reviews (e.g., Butler and Hodos, 1996; Carpenter, 1976; Jones, 1985; Jones and Peters, 1990; Paxinos, 1995).

Lemnothalamo-telencephalic pathways. There are at least five distinct cell groups in the rostral thalamus (lemnothalamus): the dorsal lateral geniculate nucleus and the ventral, anterior, medial, and intralaminar nuclear groups (Fig. 5.9). These groups give rise to projections primarily to the dorsal part of the ipsilateral isocortex via the lateral forebrain bundle (Butler, 1994a,b) (Fig. 5.11). Briefly, the projections of each of these groups are discussed below.

In eutheria (placentals), the dorsal lateral geniculate nucleus (LG in Fig. 5.9) receives a major projection from the retina (Campbell et al., 1967; Guillery, 1970; Kaas et al., 1978). The nucleus sends a projection primarily to layer 4 of the ipsilateral striate cortex via the optic radiations (Allman, 1977; Guillery, 1967; Hendrickson et al., 1978). In prototheria (monotremes), the nucleus also receives retinal input and projects to the visual cortex (Campbell and Hayhow, 1971, 1972;

Rowe, 1990; Welker and Lende, 1980). The lateral geniculate nucleus of many mammals, especially primates, is well differentiated and contains multiple subdivisions that can be classified on the basis of ipsilateral and contralateral projections from the retina, response characteristics, and cell sizes (Jones, 1985). A strictly retinotopic organization is found in the lateral geniculate nucleus and is maintained in the striate cortex.

In therian mammals, the ventral nuclear group (V in Fig. 5.9) appears to be associated with the processing of somatosensory and motor functions (Jones, 1985). This nuclear group includes the ventralis lateralis, the ventralis medialis and the ventralis posterior nuclei. The first two nuclei—the ventral lateralis and the ventral medialis—have usually been considered to be involved in motor functions (Price, 1995). The ventral lateralis receives projections from many motor centers, including the globus pallidus and cerebellar nuclei, and sends projections to the premotor and motor cortices. The ventral medialis receives input from the substantia nigra and sends a projection to part of the medial and frontal cortex (Herkenham, 1979; Krettek and Price, 1977). In contrast, the ventral posterior nucleus is involved in processing somatosensory input and receives projections from the spinal cord, trigeminal nuclei, and dorsal column nuclei (Kalil, 1981; Krubitzer and Kaas, 1992; Rainey and Jones, 1983). It gives rise to a topographically organized projection to the somatosensory isocortex (Jones and Powell, 1970; Krubitzer and Kaas, 1992; Welker, 1973).

The anterior group (A in Fig. 5.9) is deemed to be part of the limbic system. Although the existence of the anterior group is not yet clear in monotremes (Regidor and Divac, 1987; Welker and Lende, 1980), there are multiple nuclei in marsupial and eutherian mammals (Jones, 1985; Haight and Neylon, 1978). The anterior group receives projections from a variety of sources, including raphe nuclei and even a minor retinal input (Cropper et al., 1984; Itaya et al., 1986). The major sources of afferents are, however, the medial pallium (limbic cortex) and the mammillary body of the hypothalamus (Swanson, 1987). The anterior group sends a projection to the ipsilateral medial cortex (Krettek and Price, 1977; Vogt et al., 1992).

The medial group (Mc in Fig. 5.9) is also associated with the limbic system, as well as olfactory function, in marsupials and eutherian mammals (Haight and Neylon, 1978; Jones, 1985). It includes at least three nuclei: the mediodorsal, medioventral, and parataenial nuclei. The largest, the mediodorsal nucleus, is in receipt of a projection from limbic structures in the ventral forebrain, including the lateral pallium (olfactory cortex), amygdala, and ventral pallidum, and projects to the frontal and prelimbic cortices (Höhl-Abrahao and Creutzfeldt, 1991; Krettek and Price, 1977; Price, 1995). The medioventral nucleus receives projections from diverse areas of the limbic systems—septum, amygdala, and medial pallium—and projects to the limbic cortex (Baisden and Hoover, 1979; Herkenham, 1978). The parataenial nucleus has diffuse projections to the cortical areas (Jones, 1985).

In therian mammals, the intralaminar group (Int in Fig. 5.9) is known to receive projections from diverse sources, including various sensory cortices, pretectum, superior colliculi, basal ganglia, cerebellum, and brain stem reticular formation (Berman, 1977; Graham, 1977; Graybiel, 1977; Parent, 1986; Royce, 1983). This group in turn gives rise to diffuse projections to the widespread cortical areas and the striatum (Jones and Leavitt, 1974; Parent, 1986; Sadikot et al., 1992). Several lines of evidence indicate that the nuclear group is involved in regulation of the state of arousal and attention (Jones, 1985). The intralaminar group has not been found in monotremes (Ulinski, 1984; Welker and Lende, 1980).

Collothalamo-telencephalic pathways. There are at least three nuclear groups in the collothalamus, which send projections primarily to the lateral part of the isocortex: the lateral posterior and/or pulvinar complex, the medial geniculate nucleus, and the posterior nuclear group (Fig 5.9). The superior colliculus of therian mammals projects to the lateral posterior and/or pulvinar complex (LP/P in Fig. 5.9), which in turn sends projections to the extrastriate visual cortex and the striatum (Abramson and Chalupa, 1988; Beckstead, 1984; Benevento and Fallon, 1975; Graybiel, 1972; Lin et al., 1984; Symonds et al., 1981; Takada, 1992). The lateral posterior–pulvinar complex also receives input from the pretectum, striate cortex, and extrastriate cortex (Kawamura et al., 1974; Robertson et al., 1983; Thompson and Robertson, 1987; Updyke, 1981). In monotremes, it is not known whether a tectorecipient nucleus exists (Ulinski, 1984).

The therian medial geniculate nucleus (MG in Fig. 5.9) receives auditory information ascending from the hindbrain via the inferior colliculus and relays it to the auditory cortex (Andersen et al., 1980; Casseday et al., 1976; Oliver and Hall, 1978). In monotremes, although a corresponding nucleus has been identified (Jones, 1985), its connections are not known.

The posterior group (Po in Fig. 5.9) includes multiple subnuclei. Part of the posterior group is characterized by its polysensory (i.e., somatosensory, auditory, and visual) afferent from the deeper layers of the superior colliculus (Benevento and Fallon, 1975; Graham, 1977). The area sends projections to the secondary sensory areas of the isocortex and the striatum (Burton and Jones, 1976; Druga et al., 1991). The somatosensory, as well as auditory, projections from the midbrain terminate in the lateral part of the posterior nuclear group (Itoh et al., 1984; Kudo and Niimi, 1980). The part in turn sends a projection to areas in the isocortex adjacent to the primary sensory areas (Andersen et al., 1980; Burton and Jones, 1976). The medial part of the posterior group, located medially adjacent to the ventral medialis, may belong to the lemnothalamus, because it receives direct spinothalamic and trigeminal inputs (Diamond et al., 1992; Jones, 1985). This area sends a projection to the somatosensory cortex (Rausell and Jones, 1991). In monotremes, a posterior group has been recognized based on cytoarchitecture (Jones, 1985).

Basal ganglia. The principal components of the basal ganglia of mammals most frequently include the caudate-putamen (striatum) and globus pallidus or pallidum. The olfactory tubercle, the nucleus accumbens, and other closely related structures (e.g., the subthalamic nucleus and the substantia nigra) are sometimes included in this term as well (Heimer et al., 1995; Parent, 1986; Parent and Hazrati, 1995a,b). As in amphibians, the mammalian basal ganglia has routes that influence motor behavior via the tegmental structures and the midbrain roof. The mammalian striatum has reciprocal connections with dopaminergic cell groups in the tegmentum (e.g., substantia nigra pars compacta and ventral tegmental area) (Heimer et al.,

1995). The mammalian striatum also influences the midbrain tectum, yet it is accomplished only indirectly and exclusively via the substantia nigra pars reticulata (Bentivoglio, et al., 1979; Faull and Mehler, 1978; Graybiel, 1978). Mammals do not possess another indirect route to the midbrain roof via a pretectal cell group, which is found in amphibians, some reptiles, and birds.

In addition, the basal ganglia of mammals have two significant circuitries in the forebrain. First, a cell group situated in the descending striatal efferents (subthalamic nucleus) is reciprocally connected with the globus pallidus (Parent and Hazrati, 1995b). Neural circuits corresponding to such a loop are also found in sauropsids. The second circuit is based on a corticobasal ganglia-thalamo-cortical loop (Parent and Hazrati, 1995a). The mammalian striatum receives extensive projections from the sensorimotor cortex, as well as the intralaminar nucleus of the dorsal thalamus and tegmental nuclei (Heimer et al., 1995; Jones, 1985). The basal ganglia then have heavy projections to thalamic nuclei (i.e., ventral nuclear group) via the globus pallidus and the substantia nigra pars reticulata (Heimer et al., 1995; Parent and Hazrati, 1995a). The thalamic nuclei in turn send projections to motor-related cortical areas (e.g., premotor and motor cortices), but probably to nonmotor cortical areas as well (Parent and Hazarati, 1995a). Because this loop is well-developed especially in mammals, Ulinski (1983) suggests that the evolution of extensive basal ganglia–thalamic connections occurred during the therapsid to mammal transition.

Amygdala and claustrum. The amygdala of mammals is located in the tip of the temporal lobe and has extensive connections with the basal ganglia, olfactory system, limbic system, and diverse isocortical areas (Butler and Hodos, 1996). The amygdala consists of three parts—basolateral nuclear group, superficial cortexlike nuclear group, and centromedial nuclear group—each of which has multiple subnuclei (Alheid et al., 1995; McDonald, 1998).

The basolateral nuclear group consists of the lateral, basal, and accessory basal nuclei (Price et al., 1987). The basolateral group is characterized by strong reciprocal connections with many isocortical areas, including sensory areas and the hippocampus (Alheid et al., 1995; McDonald, 1998). The superficial cortex-like nuclear group contains the cortical nucleus (anterior and posterior subdivisions), the nucleus of the lateral olfactory tract, and the periamygdaloid cortex (the posterolateral subdivision of the cortical nucleus in the rat). In the rat, the bed nucleus of the accessory olfactory tract is also included in this group. These nuclei receive direct input from the main olfactory bulb via the lateral olfactory tract and send the information to the hypothalamus and brain stem structures via the stria terminalis (Alheid et al., 1995; McDonald, 1998). The centromedial nuclear group consists of the central and medial nuclei. The central nucleus receives the gustatory and visceral information from the insular cortex, whereas the medial nucleus (and the posterior division of the cortical nucleus) receives vomeronasal projections from the accessory olfactory bulb (Alheid et al., 1995; McDonald, 1998).

Between the temporal cortical area and the basal ganglia, a small structure called the *claustrum* is found in therian mammals (Sherk, 1986). It is still not clear whether the claustrum belongs to the pallium or to the basal ganglia. The claustrum is known to receive reciprocal connections with the cerebral cortex, as well as thalamic projections from the intralaminar nuclei of the dorsal thalamus and hypothalamus (Carey et al., 1980; LeVay and Sherk, 1981; Sherk, 1986). It does not, however, receive input from the sensory thalamus.

Sauropsid Pattern

Overview. In many reptiles and birds, the caudal collothalamic group has undergone greater expansion and differentiation than the rostral lemnothalamic group (Fig. 5.9). Similarly, the corresponding telencephalic area receiving input from the collothalamic divisions—the collothalamic-recipient region—has become more expanded than the lemnothalamic-recipient region.

The pallium of sauropsids, as in amphibians and mammals, can be divided into dorsal, medial, and lateral divisions (Fig. 5.10). The reptilian dorsal pallium is called the *dorsal cortex*, including pallial thickening when present, whereas the avian dorsal pallium is called the *Wulst* (German word for "bulge") or the *hyperstriatum accessorium* (Northcutt, 1981; Striedter, 1997; Ulinski, 1983, 1990b: Ulinski and Margoliash, 1990). As in the mammalian isocortex, the dorsal pallium in sauropsids is known to receive lemnothalamic sensory input. The medial pallium (cortex) of sauropsids contains equivalents to at least part of the mammalian hippoccampal complex. It receives secondary sensory input from the dorsal pallium, and thus it is suggested to be involved in a higher level of processing. The lateral pallium (cortex) receives secondary olfactory projections, as in other tetrapods (Bruce and Neary, 1995c; Lohman and Smeets, 1993).

In addition to these three pallial divisions, however, the reptilian and avian telencephalon is clearly differentiated from other tetrapods by a voluminous cellular mass called the *dorsal ventricular ridge* (DVR), which is associated with an enlarged telencephalon (Fig. 5.8B,C). The DVR is located in the lateral wall, adjacent to the lateral pallium and the basal ganglia, and protrudes into the lateral ventricle. The DVR consists of multiple nuclear cell clusters instead of a laminar organization, as in the mammalian pallium. For decades, the DVR had been regarded as a part of the basal ganglia (e.g., Ariëns Kappers et al., 1967). More recent comparative studies, however, have shown that only a portion of the telencephalon, which is situated ventral to the DVR, is truly equivalent to the mammalian basal ganglia in terms of phyletic ancestry, connections, and chemistry (Källén, 1962; Karten and Dubbeldam, 1973; Northcutt, 1981). What, then, is the DVR? The DVR includes cell populations that receive visual, somatosensory, and auditory projections from the collothalamus, and efferents of DVR are sent to other brain regions that are involved in modulating behaviors. Based on the pattern of this circuitry, the DVR often is compared with a part of the mammalian isocortex, as described later in detail.

Lemnothalamo-telencephalic pathways. In reptiles and birds, nuclei in the rostral dorsal thalamus correspond with those in the mammalian lemnothalamus and the nucleus anterior of anamniotes in terms of connections. There are at least four groups of nuclei that can be categorized in the lemnothalamic group in reptiles and birds–

dorsal lateral optic nucleus, nucleus dorsalis intermedius ventralis anterior, nucleus dorsolateralis anterior, and dorsomedialis (Fig. 5.9). All these nuclei send projections to the dorsal pallium, as well as other cortical areas, via both the lateral and medial forebrain bundles (Butler, 1994a,b) (Fig. 5.11).

In all amniotes, there are cell groups located in the dorsolateral portion that receive direct retinal input and send projections to the dorsal pallium (Bruce and Butler, 1984a; Hall and Ebner, 1970a,b; Karten et al., 1973; Miceli et al., 1975). The nomenclature of these visual nuclei are quite diverse in different groups of animals. Butler (1994a) therefore proposed the term *dorsal lateral optic nucleus* (DLO in Fig. 5.9) to refer to these cell groups in all nonmammalian amniotes. Primarily on the basis of the retino-thalamo-telencephalic connection, the dorsal lateral optic nucleus has been compared with the nucleus anterior of amphibians and to the dorsal lateral geniculate nucleus of mammals. The telencephalic target of the dorsal lateral optic nucleus has been considered to be the equivalent of the mammalian striate cortex. The reptilian dorsal lateral optic nucleus sends an ipsilateral projection to the lateral part of the dorsal pallium—the pallial thickening—whereas the avian nucleus sends a bilateral projection to the Wulst. As in the mammalian striate cortex, the Wulst is retinotopically organized (Pettigrew and Konishi, 1976) and sends a projection back to visual nuclei in the brain stem, including the optic tectum and dorsal lateral optic nucleus (Karten et al., 1973). The reptilian pallia, however, including the dorsal cortex, do not possess such long descending projections.

In birds, somatosensory projections from the spinal cord and the dorsal column nuclei terminate in the nucleus dorsalis intermedius ventralis anterior (DIVA in Fig. 5.9), which in turn project bilaterally to the anterodorsal part of the Wulst (Delius and Bennetto, 1972; Wild 1987b, 1989). This avian nucleus, therefore, corresponds to the mammalian ventral nuclear group in terms of the thalamo-telencephalic connection. A distinct somatosensory nucleus has not yet been identified in reptiles.

The rostral lemnothalamus also contains cell groups that are not directly associated with specific sensory processing. These nuclei, including the nucleus dorsolateralis anterior (DLA in Fig. 5.9) and nucleus dorsomedialis (DM), surround a large dorsal nucleus called *rotundus* (Butler and Hodos, 1996). In reptiles, the nucleus dorsolateralis anterior receives projections from a wide variety of structures, including the spinal cord, hypothalamus, other thalamic nuclei, and torus semicircularis (Hoogland, 1981, 1982).

The nucleus dorsolateralis anterior of reptiles sends widespread projections to the bilateral telencephalon, including medial, dorsal, and lateral cortices, as well as the pallial thickening (Bruce and Butler, 1984a). This connection pattern is compared with that of the anterior group of mammals. In birds, two nuclei, nucleus dorsolateralis anterior (DLA) and nucleus dorsolateralis anterior, pars medialis, can be compared with the nucleus dorsolateralis anterior of reptiles in terms of connections. The nucleus dorsolateralis anterior and nucleus dorsolateralis anterior, pars medialis, also receive projections from multiple sources, such as the dorsal column nuclei and hypothalamus (Berk and Butler, 1981; Wild, 1989). These avian nuclei send projections to the medial and lateral basal ganglia (i.e., lateral lobus parolfactorius and paleostriatum augmentatum) and the Wulst (Miceli et al., 1990; Wild, 1987a).

The nucleus dorsomedialis (DM in Fig. 5.9) is found in reptiles and birds. In reptiles, the nucleus dorsomedialis also receives projections from the spinal cord and the nucleus raphe and sends diffuse projections to the ipsilateral pallium, the DVR, and the basal ganglia (Balaban and Ulinski, 1981; González and Russchen, 1988). In birds, the nucleus dorsomedialis receives projections from the external cuneate nucleus, parabrachial nuclei, preoptic area, and hypothalamus (Berk and Butler, 1981; Wild, 1987a) and sends ipsilateral projections to the medial lobus parolfactorius, paleostriatum, medial neostriatum, and the Wulst (Karten et al., 1973; Kitt and Brauth, 1982; Wild, 1987a). The dorsomedial nuclear group is often compared with the intralaminar group of mammals based on these connections, including diffuse projections to the telencephalon (Butler, 1994a; Veenman et al., 1997).

Collothalamo-telencephalic pathways. The DVR can be roughly divided into anterior and posterior regions (Northcutt, 1981; Ulinski, 1983). The anterior DVR receives the ipsilateral collothalamic input via the lateral forebrain bundle (Figs. 5.9 and 5.11), whereas the posterior DVR receives a direct projection from the olfactory system. The reptilian anterior DVR includes at least three distinct divisions—medial, intermediate, and lateral zones. Similarly, the anterior DVR of birds, which is even more massive than the reptilian one, contains several cytoarchitectonically distinct areas, including the hyperstriatum ventrale and the neostriatum. Only limited information is available about the connections and functions of the former (Horn, 1985; Husband and Shimizu, 1999). As for the latter, at least three sensory-specific structures are embedded in the avian neostriatum: Field L (auditory), ectostriatum (visual), and nucleus basalis (somatosensory).

In all tetrapods (except monotremes), a specific thalamic nucleus in the dorsal thalamus receives axons from the optic tectum (superior colliculus) and in turn projects to the telencephalon. In reptiles and birds, this nucleus is called the *nucleus rotundus* (Rt in Fig. 5.9); it is the largest nucleus of the dorsal thalamus in these classes. The nucleus rotundus receives a bilateral projection from the optic tectum (Benowitz and Karten, 1976; Butler and Northcutt, 1971; Hall and Ebner, 1970a; Karten and Revzin, 1966) and sends a projection to a specific area in the DVR in the sauropsid telencephalon. In reptiles, a lateral part of the anterior DVR, as well as the basal ganglia, receives the ipsilateral rotundal projection (Hall, 1972; Hall and Ebner, 1970b; Pritz, 1975). The avian rotundal projection also terminates ipsilaterally in the telencephalic area called the *ectostriatum* in the DVR (Benowitz and Karten, 1976; Karten and Hodos, 1970). Based on the tecto-thalamo-telencephalic connection pattern, the nucleus rotundus in sauropsids is comparable with the lateral posterior–pulvinar complex in mammals and the anterior lateral nucleus and posterior lateral nucleus in frogs.

All tetrapods possess a dorsal thalamic nucleus that receives input from the auditory mesencephalic region (torus semicircularis or acoustic tectum) and sends a projection to the telencephalon. In reptiles, the nucleus reuniens pars compacta (RC in Fig. 5.9; also called the *nucleus medialis*), located ventromedial to the nucleus rotundus, receives a projection from the torus semicircularis (Foster and Hall, 1978; Pritz, 1974a). The nucleus reuniens sends a projection to the medial zone of the anterior DVR and the basal ganglia (Balaban and Ulinski, 1981; Bruce and Butler,

1984b; Foster and Hall, 1978; Pritz, 1974b). In birds, a projection from the acoustic tectum (the nucleus mesencephalicus lateralis, pars dorsalis) terminates in the nucleus ovoidalis (OV in Fig. 5.9), which is located dorsomedial to the nucleus rotundus (Karten, 1967). The nucleus ovoidalis in turn sends a projection to Field L, which lies caudomedially to the ectostriatum (Bonke et al., 1979; Brauth et al., 1987; Karten, 1968). The nucleus reuniens and nucleus ovoidalis are comparable with the central nucleus in amphibians and the medial geniculate nucleus in mammals in terms of midbrain–thalamo-telencephalic connections.

In crocodiles, the region receiving a somatosensory tectal projection is designated as the medialis complex (MC in Fig. 5.9; Pritz and Stritzel, 1990), which is located between the visual nucleus (nucleus rotundus) and the auditory nucleus (nucleus reuniens pars compacta/nucleus ovoidalis), both of which receive the tectal input. The medialis complex also receives the spinal and dorsal column projections (Pritz and Northcutt, 1980) and gives rise to a projection to the intermediate zone in the anterior DVR, which is interposed between the visual and auditory recipient regions (Balaban and Ulinski, 1981; Bruce and Butler, 1984b; Pritz and Northcutt, 1980; Pritz and Stritzel, 1994). In birds, the caudal part of the nucleus dorsolateralis posterior receives somatosensory input from the dorsal column nuclei in the medulla and visual input from the deeper layers of the tectum (Gamlin and Cohen, 1986; Korzeniewska and Güntürkün, 1990; Wild, 1989). Neurons of this nucleus are known to respond to multimodal (i.e., somatosensory, visual, and auditory) stimulations (Korzeniewska and Güntürkün, 1990; Wild, 1987b). The caudal part of the nucleus dorsolateralis posterior projects to a restricted area between the medial edge of the ectostriatum (visual) and the lateral edge of Field L (auditory) in the neostriatum (Gamlin and Cohen, 1986; Kitt and Brauth, 1982; Wild, 1987a,b). The pattern of connections suggests that the medialis complex in crocodiles and the caudal part of nucleus dorsolateralis posterior in birds are comparable with part of the posterior group of the mammalian dorsal thalamus.

In the avian DVR, there is an anterolateral cell group called the *nucleus basalis*. The nucleus receives direct bilateral input from the principal nucleus of the trigeminal nerve in the pons via the quintofrontal tract (Zeigler and Karten, 1973). In this respect, the avian telencephalic nucleus may be compared with part of the ventralis posterior nucleus of the mammalian thalamus. No corresponding nucleus in the reptilian telencephalon has been reported.

The posterior DVR. In both reptiles and birds, visual, auditory, and somatosensory output from the anterior DVR terminate in the ipsilateral posterior DVR. Also, the striatum, nucleus accumbens, anterior olfactory nucleus, and lateral pallium receive a direct projection from the anterior DVR (Ulinski, 1983).

The posterior DVR of reptiles additionally receives a projection from the main olfactory bulb (Lohman and Smeets, 1993; Ulinski, 1983) and gives rise to a projection to the hypothalamus (Bruce and Neary, 1995a,b). In contrast, birds do not have secondary olfactory input to the posterior DVR. The posterior DVR of snakes and lizards contains a large nucleus called the *nucleus sphericus* or *vomeronasal amygdala* (Northcutt, 1981). This nucleus receives its major input from the accessory olfactory bulb, which is innervated by the vomeronasal nerve (Halpern, 1980; Ulinski and Peterson, 1981). The nucleus sends projections predominantly to the hypothalamus, at least in snakes (Halpern, 1980). Based on these connections, at least part of the reptilian posterior DVR has been compared with the mammalian amygdala (Bruce and Neary, 1995c, Northcutt, 1981; Ulinski, 1983).

In birds, the posterior DVR is represented by the archistriatum. The archistriatum is a cytoarchitectonically distinct multinucleate formation (Zeier and Karten, 1971). The caudal and medial parts (archistriatum mediale, archistriatum posterior, and nucleus taeniae) are often compared with part of the amygdala of mammals based on connections with the medial and lateral hypothalamus via the tractus occipito-mesencephalicus pars hypothalami (Zeier and Karten, 1971). In contrast, the anterior and intermediate archistriatum are compared with parts of the mammalian sensorimotor fields of the isocortex because they send projections to the brain stem via the tractus occipito-mesencephalicus. The targets of this extratelencephalic projection include the dorsal thalamus, pretectum, midbrain roof, lateral reticular formation, lateral pontine nuclei, and rostral spinal cord (Nottebohm et al., 1976; Wild et al., 1993; Zeier and Karten, 1971). Reptiles do not have such a motor area sending long descending efferents to the brain stem or spinal cord.

Basal ganglia. As in mammals, the basal ganglia of sauropsids interconnect between pallial telencephalic structures and motor centers in the brain stem (Parent, 1986; Reiner et al., 1984; Ulinski, 1983). In reptiles, the basal ganglia receives intratelencephalic projections from the dorsal cortex and the DVR (González and Russchen, 1988, 1990; Hoogland and Vermeulen-Van der Zee, 1989) and ascending projections from all the collothalamic nuclei (Northcutt, 1981). As in mammals, the reptilian basal ganglia sends massive descending pathways to the brain stem nuclei, including tegmental dopamine-containing cell groups (ventral tegmental area and substantia nigra), ventral thalamus (anterior entopeduncular nucleus), and dorsal thalamus. In addition to these projections, turtles and crocodiles have striatal efferents to the pretectum (dorsal nucleus of the posterior commissure in diapsid reptiles), which in turn projects upon the optic tectum (Medina and Smeets, 1981; Reiner et al., 1980; ten Donkelaar and de Boer-van Huizen, 1981).

In birds, many telencephalic structures had been assumed to be equivalent to components of the subcortical basal ganglia of mammals (e.g., Ariëns Kappers et al., 1967). Major telencephalic structures were thus named with the suffix "striatum," such as paleostriatum, archistriatum, neostriatum, and hyperstriatum. Subsequent comparative studies have shown that only a small portion of the avian telencephalon corresponds to the basal ganglia. The avian basal ganglia are called the paleostriatal complex, which includes the paleostriatum augmentatum (caudate-putamen), paleostriatum primitivum and intrapeduncular nucleus (globus pallidus), and rostral lobus parolfactorius (nucleus accumbens). The paleostriatum augmentatum receives projections from the DVR and the Wulst (Brauth et al., 1978; Shimizu et al., 1995; Veenman et al., 1995) and projects to the paleostriatum primitivum and intrapeduncular nucleus. As in mammals and reptiles, a descending fiber system from the avian globus pallidus terminates in the dorsal thalamus (e.g., nucleus dorsalis intermedius posterior), ventral thalamus (anterior nucleus of the ansa lenticularis), dopaminergic tegmentum (nucleus tegmenti pedunculopontinus), and pretectum (nucleus spiriformis lateralis) (Brauth et al., 1978; Karten and Dubbeldam, 1973; Reiner et al., 1982a,b). As in reptiles and amphibians, the pretectal nucleus sends a massive and exclusive projection to the ipsilateral optic tectum—in particular to the deeper layers (Reiner et al., 1982a, 1984).

Conclusion

In tetrapods, there are three distinct patterns of forebrain organization. The anamniote (amphibian) pattern is differentiated from the amniote (mammalian and sauropsid) patterns by the smaller size of the forebrain and its less complex organization. The significant structural and organizational resemblance between amphibians and other anamniotes suggests that major changes in forebrain organization occurred during the ancestral tetrapod to amniote transition instead of the crossopterygian to tetrapod transition (Northcutt, 1981).

The amniote patterns—both the mammalian and sauropsid patterns—are characterized by an enlarged, differentiated dorsal thalamus and telencephalon in comparison with the narrow, elongated forebrain of amphibians (Fig. 5.8). Between the mammalian and sauropsid patterns, there are many thalamic nuclei that are comparable based on their connections. More studies are necessary, however, to clarify the functional similarities and differences of these thalamic structures. The mammalian and sauropsid patterns are clearly differentiated based on distinct elaborated patterns of the telencephalon: the mammalian cerebral cortex and the sauropsid DVR. Nevertheless, both the cerebral cortex and the DVR are involved in processing sensory information via the thalamo-telencephalic pathways.

In terms of development of the lemno-thalamus and collo-thalamus, the amphibian collothalamus is more differentiated (with at least three nuclei) than the lemnothalamus (with a single nucleus). Similarly, the sauropsid collothalamus occupies a larger portion of the dorsal thalamus than the lemnothalamus. In mammals, placentals in particular, both the lemnothalamus and the collothalamus are highly differentiated and reach their greatest expansion of all amniotes.

The lemnothalamic projections to the telencephalon are found in all extant tetrapods. The projection patterns, however, can be differentiated into at least two groups based on the telencephalic targets (Fig. 5.11). Thus, the lemnothalamus in the typical anamniote (amphibian) pattern sends ascending sensory projections to the medial pallium and the medial part of the dorsal pallium, whereas those of the mammalian and sauropsid patterns send major sensory input to the dorsal pallium in addition to projections to the medial pallium (hippocampus). The collothalamo-telencephalic projections are also found in all tetrapods, and the targets of the pathways are distinct for each of the three patterns. In amphibians, the collothalamic projection terminates in the basal ganglia. Whereas both the mammalian and sauropsid groups also have such direct projections to the basal ganglia, the isocortex and the DVR receive strong projections from the collothalamus as well.

In all tetrapods, direct or indirect projections have been found from the sensory-recipient pallial regions to the basal ganglia. Although there are differences in connective patterns, all tetrapods possess circuits interconnecting the basal ganglia, sensory centers in the tectum/thalamus, and the tegmental motor centers. As for the amygdala, as well as the claustrum of mammals, corresponding structures among amphibians, sauropsids, and mammals have not been clearly determined. Some hypotheses regarding the origin of these structures are introduced in the next section.

EVOLUTIONARY HISTORY OF THE TETRAPOD FOREBRAIN

For a long period of time, the understanding of forebrain evolution had been largely dominated by the idea of *scala naturae*. In the 1960s, however, new views of brain evolution emerged, some of which are described in this section. The emergence of new views about evolution owes greatly to the dramatic methodological and theoretical advancements that have occurred in comparative neurology. Methodologically, modern neuroanatomical techniques—specifically, tracing methods—were introduced to explore the connections within the brain structures. Studies using these techniques revealed then-unknown connections, including the ascending sensory thalamo-telencephalic projections in all tetrapods, as described in the previous section.

The theoretical basis of a comparative approach to brain evolution was reconceived at the same time. Through this process, the erroneous nature of *scala naturae* became manifest in the context of comparative neural and behavioral studies (Hodos, 1970; Hodos and Campbell, 1969). Furthermore, identifying the nature of neuroanatomical similarities between different taxa became acknowledged as the first step in reconstructing brain evolution (Campbell and Hodos, 1970). Regardless of the degree of similarity, if a particular character of two or more taxa has been inherited from a common ancestor of these taxa, the character is called *homologous* (Campbell and Hodos, 1970). If, however, there is no phyletic continuity and the resemblance is a consequence of independent evolution from different ancestral origins, the character is called *homoplastic* (Campbell and Hodos, 1970). Depending on whether the character is similar to that of the ancestral stock or derived specializations within a particular taxon, it is called *plesiomorphic* or *apomorphic*, respectively (Butler and Hodos, 1996). Identification of homologous and homoplastic features provides critical clues for comprehending the evolution and adaptation of the nervous system (Northcutt, 1981). If two particular structures are recognized as homologous, their similarities and differences indicate how the same neural structure from the common ancestor has diverged through adaptation to a different series of biological problems. In contrast, if two structures are homoplastic, a comparison between them provides information about how the nervous systems of different taxa have dealt with a similar series of biological problems. Basically, two structures are inferred to be homologous based on the degree of similarities in multiple features (Simpson, 1961). In neuroanatomical studies, these similarities include the topological, topographical, hodological (connection), embryological, morphological, neurochemical, physiological, behavioral (functional), and genetic features of neural characteristics (Butler and Hodos, 1996). At the same time, however, it is important to note that similarity alone is not sufficient to determine homology. To reconstruct the phylogenetic continuity of a given trait, one must analyze the systematic distribution of characters among different taxa (Northcutt, 1984).

Early Tetrapods

The evolution of the forebrain within extinct tetrapods is, to some degree, traced by examining the endocast, in which mineral fillings replaced brain tissues within the cranial bones (Hopson, 1979). Because soft brain tissues decay rapidly, available information from the endocast data is limited to general brain morphology. The endocasts of labyrinthodonts (*Edops* and *Eroyps*) indicate an extremely narrow forebrain in the early tetrapods (Jerison, 1973). The shape of these brains is similar to that of cartilaginous fish, bony fish (other than teleosts), and living amphibians (Jerison, 1973). The fossil record, however, does not provide information about internal neural organizations. Although it is tempting to assume that the organization of the early tetrapods is similar to that of the modern amphibians based on their gross similarity in shape, caution must be taken before making such an assumption. As described in the first section, there are major skeletal differences between the Paleozoic amphibians and their modern counterparts.

Based on comparative studies of different groups of vertebrates, however, at least two important characteristics in the internal organization are generally conceived of as plesiomorphic (ancestral) for all tetrapods. First, basic subdivisions of the telencephalon (a pallium and a subpallium) exist in every vertebrate radiation, including tetrapods, and thus the characteristic is probably plesiomorphic for all vertebrates (Northcutt, 1981). The pallium can be further divided into at least three parts (medial, dorsal, and lateral), and the subpallium includes septum and basal ganglia. Second, the dorsal thalamus of all tetrapods is divided into rostral and caudal zones based on connections, and thus these subdivisions are most likely plesiomorphic (Butler, 1994a). As for the lemnothalamus, the nucleus anterior of amphibians appears to be homologous as a field to multiple nuclei of the rostral thalamus in amniotes. Similarly, cell groups situated in the caudal thalamus (collothalamus) may also be plesiomorphic in terms of connections with the roof of the midbrain. The early tetrapods, therefore, probably possessed a tubular brain with these forebrain characteristics.

Early Amniotes

Endocasts of the early amniotes are not known except for that of *Diadectes*, which is closely related to the earliest amniotes (Hopson, 1979). Its endocast shows a very narrow, elongated forebrain and midbrain (Fig. 5.12A). The early synapsids (pelycosaurs and therapsids) of the Triassic show a diminutive cerebral expansion comparable to that of *Diadectes* (Quiroga, 1980) (Fig. 5.12B,C). The significant

164   5 Evolution of the Forebrain in Tetrapods

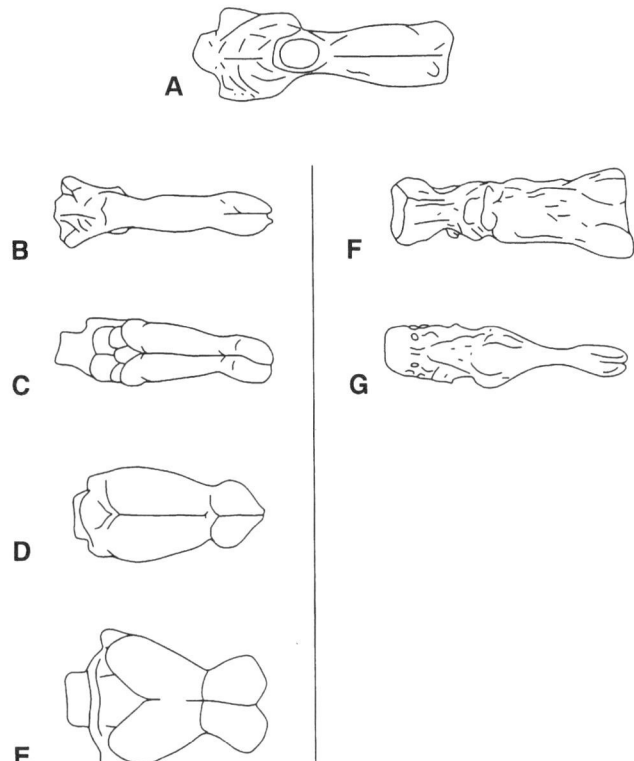

Figure 5.12. Endocasts of fossil reptiles and mammals, including *Diadectes* (*A*, a genus close to the earliest amniotes), therapsids (*B*, cynodonts *Trirachodon*; *C*, *Probainognathus*), protherian mammals (*D*, triconodont *Triconodon*; *E*, multituberculate *Ptilodus*), and archosaurs (*F*, aetosaur *Desmatosuchus*; *G*, crocodile *Sebecus*). (Adapted from Hopson [1979], Quiroga [1980], and Ulinski [1983].)

forebrain enlargement of the synapsid line became evident only in the endocasts of early mammals of the Jurassic (Hopson, 1979; Quiroga, 1980) (Fig. 12D, E), probably due to the development of the cerbral cortex (Ulinski, 1983). Similarly, the small transverse diameter of the forebrain characterizes the endocasts of the early archosaurs (thecodonts) in the middle Triassic. A gradual expansion of the reptilian forebrain became manifest only in the Late Triassic (Hopson, 1979), most likely due to the development of the DVR (Ulinski, 1983). The endocasts of the aerosaur *Desmatosuchus* and crocodile *Sebecus* show developed forebrains (Fig. 5.12F,G), which are comparable to the modern crocodilians (Hopson, 1979; Ulinski, 1983) (see also Fig. 5.8B).

The existence of lemnothalamo-telencephalic connections in both amphibians and amniotes suggests that such pathways already existed in the early amniotes, the Captorhinida. This route travels bilaterally through the medial forebrain bundle in amphibians, whereas mammals have a unilateral (ipsilateral) path through the lateral forebrain bundle. In contrast, many sauropsids have both the bilateral and ipsilateral projections via both the lateral and medial forebrain bundles. Based on these distributions, unilateral ascending fibers through the lateral forebrain bundle are apomorphic for amniotes (Butler, 1994b). In all living amniotes, the dorsal pallium, as well as the medial pallium, are primary targets of the lemnothalamic projections. In living amphibians, however, only the medial aspect of the dorsal pallium receives the lemnothalamic projections. The difference in the projection patterns between extant amniotes and anamniotes suggests the possibility that the dorsal pallium might not be the primary target of the lemnothalamic projection in the ancestral amniotes. Rather, the significant development of the lemnothalamo-dorsal pallial route might have occurred after synapsids and sauropsids diverged.

In all extant tetrapods, the collothalamic projection to the telencephalon is ipsilateral through the lateral forebrain bundle. The early amniotes, thus, most likely had the same characteristic. Furthermore, the projection in all tetrapods sends sensory input to the basal ganglia, which forms an extensive interconnection involving the tegmentum and midbrain roof. The tectum plays an important role in controlling motor output through the tectoreticular and reticulospinal pathways. The collothalamo-basal ganglia connections, descending basal ganglia efferents, and their significance in motor output via the tectum, therefore, appear to be plesiomorphic for amniotes. A marked difference, however, is also found in the collothalamic-telencephalic projection pattern of different lineages of tetrapods. In amphibians, the collothalamic projection terminates exclusively and directly in the basal ganglia. In contrast, the collothalamic input to the amniote basal ganglia is conveyed both directly from the thalamus and indirectly via sensory-specific fields of the anterior DVR of sauropsids or the isocortex of mammals (Ulinski, 1983). The issue of whether the earliest known amniotes, the Captorhinida, possessed pallial telencephalic areas that received collothalamic input will never be resolved satisfactorily because of the fossil nature of the group. Several hypotheses regarding the origins and evolution of the DVR and isocortex are, however, described next.

In addition to the characteristics above, an amygdalo-hypothalamic projection can probably be traced back to the ancestral amniotes. In all tetrapods, the hypothalamus receives projections from the amygdala (or its equivalent structure) in the telencephalon. The amygdala in turn receives various sensory signals through the medial pallium (in amphibians), anterior DVR (in sauropsids), or isocortex (in mammals).

Synapsids and Sauropsids

The fossil record shows that the reptilian ancestors of archosaurs, pelycosaurs, and therapsids had narrow tubular brains, showing no signs of the forebrain expansion (Fig. 5.12). The forebrain enlargement of amniote lineages thus must have occurred independently and separately in sauropsids and mammals (Hopson, 1979; Ulinski, 1983). The parallel forebrain expansion of reptiles, birds, and mammals is most likely correlated with the development of the DVR and the isocortex for each lineage.

What is the origin of the isocortex? Is the sauropsid DVR equivalent to the mammalian isocortex? If so, are they homologous or homoplastic? These have been some of the most debated questions in the field of comparative neurobiology for the last 30 years. They are not only important questions that have intrinsic merit for comparative biologists in order to understand forebrain evolution, but they also have a significant impact on the comprehension of the origin and evolutionary history of human intelligence, which overwhelmingly relies on the functions of the isocortex (Jerison and Jerison, 1988). Widely diverse hypotheses have been presented concerning the origins of the DVR and isocortex (e.g., Hall and Ebner, 1970a,b; Halpern, 1980; Parent, 1986). In this section, five of the current hypotheses on this issue are introduced: an equivalent-cell hypothesis (Karten, 1969, 1991, 1997), an out-group hypothesis (Northcutt and Kaas, 1995), a dual-expansion hypothesis (Butler, 1994b; Reiner, 1991, 1993), a claustrum hypothesis (MacLean, 1990; Striedter, 1997), and an amygdala hypothesis (Bruce and Neary, 1995c; Fernandez et al., 1998). Consistent with the previous sections, the emphasis here is placed on the hypotheses based on voluminous data from connection studies.

Equivalent-cell hypothesis. The equivalent-cell hypothesis is based primarily on the connection patterns of the sensory information processing system in the avian telencephalon (Karten, 1969, 1991, 1997; Nauta and Karten, 1970; Karten and Shimizu, 1989). The hypothesis has three components. First, the existence of the lemnothalamic-pallial pathway in all amniotes suggests that the dorsal division of the dorsal pallium in sauropsids—including the lateral part of the dorsal cortex (or pallial thickening) of reptiles and the visual Wulst in birds—contains cell groups that are homologous to those in the dorsal part of the mammalian isocortex (including the striate cortex). This point has been widely accepted by other authors (Butler, 1994b; Reiner, 1991, 1993).

The second part of the hypothesis deals with the origin of the DVR. In the avian and reptilian DVR, which is composed of a complex multinucleate formation, neurons processing sensory signals are clustered as distinct modality-specific nuclei in a nonlaminated DVR. The hypothesis proposes that neurons of these individual cell populations in the DVR are comparable with those in distinct layers of the lateral portion of the mammalian isocortex, despite the lack of a laminar organization of the DVR as a whole. For instance, in birds, the visual thalamic nucleus (nucleus rotundus) sends a projection to the ectostriatum of the DVR. Thus, those thalamo-recipient neurons of the ectostriatum are equivalent to those in layer 4 of the mammalian extrastriate cortex in receipt of the collothalamic visual pathways. Neurons of the ectostriatum further project on nuclei in the neostriatum, which in turn send projections to the archistriatum intermediale, which then gives rise to a projection to various nuclei in the brain stem and mesencephalon, including the optic tectum (Karten and Shimizu, 1989; Ritchie, 1979). The basic pattern of this internuclear circuit of the avian brain is compared with that of the interlaminar circuit in the extrastriate cortex of mammals, in which layer 4 sends a projection to cells in layers 2 and 3, which project to cells in layers 5 and 6, which in turn project to the brain stem nuclei and mesencephalon, including the superior colliculus. Thus, the hypothesis maintains that neurons of these DVR nuclei correspond with those of distinct cortical layers. Similarly, neurons of distinct auditory and somatosensory nuclei in the DVR have corresponding neurons in different layers of the auditory and somatosensory areas in the isocortex.

The third part of the hypothesis proposes that ancestral amniotes possessed cell populations that had subsequently evolved into either the nonlaminated nuclei in the DVR or distinct layers in the lateral isocortex. Thus, neurons of these nuclei of the DVR and parts of the isocortex are homologous as derivatives of the same cell populations in the plesiomorphic neural circuits for processing sensory information. Characteristics in cellular organizations—nuclei or lamination—are thus apomorphic for sauropsids and synapsids, respectively.

Out-group hypothesis. The second hypothesis is proposed by Northcutt and Kaas (1995). The hypothesis can also be organized into three aspects. The first aspect of the hypothesis suggests that, based on the information available from the fossil record (endocasts), the ancestral tetrapods had a telencephalic organization comparable with that of modern amphibians rather than reptiles. The expansion of the forebrain, the pallium in particular, thus occurred independently and separately in nonsynapsids and synapsids. The hypothesis maintains that the early therapsids leading to mammals might have had only a small dorsal pallium and no DVR, as in living amphibians.

The second aspect of the hypothesis deals with the comparison between the mammalian isocortex and amphibian pallium. Although the dorsal pallium of modern amphibians is traditionally compared with the mammalian isocortex, Northcutt (1981) points out that the amphibian lateral pallium also possesses an important hodological feature that is similarly found in the isocortex. Thus, the source of the long descending palliomedullar/spinal projections in mammals is located in the isocortex. In amphibians, however, descending brain stem projections originate in the caudal ventrolateral hemispheric wall (lateral pallium and amygdala) instead of the dorsal pallium (Kokoros and Northcutt, 1977). Consequently, this viewpoint maintains that the mammalian isocortex may be homologous to the dorsal and, possibly, part of the lateral pallium of modern amphibians.

In the third aspect, the hypothesis discusses a comparison of the sauropsid telencephalon with the mammalian counterparts. It holds that both the sauropsid DVR and the mammalian isocortex are pallial in origin, based on their position, internal organization, and connections with other forebrain structures. According to this view, however, they arose from different pallial divisions. The DVR was derived from the ancestral lateral pallium, whereas the isocortex evolved from the ancestral dorsal pallium and, possibly, parts of the lateral pallium (Northcutt and Kaas, 1995; Striedter, 1997). Thus, the DVR and the isocortex are not homologous as cell populations, but homoplastic by convergent evolution.

Dual-expansion hypothesis. The third hypothesis was developed and formulated by Butler (1994b), and a similar hypothesis was formed independently by Reiner (1991, 1993). The hypothesis maintains that the ancestral amniotes did not possess the DVR nor the lateral portions of isocortex based on comparative studies of these traits within living amniotes and anamniotes. It argues, however, that the DVR and the lateral isocortex are derived from the dorsal pallium of the early amniotes.

The hypothesis points out that the dorsal pallium of all amniotes has two subdivisions, a medial (Dm) and a lateral (Dl) one. The medial division (Dm) primarily receives thalamic input from the lemnothalamic nuclei, whereas the lateral division (Dl) receives the collothalamic input. According to the hypothesis, before the divergence of synapsid and nonsynapsid lines, the common ancestral amniote stock, the Captorhinida, already had these two pallial subdivisions and specific thalamic input to each region.

Both the medial (Dm) and lateral (Dl) divisions expanded in synapsids, whereas primarily the lateral division expanded in nonsynapsids. The medial division (Dm) is further subdivided into two portions, which are the medial (Dmm) and lateral (Dml) parts. In mammals, as the lemnothalamus expanded, the medial part (Dmm) formed the subicular, cingulate, prefrontal, primary sensorimotor, and related cortices, whereas the lateral part (Dml) became the striate cortex. In nonsynapsids, the medial part (Dmm) formed the medial part of the dorsal cortex, and the lateral part (Dml) became the lateral part of the dorsal cortex (the pallial thickening of reptiles and the visual Wulst in birds). The mammalian lateral division (Dl) became expanded to include the extrastriate visual, auditory, somatosensory-multisensory, and related cortices, which are characterized by the collothalamic inputs. In contrast, the nonsynapsid lateral division (Dl) formed areas of the DVR with similar thalamic afferents. Corresponding areas in the DVR and isocortex, thus, are homologous as a field receiving the collothalamic input. However, specific morphological and chemical characteristics of cells in the DVR and the isocortex are probably homoplastic.

Claustrum hypothesis. The three hypotheses described above agree that the DVR and the dorsal cortex of sauropsids are related to the mammalian isocortex. There are authors who express opposing views by pointing out cytological and hodological differences between the DVR and the isocortex (Lohman and Smeets, 1991; Smeets and González, 1994). One view suggests that the DVR is comparable with the mammalian claustrum (Díaz et al., 1990; MacLean, 1990; Striedter, 1997).

The claustrum has extensive reciprocal connections with many diverse areas of the isocortex and a projection from the dorsal thalamus, although it does not have direct projections to the brain stem or thalamus (LeVay and Sherk, 1981). The patterns of these connections are ostensibly similar to those of the DVR. This comparison needs to be viewed with caution. The thalamic input to the claustrum originates in the intralaminar nuclei, whereas the DVR receives modality-specific sensory projections. Based on connections, the intralaminar nuclear group should be comparable only with limited cell groups in sauropsids, as described in the previous section. Furthermore, the claustrum receives a projection from the hypothalamus, which does not directly project on the DVR. Finally, the DVR sends a major projection to the striatum, and the claustrum lacks such a projection. According to Butler (1994b), it is possible that, although a part of the DVR may correspond to the claustrum, most (or even all) of the DVR cannot be homologous to the claustrum based on currently available connection data.

Striedter (1997) points out, however, that although the connection patterns are different between the sauropsid DVR and the mammalian claustrum, these differences might have developed after they were separated from the ancestral amniote stock. By analyzing embryological patterns of telencephalic organization, he proposes another claustrum hypothesis in which he divides the claustrum into a ventrally located endopiriform nucleus and a dorsally situated claustrum proper (Striedter, 1997). The author suggests that the endopiriform nucleus and the anterior DVR derive from the embryonic lateral pallium of mammals and sauropsids, respectively. He thus proposes that the anterior DVR of reptiles is homologous to the avian DVR (both the neostriatum and the hyperstriatum ventrale) and the mammalian endopiriform nucleus. Moreover, he proposes that the posterior DVR of reptiles is homologous to the archistriatum of birds and to the pallial amygdala of mammals (Striedter, 1997).

Amygdala hypothesis. Bruce and Neary (1995c) introduced the hypothesis that the anterior DVR is homologous to the lateral amygdala of the basolateral complex of mammals. They point out that the isocortex has significant connections that the anterior DVR does not possess, such as interhemispheric connections and long descending efferents to the brain stem. In contrast, the anterior DVR and the basolateral amygdalar complex have many similarities, including (1) ascending sensory thalamic projections (LeDoux et al., 1990; Turner and Herkenham, 1991); (2) projections to the striatum; (3) similar cell morphology; (4) comparable position related to the olfactory cortex and ventricular surface; and (5) absence of interhemispheric and long descending connections (Bruce and Neary, 1995c). In addition, whereas the isocortex has an "inside-out" pattern of neurogenesis, the DVR and amygdala have an "outside-in" pattern (Tsai et al., 1981a,b).

A similar hypothesis is proposed based on a study analyzing the expression of homeobox genes (i.e., *Emx* and *Dlx*) during the embryogenesis of mice, chicks, turtles, and frogs (Fernandez et al., 1998). The authors found three main telencephalic subdivisions in all species: the pallial, intermediate, and striatal neuroepithelial domains. Based on their findings, they propose that the reptilian DVR and part of the avian DVR (i.e., the neostriatum) likely derive from the intermediate territory, whereas the hyperstriatum ventrale of the avian DVR is a pallial derivative. Because the basolateral amygdalar complex of mammals could also derive from the intermediate territory, the authors further suggest that the reptilian DVR and the avian neostriatum are homologous to the basolateral amygdalar complex. Meanwhile, the posterior DVR of reptiles and the avian archistriatum are compared with the corticomedial and central parts of the amygdala (Fernandez et al., 1998).

Conclusion

To compare the DVR and isocortex, it is important to remember that neither the DVR nor the isocortex is a unitary, homogeneous structure. The DVR can be divided into many hodologically and functionally distinct subdivisions. Many of the above hypotheses have been formulated based on studies of connections with other brain regions, emphasizing ascending sensory input. Although the sensory-specific areas occupy the major parts of the DVR (e.g., the neostriatum of birds), there are still regions for which connections and/or functions are not known (e.g., the hyperstriatum ventrale of birds). For instance, the medial portion of the hyperstriatum ventrale is associated with imprinting learning in birds (Horn, 1985). The area, however, does not receive the primary ascending sensory input, nor do they send direct motor output to the brain stem. The caudal hyperstriatum and archistriatum are also suggested to be involved in attention and arousal, although direct associations with the sensory and motor connections are not known. Do these regions within the DVR also have homologous (or homoplastic) counterparts in the mammalian brain? Or are these cell populations apomorphic as a result of adaptation to unique selective pressures? The arguments developed in the hypotheses above may be valid for a particular part of the DVR. However, more studies are essential to provide critical information for delineating the whole picture of the evolution of the DVR.

One of the most objective approaches to evolutionary neurobiology is the method of cladistic analysis, which uses out-group comparison (Butler and Hodos, 1996; Northcutt, 1984). Thus, whether a particular structure is plesiomorphic or apomorphic in a particular group is inferred based on comparisons of the trait in out groups, as well as the group in question. Comparative studies of living amphibians and cartilaginous and bony fishes are critical, but as yet insufficient for such an analysis in order to understand the evolution of the tetrapod and amniote forebrain (Northcutt, 1981). Moreover, many comparative analyses, including cladistic analysis, have been conducted based on the cytoarchitectonic and histochemical studies of different brains. Some gene expressions cannot, however, be revealed by such levels of study. Investigations with in situ hybridization, such as the study by Fernandez et al. (1998), will perhaps provide us with more information about similarities of brain structures between sauropsids and mammals than will studies at the higher organizational levels alone (Butler and Hodos, 1996; Reiner, 1991).

ENVIRONMENTAL PRESSURES ON THE TETRAPOD FOREBRAIN

This last section lays out the major external and internal events that occurred through the evolution of tetrapods, possibly affecting differential elaborations of the forebrain organization. Our understanding of what these environmental pressures were remains underdeveloped (Northcutt, 1984). In considerations of forebrain evolution in tetrapods, two major concepts have confused much of the discussion about the selective pressures on forebrain evolution. One is, under the influence of *scala naturae*, the failure to discern independent development of the forebrain in various tetrapod lineages. Consequently, misguided attempts have been made to identify a single, continuing selective pressure that would explicate a unilinear progression of the expansion and differentiation of the forebrain in tetrapods. The other reason, which has often marred an understanding of the selective pressures, is the failure to acknowledge that the brain is not a unitary organ. It is important to appreciate that discrete neural divisions and their connections are associated with multifarious roles, including visceral, musculoskeletal, arousal, sensory, emotion, motor coordination, and limbic functions (Hodos, 1988). These various systems are subject to different selective pressures, resulting in a differential development of individual systems.

Systematic comparative analyses should be undertaken to determine what selective pressures are associated with differential evolution of various neural subdivisions and connections in different species. However, the purview of this section has to be restricted. A special focus here is on the conjecture of what factors had a significant impact on the differentiation of the three forebrain organizations—amphibian, sauropsid, and mammalian patterns.

Anamniote Pattern Versus Amniote Pattern

In comparison with amphibians, one of the most distinct characteristics of the amniote brain is expansion of the forebrain—both the diencephalon and telencephalon. The brain–body ratio of amphibians is comparable with that of the living crossopterygian fish *Latimeria chalumnae* (Northcutt, 1981). If the body sizes are comparable, the forebrains of reptiles are one to two times larger than those of anamniotes (at least of amphibians and bony fishes; Northcutt, 1981). In the cases of birds and mammals, their brains are 5 to 20 times larger than those of the anamniotes (Northcutt, 1981). The amphibian thalamus is not well differentiated and contains only a limited number of nuclei. The thalamo-recipient pallium also remains underdeveloped in amphibians. In contrast, the lemnothalamus and collothalamus of amniotes consist of many distinct cell groups, and the pallium is well developed along with the hypertrophy of the thalamo-telencephalic pathways.

Aquatic to terrestrial habitat. The development of the forebrain in amniotes can be ascribed to at least two major changes that took place during the early tetrapod to amniote transition. The first significant change from anamniotes to amniotes was a shift from an aquatic to a fully terrestrial habitat. This change affected many aspects of the way of life of amniotes, including two important features: dietary pattern and locomotion. According to Carroll (1988), many Paleozoic amphibians tended to have a large body and disproportionally large head with large sharp teeth (Fig. 5.3A). These characteristics suggest that they were predators preying on relatively large animals—fish in water or invertebrates on land. In contrast, the early amniotes were similar to extant lizards with a similar body and skull size, jaw musculature arrangement, and dental features (Fig. 5.3B). The early amniotes are thus considered to be insectivorous—feeding on small, fast-moving, terrestrial arthropods. Their locomotive functions also became adapted to the new environment. All living amniotes have stretch receptors in the trunk and limb muscles that allow them to effectively coordinate locomotion. Living amphibians, however, do not have well-developed stretch receptors, suggesting the lack of the system in the early tetrapods (Carroll, 1988). These dramatic changes in the dietary and locomotive patterns in new terrestrial niches must be related to the expansion and development of the sensorimotor systems in the amniote brain.

Reproductive pattern. The second major change is in the reproductive pattern of amniotes. As living amphibians, the early tetrapods had external fertilization, laid numerous eggs in the water, and had an aquatic larval stage (Carroll, 1988). This reproductive pattern contrasts markedly with that of amniotes. Amniotes have internal fertilization, lay fewer eggs or retain them within their body, and have no aquatic larval stage. Owing to these reproductive features, amniotes have greatly increased parental investment. Parental investment is any behavioral effort by the parent in order to increase an individual offspring's chance of survival (Tivers, 1972). The degree and extent of parental investment controls many aspects of the animals' way of life beyond obvious parenting behaviors (Tivers, 1972). For instance, energy and time must be expended for finding stronger and healthier mates (intersexual selection), competing more vigorously with members of the same sex for access to the other sex (intrasexual selection), and protecting more attentively mates or offspring from predators (Alcock, 1993). Both males and females may exhibit unique and species-specific sexual displays to attract potential mates, and at the same time they may need to compete with rivals in dangerous fights. They also need to localize, identify, and evaluate potential mates, nearby rivals, possible nest sites, nutritious food, and approaching predators. These changes must be correlated with the dramatic development in the sensory, motor, and integrative systems.

Sauropsid Pattern Versus Mammalian Pattern

In the sauropsid brain, the collothalamus (and the collothalamic-recipient DVR) is much more developed than the lemnothalamus (and the lemnothalamic-recipient dorsal pallium; Butler, 1994a,b). In contrast, the mammalian brain possesses an equally well-developed lemnothalamus and collothalamus (Butler, 1994a,b). In general, the brains of mammals and birds are comparable in size, roughly ten times larger than those of modern reptiles with similar body weights (Jerison, 1973). What selective pressures launched the hypertrophy of the optic tectum and subsequent neural structures (i.e., collothalamus and collothalamic-recipient DVR) in sauropsids? Why did both divisions greatly expand in mammals? At least two important factors clearly differentiate the lifestyles between sauropsids and mammals; these factors may be related to the differential development of these two groups (Fig. 5.13).

Metabolic pattern. One factor is the difference in the metabolic pattern between synapsids and sauropsids. In comparison with the early amniotes, the expanded adductor chamber, complex cheek teeth, and secondary palate in early therapsids indicate that therapsids were characterized by an increased metabolic rate (Carroll, 1988). Such signs associated with characteristic changes in metabolism became further manifest in the early mammals. Metabolic rate can be measured by the amount of oxygen used per unit of weight. The resting metabolic rate of living mammals is about 10 times higher than that of modern reptiles of comparable size (Carroll, 1988). The brain is metabolically a very active organ, which requires a large supply of oxygen and glucose. The development of the brain is therefore inevitably constrained by the metabolic characteristics (Armstrong, 1983, 1990; Armstrong and Bergeron, 1985).

Environmental Pressures on the Tetrapod Forebrain 173

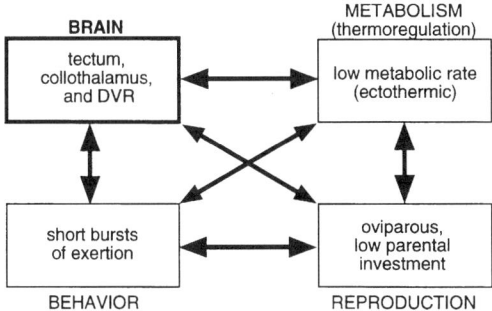

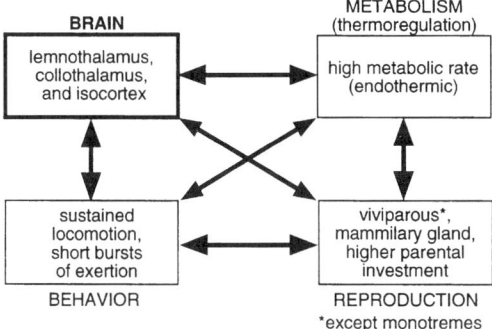

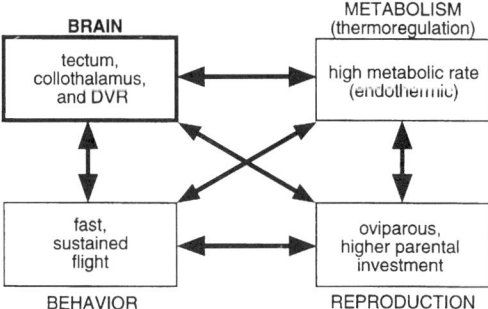

Figure 5.13. Schematic figures showing the relationships between the forebrain evolution and the internal and external pressures that distinguish the reptilian, avian, and mammalian patterns. The arrows indicate possible influence of the metabolic, reproductive, behavioral, and brain characteristics.

The metabolism of living mammals (as well as birds) is quite different from that of the ancestral reptiles in many features, including metabolic rate, body temperature control, and source of body heat. Mammals and birds are homeotherms (maintaining constant body temperature): The body heat source is their high metabolic rate, and thus mammals and birds are called *endotherms*. In contrast, amphibians and most reptiles are poikilotherms (with temperatures that fluctuate). They depend on external sources (e.g., the radiant heat from the sun), and thus they are termed *ectotherms*.

Energy for muscles can be generated by aerobic (oxidative) metabolism or anaerobic (fermentative) metabolism. Reptiles depend mainly on anaerobic glycosis, the degradation of glycogen or glucose to lactic acid, because they have limited capacities for oxygen transport. When electrical stimulation is applied to lizards, they struggle most vigorously only for the first 30 seconds (Bennett and Dawson, 1976). During this first half minute, over 80 to 90% of the total energy used by many lizards is associated with lactate formation and thus based on anaerobic metabolism (Bennett and Licht, 1972). The major disadvantage of the anaerobic metabolism is considerable accumulation of lactic acid. The large amount of lactic acid in the blood results in rapid muscle fatigue and exhaustion. To eliminate the lactate, reptiles need to take long periods of rest: several hours to a day in some cases (Bennett and Dawson, 1976). The activity patterns of reptiles thus are characterized by short bursts of exertion and subsequent quiet periods (Fig. 5.13A).

The reptilian (and amphibian) activity pattern—short bursts of strenuous exertion, but inability for sustained locomotion—affects every aspect of their lives: foraging, courting, mating, and avoiding predators. They have to accurately detect and analyze external stimuli (i.e., prey, food, potential mate, predators) and move in an appropriate direction quickly. This type of behavioral pattern is probably correlated with the development of an optic tectum that contains an extremely accurate map of the external world and a system for direct control on the skeletal muscles (Butler and Hodos, 1996). Although the tectum tends to be considered as a sensory structure, it also has extensive descending projections to the brain stem reticular formation, which in turn give rise to a projection to the motor neurons in the spinal cord. Along with the hypertrophy of the optic tectum, there is an expansion of the collothalamus and the DVR, which are also related to functions of encoding the multisensory signals in the internal map and generating quick orienting behaviors.

In contrast, the endothermic condition in mammals necessitates a higher metabolic rate, which in turn forces mammals to rely primarily on the aerobic process, the oxidation of foodstuffs. Although they also use anaerobic processes for initial quick movements, homeothermic animals do not endure anaerobic conditions very well. Mammals are able to maintain sustained locomotion for long periods without rapid fatigue, owing to oxidative metabolism (Fig. 5.13B). Because the metabolic rate of mammals is so high, however, it necessitates a constant food supply to raise body temperature. This activity pattern is correlated with the development of a neural system that is different from that required for the reptilian type of behavior patterns. They still need the ability for quick detection of stimuli and swift movements, and yet, in comparison with reptiles, mammals do not face urgency as restrained by the anaerobic metabolism. Instead, detailed analysis of stimuli and fine control of lasting locomotion is essential for their way of life, which is probably associated with the development of the lemnothalamic division and the lemnothalamic recipient cortical areas.

Reproductive pattern. The other dramatic difference between sauropsid and mammals is found in the reproductive patterns between the two classes. The reproductive patterns of the early mammals probably were similar to living monotremes (Carroll, 1988). They were hatched from eggs at a very immature stage of development (Griffiths, 1978). Nevertheless, all mammals (including monotremes) are unique in the presence of mammary glands, which evolved before the end of the Triassic (Carroll, 1988). Feeding young with maternal milk becomes absolutely necessary for them because the young cannot maintain their own high metabolic rate and body temperature without depending on parents. Mammals, therefore, have a longer period for nurturing young, and they are burdened with a much higher parental investment in comparison with reptiles. An increase in parental investment is particularly evident for placental mammals.

The higher the parental investment becomes, the greater the changes in behavioral patterns and underlying neural systems. As caring for offspring becomes more time and energy consuming, intersexual and intrasexual selections become more vigorous and competitive. Sensory and motor systems are required to adapt to these demands. In addition, a highly developed limbic system emerges in order to control the more sophisticated learning and motivational functions that are associated with these changes. As a result, the lemnothalamic nuclei in the dorsal thalamus, including the limbic nuclei, and their target in the dorsal pallium may become more elaborated and differentiated.

In many aspects, birds are unique in that they share a similar pattern of metabolism with mammals and a similar reproductive condition with reptiles (Fig. 5.13C). Their forebrain pattern, however, clearly belongs to the sauropsid pattern with the hypertrophy of the optic tectum and the DVR. It is important to note the following two issues to understand the forebrain evolution of birds. First, the avian lineage was derived probably from theropod dinosaurs in the Jurassic period about 100 million years ago (Carroll, 1988). At this point, the reptilian brain already included a developed optic tectum and probably enlarged collothalamus and DVR. Second, birds live in the aerial environment where they move extremely fast—much faster than any other terrestrial animals. As such, birds require a neural system that enables them to maneuver smoothly and rapidly in their three-dimensional environment. At the same time, their aerial habitat necessitates the aerobic metabolism to sustain long flight and a high brain–body ratio to maintain light body weight. These factors may be intertwined to generate the development of the optic tectum, collothalamus, and DVR in the avian brain. The well-developed cerebellum of birds must also be a result of adaptation to these environmental pressures.

Conclusion

The brain is the organ of behavior, and behavior is expressed by living animals. The brain needs to be studied not merely as an isolated, fixed object but also as an active machine that detects diverse stimuli and dynamically controls various motor behaviors. Thus, studies of selective pressures on brain evolution should be approached from a point of view in which dynamic behavioral patterns and the lifestyles of ancestral and living animals are taken into consideration.

In light of this view, the proposal of two forebrain subdivisions (i.e., collothalamic and lemnothalamic systems) by Butler (1994a,b) provides a conceptually important and practically useful framework to study the evolution of the forebrain. By extending this distinction to the functional aspects of the two forebrain divisions, it is my belief that we will have another interesting approach to understanding the evolutionary histories of forebrain organization. Consideration of the functional aspects involves at least two levels of analyses: the sensory and behavioral significance of the two divisions.

At the sensory level, the question should be addressed as to what kind of information was sent to the telencephalon via the lemnothalamus and the collothalamus in the earliest amniotes, the Captorhinida. The ancient collothalamus was probably involved in processing sensory information concerning the localization of external stimuli and quick recognition of the nature of the stimuli, as in all extant tetrapods. In contrast, the functional significance of the ancient lemnothalamus in the sensory process is difficult to speculate on because of its diverse roles in different living species. Although it might be related to the detailed analysis of stimulus characteristics, such a speculation warrants further comparative studies.

At the behavioral level, the question is which types of behaviors depend heavily on lemnothalamic and the collothalamic information. In the collothalamus, the initial control of short-term motor activities, such as orienting reflex, may have been plesiomorphic for amniotes. As described in the previous section, this feature is particularly important for amphibians and reptiles that rely on anaerobic metabolism. In contrast, the lemnothalamic information may have been processed and used in order to generate the fine control of long-term motor activities. Systematic and extensive comparative analyses of the actual behavioral patterns of living vertebrates need to be conducted. Furthermore, the fossil record has provided a significant amount of information about the behavioral patterns of extinct species. When the functional level of analysis is interwoven with the neuroanatomical, embryological, genetic, and paleontological analyses, we will be one step closer to truly understanding the evolution of the forebrain.

ACKNOWLEDGMENTS

The author thanks Drs. Cesario, V. Borlongan, William Hodos, Scott A. Husband, Erich D. Jarvis Kent T. Keyser, Anton J. Reiner, and Mario F. Wullimann for critically reading the manuscript and providing helpful suggestions. This work was partly supported by grants from the NSF, NASA, and University of South Florida (Research and Creative Scholarship Award).

REFERENCES

Abramson, B.P., and L.M. Chalupa (1988) Multiple pathways from the superior colliculus to the extrageniculate visual thalamus of the cat. *J. Comp. Neurol.* 271:397–418.

Alcock, J. (1993) *Animal Behavior: An Evolutionary Approach*, 5th ed. Sinauer Associates, Sunderland, MA.

References

Alheid, G.F., J.S. de Olmos, and C.A. Beltramino (1995) Amygdala and extended amygdala. In G. Paxinos (ed.); *The Rat Nervous System* 2nd ed. Academic Press, New York, pp. 495–578.

Allman, J. (1977) Evolution of the visual system in the early primates. In J.M. Sprague and A.N. Epstein (eds.); *Progress in Psychobiology and Physiological Psychology*, vol. VII. Academic Press, New York, pp. 1–53.

Andersen, R.A., P.L. Knight, and M. Merzenich (1980) The thalamocortical and corticothalamic connections of AI, AII and the anterior auditory field (AAF) in the cat: evidence for two largely segregated systems of connections. *J. Comp. Neurol.* 194:663–701.

Ariëns Kappers, C.U., G.C. Huber, and E.C. Crosby (1967) *The Comparative Anatomy of the Nervous System of Vertebrates, Including Man.* Hafner, New York.

Armstrong, E. (1983) Metabolism and relative brain size. *Science* 220:1302–1304.

Armstrong, E. (1990) Brains, bodies and metabolism. *Brain Behav. Evol.* 36:166–176.

Armstrong, E., and R. Bergeron (1985) Relative brain size and metabolism in birds. *Brain Behav. Evol.* 26:141–153.

Baisden, R.H., and D.B. Hoover (1979) Cells of origin of the hippocampal afferent projections from the nucleus reuniens thalami: a combined Golgi-HRP study in the rat. *Cell Tissue Res.* 203:387–391.

Balaban, C.D., and P.S. Ulinski (1981) Organization of thalamic afferents to anterior dorsal ventricular ridge in turtles. I. Projections of thalamic nuclei. *J. Comp. Neurol.* 200:95–129.

Beckstead, R.M. (1984) The thalamostriatal projection in the cat. *J. Comp. Neurol.* 223:313–346.

Benevento, L.A., and J.A. Fallon (1975) The ascending projections of the superior colliculus in the rhesus monkey *(Macaca mulatta) J. Comp. Neurol.* 160:339–362.

Bennett, A.F., and W.R. Dawson (1976) Metabolism. In C. Gans (ed.); *Biology of Reptilia*, vol. 5. Academic Press, New York, pp. 127–223.

Bennett, A.F., and P. Licht (1972) Anaerobic metabolism during activity in lizards. *J. Comp. Physiol.* 81:277–288.

Benowitz, L.I., and H.J. Karten (1976) Organization of the tectofugal visual pathway in the pigeon. *J. Comp. Neurol.* 167:503–520.

Bentovoglio, M., D. VanderKooy, and H.G.J.M. Kuypers (1979) The organization of the efferent projections of the substantia nigra in the cat. A retrograde fluorescent double labeling study. *Brain Res.* 174:1–17.

Berk, M.L., and A.B. Butler (1981) Efferent projections of the medial preoptic nucleus and medial hypothalamus in the pigeon. *J. Comp. Neurol.* 203:379–399.

Berman, N. (1977) Connections of the pretectum in the cat. *J. Comp. Neurol.* 174:227–254.

Bonke, B. A., D. Bonke, and H. Scheich (1979) Connectivity of the auditory forebrain nuclei in the guinea fowl *(Numida meleagris). Cell Tissue Res.* 200:101–121.

Brauth, S.E., J.L. Ferguson, and C.A. Kitt (1978) Prosencephalic pathways related to the paleostriatum of the pigeon, *Columba livia. Brain Res.* 147:205–221.

Brauth, S.E., C. M. McHale, C. A. Brasher, and R.J. Dooloing (1987) Auditory pathways in the budgerigar. I. Thalamo-telencephalic projections. *Brain Behav. Evol.* 30:174–199.

Bruce, L.L., and A.B. Butler (1984a) Telencephalic connections in lizards. I. Projections to cortex. *J. Comp. Neurol.* 229:585–601.

Bruce, L.L., and A.B. Butler (1984b) Telencephalic connections in lizards. II. Projections to anterior dorsal ventricular ridge. *J. Comp. Neurol.* 229:602–615.

Bruce, L.L., and T.J. Neary (1995a) Afferent projections to the ventromedial hypothalamus in a lizard, *Gekko gecko. Brain Behav. Evol.* 46:14–29.

Bruce, L.L., and T.J. Neary (1995b) Afferent projections to the lateral and dorsomedial hypothalamus in a lizard, *Gekko gecko. Brain Behav. Evol.* 46:30–42.

Bruce, L.L., and T.J. Neary (1995c) The limbic system of tetrapods: a comparative analysis of cortical and amygdalar populations. *Brain Behav. Evol.* 46:224–234.

Burton, H., and E.G. Jones (1976) The posterior thalamic region and its cortical projection in New World and Old World monkeys. *J. Comp. Neurol.* 168:249–301.

Butler, A.B. (1994a) The evolution of the dorsal thalamus of jawed vertebrates, including mammals: cladistic analysis and a new hypothesis. *Brain Res. Rev.* 19:29–65.

Butler, A.B. (1994b) The evolution of the dorsal pallium in the telencephalon of amniotes: cladistic analysis and a new hypothesis. *Brain Res. Rev.* 19:66–101.

Butler, A.B., and W. Hodos (1996) *Comparative Vertebrate Neuroanatomy: Evolution and Adaptation.* Wiley-Liss, New York.

Butler, A.B., and R.G. Northcutt (1971) Ascending tectal efferent projections in the lizard *Iguana iguana*. *Brain Res.* 35:597–601.
Campbell, C.B.G., and W.R. Hayhow (1971) Primary optic pathways in the echidna *Tachyglossus aculeatus*: an experimental degeneration study. *J. Comp. Neurol.* 143:119–136.
Campbell, C.B.G., and W.R. Hayhow (1972) Primary optic pathways in the duckbill platypus *Ornithorynchus anatinus*: an experimental degeneration study. *J. Comp. Neurol.* 145:195–208.
Campbell, C.B.G., and W. Hodos (1970) The concept of homology and the evolution of the nervous system. *Brain Behav. Evol.* 3:353–367.
Campbell, C.B.G., J.A. Jane, and D. Yashon (1967) The retinal projections of the tree shrew and hedgehog. *Brain Res.* 5:406–418.
Carey, R.G., M.F. Bear, and I.T. Diamond (1980) The laminar organization of the reciprocal projections between the claustrum and striate cortex in the tree shrew *(Tupaia glis)*. *Brain Res.* 184:193–198.
Carpenter, M.B. (1976) *Human Neuroanatomy*, 7th ed. Williams and Wilkins, Baltimore.
Carroll, R.L. (1988) *Vertebrate Paleontology and Evolution*. W.H. Freeman, New York.
Caroll, R. L., and Baird, D. (1972). Carboniferous stem-reptiles of the family Romeriidae. Bull. *Mus. Comp. Zool.*, 143:321–363.
Casseday, J.H., I.T. Diamond, and J.K. Harting (1976) Auditory pathways to the cortex in *Tupaia glis*. *J. Comp. Neurol.* 166:303–340.
Cropper, E.C., J.S. Eisenman, and E.C. Asmitia (1984) An immunocytochemical study of the serotoninergic innervation of the thalamus of the rat. *J. Comp. Neurol.* 224:38–50.
Delius, J.D., and K. Bennetto (1972) Cutaneous sensory projections to the avian forebrain. *Brain Res.* 37:205–221.
Diamond, M.E., M. Armstrong-James, and F.F. Ebner (1992) Somatic sensory responses in the rostral sector of the posterior group (POm) and in the ventral posterior medial nucleus (VPM) of the rat thalamus. *J. Comp. Neurol.* 318:462–476.
Díaz, C., C. Yanes, L. Medina, M. Monzon, C.M. Trujillo, and L. Puelles (1990) Golgi study of the anterior dorsal ventricular ridge in a lizard. I. Neuronal typology in the adult. *J. Morphol.* 203:293–300.
Druga, R., R. Rokyta, and V. Benes, Jr. (1991) Thalamocaudate projections in the macaque monkey (a horseradish peroxidase study). *J. Hirnforsch.* 32:765–774.
Ebbesson, S.O.E. (ed.). (1980) *Comparative Neurology of the Telencephalon*. Plenum Press, New York.
Faull, R.L.M., and W.R. Mehler (1978) The cells of origin of nigrotectal, nigrothalamic and nigrostriatal projections in the rat. *Neuroscience* 3:989–1002.
Feduccia, A. (1996) *Origin and Evolution of Birds*. Yale University Press, New Haven, CT.
Fernandez, A.S., C. Pieau, J. Repérant, E. Boncinelli, and M. Wassef (1998) Expression of the *Emx-1* and *Dlx-1* homeobox genes define three molecularly distinct domains in the telencephalon of mouse, chick, turtle and frog embryos: implications for the evolution of telencephalic subdivisions in amniotes. *Development* 125:2099–2111.
Foster, R.E., and W.C. Hall (1978) The connections and laminar organization of the optic tectum in a reptile *(Iguana iguana)*. *J. Comp. Neurol.* 178:783–832.
Gamlin, P.D.R., and D.H. Cohen (1986) A second ascending visual pathway from the optic tectum to the telencephalon in the pigeon *(Colombia livia)*. *J. Comp. Neurol.* 250:296–310.
González, A., and F.T. Russchen (1988) Connections of the basal ganglia in the lizard *Gekko gecko*. In W.K. Schwerdtfeger and W.J.A.J. Smeets (eds.): *The Forebrain of Reptiles: Current Concepts of Structure and Function*. Karger, Basel, pp. 50–59.
González, A., and F.T. Russchen (1990) Afferent connections of the striatum and the nucleus accumbens in the lizard *Gekko gecko*. *Brain Behav. Evol.* 36:39–58.
Graham, J. (1977) An autoradiographic study of the efferent connections of the superior colliculus in the cat. *J. Comp. Neurol.* 173:629–654.
Graybiel, A.M. (1972) Some fiber pathways related to the posterior thalamic region in the cat. *Brain Behav. Evol.* 6:363–393.
Graybiel, A.M. (1977) Direct and indirect preoculomotor pathways of the brainstem: an autoradiographic study of the pontine reticular formation in the cat. *J. Comp. Neurol.* 175:37–78.
Graybiel, A.M. (1978) The organization of the nigrotectal connection: an experimental tracer study in the cat. *Brain Res.* 143:339–348.
Griffiths, M. (1978) *The Biology of the Monotrems*. Academic press, London.
Gruberg, E.R. (1972) Optic fiber projections of the tiger salamander, *Ambystoma tigrinum*. *J. Hirnforsch.* 14:399–411.

Gruberg, E.R., and V.R. Ambros (1974) A forebrain visual projection in the frog *(Rana pipiens)*. *Exp. Neurol.* 44:187–197.

Guillery, R.W. (1967) Patterns of fiber degeneration in the dorsal lateral geniculate nucleus of the cat following lesions in the visual cortex. *J. Comp. Neurol.* 130:197–222.

Guillery, R.W. (1970) The laminar distribution of retinal fibers in the dorsal lateral geniculate nucleus of the cat: a new interpretation. *J. Comp. Neurol.* 138:339–367.

Haight, J.R., and L. Neylon (1978) An atlas of the dorsal thalamus of the marsupial brush-tailed possum *Trichosurus vulpecula*. *J. Anat.* 126:225–245.

Hall, J.C., and A.S. Feng (1987) Evidence for parallel processing the frog's auditory thalamus. *J. Comp. Neurol.* 258:407–419.

Hall, W.C. (1972) Visual pathway to the telencephalon in reptiles and mammals. *Brain Behav. Evol.* 5:95–113.

Hall, W.C., and F.F. Ebner (1970a) Parallels in the visual afferent projections of the thalamus in the hedgehog *(Paraechinus hypomelas)* and the turtle *(Pseudemys scripta)*. *Brain Behav. Evol.* 3:135–154.

Hall, W.C., and F.F. Ebner (1970b) Thalamotelencephalic projections in the turtle *(Pseudemys scripta)*. *J. Comp. Neurol.* 140:101–122.

Halpern, M. (1972) Some connections of the telencephalon of the frog, *Rana pipiens*. *Brain Behav. Evol.* 6:42–68.

Halpern, M. (1980) The telencephalon of snakes. In. S.O.E. Ebbesson (ed.); *Comparative Neurology of the Telencephalon*. Plenum Press, New York, pp. 257–295.

Harland, W.B., Cox, A.V., Llewellyn, P.G., Pickton, C.A.G., Smith, A.G., and Walters, R. (1982). A Geologic Time Scale. Cambridge University Press, New York.

Heimer, L., D.S. Zahm, and G.F. Alheid (1995) Basal ganglia. In G. Paxinos (ed.); *The Rat Nervous System*, 2nd ed. Academic Press, New York, pp. 579–628.

Hendrickson, A.E., J.R. Wilson, and M.P. Ogren (1978) The neuroanatomical organization of pathways between the dorsal lateral geniculate nucleus and visual cortex in Old World and New World primates. *J. Comp. Neurol.* 182:123–135.

Herkenham, M. (1978) The connections of the nucleus reuniens thalami: evidence for a direct thalamo-hippocampal pathway in the rat. *J. Comp. Neurol.* 177:589–610.

Herkenham, M. (1979) The afferent and efferent connections of the ventromedial thalamic nucleus in the rat. *J. Comp. Neurol.* 183:487–518.

Hodos, W. (1970) Evolutionary interpretation of neural and behavioral studies of living vertebrates. In F.O. Schmitt (ed.); *The Neurosciences: Second Study Program*. Rockefeller University Press, New York, pp. 26–38.

Hodos, W. (1988) Comparative neuroanatomy and the evolution of intelligence. In H.J. Jerison and I.J. Jerison (eds.); *Intelligence and Evolutionary Biology*. Springer-Verlag, Berlin, pp. 93–107.

Hodos, W., and C.B.G. Campbell (1969) *Scala naturae*: why there is no theory in comparative psychology. *Psychol. Rev.* 76:337–350.

Hohl-Abrahao, J.C., and O.D. Creutzfeldt (1991) Topographical mapping of the thalamocortical projections in rodents and comparison with that in primates. *Exp. Brain Res.* 87:283–294.

Hoogland, P.V. (1981) Spinothalamic projections in a lizard, *Varnus exanthematicus*: an HRP study. *J. Comp. Neurol.* 198:7–12.

Hoogland, P.V. (1982) Brainstem afferents to the thalamus in a lizard, *Varnus exanthematicus*. *J. Comp. Neurol.* 210:152–162.

Hoogland, P.V., and E. Vermeulen-Van der Zee (1989) Efferent connections of the dorsal cortex of the lizard *Gekko gecko* studied with *Phaseolus vulgaris–leucoagglutinin*. *J. Comp. Neurol.* 285:289–303.

Hopson, J.A. (1979) Paleoneurology. In C. Gans, R.G. Northcutt, and P. Ulinski (eds.); *Biology of the Reptilia*, vol. 9. Academic Press, New York, pp. 39–146.

Horn, G. (1985) *Memory, Imprinting, and the Brain*. Oxford University Press, New York.

Husband, S.A., and T. Shimizu (1999) Efferent connections of the ectostriatum in the pigeon *(Columba livia)*. *J. Comp. Neurol.* 406, 329–345.

Itaya, S.K., G.W. Van Hoesen, and L.A. Benevento (1986) Direct retinal pathways to the limbic thalamus of the monkey. *Exp. Brain. Res.* 61:607–613.

Itoh, K., T. Kaneko, M. Kudo, and N. Mizuno (1984) The intercollicular region in the cat: a possible relay in the parallel somatosensory pathways from the dorsal column nuclei to the posterior complex of the thalamus. *Brain Res.* 308:166–171.

5 Evolution of the Forebrain in Tetrapods

Jarvik, E. (1955) The oldest tetrapods and their forerunners. *Sci. Monthly*, 80:141–154.
Jenkins, F.A. Jr., and F.R. Parrington (1976) The postcranial skeletons of the Triassic mammals *Eozostrodon*, *Megazostrodon*, and *Erythrotherium*. *Philos. Trans. R. Soc. Lond. Biol.* 273:387–431.
Jerison, H.J. (1973) *Evolution of the Brain and Intelligence*. Academic Press, New York.
Jerison, H.J., and I. Jerison (1988) *Intelligence and Evolutionary Biology*. Springer-Verlag, Berlin.
Ji, Q., P.J. Currie, M. Norell, and S.A. Ji (1998) Two feathered dinosaurs from northeastern China. *Nature* 393:753–761.
Jones, E.G. (1985) *The Thalamus*. Plenum Press, New York.
Jones, E.G., and R.Y. Leavitt (1974) Retrograde axonal transport and the demonstration of non-specific projections to the cerebral cortex and striatum from thalamic intralaminar nuclei in the rat, cat and monkey. *J. Comp. Neurol.* 154:349–378.
Jones, E.G., and A. Peters (eds.) (1990) *Cerebral Cortex, vol. 8A and B, Comparative Structure and Evolution of Cerebral Cortex, Part I and II*. Plenum Press, New York.
Jones, E.G., and T.P.S. Powell (1970) Connections of the somatic sensory cortex of the rhesus monkey. III. Thalamic connections. *Brain* 93:37–56.
Kaas, J.H., M.F. Huerta, J.T. Weber, and J.K. Harting (1978) Patterns of retinal terminations and laminar organization of the lateral geniculate nucleus of primates. *J. Comp. Neurol.* 182:517–554.
Kalil, K. (1981) Projections of the cerebellar and dorsal column nuclei upon the thalamus of the rhesus monkey. *J. Comp. Neurol.* 195:25–50.
Källén, B. (1962) Embryogenesis of brain nuclei in the chick telencephalon. *Ergebn. Anat. Entwgesch.* 36:62–82.
Karten, H.J. (1967) The ascending auditory pathway in the pigeon (*Colombia livia*). I. Diencephalic projections of the inferior colliculus (nucleus mesencephali lateralis, pars dorsalis). *Brain Res.* 6:409–427.
Karten, H.J. (1968) The ascending auditory pathway in the pigeon (*Colombia livia*). II. Telencephalic projections of the nucleus ovoidalis thalami. *Brain Res.* 11:134–153.
Karten, H.J. (1969) The organization of the avian telencephalon and some speculations on the phylogeny of the amniote telencephalon. *Ann. N.Y. Acad. Sci.* 167:164–179.
Karten, H.J. (1991) Homology and evolutionary origin of the "neocortex". *Brain Behav. Evol.* 38:264–272.
Karten, H.J. (1997) Evolutionary developmental biology meets the brain: the origins of mammalian cortex. *Proc. Natl. Acad. Sci. U.S.A.* 94:2800–2804.
Karten, H.J., and J.L. Dubbeldam (1973) The organization and projections of the paleostriatal complex in the pigeon *(Columba livia)*. *J. Comp. Neurol.* 148:61–90.
Karten, H.J., and Hodos, W. (1970) Telencephalic projections of the nucleus rotundas in the pigeon *(Colombia livia)*. *J. Comp. Neurol.* 140:35–52.
Karten, H.J., W. Hodos, W.J.H. Nauta, and A.M. Revzin (1973) Neural connections of the "visual Wulst" of the avian telencephalon. Experimental studies in the pigeon *(Colombia livia)* and owl *(Speotyto cunicularia)*. *J. Comp. Neurol.* 150:253–278.
Karten, H.J., and A.M. Revzin (1966) The afferent connections of the nucleus rotundus in the pigeon. *Brain Res.* 2:368–377.
Karten, H.J., and T. Shimizu (1989) The origins of neocortex: connections and lamination as distinct events in evolution. *J. Cogn. Neurosci.* 1:291–301.
Kawamura, S., J.M. Sprague, and K. Niimi (1974) Corticofugal projections from the visual cortices to the thalamus, pretectum and superior colliculus in the cat. *J. Comp. Neurol.* 158:339–362.
Kicliter, E. (1979) Some telencephalic connections in the frog, *Rana pipiens*. *J. Comp. Neurol.* 185:75–86.
Kitt, C.A., and S.E. Brauth (1982) A paleostriatal-thalamic-telencephalic path in pigeons. *Neuroscience* 7:2735–2751.
Kokoros, J.J., and R.G. Northcutt (1977) Telencephalic efferents of the tiger salamander *Ambystoma tigrinum* (Green). *J. Comp. Neurol.* 178:613–628.
Korzeniewska, E., and O. Güntürkün (1990) Sensory properties and afferents of the n. dorsolateralis posterior thalami of the pigeon. *J. Comp. Neurol.* 292:457–479.
Krettek, J.E., and J.L. Price (1977) The cortical projections of the mediodorsal nucleus and adjacent thalamic nuclei in the rat. *J. Comp. Neurol.* 171:157–191.
Krubitzer, L.A., and J.H. Kaas (1992) The somatosensory thalamus of monkeys: cortical connections and a redefinition of nuclei in marmosets. *J. Comp. Neurol.* 319:123–140.
Kudo, M., and K. Niimi (1980) Ascending projection of the inferior colliculus in the cat: an autoradiographic study. *J. Comp. Neurol.* 191:545–556.

LeDoux, J.E., C. Farb, and D.A. Ruggiero (1990) Topographic organization of neurons in the acoustic thalamus that project to the amygdala. *J. Neurosci.* 10:1043–1054.
LeVay, S., and H. Sherk (1981) The visual claustrum of the cat. I. Structure and connections. *J. Neurosci.* 1:956–980.
Lin, C.S., P.J. May, and W.C. Hall (1984) Nonintralaminar thalamostriatal projections in the gray squirrel (*Sciurus carolinensis*) and tree shrew *(Tupaia glis). J. Comp. Neurol.* 230:33–46.
Lohman, A.H.M., and W.J.A.J. Smeets (1991) The dorsal ventricular ridge and cortex of reptiles in historical and phylogenetic perspective. In B.L. Finlay, G. Innocenti, and H. Scheich (eds.); *The Neocortex: Ontogeny and Phylogeny*. Plenum Press, New York, pp. 59–74.
Lohman, A.H.M., and W.J.A.J. Smeets (1993) Overview of the main and accessory olfactory bulb projections in reptiles. *Brain Behav. Evol.* 41:147–155.
MacLean, P.D. (1990) *The Triune Brain in Evolution*. Plenum Press, New York.
Macphail, E.M. (1982) *Brain and Intelligence in Vertebrates*. Oxford University Press, New York.
Marín, O., A. Gonzalez, and W.J. Smeets (1997a) Basal ganglia organization in amphibians: afferent connections to the striatum and the nucleus accumbens. *J. Comp. Neurol.* 378:16–49.
Marín, O., A. Gonzalez, and W.J. Smeets (1997b) Basal ganglia organization in amphibians: efferent connections to the striatum and the nucleus accumbens. *J. Comp. Neurol.* 380:23–50.
Marín, O., A. Gonzalez, and W.J. Smeets (1997c) Anatomical substrate of amphibian basal ganglia involvement in visuomotor behaviour. *Eur. J. Neurosci.* 9:2100–2109.
McDonald, A.J. (1998) Cortical pathways to the mammalian amygdala. *Prog. Neurobiol.* 55:257–332.
Medina, L., and W.J.A.J. Smeets (1981) Comparative aspects of the basal ganglia–tectal pathways in reptiles. *J. Comp. Neurol.* 308:614–629.
Miceli, D., L. Marchand, J. Repérant, and J.-P. Rio (1990) Projections of the dorsolateral anterior complex and adjacent thalamic nuclei upon the visual Wulst in the pigeon. *Brain Res.* 518:317–323.
Miceli, D., J. Peyrichoux, and J. Repérant (1975) The retinothalamo-hyperstriatal pathway in the pigeon *(Colombia livia). Brain Res.* 100:125–131.
Montgomery, N.M., and K.V. Fite (1991) Organization of ascending projections from the optic tectum and mesencephalic pretectal gray in *Rana pipiens. Vis. Neurosci.* 7:459–478.
Nauta, W.J.H., and H.J. Karten (1970) A general profile of the vertebrate brain, with sidelights on the ancestry of cerebral cortex. In F.O. Schmitt (ed.); *The Neurosciences: Second Study Program*. Rockefeller University Press, New York, pp. 7–26.
Neary, T.J. (1974) Diencephalic efferents of the torus semicircularis in the bullfrog, *Rana catesbeiana. Anat. Rec.* 425.
Neary, T.J. (1984) Anterior thalamic nucleus projections to the dorsal pallium in ranid frogs. *Neurosci. Lett.* 51:213–218.
Neary, T.J. (1990) The pallium of anuran amphibians. In E.G. Jones and A. Peters (eds.) *Cerebral Cortex, vol. 8A: Comparative Structure and Evolution of Cerebral Cortex, Part I*. Plenum Press, New York, pp. 107–138.
Neary, T.J. (1995) Afferent projections to the hypothalamus in ranid frogs. *Brain Behav. Evol.* 46:1–13.
Neary, T.J., and W. Wilczynski (1977) Ascending thalamic projections from the obex region in ranid frogs. *Brain Res.* 138:529–533.
Northcutt, R.G. (1981) Evolution of the telencephalon in nonmammals. *Annu. Rev. Neurosci.* 4:301–350.
Northcutt, R.G. (1984) Evolution of the vertebrate central nervous system: patterns and processes. *Am. Zool.* 24:701–716.
Northcutt, R.G., and J.H. Kaas (1995) The emergence and evolution of mammalian neocortex. *TINS*, 18:373–379.
Northcutt, R.G., and E. Kicliter (1980) Organization of the amphibian telencephalon. In S.O.E. Ebbesson (ed.); *Comparative Neurology of the Telenchepalon*. Plenum Press, New York, pp. 203–255.
Northcutt, R.G., and M. Ronan (1992) Afferent and efferent connections of the bullfrog medial pallium. *Brain Behav. Evol.* 40:1–16.
Northcutt, R.G., and G.J. Royce (1975) Olfactory bulb projections in the bullfrog, *Rana catesbeiana. J. Morphol.* 145:251–268.
Nottebohm, F., T.M. Stokes, and C.M. Leonard (1976) Central control of song in the canary, *Serinus carius. J. Comp. Neurol.* 165:457–486.
Oliver, D.L., and W.C. Hall (1978) The medial geniculate body of the tree shrew *Tupaia glis*. II. Connections with the neocortex. *J. Comp. Neurol.* 182:459–494.

Ostrom, J.H. (1976) Archaeopteryx and the origin of birds. *Biol. J. Linn. Soc.* 8:91–182.
Parent, A. (1986) *Comparative Neurobiology of the Basal Ganglia.* John Wiley, New York.
Parent, A., and L.N. Hazrati (1995a) Functional anatomy of the basal ganglia. I. The cortico-basal ganglia-thalamo-cortical loop. *Brain Res. Rev.* 20:91–127.
Parent, A., and L.N. Hazrati (1995b) Functional anatomy of the basal ganglia. II. The place of subthalamic nucleus and external pallidum in basal ganglia circuitry. *Brain Res. Rev.* 20:128–154.
Paxinos, G. (ed.) (1995) *The Rat Nervous System*, 2nd ed. Academic Press, New York.
Pettigrew, J.D., and M. Konishi (1976) Neurons selective for orientation and binocular disparity in the visual Wulst of the barn owl *(Tyto alba). Science* 193:675–678.
Price, J.L. (1995) Thalamus. In G. Paxinos (ed.); *The Rat Nervous System* 2nd ed. Academic Press, New York, pp. 629–648.
Price, J.L., and F.T. Russchen, and D.G. Amaral (1987) The limbic region. II. The amygdaloid complex. In A. Björklund, T. Hökfelt, and L.W. Swanson (eds.); *Handbook of Chemical Neuroanatomy*, vol. 5. Elsevier, Amsterdam, pp. 279–388.
Pritz, M.B. (1974a) Ascending connections of a midbrain auditory area in a crocodile, *Caiman crocodilus. J. Comp. Neurol.* 153:179–198.
Pritz, M.B. (1974b) Ascending connections of a thalamic auditory area in a crocodile, *Caiman crocodilus. J. Comp. Neurol.* 153:199–214.
Pritz, M.B. (1975) Anatomical identification of a telencephalic visual area in crocodiles: ascending connections of nucleus rotundus in *Caimen crocodilus. J. Comp. Neurol.* 164:323–338.
Pritz, M.B., and R.G. Northcutt (1980) Anatomical evidence for an ascending somatosensory pathway to the telencephalon in crocodiles, *Caiman crocodilus. Exp. Brain Res.* 40:342–345.
Pritz, M.B., and Stritzel, M.E. (1990) Thalamic projections from a midbrain somatosensory area in a reptile, *Caiman crocodilus. Brain Behav. Evol.* 36:1–13.
Pritz, M.B., and M.E. Stritzel (1994) Anatomical identification of a telencephalic somatosensory area in a reptile. *Brain Behav. Evol.* 43:107–127.
Quiroga, J.C. (1980) The brain of the mammal-like reptile *Probainognathus jensini* (Therapsida, Cynodontia). A correlative paleo-neonurological approach to the neocortex at the reptile-mammal transition. *J. Hirnforsch.* 21:299–336.
Rainey, W.T., and E.G. Jones (1983) Spatial distribution of individual medial lemniscal axons in the thalamic ventrobasal complex of the cat. *Exp. Brain Res.* 49:229–246.
Rausell, E., and E.G. Jones (1991) Chemically distinct compartments of the thalamic VPM nucleus in monkeys relay principal and spinal trigeminal pathways to different layers of the somatosensory cortex. *J. Neurosci.* 11:226–237.
Regidor, J., and I. Divac (1987) Architectonics of the thalamus in the echidna *(Tachyglossus aculeatus)*: search for the mediodorsal nucleus. *Brain Behav. Evol.* 30:328–341.
Reiner, A. (1991) A comparison of neurotransmitter-specific and neuropeptide-specific neuronal cell types in turtle cortex to those present in mammalian isocortex: implications for the evolution of isocortex. *Brain Behav. Evol.* 38:53–91.
Reiner, A. (1993) Neurotransmitter organization and connections of turtle cortex: implications for the evolution of mammalian isocortex. *Comp. Biochem. Physiol.* 104A:735–748.
Reiner, A., S.A. Brauth, and H.J. Karten (1984) Evolution of the amniote basal ganglia. *TINS* 7:320–325.
Reiner, A., S.E. Brauth, C.A. Kitt, and H.J. Karten (1980) Basal ganglionic pathways to the tectum: studies in reptiles. *J. Comp. Neurol.* 193:565–589.
Reiner, A., N.C. Brecha, and H.J. Karten (1982a) Basal ganglia pathways to the tectum: the afferent and efferent connections of the lateral spiriformi nucleus of the pigeon. *J. Comp. Neurol.* 208:16–36.
Reiner, A., H.J. Karten, and N.C. Brecha (1982b) Enkephalin-mediated basal ganglia influences over the optic tectum: immunohistochemistry of the tectum and the lateral spiriform nucleus in the pigeon. *J. Comp. Neurol.* 208:37–53.
Reisz, R. (1981). A diapsid reptile from the Pennsylvanian of Kansas. Univ. Kansas, *Mus. Nat. Hist., Spec. Publ.*, 7: 1–74.
Ritchie, T.L.C. (1979) *Intratelencephalic Visual Connections and Their Relationship to the Archistriatum in the Pigeon (Columba livia).* Unpublished Ph.D. dissertation, University of Virginia.
Robertson, R.T., S.M. Thompson, and S.S. Kaitz (1983) Projections from the pretectal complex to the thalamic lateral dorsal nucleus of the cat. *Exp. Brain Res.* 51:157–171.
Romer, A.S. (1959) *Vertebrate Story*, 4th ed. University of Chicago Press, Chicago.
Romer, A.S. (1966) *Vertebrate Paleontology*, 3rd ed. University of Chicago Press, Chicago.

References 183

Romer, A.S. (1970) *Vertebrate Body*, 4th ed. W. B. Saunders, Philadelphia.
Rowe, M. (1990) Organization of the cerebral cortex in monotermes and marsupials. In E.G. Jones and A. Peters (eds.); *Cerebral Cortex, vol. 8B, Comparative Structure and Evolution of Cerebral Cortex, Part II*. Plenum Press, New York, pp. 263–334.
Royce, G.J. (1983) Cortical neurons with collateral projections to both the caudate nucleus and the centromedian-parafascicular thalamic complex: a fluorescent retrograde double labeling study in the cat. *Exp. Brain Res.* 50:157–165.
Rubinson, K. (1968) Projections of the tectum opticum of the frog. *Brain Behav. Evol.* 1:529–561.
Sadikot, A.F., A. Parent, Y. Smith, and J.P. Bolam (1992) Efferent connections of the centromedian and parafascicular thalamic nuclei in the squirrel monkey: a light and electron microscopic study of the thalamostriatal projection in relation to striatal heterogeneity. *J. Comp. Neurol.* 320:228–242.
Sarnat, H.B., and M.G. Netsky (1981) *Evolution of the Nervous System*. Oxford University Press, New York.
Scalia, F. (1972) The projection of the accessory olfactory bulb in the frog. *Brain Res.* 36:409–411.
Scalia, F., G. Gallousis, and S. Roca (1991) Differential projections of the main and accessory olfactory bulb in the frog. *J. Comp. Neurol.* 305:443–461.
Scalia, F., and K. Gregory (1970) Retinofugal projections in the frog. Location of postsynaptic neurons. *Brain Behav. Evol.* 3:16–29.
Scalia, F., M. Halpern, H. Knapp, and W. Riss (1968) The efferent connexions of the olfactory bulb in the frog, a study of degenerating unmyelinated fibers. *J. Anat.* 103:245–262.
Seeley, K. (1888). Researches on the structure, organization and classification of the fossil Reptilia. 1. On *Protorosaurus speneri* (von Meyer) *Phil. Trans. Roy. Soc. London.*, B, 178: 187–213.
Sherk, H. (1986) The calustrum and the cerebral cortex. In E.G. Jones and A. Peters (eds.); *Cerebral Cortex, vol. 5: Sensory-Motor Areas and Aspects of Cortical Connectivity*. Plenum Press, New York, pp. 467–499.
Shimizu, T., K. Cox, and H.J. Karten (1995) Intratelencephalic projections of the visual Wulst in pigeons *(Columba livia)*. *J. Comp. Neurol.* 359:551–572.
Simpson, G.G. (1961) *Principles of Animal Taxonomy*. Columbia University press, New York.
Smeets, W.J.A.J., and A. González (1994) Sensorimotor integration in the brain of reptiles. *Eur. J. Morphol.* 32:299–302.
Smeets, W.J.A.J., and A. Reiner (1994) *Phylogeny and Development of Catecholamine Systems in the CNS of Vertebrates*. Cambridge University Press, New York.
Striedter, G.F. (1997) The telencephalon of tetrapods in evolution. *Brain Behav. Evol.* 49. 179–213.
Swanson, L.W. (1987) The hypothalamus. In A. Björklund, T. Hökfelt, and L.W. Swanson (eds.); *Handbook of Chemical Neuroanatomy*, vol. 5. Elsevier, Amsterdam, pp. 1–124.
Symonds, L.L., A.C. Rosenquist, S.B. Edwards, and L.A. Palmer (1981) Projections of the puvinar–lateral posterior complex to visual cortical areas in the cat. *Neuroscience* 6:1995–2020.
Takada, M. (1992) The lateroposterior thalamic nucleus and substantia nigra pars lateralis: origin of dual innervation over the visual system and basal ganglia. *Neurosci. Lett.* 139:153–156.
ten Donkelaar, H.J., and R. de Boer-van Huizen (1981) Basal ganglia projections to the brain stem in the lizard *Varanus exanthematicus* as demonstrated by retrograde transport of horseradish peroxidase. *Neuroscience* 6:1567–1590.
ten Donkelaar, H.J., R. de Boer-van Huizen, F.T.M. Schouten, and S.J.H. Eggen (1981) Cells of origin of descending pathways to the spinal cord in the clawed toad *(Xenopus laevis)*. *Neurosciences* 6:2297–2312.
Thompson, S.M., and T.R. Robertson (1987) Organization of subcortical pathways for sensory projections to the limbic cortex. II. Afferent projections to the thalamic lateral dorsal nucleus in the rat. *J. Comp. Neurol.* 265:189–202.
Tivers, R.L. (1972) Parental investment and sexual selection. In B. Campbell (ed.); *Sexual Selection and the Descent of Man*. Aldine de Gruyter, New York.
Tsai, H.M., B.B. Garber, and L.M.H. Larramendi (1981a) Thymidine autoradiographic analysis of telencephalic histogenesis in the chick embryo: I. Neuronal birthdates of telencephalic compartments in situ. *J. Comp. Neurol.* 198:275–292.
Tsai, H.M., B.B. Garber, and L.M.H. Larramendi (1981b) Thymidine autoradiographic analysis of telencephalic histogenesis in the chick embryo: II. Dynamics of neuronal migration, displacement, and aggregation. *J. Comp. Neurol.* 198:293–306.
Turner, B.H., and M. Herkenham (1991) Thalamoamygdaloid projections in the rat: a test of the amygdala's role in sensory processing. *J. Comp. Neurol.* 313:295–325.

Ulinski, P.S. (1983) *Dorsal Ventricular Ridge.* John Wiley, New York.
Ulinski, P S (1984) Thalamic projections to the somatosensory cortex of the echidna *Tachyglossus aculeatus. J. Comp. Neurol.* 229:153–170.
Ulinski, P.S. (1990a) Nodal events in forebrain evolution. *Neth. J. Zool.* 40:215–240.
Ulinski, P.S. (1990b) The cerebral cortex of reptiles. In E.G. Jones and A. Peters (eds.); *Cerebral Cortex, vol. 8A: Comparative Structure and Evolution of Cerebral Cortex, Part I.* Plenum Press, New York, pp. 139–215.
Ulinski, P.S., and D. Margoliash (1990) Neurobiology of the reptile-bird transition. In E.G. Jones and A. Peters (eds.); *Cerebral Cortex, vol. 8A: Comparative Structure and Evolution of Cerebral Cortex, Part I.* Plenum Press, New York, pp. 217–265.
Ulinski, P.S., and E.H. Peterson (1981) Patterns of olfactory projections in the desert iguana, *Dipsosaurus dorsalis. J. Morphol.* 168:189–228.
Updyke, B.V. (1981) Projections from visual areas of the middle suprasylvian sulcus onto the lateral posterior complex and adjacent thalamic nuclei in the cat. *J. Comp. Neurol.* 201:477–506.
Veenman, C.L., L. Medina, and A. Reiner (1997) Avian homologues of mammalian intralaminar, mediodorsal, and midline thalamic nuclei: immunohistochemical and hodological evidence. *Brain Behav. Evol.* 49:78–98.
Veenman, C.L., J.M. Wild, and A. Reiner (1995) Organization of the avian "corticostriatal projection system: a retrograde and anterograde pathway tracing study in pigeons. *J. Comp. Neurol.* 354:87–126.
Vogt, L.J. B.A., Vogt, and R.W. Sikes (1992) Limbic thalamus in rabbit: architecture, projections to cingulate cortex and distribution of muscarinic acetylcholine, GABA $_A$ and opioid receptors. *J. Comp. Neurol.* 319:205–217.
Welker, W.I. (1973) Principles of organization of the ventrobasal complex in mammals. *Brain Behav. Evol.* 7:253–336.
Welker, W., and R.A. Lende (1980) Thalamocortical relationships in echidna *(Tachyglossus aculeatus).* In S.O.E. Ebbesson (ed.); *Comparative Neurology of the Telencephalon.* Plenum Press, New York, pp. 449–481.
Wellnofer, P. (1978). Pterosauria. In P. Wellnofer (ed.), *Handbuch der Paläoherpetologie.* Part 19; pp. 1–82.
Wicht, H., and W. Himstedt (1988) Topologic and connectional analysis of the dorsal thalamus of *Triturus alpestris* (Amphibia, Urodela, Salamandridae). *J. Comp. Neurol.* 267:545–561.
Wilczyniski, W. (1981) Afferents to the midbrain auditory center in the bull frog, *Rana catesbeiana. J. Comp. Neurol.* 198:421–433.
Wilczyniski, W., and R.G. Northcutt (1977) Afferents to the optic tectum in the leopard frog: an HRP study. *J. Comp. Neurol.* 173:219–229.
Wilczyniski, W., and R.G. Northcutt (1983a) Connections of the bullfrog striatum: afferent organization. *J. Comp. Neurol.* 214:321–332.
Wilczyniski, W., and R.G. Northcutt (1983b) Connections of the bullfrog striatum: efferent organization. *J. Comp. Neurol.* 214:333–343.
Wild, J.M. (1987a) Thalamic projections to the paleostriatum and neostriatum in the pigeon *(Colombia livia). Neuroscience* 20:305–327
Wild, J.M. (1987b) The avian somatosensory system: connections of regions of body representation in the forebrain of the pigeon. *Brain Res.* 412:205–223.
Wild, J.M. (1989) Avian somatosensory system. II. Ascending projections of the dorsal column and external cuneate nuclei in the pigeon. *J. Comp. Neurol.* 287:1–18.
Wild, J.M., H.J. Karten, and B.J. Frost (1993) Connections of the auditory forebrain in the pigeon *(Columba livia). J. Comp. Neurol.* 337:32–62.
Zeier, H.J., and H.J. Karten (1971) The archistriatum of the pigeon: organization of afferent and efferent connections. *Brain Res.* 31:313–326.
Zeigler, H.P., and H.J. Karten (1973) Brain mechanisms and feeding behavior in the pigeon *(Columba livia).* Quinto-frontal structures. *J. Comp. Neurol.* 152:59–81.
Zilles, K., and A. Wree (1995) Cortex: areal and laminar structure. In G. Paxinos (ed.); *The Rat Nervous System*, 2nd ed. Academic Press, New York, pp. 649–688.

Chapter 6

NEOCORTICAL MACROCIRCUITS

Rudolf Nieuwenhuys, Hanse Institute for Advanced Study, Delmenhorst

INTRODUCTION

The origin, expansion, and differentiation of the neocortex are doubtless major events in the evolution of the vertebrate brain. Although numerous authors (for review, see Reiner, 1991) have claimed that the dorsal or general cortex of reptiles represents, or at least contains, a primordial neocortex, it is generally agreed that a fully developed neocortex, to be defined as a superficial, six-layered structure, situated within the pallial part of the telencephalic hemispheres, is only present in mammals.

The size of the neocortex varies greatly among the various mammalian groups (cf. Nieuwenhuys et al., 1998, Chapters 22 and 23). In insectivores, its size does not exceed that of the "older" parts of the cortex, but in primates and cetaceans it attains remarkable dimensions, becoming by far the largest center in the brain. As regards the differentiation of the neocortex, it is known that in primitive mammals much of the neocortex is occupied by areas that either receive, via the thalamus, impulses directly related to the various special senses (somatic sensibility, vision, audition) or are concerned with the steering of motor activity.

There is evidence suggesting that already in primitive mammals the various sensory projection areas are separated from each other by strips of nonprojection cortex (cf. Ramon y Cajal, 1911, p. 830 and Fig. 531). If we study the functional differentiation of the neocortex in the series insectivores/prosimians/simians/humans, it appears that the initially narrow strips of nonprojection cortex expand to form a large area known as the *parieto-occipito-temporal association cortex*. Another area of association cortex develops in front of the motor cortical areas. This region is designated as the *prefrontal association cortex*. In humans the association areas are much more extensive than the sensory and motor projection areas. All cortical areas maintain afferent and efferent connections with subcortical centers. It should be emphasized, however, that the various association areas are primarily connected with other neocortical fields.

This Chapter reviews the functional organization of the human neocortex at the macrocircuit level (for discussion of the neocortical microcircuitry, see Nieuwenhuys, 1994; and Nieuwenhuys et al., 1998, Chapter 22). The major sensorimotor projections are considered first. It is shown that the various association areas represent important way stations in these projections. Next, the sensorimotor projections are placed within the wider context of cortical and cortico-subcortical circuitry. It is pointed out that many of the neuronal links, composing the sensorimotor projections, are reciprocated by feedback loops and that several other functional systems, including the ascending reticular system and the greater limbic system, have access to the neocortical circuitry. Finally, attention is drawn to the remarkable fact that certain parts of the thalamus, the caudate nucleus, and the cerebellum receive their principal afferents from the neocortex and project back to neocortical association areas. Functionally, these structures have to be considered as neocortical dependencies.

MAJOR SENSORIMOTOR PROJECTIONS

Sensory pathways within the central nervous system connect primary afferents with specific areas of the contralateral cerebral cortex (Fig. 6.1). The somatosensory projections, which relay impulses originating from sensors situated on the body surface, from muscle spindles and joint receptors, pass, via the dorsal column nuclei in the lower medulla oblongata, and the ventral posterior nucleus of the thalamus, to the primary somatosensory area of the neocortex, situated directly behind the central sulcus, in the parietal lobe. The conscious component of this somatosensory projection, which subserves what is called *gnostic sensibility*, is first and foremost involved in active tactile exploration. The auditory projection reaches the primary auditory cortex on the upper surface of the temporal lobe via the cochlear nuclei, the superior olivary complex, and the medial geniculate body. The visual projection, finally, extends from the retina to the primary visual cortex in the occipital lobe and is synaptically interrupted in the lateral geniculate body. The three primary sensory cortical areas, which lie far apart in the posterior half of the cerebral hemispheres, all display a typical granular or koniocortex and, hence, are easily delineated on cytoarchitectonic grounds.

The central sulcus, or sulcus Rolandi, represents a very important landmark in the human brain because it divides the cerebral hemispheres into an anterior or pre-Rolandic, primarily motor, and a posterior or post-Rolandic, primarily sensory, region. The surface of the latter, which encompasses the parietal, the temporal, as well as the occipital lobes of the cerebral hemispheres, is mainly occupied by sensory association areas.

Experimental studies carried out in monkeys and extrapolated here to the human (Pandya and Kuypers, 1969; Jones and Powell, 1970; Pandya and Yeterian, 1985) have revealed that each primary sensory area is flanked by a cortical belt, which receives its main input from cascades of short association fibers originating from the same adjoining primary sensory cortical regions. These cortical belts, which are concerned with the further processing of modality-specific inputs, are termed *unimodal association areas*. The unimodal association areas can be divided into upstream and downstream sectors. The former are only one synapse away from the corresponding primary sensory area, whereas the latter are at a distance of two or more synapses from the relevant primary sensory area (Hackett et al., 1998a,b;

Major Sensorimotor Projections 187

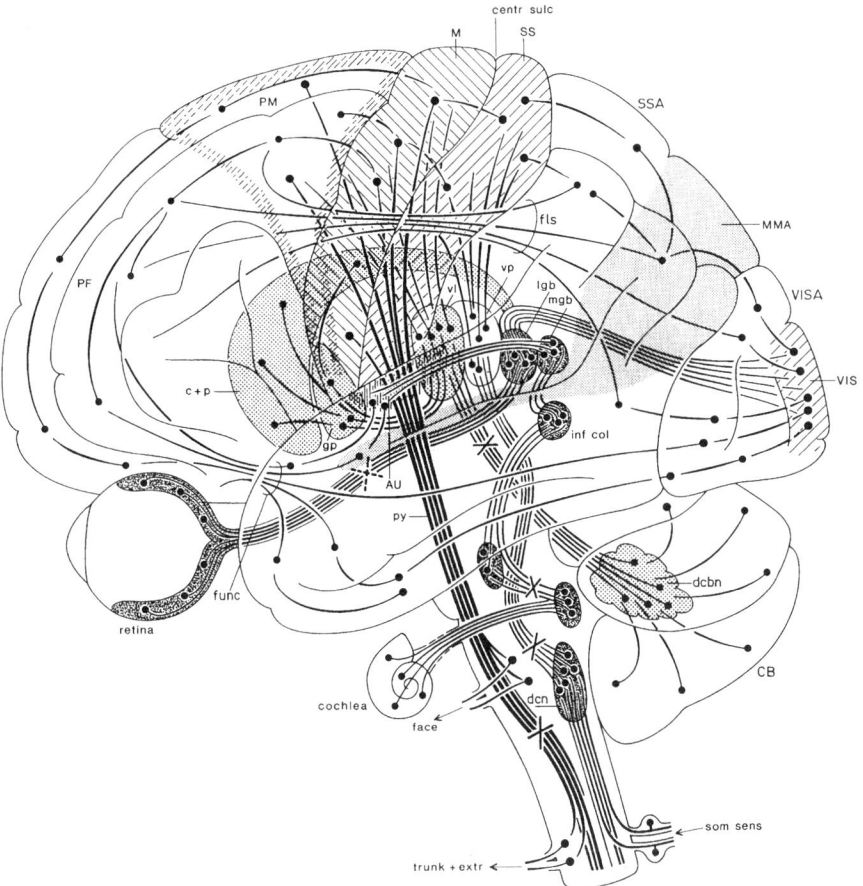

Figure 6.1. Diagrammatic representation of the great sensory and motor systems in the human brain. Some pathways related to the cortical association system, the basal ganglia, and the cerebellum are also shown. AU, primary auditory cortex; c+p, caudate nucleus + putamen; CB, cerebellum; centr sulc, central sulcus; dcn, dorsal column nuclei; dcbn, deep cerebellar nuclei; extr, extremities; fls, fasciculus longitudinalis superior; func, fasciculus uncinatus; gp, globus pallidus; inf col, inferior colliculus; lgb, lateral geniculate body; M, primary motor cortex; MMA, multimodal association cortex; mgb, medial geniculate body; PF, prefrontal cortex; PM, premotor cortex; pcn, posterior column nuclei, py, pyramidal tract; SS, primary somatosensory cortex; SSA, somatosensory association cortex; som sens, somatic sensibility; VIS, primary visual cortex; VISA; visual association cortex; vl, ventral lateral thalamic nucleus; vp, ventral posterior thalamic nucleus. (Modified from Nieuwenhuys, 1996.)

Mesulam, 1998). The upstream sectors of unimodal association areas encode basic features of sensation such as texture, tone, motion and color, whereas the downstream sectors of these areas serve more complex functions, like the detection and recognition of specific objects, sound sequences, and faces.

The somatosensory association cortex is situated in the parietal lobe directly behind the postcentral gyrus; the auditory association cortex occupies much of the superior temporal gyrus, whereas the visual association area extends far rostrally into the lower parts of the temporal lobe.

In the sensory association areas not only sequential but also parallel processing of information takes place. Thus, within the visual association area, the occipitofugal flow of information takes the form of two divergent multisynaptic pathways, a relatively short, dorsal pathway directed toward the caudal parietal lobe and a long, ventral pathway directed toward the downstream visual association area in the rostral inferior temporal cortex. The dorsal pathway is specialized for encoding spatial attributes of visual information. The ventral pathway is mainly concerned with the identification of objects and faces (Ungerleider and Mishkin, 1982; Mesulam, 1994).

Interestingly, at the junction of the three unimodal or modality-specific sensory association areas a multimodal association area is found, which receives converging afferents from its surrounding cortical fields. This multimodal association area forms a strip, extending forward from the junction of the occipital and parietal lobes along the superior temporal sulcus into the anterior part of the temporal lobe (MMA in Fig. 6.1).

The next step of sensorifugal processing may be characterized as "the great leap forward" from the post-Rolandic to the pre-Rolandic cortical region. The pre-Rolandic region, which coincides with the cortex of the frontal lobe, can be divided into the primary motor cortex, the premotor cortex, and the prefrontal cortex. The motor cortex, which corresponds to area 4 of Brodmann, is located in the rostral wall of the central sulcus and in the caudal part of the precentral gyrus. The premotor cortex lies, as its name implies, in front of the motor cortex. It includes areas 6 and 8. The motor portion of the pyramidal tract arises largely from the motor and premotor areas. The vast prefrontal cortex, which occupies the remainder of the frontal lobe neither receives projections from subcortical sensory centers, nor sends out fibers to lower motor nuclei and should, hence, be characterized as an association area. The premotor and motor areas participate in the preparation and execution of voluntary movements. The prefrontal cortex is critically involved in the planning and in the temporal organization of action, whether in the form of somatic movement, ocular motility, or spoken language (Fuster, 1993).

The morphological substrate of "the great leap forward" mentioned above is formed by two large fiber systems, the longitudinal superior and uncinate fascicles. By way of these fascicles, fibers arising from the various unimodal association areas as well as from the multimodal association area pass rostrally to terminate in the prefrontal and premotor areas (Pandya and Kuypers, 1969; Pandya and Yeterian, 1985; Petrides and Pandya, 1984, 1988; Neal et al., 1990; Matelli et al., 1998; Hackett et al., 1999; Romanski et al., 1999). An important output system of the prefrontal cortex is formed by sequences of short association fibers, which successively link the orbital frontal cortex (areas 11 and 12), the various prefrontal areas (10, 45, 46, and 9), the premotor areas 6 and 8, and the primary motor area 4 (Pandya and Yeterian, 1985; Morelli et al., 1986; Leichnetz, 1986; Lu et al., 1994). This suggests that highly processed somatosensory, visual, auditory, and multimodal sensory information is transferred to the frontal lobe and that this lobe participates via a stream of short association fibers in the planning, timing, and sequencing of complex motor tasks (Fuster, 1991, 1993). Thus, it requires a long circuitous route to get from the various sensory systems and their central representations to the area where the large highway of voluntary motor control originates (i.e., the motor part of the pyramidal tract). The motor and premotor cortices and their outflow via the pyramidal tract are mainly concerned with the programming and execution of skilled movements. Movements of this type require detailed control of the distal limb muscles (Porter, 1985; Kuypers, 1987).

The motor and premotor cortices are supported during both the programming and the execution phases of their tasks by two large control systems, the extrapyramidal and the cerebellar systems. After signals, originating mainly from the neocortex, have been processed through the basal ganglia (caudate nucleus, putamen, and globus pallidus) and the cerebellum (cerebellar cortex and central cerebellar nuclei), they converge via the ventral lateral thalamic nucleus on the motor and premotor cortices. Both systems play an important role in motor integration. Whereas the cerebellum is involved in the initiation and proper timing of movements, the basal ganglia play a role in the speed of movements. The two motor control systems just touched on are shown diagrammatically in Figure 6.1. For the sake of clarity, however, the large corticostriatal projection, terminating in the caudate nucleus and the putamen, as well as the cerebrocerebellar projection, which is relayed in the pons, have been omitted. (Until recently, it was generally believed that the basal ganglia and the cerebellum are entirely and exclusively concerned with motor control and that, hence, the large corticostriatal and cortico-ponto-cerebellar projections represent the afferent links of motor control systems. As is pointed out in a later section of this chapter, it now has become clear that large parts of the basal ganglia and of the cerebellum, including their neocortical afferents and efferents, are subserving nonmotor, mainly cognitive, functions.)

CONTROL SYSTEMS

The overview of the principal sensory and motor pathways presented in the preceding section gives an impression of the canalization of the flow of information through the human brain. It appeared that the cerebral cortex can globally be subdivided into a sensory post-Rolandic and a motor pre-Rolandic domain and that within the latter a number of hierarchically organized, parallel processing streams can be distinguished. The transcortical pathways discussed should not, however, be envisioned as multisynaptic reflex loops along which given ensembles of external stimuli lead to predictable, stereotyped action patterns. Rather, these pathways are embedded in a dynamic network in which an enormous capacity for plastic changes is built in (Gilbert, 1998). This network includes, apart from serial and parallel sensorifugal connections, shunts or "bypasses" that skip over certain intermediate levels*, lateral pathways forming (for the most part reciprocal) links with neural nodes of the same synaptic level, and top-down or sensory-petal connections, enabling higher synaptic levels to exert feedback influence on earlier levels (Felleman and van Essen, 1991; van Essen et al., 1992) (Fig. 6.2).

---

* As, for instance the strong, monosynaptic projection from the primary somatosensory to the primary motor area.

6 Neocortical Macrocircuits

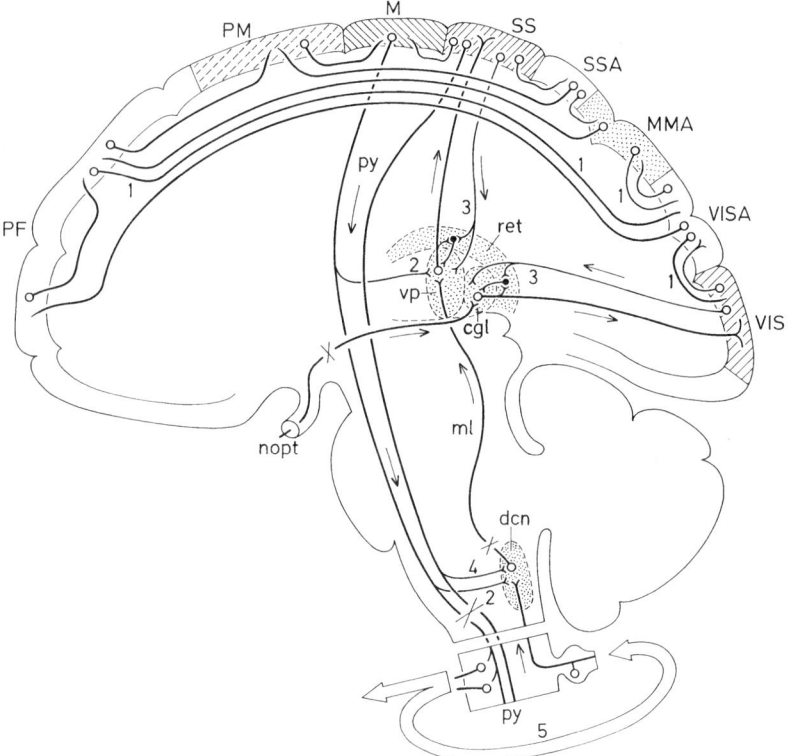

Figure 6.2. Diagrammatic representation of some control systems. 1, cortical feedback systems; 2, control of motor cortex over the somatosensory system; 3, corticothalamic fibers reciprocating thalamo-cortical projections; 4, control of somatosensory cortex over its own ascending system; 5, somatomotor output, used to direct sense organs. Further explanation in text. ml, medial lemniscus; nopt, nervus opticus; ret, thalamic reticular nucleus; cgl, dcn, dorsal column nuclei; MMA, multimodal association cortex; PF, prefrontal cortex; PM, premotor cortex; py, pyramidal tract; SS, primary Somatosensory cortex; VIS, primary visual cortex; VISA, visual association cortex.

The preparation and execution of skilled, purposive movements requires continual processing of the incoming sensory information. This processing includes the intervention of the mechanism of selective attention and of other control systems.

Selective attention allows the extraction and enhancement of information relevant to current behavioral demands and goals and the suppression or complete neglect of irrelevant information. The neural correlate of selective attention is still largely unknown (cf. Parasuraman, 1998); it seems reasonable to assume that the lateral projections and the feedback pathways discussed above form part of it. The mechanisms by which the neocortex exerts control over "its own" sensory information are, however, by no means confined to the cortical level. To give an example, the primary motor cortex and its outflow via the pyramidal tract not only plays a prominent role in the initiation of differentiated volitional movements but also is involved in the control of the sensory ascendant signal transmission. Collaterals of pyramidal tract neurons project to the areas of termination of primary somatosensory fibers (the spinal dorsal horn, the dorsal column nuclei, the sensory trigeminal nucleus) as well as the ventral posterior thalamic nucleus (i.e., the end station of the medial and trigeminal lemnisci) (Canedo, 1997). It is known that the outflow of a focus in the motor cortex, inducing movement of a given limb joint, selectively facilitates the transmission of exteroceptive messages originating from the body segment corresponding to the same joint and simultaneously depresses the flow of information from the neighboring zones in the cortex (Palmeri et al., 1999). These selective excitatory and inhibitory cortical influences, which recall a scheme of "surrounding inhibition," are exerted at the dorsal column nuclear levels as well as the thalamic levels (Palmeri et al., 1999) (Fig. 6.2).

The thalamic nuclei receive a massive input from their cortical target regions. The corticothalamic fibers involved terminate, contrary to the ascending thalamic afferents, mainly on distal segments of the thalamic projections, neurons. The ascending thalamocortical fibers and the descending corticothalamic fibers both give off collaterals to the thalamic reticular nucleus, a thin sheet of cells that encapsulates the thalamus. The thalamic reticular nucleus is composed of inhibitory GABAergic neurons (Houser et al., 1980), which project back in a strictly reciprocal fashion to the thalamic nucleus from which they receive afferents. The collaterals of the thalamocortical and corticothalamic fibers excite the reticular neurons, and these exert recurrent inhibition on the thalamic projection neurons (Fig. 6.2). The thalamic reticular nucleus is clearly involved in modifying thalamocortical signal transmission, but its exact function is still rather mysterious. Sillito et al. (1994) studied the influence exerted by neurons projecting from the primary visual cortex on relay cells in the lateral geniculate body. They found that, depending on the stimulus present, the cortical neurons synchronize the activity of a precisely selected subpopulation of thalamic relay cells. The stimulus characteristics determine which neurons are selected to become synchronized. This synchronized firing of selected thalamic relay cells increases the probability of some special stimulus features to be detected. These findings suggest that the reciprocal relations between the visual cortex and the lateral geniculate body are involved in pattern recognition.

From the foregoing it appears that the neocortex by way of direct cortico-subcortical projections exerts control over its own input and that within the somatosensory system such feedback fibers terminate in the thalamic ventral posterior nucleus as well as in the centers of termination of the primary afferent fibers. Similar cortical influences are exerted on cell masses intercalated in the other sensory systems. For example, the primary auditory cortex projects directly to the medial geniculate body as well as to the inferior colliculus (cf. Fig. 6.1), and it is known that the latter projection can both facilitate and suppress collicular activity (Huffman and Henson, 1990).

The control systems discussed thus far, however extensive some of them may be, are all confined to the central nervous system. Other control systems are still more extensive and include motor effector organs (striated muscles) as well as sense organs. Much if not most of the skeletomotor activity is not directed toward the external world, but rather to the organism itself to direct the sense organs as "windows of attention" to features currently relevant to behavior (Fig. 6.2).

RETICULAR, GREATER LIMBIC AND GENERAL MODULATORY INPUTS TO NEOCORTICAL CIRCUITRY

We have seen that the sensory as well as the motor poles of the principal neocortical processing stream (Fig. 6.1) are in receipt of major afferent inputs. The sensory pole, which is formed by the primary sensory cortices, receives information originating from the external world via the so-called specific sensory or lemniscal projections. Two large control systems, the extrapyramidal and cerebellar systems, converge, via the ventral lateral thalamic nucleus, on the motor pole; the latter consists of the primary motor and premotor cortical areas. It is important that the impulse flow through the long, multisynaptic channels intercalated between the sensory and motor poles is influenced, throughout its extent, by side inputs from many sources. The most important of these sources include (1) the ascending reticular system, (2) the greater limbic system, (3) the monoaminergic and cholinergic modulatory systems, and (4) the cortico-subcortico-cortical association systems. Brief consideration is now given to the first three sources; the fourth source is discussed in the next section.

The Ascending Reticular System

After having entered the central nervous system, stimuli gathered by the various kinds of sensors may reach the neocortex either via modality-specific lemniscal systems or via what is traditionally called the nonspecific afferent or extralemniscal system. Because the reticular formation is a crucial part of the latter system, it is also known as the *ascending reticular system*. The structural components of this system are (1) certain "segments" of the rhombencephalic and mesencephalic reticular formation; (2) the intralaminar thalamic nuclei; (3) spinoreticular projections, conveying general somatosensory impulses of various modalities, including pain; (4) afferents from relay centers of most sensory cranial nerves; and (5) some spinothalamic fibers, and a much larger contingent of direct and indirect reticulothalamic fibers. All of these ascending fibers converge on the intralaminar thalami nuclei, which represent the rostral poles of the ascending reticular system. The intralaminar nuclei project massively to the striatum and more sparsely to the neocortex.

Until recently, the thalamocortical projection was described as diffusely arranged and widespread. Electrical stimulation of the reticular formation produces a general cortical activation, associated with the well-known behavioral and corticoelectrical arousal reaction. It was believed that the diffusely arranged thalamocortical fibers arising from the intralaminar nuclei represent the final link in the ascending reticular activating system. Studies with modern tracing techniques, however, summarized by Groenewegen and Berendse (1994), have convincingly shown that each of the individual intralaminar nuclei has a restricted field of termination that overlaps only slightly with the projections of adjacent nuclei. Moreover, it has become clear that the targets of the thalamocortical and thalamostriatal projections of a given nucleus are interconnected through corticostriatal projections. The functional significance of these thalamo-cortico-striatal circuits is unknown. As for the ascending reticular activating mechanism, an alternative route to the cortex, passing via cholinergic neurons in the basal forebrain (see Monoaminergic and Cholinergic Modulatory Systems, below), has been suggested.

The Greater Limbic System

The greater limbic system (Fig. 6.3) consists of an array of strongly interconnected grisea extending throughout the length of the brain that is directly concerned with the maintenance of homeostasis and with the organization of behaviors aimed at the survival of the individual organism and of the species as a whole (for references and details, see Nieuwenhuys, 1996; Nieuwenhuys et al., 1988, 1998). It monitors the internal state of the organism on the basis of humoral signals and interoceptive inputs, and it also receives direct projections conveying nociceptive and thermoreceptive information. It organizes the specific motivated or goal-oriented behaviors, related to its central task, via its own motor system. This limbic or emotional motor system (Holstege 1992) is completely distinct from the voluntary somatomotor system. All of the specific behaviors organized by the limbic motor system include integrated endocrine, autonomic, and skeletomotor responses, and the latter pass generally through three sequential phases: initiation, procurement, and consummatory. Two large telencephalic structures, the hippocampal formation and the amygdaloid complex, constitute together the rostral pole of the limbic domain. It is important that these structures, and therewith the entire limbic system, are under the control of the neocortex.

We have seen (Fig. 6.1) that the primary sensory cortices and the primary motor cortex are connected by a long, circuitous processing stream. It may be added that an important branch of this stream, composed of fibers, originating from unimodal sensory association areas, the multimodal association area, as well as the prefrontal cortex, converge on the amygdala and the hippocampus. Most of these corticolimbic projections are synaptically interrupted in the cingulate and/or parahippocampal gyri, which on that account are designated as *paralimbic cortical areas* (Mesulam, 1985; Pandya, 1987). Along this route, highly processed information concerning the external environment is fed into the circuitry of the greater limbic system. This information is of great importance for an adequate execution of the various motivated behaviors, particularly for their often highly complex procurement phases. The descending corticolimbic projections are reciprocated by substantial ascending limbicocortical projections. These ascending projections are, just like the descending ones, largely funneled through and synaptically interrupted in the amygdalo-hippocampal complex. They terminate mainly in the prefrontal cortex and in the various sensory association areas. Impulses traveling along these projections may be instrumental in adapting the activities of the cognitive brain to the prevailing motivational state of the organism.

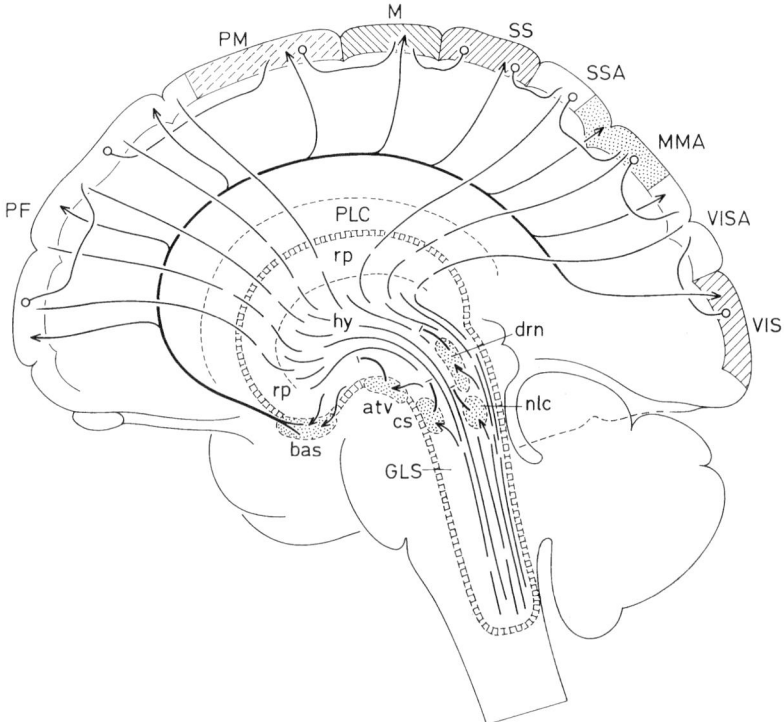

Figure 6.3. Diagrammatic representation of the greater limbic system (GLS) and of some transmitter-specific cell masses. The caudoventral rotation, by which the hippocampal formation and the amygdaloid complex are displaced toward the temporal lobe, has been omitted. Thus, the rostral pole (rp) of the greater limbic system represents the hippocampus and the amygdala in their "original" position. The paralimbic cortex (PLC) flanks the rostral pole of the GLS. The transmitter-specific nuclei depicted are bas, the cholinergic basal nucleus of Meynert; atv, the dopaminergic area tegmentalis ventralis; drn and cs, the (largely) serotoninergic dorsal raphe and central superior nuclei; nlc, the noradrenergic nucleus locus coeruleus. All of these nuclei receive their afferents mainly from limbic structures (arrows), and all project diffusely to the neocortex; however, to avoid crowding, only the cholinergic projection from the basal nucleus has been included. hy, ; M, primary motor cortex; MMA, multimodal association complex; PF, prefrontal cortex; PM, premotor cortex; SS, primary somatosensory cortex; SSA, somatosensory association cortex; VIS, primary visual cortex; VISA, visual association cortex.

Monoaminergic and Cholinergic Modulatory Systems

The basal telencephalon and brain stem contain a number of relatively small cell groups that can be characterized on the basis of their neurotransmitter. The axonal systems of these cell groups ramify widely and may reach large parts of the brain. Some of these cell groups project to the neocortex. Their cortical afferents, which are not synaptically interrupted in the thalamus, project diffusely to large parts of the neocortex, with no distinct topographical pattern and without respecting cytoarchitectonic boundaries. The cortically projecting, transmitter-specific cell groups include (1) the noradrenergic nucleus locus coeruleus, situated in the most rostral part of the rhombencephalic tegmentum; (2) the (mostly) serotoninergic mesencephalic raphe nuclei; (3) the mesencephalic, dopaminergic area tegmentalis ventralis; and (4) some groups of large, cholinergic neurons embedded in the substantia innominata in the basal telencephalon (Fig. 6.3). The cortical noradrenergic, serotoninergic, and cholinergic innervations reach all cortical regions, but the dopaminergic projection is mainly confined to the prefrontal cortex.

The cell groups under discussion are situated in the border zone between the classic reticular formation and the greater limbic system, and this intermediate position is also reflected in their (alleged) functions. Thus, it is stated that these cell groups, by way of their diffuse cortical projections, regulate general brain states such as sleep and wakefulness, attention, and arousal (e.g., Windhorst, 1996). It has already been mentioned that the cholinergic cortical projections arising from the basal telencephalon are currently considered to form the final link of the ascending reticular activating system. There is also morphological and physiological evidence, however, indicating that the activities of the various cortically projecting, transmitter-specific cell groups should be placed in a limbic context. Most of these cell masses receive their principal afferents from limbic domains. The large cholinergic neurons in the basal telencephalon have been shown to be particularly sensitive to novel and motivationally relevant stimuli (Wilson and Rolls, 1990). Similar findings have been reported for noradrenergic locus coeruleus neurons (Aston Jones et al., 1996, 1997).

CORTICO-SUBCORTICO-CORTICAL ASSOCIATION SYSTEMS

From the study of the brains of extant tetrapods, it may be inferred that in the line from synapsid amniotes to mammals a neocortex has developed, that the highest centers for sensory and motor control became established within this new domain, and that in some mammalian lines (ferungulates, cetaceans, primates) the processing capacity of the neocortex has become considerably increased by the development and expansion of association areas. Another feature involving neocortical development is that many subcortical structures, which originally operated independently, have become subordinated to the neocortex. They have become invaded by neocortical afferents and have gone to direct part of their output to the neocortex. The basal ganglia and the greater limbic system represent clear cases in point, and it may be added that the reticular formation, which, by way of the cholinergic basal telencephalon, projects to the cortex, is also in receipt of direct neocortical afferents. It is remarkable that the subordination process just discussed has led to the total annexation and functional incorporation of some subcortical structures. Certain parts of the thalamus and of the striatal and cerebellar circuitry receive their principal input from the neocortex and project exclusively to neocortical association areas. By the formation of these cortico-subcortico-cortical association systems, the neocortex has further increased its processing capacity. I conclude this chapter with a brief discussion of the three association systems mentioned (Fig.6.4).

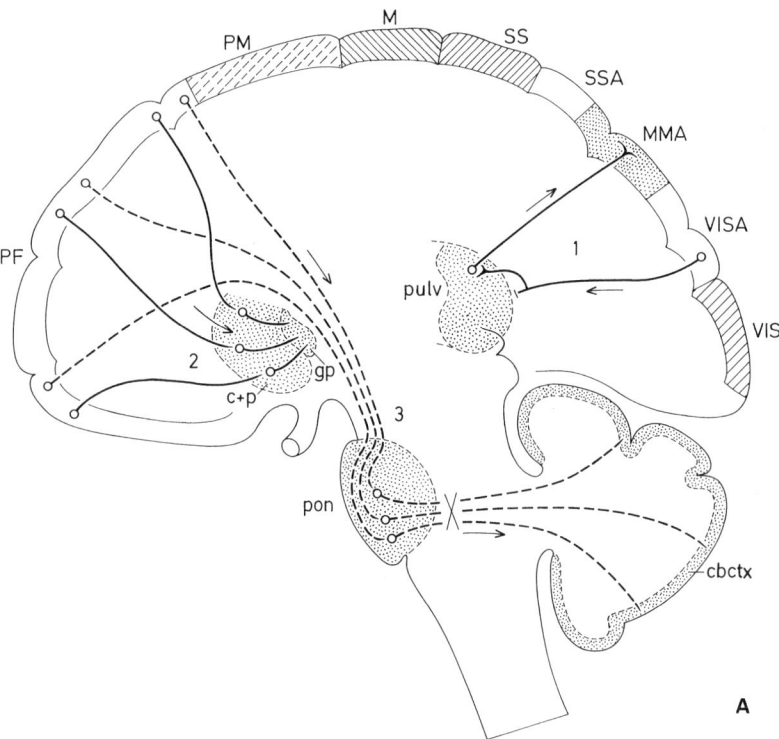

Figure 6.4. Cortico-subcortico-cortical association systems. 1, The thalamic association system; 2, the striatal association system; 3, the cerebellar association system. (*A*) System 1 and afferent loops of systems 2 and 3. *Continued on the opposite page.*

The Thalamic Association System [for references and further details, the reader is referred to Guillery (1995) and to Steriade et al., (1997)]

The fibers passing from the neocortex to the thalamus are of two different kinds: (1) thin fibers originating from layer-VI cells, which reciprocate the thalamocortical projection systems (Fig. 6.2), and (2) coarse afferents formed by collateral branches of layer V pyramidal neurons, whose main axons continue on to other subcortical sites in the midbrain, medulla oblongata, and spinal cord. These coarse cortical efferents do not reciprocate thalamocortical afferent systems, but rather connect the site of termination of one thalamocortical projection to the area of origin of another one. They terminate in grapelike clusters of large boutons, which form excitatory synapses on the somata and proximal dendrites of thalamocortical relay cells. Remarkably, these endings are indistinguishable from those of the principal afferents of the sensory and motor thalamic relay nuclei. As already mentioned, the terminals of the thin corticothalamic fibers are concentrated on the distal dendrites of the thalamocortical projection neurons.

Cortico-Subcortico-Cortical Association Systems 197

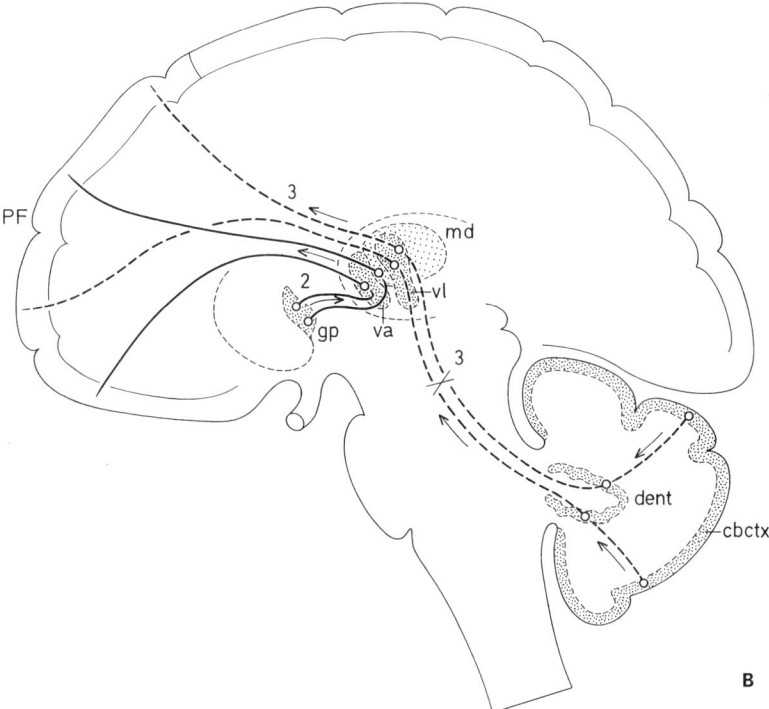

Figure 6.4. contd.
(*B*) Efferent loops of systems 2 and 3. Abbreviations: c+p, caudate nucleus + putamen; cbctx, cerebellar cortex; dent, dentate nucleus; gp, globus pallidus; md, mediodorsal thalamic nucleus; pon, pontine nuclei; pulv, pulvinar thalami; va, ventral anterior thalamic nucleus; vl, ventral lateral thalamic nucleus. M, primary motor cortex; MMA, multimodal association complex; PF, prefrontal cotex; PM, premotor cortex; SS, primary somatosensory cortex; SSA, somatosensory cortes; VIS, primary visual cortex; VISA, visual association cortex.

Two thalamic nuclei, the pulvinar and the dorsomedial nucleus (both represent in fact nuclear complexes) are specifically related to cortical association areas. The pulvinar projects in a point-to-point fashion to the parieto-temporo-occipital association area, intercalated between the various primary sensory cortical areas, while the dorsomedial nucleus projects in a similar way to the cortex of the frontal lobe. The pulvinar and the dorsomedial thalamic nucleus receive both layer V– and layer VI–originating fibers. Both nuclei receive, apart from these cortical afferents, inputs from several subcortical sources. Thus, it is known that the superior colliculus and the pretectum project to the pulvinar and that the dorsomedial nucleus is in receipt of afferents from olfactory structures and from the basal forebrain. These subcortical projections are, however, much less massive than those to the sensory and motor relay nuclei and do not attain all parts of the two nuclei under discussion. Hence, it is plausible that at least certain parts of the pulvinar and of the dorsomedial nucleus receive most or all of their afferents from the neocortex. Guillery (1995) proposed that these nuclei are largely concerned with transmitting information about the output of one cortical area to another cortical area and that they play a key role in cortico-cortical communication and higher cortical functions.

The Striatal Association System

Classically, the striatum has been regarded as a part of the motor system, particularly because disturbances of its functions can lead to severe movement disorders. During the first decades of the twentieth century, it was generally believed that the striatum influences motor activity quite independently from the control exerted by the motor cortex via the pyramidal tract (hence the term *extrapyramidal motor system*). Later, it became clear that the basal ganglia do not operate independently from the cortex. It appeared that the striatum (i.e., the caudate-putamen complex) receives a massive direct projection from the entire neocortex and that this complex, via the globus pallidus (another basal ganglion) and the ventral lateral thalamic nucleus, projects back to the primary motor and premotor cortical areas (Fig. 6.1).

The realization that the basal ganglia receive their principal input from the neocortex and that the main outflow of these ganglia is directed toward the motor and premotor cortices represented a significant departure from the concept of separately operating cortical, pyramidal and subcortical, extrapyramidal motor systems. Moreover, experimental neuroanatomical studies on monkeys during the 1980s and 1990s have shown that the striatum does not participate in one, but in several cortico-striato-thalamocortical loops. Thus, DeLong and Georgopoulos (1981) suggested the presence of two separate loops through the striatum: (1) a "motor" loop passing largely through the putamen, which receives input from the sensorimotor cortex converging on certain premotor cortical areas; and (2) a "complex" loop passing through the caudate nucleus, which receives input from the association areas and whose influences are ultimately returned to certain portions of the prefrontal cortex.

Somewhat later, Alexander et al. (1986) suggested the presence of five parallel circuits: motor, oculomotor, orbitofrontal, dorsolateral prefrontal, and anterior cingulate. Each of these five striato-thalamocortical circuits was thought to receive inputs from separate, but functionally related cortical areas and to be centred on a separate part of the frontal lobe. Parent and Hazrati (1995) reported that the striatum, on the basis of its spatial arrangement of the cortical afferents, may be subdivided into separate somatomotor, associative, and limbic territories and that this segregation is maintained at the level of the next processing station (i.e., the inner segment of the globus pallidus).

Finally, Middleton and Strick (1994), using a transsynaptic retrograde tracer, demonstrated that in the monkey a dorsomedial sector of the internal pallidal segment projects, via thalamic relays, to area 46 of the prefrontal cortex. It will be clear that the concept, according to which the striatum is considered to form an integral part of the motor system, is hard to reconcile with the existence of the parallel processing circuits discussed. It has been suggested that the circuits of which the motor and premotor cortices form part are most probably primarily involved in motor control but that those centred on the prefrontal association cortex subserve a cognitive rather than a motor function (Nauta, 1986; Middleton and Strick, 1994). This extension of the function of the striatum is supported by clinical evidence. Individuals affected by Parkinson's disease, a well-known striatal disorder, show, apart from their motor symptoms, distinct cognitive deficits (Cools et al., 1984; Taylor et al., 1986).

The Cerebellar Association System

The history of the cerebellar association system runs parallel to that of the striatal sytem. Until recently, it was generally believed that functionally the cerebellum is devoted entirely to motor control. As mentioned in a previous section of the present chapter, a complex cerebrocerebellar circuit, comprising a feedforward or afferent limb and a feedback or efferent limb, was considered to represent an essential component of the cerebellar motor control system. Topographically organized corticopontine and pontocerebellar projections form the feedforward limb, whereas the feedback is comprised of the cerebellar corticonuclear projection, the efferents from deep cerebellar nuclei to the thalamus, and the thalamocortical relay (Fig. 6.1). It was held that, along the consecutive neuronal links in this circuit, information derived from widespread regions of the cerebral cortex (including sensorimotor, prefrontal and parietal association areas) is funneled through the motor thalamus (i.e., the ventral lateral thalamic nucleus) to the primary motor cortex.

During the 1990s, the idea that the cerebellum is exclusively involved in motor control has been challenged by neuroanatomical, neurophysiological, and clinical evidence, as well as by functional neuroimaging results.

Experimental neuroanatomical studies in monkeys revealed that cerebellar output is not limited to the primary motor cortex. Thus, the temporal and posterior parietal lobes have been shown to receive projections from the cerebello-recipient ventral lateral thalamic nucleus (Yeterian and Pandya, 1989; Schmahmann and Pandya, 1990), and the transsynaptic retrograde tracer studies of Middleton and Strick (1994, 1998) revealed that distinct regions within the deep cerebellar nuclei form the origin of projections to different cortical areas, among which are not only motor, premotor, oculomotor, and premotor areas but also the prefrontal areas 9 and 46 and parietal and temporal association areas. The cerebellar neurons, labeled following injection of tracer in the prefrontal areas, were confined to the most ventral portion of the contralateral dentate nucleus. This region of the dentate nucleus appeared to differ clearly from the more dorsal regions of this nucleus, which were labeled by retrograde transneural transport from the primary motor cortex. On the basis of these findings, Middleton and Strick concluded that the cerebrocerebellar circuit, just like the corticostriatal one, is not converging on the primary motor cortex, but is rather composed of a number of parallel loops. They suggested that the loop involving the prefrontal cortex operates in parallel with that serving the motor areas of the cerebral cortex, but has a cognitive rather than a motor function.

Although there is still uncertainty about the matching and topical correspondence of the corticopontine and pontocerebellar projections (cf. Schmahmann, 1996), there can be little doubt that in primates highly organized, substantial cerebrocerebellar association systems are present. In the course of hominoid evolution not only the neocortical association areas but also the cerebellar hemispheres increased dramatically in size. The latter send their output mainly to the dentate nuclei. Dow (1942, 1988) reported that in the dentate nucleus of primates separate dorsomedial and ventrolateral parts can be distinguished and that the latter part—designated by him as the neodentate—expanded enormously when hominoids evolved. Indeed, in the anthropoid apes and in humans the "neodentate" represents the bulk of the dentate nucleus. These data and the finding that the ventral part of the dentate nucleus projects specifically to the prefrontal cortex (Middleton and Strick, 1994, 1998) indicate that the prefrontal cerebrocerebellar association system is particularly strongly developed in anthropoids and humans.

The hypothesis that the cerebellum is involved in cognitive processes has received support from physiological, neuroimaging, and clinical studies. As regards physiology, Middelton and Strick (1998), who recorded the activity of single neurons in the dentate nucleus in awake trained monkeys, found that units located in ventral regions of the nucleus are involved in working memory. Neuroimaging studies (summarized by Leiner et al., 1995; Schmahmann, 1996; Desmond and Fiez, 1998) indicate that the cerebellum (particularly the lateral cortex and the dentate nucleus) is involved in such diverse activities as working memory, implicit and explicit learning, linguistic processing, and mental imagery.

Finally, evidence has been presented that patients with cerebellar diseases have cognitive dysfunction related to the cerebellar disorder itself. Drepper et al. (1999) reported that patients with isolated degenerative cerebellar disease show deficits in cognitive associative learning. Schmahmann and Sherman (1998), who examined a cohort of patients with diseases confined to the cerebellum, found that behavioral changes were clinically prominent in patients with lesions involving the posterior lobe of the cerebellum and the vermis. According to Schmahmann and Sherman, these deficits conformed to an identifiable syndrome, which they termed the *cerebellar cognitive affective syndrome*. Its defining features are disturbances of executive planning, impaired spatial cognition, linguistic difficulties, and personality change characterized by flattening or blunting of affect. Schmahmann (1998) pointed out that these disturbances are similar to the functional affiliations of the cerebral cortical regions with which the cerebellum has reciprocal interconnections. He proposed that disruption of the neural circuitry linking the cerebellum with the associative and paralimbic neocortical regions produce the observed cognitive and affective deficits.

Drawing an analogy with the disturbances observed in patients with lesions in the motor parts of the cerebellum, he characterized the disorders of intellect and emotion detected as "dysmetria of thought". "In the same way as the cerebellum regulates the rate, force, rhythm, and accuracy of movement, so might it regulate the speed, capacity, consistency, and appropriateness of mental or cognitive processes" (Schmahmann, 1998, p. 367).

SUMMARY

Information related to happenings in the external world enter the brain via the somatosensory, auditory, and visual systems. This information from the extrapersonal space is subjected to a detailed analysis in the sensory association and multimodal cortices and transferred from there to the prefrontal association cortex. Among other things, the latter is concerned with the planning and sequencing of complex and skilled behavior aimed at manipulation of the external world. The premotor and motor cortices and the large pyramidal tract are instrumental in the planning and execution of the movements related to this behavior. The various sensory projections or lemniscal systems attain their respective cortical territories via a synaptic relay in the dorsal thalamus. The output from the primary motor cortex is not only directed to the various efferent centers but also to two large subcortical complexes, the basal ganglia and the cerebellum. These complexes project back to the primary motor cortex, and they do so, just like the sensory projections, via a synaptic relay in the dorsal thalamus.

Much of the intrinsic and extrinsic wiring of the neocortex forms part of sensory, motor, or sensorimotor control systems. Sensory control systems include the various corticocortical and corticosubcortical "top-down" connections, enabling higher synaptic levels to exert feedback influence on earlier levels. The parts of the basal ganglia and the cerebellum that are in receipt of afference from the primary motor cortex represent motor control systems, the former being involved in the selection of the most appropriate motor responses in relation to current behavioral demands, whereas the latter is concerned with optimizing movements by monitoring their outcome (Jueptner and Weiller, 1998). Sensorimotor control, finally, may be exemplified by collaterals of pyramidal tract fibers, which exert selective excitatory and inhibitory influences on somatosensory relay centers.

The vast neocortical network intercalated between the various primary sensory areas on the one hand and the primary motor cortex on the other is throughout its extent influenced by side inputs from many sources. Prominent among these are the greater limbic system, a number of transmitter-specific cell groups in the basal telencephalon and the brain stem, and the ascending reticular system.

Strong ascending projections connect the rostral parts of the greater limbic system with the various neocortical association areas. Impulses traveling along these limbicocortical projections are instrumental in assessing the vital importance of particular sensory stimuli in relation to the prevailing emotional and motivational states of the individual.

Transmitter-specific nuclei, including the cholinergic basal nucleus, the noradrenergic nucleus locus coeruleus, and the (mostly) serotoninergic dorsal and central superior raphe nuclei, project diffusely to large parts of the neocortex. Connectional and functional evidence indicates that the activity of these centers is strongly influenced by the greater limbic system.

It was long held that diffusely arranged thalamocortical fibers, originating from the intralaminar thalamic nuclei, form the final link of the ascending reticular activating or "arousal" system. It seems now more likely, however, that the route from the reticular formation to the neocortex passes via cholinergic neurons in the basal telencephalon.

During evolution the information processing capacity of the neocortex is increased by not only the development and expansion of association areas but also by the accaparation of certain subcortical territories. The neocortical dependencies, thus created, include parts of the pulvinar thalami and of the dorsomedial thalami nucleus, sectors of the striatum, and the lateral parts of the cerebellar hemispheres. All of these structures receive their principal input from the neocortex and project exclusively to neocortical association areas.

Whereas the corticostriatal and cereberocerebellar loops involving the motor and premotor cortices form part of motor control systems, those centered on the association areas have been shown to participate in cognitive functions.

REFERENCES

Alexander, G.E., M.R. DeLong, and P.L. Strick (1986) Parallel organization of functionally segregated circuits linking basal ganglia and cortex. *Annu. Rev. Neurosci.* 9:357–381.

Aston-Jones, G., J. Rajkowski, and P. Kubiak (1997) Conditioned responses of monkey locus coeruleus neurons anticipate acquisition of discriminative behavior in a vigilance task. *Neuroscience* 80:697–715.

Aston-Jones, G., J. Rajkowski, P. Kubiak, R.J. Valentino, and M.T. Shipley (1996) Role of the locus coeruleus in emotional activation. *Prog. Brain Res.* 107:379–402.

Canedo, A. (1997) Primary motor cortex influences on the descending and ascending systems. *Prog. Neurobiol.* 51:287–335.

Cools, A.R., J.H.L. van den Bercken, M.W.I. Horstink, K.P.M. van Spaendonck, and H.J.C. Berger (1984) Cognitive and motor shifting aptitude disorder in Parkinson's disease. *J. Neurol. Neurosurg. Psychiatry* 47:443–453.

DeLong, M.R., and A.P. Georgopoulos (1981) Motor functions of the basal ganglia. In: J.M. Brookhart, V.B. Mountcastle, and V B. Brooks (eds.): *Handbook of Physiology, sect 1: The Nervous System, vol 2: Motor Control, part 2.* American Physiological Society, Bethesda, pp. 1017–1061.

Desmond, J.E., and J.A. Fiez (1998) Neuroimaging studies of the cerebellum: language, learning and memory. *Trends Cogn. Sci.* 2:355–362.

Dow, R.S. (1942) The evolution and anatomy of the cerebellum. *Biol. Rev.* 17:179–220.

Dow, R.S. (1988) Contribution of electrophysiological studies to cerebellar physiology. *J. Clin. Neurophysiol.* 5:307–323.

Drepper, J., D. Timmann, F.P. Kolb, and H.C. Diener (1999) Non-motor associative learning in patients with isolated degenerative cerebellar disease. *Brain* 122:87–97.

Felleman, D.J., and D.C. van Essen (1991) Distributed hierarchical processing in the primate cerebral cortex. *Cerebral Cortex* 1:1–47.

Fuster, J.M. (1991) The prefrontal cortex and its relation to behavior. *Prog. Brain Res.* 87:201–211.

Fuster, J.M. (1993) Frontal lobes. *Curr. Opin. Neurobiol.* 3:160–165.

Gilbert, C.D. (1998) Adult cortical dynamics. *Physiol. Rev.* 78:467–485.

Groenewegen, H.J., and H.W. Berendse (1994) The specificity of the "nonspecific" midline and intralaminar thalamic nuclei. *Trends Neurosci.* 17:52–57.

Guillery, R.W. (1995) Anatomical evidence concerning the role of the thalamus in corticocortical communication: a brief review. *J. Anat.* 187:583–592.

Hackett, T.A., I. Stepniewska, and J.H. Kaas (1998a) Subdivisions of auditory cortex and ipsilateral cortical connections of the parabelt auditory cortex in macaque monkeys. *J. Comp. Neurol.* 394:475–495.

Hackett, T.A., I. Stepniewska, and J.H. Kaas (1998b) Thalamocortical connections of the parabelt auditory cortex in macaque monkeys. *J. Comp. Neurol.* 400:271–286.

Hackett, T.A., I. Stepniewska, and J.H. Kaas (1999) Prefrontal connections of the parabelt auditory cortex in macaque monkeys. *Brain Res.* 817:45–58.

Holstege, G. (1992) The emotional motor system. *Eur. J. Morphol.* 30:67–79.
Houser, C.R., J.E. Vaugh, J.P. Barber, and E. Roberts (1980) GABA neurons are the major cell type of the nucleus reticularis thalami. *Brain Res.* 200:341–354.
Huffman, R.F., and O.W. Henson Jr. (1990) The descending auditory pathway and acousticomotor systems: connections with the inferior colliculus. *Brain Res.* 15:295–323.
Jones, E.G., and T.P.S. Powell (1970) An anatomical study of converging sensory pathways within the cerebral cortex of the monkey. *Brain* 93:793–824.
Jueptner, M., and C. Weiller (1998) A review of differences between basal ganglia and cerebellar control of movements as revealed by functional imaging studies. *Brain* 121:1437–1449.
Kuypers, H.G.J.M. (1987) "Pyramidal tract." In: G. Adelman (ed.): *Encyclopedia of Neuroscience*, vol. II Birkhäuser, Boston, pp. 1018–1020.
Leichnetz, G.R. (1986) Afferent and efferent connections of the dorsolateral precentral gyrus (area 4, hand/arm region) in the macaque monkey. *J. Comp. Neurol.* 254:460–492.
Leiner, H.C., A.L. Leiner, and S.R. Dow (1995) The underestimated cerebellum. *Hum. Brain Map.* 2:244–254.
Lu, M.-T., J.B. Preston, and P. L. Strick (1994) Interconnections between the prefrontal cortex and the premotor areas in the frontal lobe. *J. Comp. Neurol.* 341:375–392.
Matelli, M., P. Govoni, C. Galletti, D. F. Kutz, and G. Luppino (1998) Superior area 6 afferents from the superior parietal lobule in the macaque monkey. *J. Comp. Neurol.* 402:327–352.
Mesulam, M.-M. (1985). Patterns in behavioral neuroanatomy. In: M.-M. Mesulam (ed.); *Principles of Behavioral Neurology* F. A. Davis, Philadelphia, pp. 1–70.
Mesulam, M.-M. (1994) Higher visual functions of the cerebral cortex and their disruption in clinical practice. In: D. M. Albert and F.A. Jakobiec (eds.); *Principles and Practice of Ophthalmology* WB Saunders, Philadelphia, pp. 2640–2653.
Mesulam, M.-M. (1998) From sensation to cognition. *Brain* 121:1013–1052.
Middleton, F.A., and P.L. Strick (1994) Anatomical evidence for cerebellar and basal ganglia involvement in higher cognitive function. *Science* 266:458–461.
Middleton, F.A., and P.L. Strick (1998) Cerebellar output: motor and cognitive channels. *Trends Cogn. Sci.* 2:348–354.
Morelli, M., M. Camardi, M. Glickstein, and G. Rizzolatti (1986) Afferent and efferent projections of the inferior area 6 in the macaque monkey. *J. Comp. Neurol.* 251:281–298.
Nauta, W.J.H. (1986) Circuitous connections linking cerebral cortex, limbic system, and corpus striatum. In: B.K. Doane and K.E. Livingston (eds.): *The Limbic System: Functional Organization and Clinical Disorders* Raven, New York, pp. 43–54.
Neal, J.W., R.C.A. Pearson, and T.P.S. Powell (1990) The ipsilateral corticocortical connections of area 7 with the frontal lobe in the monkey. *Brain Res.* 509:31–40.
Nieuwenhuys, R. (1994) The neocortex. *Anat. Embryol.* 190:307–337.
Nieuwenhuys, R. (1996) The greater limbic system, the emotional motor system and the brain. *Prog. Brain Res.* 107:551–580.
Nieuwenhuys, R., H.J. ten Donkelaar, and C. Nicholson (1998) *The Central Nervous System of Vertebrates*, vol. 3 Springer-Verlag, Heidelberg.
Nieuwenhuys, R., J. Voogd, and C. van Huijzen (1988) *The Human Central Nervous System*. Springer-Verlag, Heidelberg.
Palmeri, A., M. Bellomo, R. Giuffrida, and S. Sapienza (1999) Motor cortex modulation of exteroceptive information at bulbar and thalamic lemniscal relays in the cat. *Neuroscience* 88:135–150.
Pandya, D.N. (1987) Association cortex. In: G. Adelman (ed.): *Encyclopedia of Neuroscience*, vol. 1, Birkhäuser, Boston, pp. 80–83.
Pandya, D.N., and H.G.J.M. Kuypers (1969) Cortico-cortical connections in the rhesus monkey. *Brain Res.* 13:13–36.
Pandya, D.N., and E.H. Yeterian (1985) Architecture and connections of cortical association areas. In: A. Peters and E.G. Jones (eds.): *Cerebral Cortex*. Plenum Press, New York, pp. 3–61.
Parasuraman, R. (ed.) (1998) *The Attentive Brain*. MIT Press, Boston.
Parent, A., and L.-N. Hazrati (1995) Functional anatomy of the basal ganglia. I. The cortico-basal ganglia-thalamo-cortical loop. *Brain Res. Rev.* 20:91–127.
Petrides, M., and D.N. Pandya (1984) Projections to the frontal cortex from the posterior parietal region in the rhesus monkey. *J. Comp. Neurol.* 228:105–116.

Petrides, M., and D.N. Pandya (1988) Association fiber pathways to the frontal cortex from the superior temporal region in the rhesus monkey. *J. Comp. Neurol.* 273:52–66.
Porter, R. (1985) The corticomotoneuronal component of the pyramidal tract: corticomotoneuronal connections and functions in primates. *Brain Res. Rev.* 10:1–26.
Ramón y Cajal, S. (1911) *Histologie du Système Nerveux,* vol. 2. Maloine, Paris, Reprint 1972: Consejo Sup. Invest. Cient. Inst. Ramon y Cajal, Madrid.
Reiner, A. (1991) A comparison of neurotransmitter-specific and neuropeptide-specific neuronal cell types present in the dorsal cortex in turtles with those present in the isocortex in mammals: implications for the evolution of isocortex. *Brain Behav. Evol.* 38:53–91.
Romanski, L.M., J.F. Bates, and P.S. Goldman-Rakic (1999) Auditory belt and parabelt projections to the prefrontal cortex in the rhesus monkey. *J. Comp. Neurol.* 403:141–157.
Schmahmann, J.D. (1996) From movement to thought: anatomic substrates of the cerebellar contribution to cognitive processing. *Hum. Brain Map.* 4:174–198.
Schmahmann, J.D. (1998) Dysmetria of thought: clinical consequences of cerebellar dysfunction on cognition and affect. *Trends Cogn. Sci.* 2:362–371.
Schmahmann, J.D., and D.N. Pandya (1990) Anatomical investigation of projections from thalamus to the posterior parietal association cotices in rhesus monkey. *J. Comp. Neurol.* 295:299–326.
Schmahmann, J.D., and J.C. Sherman (1998) The cerebellar cognitive affective syndrome. *Brain* 121:561–579.
Sillito, A.M., H.E. Jones, G.L. Gerstein, and D.C. West (1994) Feature-linked synchronization of thalamic relay cell firing induced by feedback from the visual cortex. *Nature* 369:479–482.
Steriade, M., E.G. Jones, and D.A. McCormick (1997) *Thalamus,* vol. I. Elsevier, Amsterdam.
Taylor, A.E., J.A. Saint-Cyr, and A.E. Lang (1986) Frontal lobe dysfunction in Parkinson's disease. *Brain* 109:845–883.
Ungerleider, L.G., and M. Mishkin (1982) Two cortical visual systems. In D.J. Ingle, R.J.W. Mansfield, and M.D. Goodale (eds.): *The Analysis of Visual Behavior.* MIT Press, Cambridge, MA, pp. 549–586.
van Essen, D.C., C.H. Anderson, and D.J. Felleman (1992) Information processing in the primate visual system: an integrated systems perspective. *Science* 255:419–423.
Wilson, F.A., and E.T. Rolls (1990) Neuronal responses related to novelty and familiarity of visual stimuli in the substantia innominata, diagonal band of Broca and periventricular region of the primate basal forebrain. *Exp. Brain Res.* 80:104–120.
Windhorst, U. (1996) Bilateral organization of the brain. In: R. Gregor and U. Windhorst (eds.): *Comprehensive Human Physiology*, vol. I. Springer-Verlag, Berlin, pp. 1137–1160.
Yeterian, E.H., and D.N. Pandya (1991) Prefrontostriatal connections in relation to cortical architectonic organization in rhesus monkeys. *J. Comp. Neurol.* 312:43–67.

Chapter 7

HUNTING IN BARN OWLS: PERIPHERAL AND NEUROBIOLOGICAL SPECIALIZATIONS AND THEIR GENERAL RELEVANCE IN NEURAL COMPUTATION

Hermann Wagner, Institut für Biologie II, Lehrstuhl für Zoologie/Tierphysiologie, RWTH Aachen

INTRODUCTION

Specialists are good models for understanding adaptations, because specialists show the amazing achievements of evolution. Although these animals are named because of conspicuous adaptations, many universal features are also found in their anatomy and physiology. Design principles and algorithms of general features often, however, appear clearer in specialists than in generalists. Humans might be regarded as *the* brain specialists, because they have one of the largest brains in the animal kingdom. Thus, it seems that higher brain functions should mainly be studied in humans. This is true to some extent. The human brain is so complex that it has escaped the analysis of many brain functions. Moreover, brains are organ systems adapted to certain functions. There is no "super brain" that lends itself to the solution of all questions concerning nervous function. Instead, for the answering of specific questions, we need specific "model brains" or "model neurons" that evolved through adaptation to specific ecological niches. Classic examples are the giant axon of the squid (Hodgkin and Huxley, 1952), the electric organ of the electric eel (Changeux, 1981), associative learning in snails (Kandel and Schwartz, 1982), and the echolocating system in bats (Suga, 1988).

Complex behavior appeared in many animals independent of their position in the evolutionary tree. Behavior is generated in the brain by neural computations that trigger muscle actions. Computations by the brain involve the extraction of sensory information, the integration of sensory cues with internal representations, and the generation of appropriate motor commands. Computations may be simple, like adding up two signals, or they may be more complex, like binding together two or more aspects of a stimulus.

Certain principles of neural computing are found in a wide variety of species and work similarly in these species. At least in some cases, as in the case of coincidence detection discussed in some detail below, it appears that neural algorithms are more conservative than brain anatomy. This allows us to study a specific question in physiology or medical application in a less complex brain than in a primate brain. I shall use hunting behavior and its neural correlates in barn owls to illustrate my points.

The aim of this chapter is, thus, to demonstrate how evolution has shaped the brain and generated a complex behavior that allows owls to survive under high selection pressure. The chapter first introduces the position of the barn owl in the evolutionary tree, then describes hunting as a complex behavior, mentions special adaptations of the owl to physical constraints in the environment, and, finally, discusses the underlying variability and constancy of neural morphology and physiology. A concluding section mentions some possible general applications of the findings presented here.

EVOLUTIONARY POSITION AND GEOGRAPHICAL DISTRIBUTION OF THE BARN OWL

Classic as well as modern taxonomy has demonstrated that owls (*Strigiformes*) form a monophyletic group within the birds (Wink, 1993). Their nearest relatives are the nightjars and the frogmouths. Similarities to hawks and falcons are due to convergent evolution. All owls are hunters. Some of the owl species, such as the little owl, the snowy owl and the burrowing owl, are more active during the day, while others, such as the Tengmalm's owl, the long-eared owl, and the barn owl, are predominantly nocturnal hunters. *Strigiformes* are further divided into two taxonomic groups, the *Tytonidae* with the barn owls (*Tytoninae*) and the bay owls (*Phodilinae*) in one group and all remaining species in the other one (*Strigidae*).

The barn owl (*Tyto alba*) is a cosmopolitan with over 30 subspecies (de Bruin, personal communication.). Barn owls are middle-sized birds. Their weight varies from about 330 to over 500 g and depends to a large extent on the subspecies (de Bruin, personal communication.). Its range comprises grassland, brush, swamp, and forest. The bird is found in most tropical zones of the world and in temperate regions wherever the winter temperature does not fall too low. It avoids deserts and dense forests and does not live in the tundra. The species shows a fair degree of adaptability to several variations in the habitat (Taylor, 1994). This makes it the most widespread land bird in the world.

HUNTING AS A COMPLEX BEHAVIOR

General Comments

Hunting is a behavior that may be subdivided into components such as a deciding to start hunting, searching for prey, localizing prey, approaching prey, grasping prey, and returning prey to a den or nest. Many of these behaviors can be described by straightforward geometrical relations. This holds especially for localization (see Fig. 7.1, below). Therefore, localization has often been regarded as a reflexlike component. Such components do not seem to qualify under the label "cognitive." This opinion was not justified, however, because by the interrelation with the other components of hunting localization is also part of a complex context. Indeed, hunting in the barn owl, and the processes involved in localizing prey, while involving reflexlike components, also exhibit very complex, cognitive characteristics.

Barn owls hunt mainly small rodents like mice or insectivores like shrews. Adult animals need about two mice a day for survival. When the nestlings are in the phase of rapid development, each of them demands up to five mice. Because there are often up to seven babies in a nest, the father—he is hunting alone when the babies are small and not yet homoiothermic—has to catch up to 30 mice a night. Indeed, the mating system of these birds is such that a female accepts a male only if he can bring enough mice for a "wedding present." That the birds are indeed very effective hunters of mice was observed in the wild: During the breeding season, the male brings a prey item to the nest every 10 to 15 minutes (Bunn et al., 1982). In this time the male has to fly out from the nest, search in an area of approximately 5 km², detect, localize, and catch a prey, and then fly back to the nest. They do this continually for several hours.

Such observations suggest some regularity in hunting and, thus, seem to emphasize the reflexlike aspects of this behavior. It could also indicate some reliance on memory to relocate places with abundant food, and indeed field observations suggest that hunting barn owls follow a favored route time after time (Bunn et al., 1982). In the laboratory, capability for memorizing sounds (Quine and Konishi, 1975) as well as locations (Knudsen and Knudsen, 1996) was demonstrated. The evolutionary success of the barn owl seems also, however, to depend on hunting flexibility. Different hunting strategies have been observed (Brandt and Seebass, 1994): Barn owls may hunt from a waiting post or by flying slowly over the foraging area. Each individual may adopt either hunting strategy. In addition, different individuals specialize in different prey in the wild. Although the main diet of most barn owls consists of small rodents, there are individuals that prefer shrews. The selection is most probably made by listening to the sounds of the shrews. Therefore, the birds must be able to recognize and select shrew sounds from the sounds of other animals. In conclusion, barn owls are not reacting stereotypically, but are able to discriminate meaningful stimuli from nonmeaningful stimuli.

What I have mentioned thus far shows that barn owls can control reactions to a stimulus in some way. If we want to study behavior, we have not only to create constant stimuli but also a situation in which the animal reacts in a reliable and constant way to such a stimulus. In quantitative experiments in the laboratory, we also see both reflexlike and cognitive features of sound-localization behavior. Untrained owls respond with a turn of the head toward novel sounds. This response may be reinforced by feeding the birds if they turn appropriately. The birds then may execute this reflexlike behavior for many trials a day. We have observed, however, that the owls might also stop responding if they fail to associate stimuli with a reward. The owl will then no longer react to the sound, even if it is hungry. In addition, in some cases, even if the owl is well trained and seemingly alert, it does not turn after sound presentation. This again shows a high flexibility in the reaction to sounds and suggests that attentional mechanisms might play an important role in sound localization. The importance of attention and neglect is meaningful, because in the wild the owls should be selective and should not make too many errors in hunting. After a failed attempt, the owl has to weigh whether it is worth trying again.

Because hunting is a complex behavior, hunting animals cannot rely on genetic information alone; they have to "train" hunting behavior. Hunting animals are usually altricial, which means that they possess a prolonged time of development. In addition, they are often seen to "play" with "toys." This is known from cats, but occurs also in birds like owls: Owl babies tend to hop onto things thrown into their vicinity. They also view new or interesting things by translating and rotating their head, which probably helps to obtain information about the three-dimensional shape of the object and its relative position in space.

Although in some hunting species the fledglings are fed by the parents or live in a pack where they can eat from the food the adults' hunt or learn to hunt in the pack, barn owl fledglings have to rely on themselves soon after they leave the nest. This leads to a high rate of casualties in the first weeks after adopting independence, especially if the food is not abundant due to bad weather. It is known from populations in Central Europe that about 60% of the yearlings die during the winter, and of the surviving birds again 60% do not make it through the second winter (Mebs, 1980). Thus, there is a high evolutionary pressure on these birds selecting effective hunters.

Formal Description of the Hunting Situation

Hunting takes place in three-dimensional space (Fig. 7.1A). Out of the possible three-dimensional coordinate systems that describe the hunting situation, the spherical coordinate system seems to be closest to the natural coordinate system the owl uses (Fig. 7.1B). A spherical coordinate system consists of two angles, azimuth and elevation, and the distance between the predator and the prey. Azimuth is the horizontal angular deviation of the prey from the midsagittal plane, while elevation is the vertical angular deviation of the prey from the horizontal plane. These two angles can easily be measured in visual or auditory space (Fig. 7.1C,D). While distance measurement is easy by vision (see below), not much is known about the third spatial parameter, distance measurement by audition in the owl. In contrast to echolocation in bats (Suga, 1988), which analyze echos in response to the actively produced search sounds, the owl listens "passively" to the sounds in the surrounding area. Passive distance measurement by auditory cues is coarse and may play a minor role in hunting. Payne (1971) has performed an experiment to test whether the owls use auditory cues for distance measurement, but the result was inconclusive. Kolb (1988) has observed different flight postures and different flight paths during hunting in the dark and when the lights were turned on. During flights in the dark, the talons were extended when the owl was about 50 cm from the prey. Thus, Kolb's data suggested that Tengmalm's owls might be able to measure distance with a precision of some 50 cm when they start from a post about 2 m from the prey.

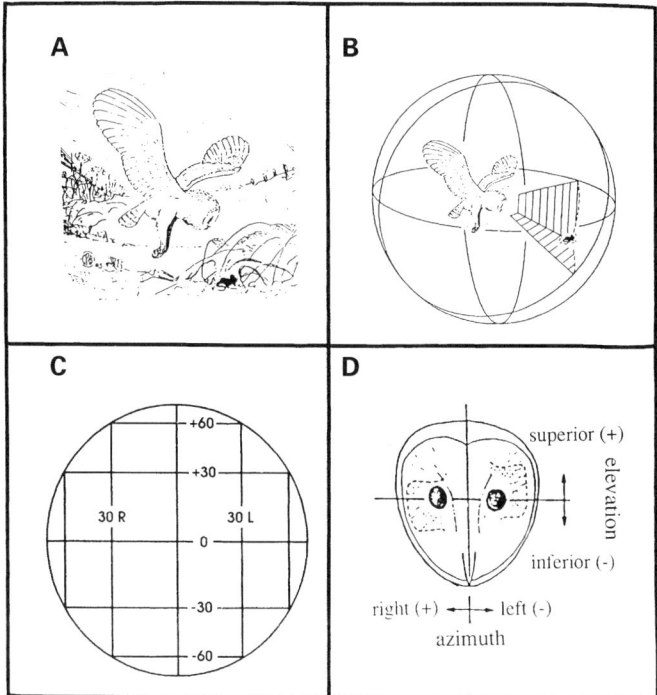

Figure 7.1. The hunting situation. (*A*) The natural situation. (*B*) Formalization in a three-dimensional spherical coordinate system with two angles, azimuth and elevation, and the distance between the owl and the mouse. (*C*) Reduction of the three-dimensional coordinate system to a two-dimensional coordinate system. Only the angles, azimuth and elevation, remain. (*D*) Centering of the two-dimensional coordinate system on the owl's head.

It should be kept in mind, however, that relative movement between predator and prey must take into account the six degrees of freedom of a moving three-dimensional body, which makes the description much more complicated. For this review, the simple situation with stationary sounds is sufficient in most cases.

Adaptations of Barn Owls to Hunting in the Night

Owls are one of only a few bird groups that have specialized for life at night. They have developed several specializations for hunting at night or for hunting in environments with reduced or lacking visibility of prey. In principle, a prey is localized by the visual and the auditory senses. However, owls can locate and catch a prey by acoustic information alone. A very convincing demonstration for the localization by hearing came from observations on great gray owls that hunt lemmings below the snow.

Payne (1962) and Konishi (1973) have performed experiments in a dark room to find out which senses the barn owl uses during hunting at night. They let a mouse with a thread tied to the tail and a leaf tied to the thread run in a darkened room. The leaf was making more noise than the mouse. The owl attacked the leaf and not the mouse. This excluded the use of visual, smell, taste, infrared, and ultrasound information. The only sense that remained was audition.

Morphological specialization for silent flight. Owls hunt from perches or from midflight (Brandt and Seebass, 1994). Because acoustic signals play such an important role, the noise produced during flight has to be reduced. This is achieved by several adaptations in the morphology of the feathers. The contour feathers of the owls have a special adaptation—the pennulae of the distal barbules are bent dorsally—which makes the plumage velvetlike and serves to reduce turbulences during flight (Sick, 1937). Apart from this general noise-reductive adaptation, the feathers at the front end of the wing are also specialized. The comblike structure found at the front edge of the wing seems to reduce noise during the starting phase of a flight (Neuhaus et al., 1973).

Morphological specializations for hearing. The next and most conspicuous specialization is the ruff (Fig. 7.2). There are two important morphological types of feathers in the ruff, the conch or ruff feathers that form the edge of the ruff (Fig. 7.2, top right inset) and the auricle feathers (Fig. 7.2, top left inset). The ruff feathers are densely ramified and have a closed vane. They reflect the sound and direct it to the ear canals. The auricle feathers, on the other hand, have a less dense ramification and an open vane. They are transparent for sound and have a protective, but not an acoustic function.

The ruff functions to amplify sounds (Coles and Guppy, 1988). Quantitative experiments in the laboratory have shown that the owl has a very low hearing threshold. Owls can react to sounds having a sound pressure level of −15 to −20 dB SPL (Konishi, 1973; Wagner, 1993; Klump, Dyson, and Gauger, personal communication). The hearing threshold of the barn owl is about 10 times lower than the hearing threshold of humans. The amplification of the ruff is approximately 15 to 20 dB (Coles and Guppy, 1988). Thus, one may say that it is the ruff that allows the owl to hear very faint sounds. In nature, each signal from a potential prey is usually embedded in noise from the environment. The relevant parameter is the signal-to-noise ratio that the predator can utilize. Here, the owl is also extremely good. Most neurons were able to sense the signal at a level 9 dB lower than the level of the background noise (Takahashi and Keller, 1992; Wagner et al., 1994).

If we remove the auricle feathers, the preaural flaps become visible (Fig. 7.3). The left flap is located higher on the head than the right one. The preaural flaps conceal the ear openings, which are also located asymmetrically on the head. This asymmetry in preaural flap position was first noticed by Streets (1870). The anatomical asymmetry is the basis of a physiological asymmetry: High-frequency sounds from below the horizon are louder in the left ear, and those from above the horizon are louder in the right ear. In animals with symmetrical ears the differences in the sound level in the two ears, the interaural amplitude difference (ILD), varies with azimuth. In contrast, due to the asymmetrical ears in the barn owl, the ILD varies more with elevation than with azimuth (Moiseff, 1989a; Brainard et al., 1992). Indeed, barn owls associate changes in ILD with changes in elevation (Moiseff, 1989b). The cue that varies with azimuth

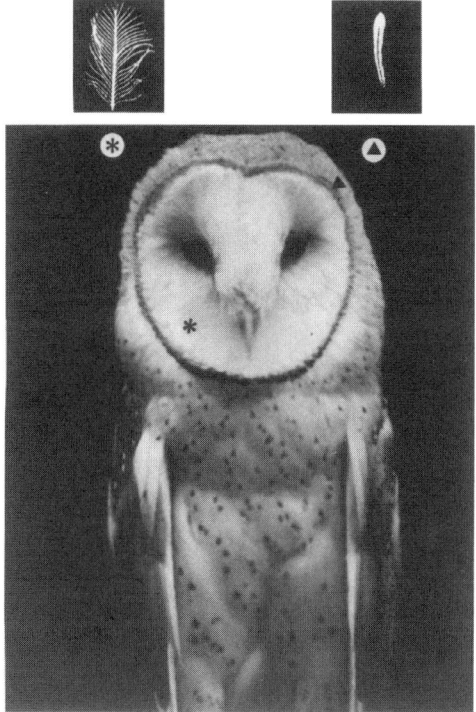

Figure 7.2. Owl viewed from front with full plumage. The asterisk is located in the facial disk, where auricle feathers (*top left*) are found. The triangle points to the edge of the ruff, where densely packed ruff feathers abound (*top right*).

is interaural time difference (ITD) (Moiseff, 1989a), and barn owls use ITD to localize the azimuthal position of a sound source. Thus, the ear asymmetry leads to a separation of the coordinates along which ITD and ILD vary and generates a two-dimensional grid, one coordinate of which is ILD and the other of which is ITD. Because both cues are good localization cues, this two-dimensional grid allows the owl to simultaneously determine the location of sounds in azimuth and elevation with high accuracy. The spatial resolution is between 1° and 2° in azimuth and elevation (Knudsen, 1984). In other words, the barn owl is able to localize sounds better than any other animal whose hearing has been tested. This precision is improved by the owl's ability to use information about the prey's motion (Payne, 1971).

Specializations of the Visual System. An eye-catching feature of barn owls is the frontally oriented eyes (Fig. 7.2). Such eyes allow for a large binocular overlap—much larger than in other birds. The binocular overlap would make the owls good candidates for depth vision by stereo. Small disparities in the two-dimensional retinal images of the left and right eyes can be used to create one three-dimensional image of the external world. Indeed, we could train owls to discriminate visual displays having disparities from those not having disparities (Willigen and Wagner, 1997).

212   7 Hunting in Barn Owls

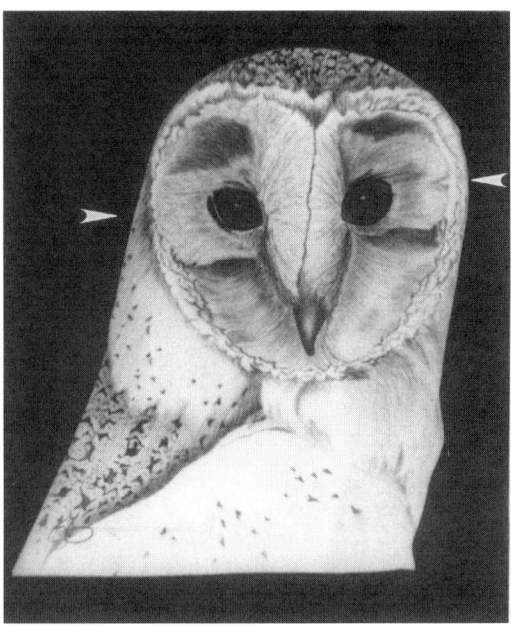

Figure 7.3. Barn owl after removal of the auricle feathers. Note the asymmetrically arranged preaural flaps (arrowheads) that conceal the ear openings. (from Volman, 1994, by permission of Karger, Basel.)

Birds with lateral eyes have both accommodation and the pupillary reflex decoupled in the two eyes. This allows them to use the two eyes independently (Andrew, 1982). For stereo vision, one would want to have accommodation in the two eyes coupled so that both eyes are focused to the same depth—indeed, accommodation is coupled in barn owls (Schaeffel and Wagner, 1992).

Frontally oriented eyes and stereo vision have other consequences as well. Animals with frontal eyes usually exhibit a symmetrical optokinetic nystagmus: If one eye is stimulated, the reaction to front-to-back optokinetic stimulation is about as strong as the reaction to stimulation from back to front. This is not so in laterally eyed animals as in most birds, which have an asymmetrical nystagmus or a stronger reaction to back-to-front motion than to front-to-back motion (Wallman and Velez, 1985). The owl's optokinetic nystagmus is much more symmetrical than that of the chicken or the pigeon and even that of the cat (Wagner et al., 1993).

THE BARN OWL'S BRAIN

Up to now we have only talked about peripheral adaptations. To be relevant for hunting, some of these peripheral specializations should have corresponding specializations in the brain. The gross morphology of the owl's brain looks much like that of other birds. Some extrusions are, however, more conspicuous than in other birds. A big dorsal telencephalic vault separated by a groove, the vallecula, from the "rest" of the telencephalon has been termed *Wulst* by early neuroanatomists (Fig. 7.4). We now know that part of the Wulst is involved in visual processing, as is outlined in more detail below. Likewise, the dorsal hindbrain has a big vault close to the pons. This is the nucleus laminaris, a hindbrain nucleus involved in auditory processing. In the following I shall describe some of these specializations in the brain in more detail. Two kinds of specializations are of interest here: morphological specializations in nerve cells and nuclei and physiological specializations such as effective neural algorithms.

Morphological Adaptations of the Owl's Brain to Hunting and Life at Night

Hypertrophy of Nuclei. The barn owl possesses the longest basilar papilla of any bird studied thus far (Köppl et al., 1993). This hearing organ contains some 30,000 hair cells (Köppl, 1997), much more than other species of a comparable size like the chicken or the pigeon.

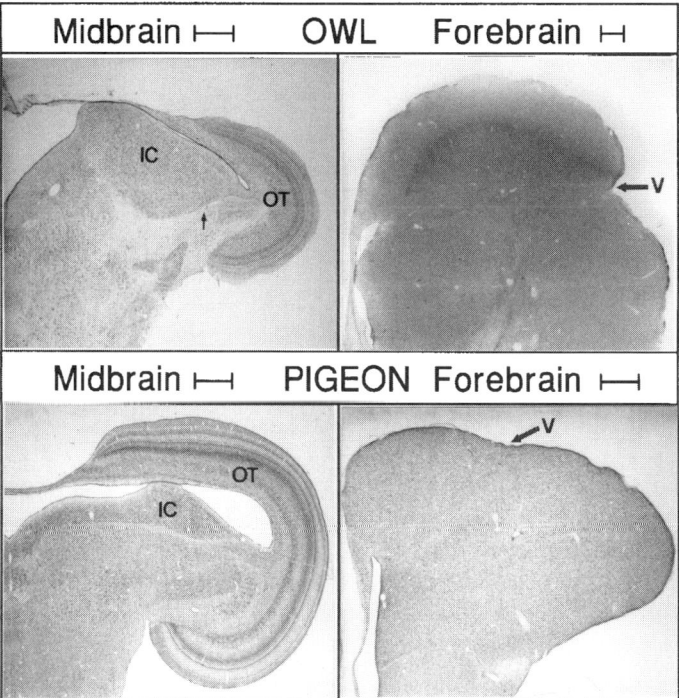

Figure 7.4. Comparison of owl and pigeon midbrains and telencephalons. The optic tectum (OT) is larger in the pigeon than in the owl, while the colliculus inferior (IC) is larger in the owl than in the pigeon. The visual Wulst and the vallecula (V) are much more outstanding in the owl than in the pigeon. Arrow in the upper left picture points to the region that separates the laterally lying external nucleus of the colliculus inferior from the medial inferior colliculus. Bars = 1 mm.

The general auditory pathway is not different from that of other birds (Fig. 7.5). A subpathway (stream) that processes ITD and its precursors ("time pathway") can be separated from a subpathway that processes ILD and its precursors ("intensity pathway") (Moiseff and Konishi, 1983; Takahashi et al., 1984). Important stages in the initial time pathway are the cochlear nucleus magnocellularis (NM) and the nucleus laminaris in the pontine region. The nucleus laminaris (NL) is the first station of binaural interaction. Further up, the anterior part of the auditory nucleus in the lateral lemniscus (VLVa) and the core of the central nucleus of the inferior colliculus (ICc Core) (Takahashi and Konishi, 1988) are part of the time pathway. The intensity pathway starts at the second cochlear nucleus, the nucleus angularis (NA), which projects to the posterior part of the auditory nucleus in the lateral lemniscus (VLVp). In the lateral shell of the central nucleus of the inferior colliculus (ICcls), the convergence of the hitherto separated pathways begins. The convergence and neural computation of ILD and ITD are completed in the next station, the external nucleus of the colliculus inferior (ICx).

While the auditory pathway in the barn owl is equivalent to the auditory pathway in other birds, the volume of the nuclei that process auditory information is enlarged in the barn owl. This holds for all nuclei of the auditory pathway. It means that more cells take part in the computation of a certain variable. This hypertrophy of the nuclei

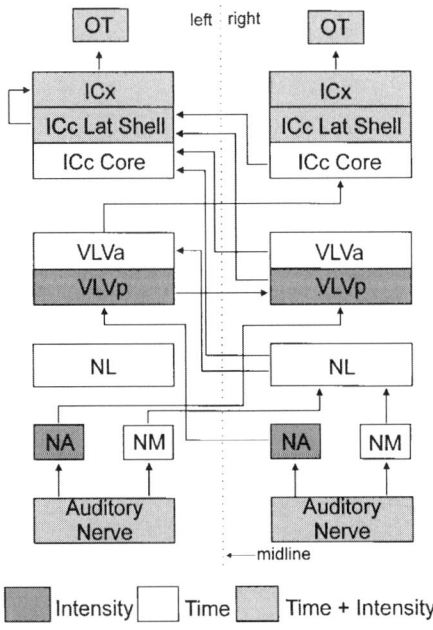

Figure 7.5. The auditory pathway of the barn owl. There are two parallel pathways, the time pathway and the intensity pathway, that separate at the level of the cochlear nucleus and converge at the level of the lateral shell of the central nucleus of the inferior colliculus (ICc Lat Shell). OT, optic tectum; ICx, external nucleus of the colliculus inferior; ICc core, core of the central nucleus of the inferior colliculus; VLVa, posterior part of the auditory nucleus in the lateral lemniscus; VLVp, posterior part of the auditory nucleus in the lateral lemniscus; NL, nucleus laminaris; NA, nucleus angularis; NM, nucleus magnocellularis.

can best be demonstrated by comparing the size of the auditory midbrain, the colliculus inferior, of the owl with that of a generalist of comparable size, the pigeon (Fig. 7.4, left). The drawings show a frontal section at the largest cross section of the inferior colliculus in both species. The owl's inferior colliculus is quite conspicuous compared with the pigeon's inferior colliculus. The volume of the owl's nucleus is at least five times larger than that of the pigeon's nucleus (Wagner and Güntürkün, unpublished data). In the lateral third of the nucleus often a region of low cell density can be seen in Nissl stains (arrow in Fig. 7.4, top left). This region lies just medial to the ICx (Knudsen and Konishi, 1978; Knudsen and Knudsen, 1983). The ICx plays an important role in sound localization, as is discussed below.

Similar enlargements in brain areas are found in parts of the visual pathway. Because owls are able to extract depth by stereo vision, they should have a neural substrate to measure disparities. The estimation of depth information from stereo vision is computationally expensive. In the owl, cells sensitive to horizontal disparities have been found in the telencephalon (Pettigrew and Konishi, 1976; Wagner and Frost, 1993). These neurons lie in the "visual Wulst." If we compare the Wulst of the barn owl with the Wulst of the pigeon, we see a similar difference as in the auditory midbrain: The owl's Wulst is large and sits on top of the brain forming an additional ridge, whereas the pigeon's Wulst is much smaller, with the vallecula barely discernible (Fig. 7.4, right).

Specializations in pathways. In the auditory system of the barn owl, the only connection not reported in other birds is the commisural projection from the ICc Core to the ICcls (Takahashi et al., 1989) (Fig. 7.5). The visual pathway seems to possess more specializations related to binocular vision and to the symmetrical optokinetic nystagmus. In owls as in all birds, there is a total decussation of the retinal fibers in the optic chiasm (Karten et al., 1973; Pettigrew and Konishi, 1976). The retinal fibers project to the contralateral optic tectum and thalamus. Thus, the thalamic relay nucleus, the nucleus opticus principalis thalami (OPT), of the owl represents the whole contralateral eye, while in the cat or primates this nucleus represents the contralateral hemifield of both eyes. To achieve binocular convergence, the thalamic fibers that represent the temporal retina recross in the supraoptic chiasm on their way to the visual Wulst. The crossing of the fibers in the supraoptic chiasm allows the owl to represent the contralateral hemifield on each side in the Wulst. In the binocular neurons of the Wulst, the functional characteristics, like disparity tuning, are similar to the functional characteristics of binocular neurons found in cat or monkey (Pettigrew and Konishi, 1976). The visual Wulst projects back to the optic tectum (Karten et al., 1973). In the owl, this projection is bilateral (Karten et al., 1973). Due to the symmetrical optokinetic nystagmus, one would also expect a bilateral projection onto the nucleus of the basal optic root (nBOR) that is involved in the optokinetic nystagmus. Such a tracing study has not yet been done in the owl, however.

In conclusion, the anatomical specializations introduced in the last section suggest that the owl's brain is especially suited to process acoustic information related to sound loci and to visual information conveying depth. The hypertrophy of the nuclei points toward a special physiological effectivity of some algorithms. Such algorithms are introduced in the following section.

Physiological Adaptations

Physiological specializations are found along the entire auditory pathway. These specializations have primarily made neural algorithms also existing in generalists more effective. I shall discuss three of these mechanisms that are important for sound localization. The first, phase locking, depends mainly on the properties of hair cells and may thus be regarded as a simple mechanism. More requirements are necessary for the second algorithm, coincidence detection. The last algorithm, across-frequency integration, is even more complex, binding together the responses of many coincidence-detecting cells in a specific manner that may be influenced by behavioral feedback. Complexity of computation thus increases as we move from phase locking to across-frequency integration.

Phase locking. As described above, barn owls and other animals use ITD to determine the azimuthal position of a sound source. To be able to compute ITD (i.e., the relative arrival time of the sound at the two ears), the animals must be equipped with a mechanism to represent time in some way in the first place. Animals possess internal clocks, for example, a diurnal clock, that provide information about time. In the task of measuring time differences, a measurement of time relative to an external signal is important. To this end, the internal clocks could be reset and then started again. This possibility is not realized, however, probably because the time measurement has to be much more precise than would be possible with the internal clocks. As mentioned before, ITDs are in the range of microseconds. Because 1° in azimuth corresponds to some 2 to 2.5 µs in ITD, the threshold lies in the range of about 2 to 5 µs (Moiseff and Konishi, 1981; Knudsen, 1984; Brainard et al., 1992). In the auditory system representation of time becomes possible through a mechanism termed *phase locking*.

To explain phase locking, let us regard a simple auditory stimulus, a tone (Fig. 7.6A). The amplitude of a tonal stimulus changes in a sinusoidal way. The same amplitude is reached after a full period or 360° of phase. If cells could now preferably respond at the highest amplitude (90° of phase) or at the time when the amplitude decreases fastest (180° of phase), then the cells could represent time relative to an external event, the tone. Whether cells are able to do this can be determined when their responses at an electrode are measured relative to the period of the external stimulus (Fig. 7.6A). By noting the arrival time in this way and by plotting the arrival time of many action potentials in histogram form, one arrives at the so-called *period histogram* (Fig. 7.6B). The period histogram can be statistically analyzed to determine whether a neuron's response is locked to the phase of a stimulus.

Phase locking is first seen in hair cell responses. These cells respond to acoustic stimulation with a change in their membrane potential. The change has two components, a DC component and an AC component (Russel and Sellick, 1983). Phase-locking seems to be correlated with a detectable AC response of a cell. It is easier to change the membrane potential in a slow rhythm. Thus, phase locking is best for low frequencies, because these frequencies have a long period (10 ms for a 100 Hz tone). The higher the frequency, the more difficult is phase locking. Research in the last 30 years has shown that normal laboratory animals such as guinea pigs are

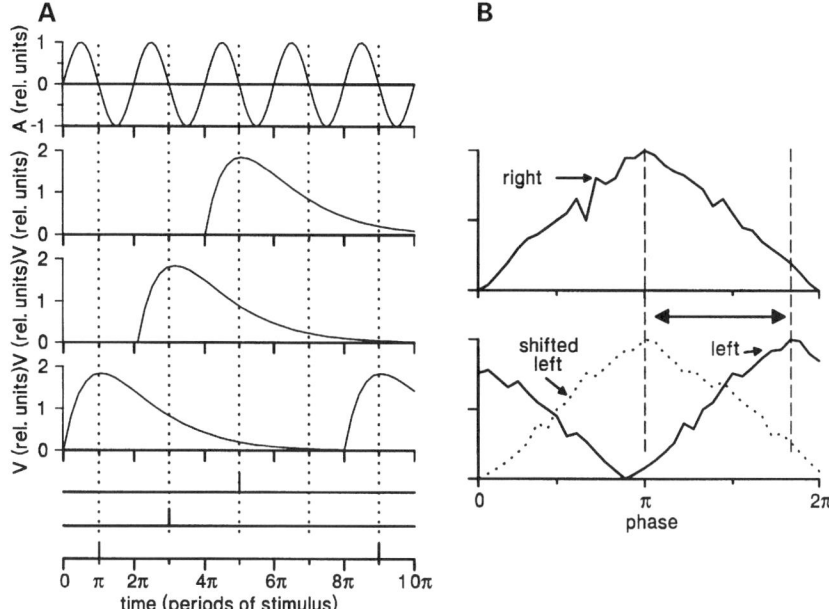

Figure 7.6. Phase locking. When the stimulus is a tone (*A*), spikes are found preferably at certain phases of the stimulus. If spike arrival time is plotted with respect to the period of the stimulus one, arrives at a period histogram (*B*). In this simulation, a stimulation with 4761 Hz was assumed, and the maxima of the period histograms obtained by stimulating the left ear (*left*) and the right ear (*right*) have been separated by about 150°, corresponding to 90 μs. If the left period histogram is advanced by about 150°, it parallels the right one. Thus, the highest response is expected for a time shift of 90 μs.

able to exhibit phase locking up to frequencies of 4 to 5 kHz (Russell and Selick, 1983). In the barn owl, phase locking is seen at frequencies one octave or more higher than in other laboratory animals. Thus, in terms of temporal precision, a single auditory nerve fiber can represent time with a precision of about 22 μs at 9 to 10 kHz, whereas in the chicken the precision is about 100 μs at 2 kHz (Warchol and Dallos, 1990). This observation supports the claim made above that existing algorithms have become more effective in specialists. To achieve this, the owl must have some specializations—probably fast ion channels—that allow for high-frequency phase locking. The underlying molecular and biochemical mechanisms are unresolved and represent an interesting topic for further research.

From a functional point of view, this high-frequency phase-locking is a precondition for the simultaneous precise analysis of localization information in two dimensions, because reasonable ILDs appear only above 5 kHz (Brainard et al., 1992). For sounds having a frequency of less than 5 kHz, the head does not cast a shadow, and, therefore, no ILDs arise. Simultaneous measurements of ITD should take place for the same frequency components. Thus, phase locking must extend above 5 kHz and indeed does so. Because a precise localization by hearing is indispensable for survival in a nocturnal hunter, it might be speculated that evolutionary pressure led to this high-precision, high-frequency phase locking (Volman, 1994).

Phase-locking in the range of 20 μs presents a formidable problem for the nervous system, because the neural signals that are used for signal transmission, action potentials and postsynaptic potentials, are 10 to 100-fold longer in normal cells. With such long potentials, phase locking in the microsecond range would be impossible. Experiments in both mammals and birds have revealed a mechanism that shortens action potentials and especially postsynaptic potentials (Reyes et al., 1996). The clue lies in a voltage-dependent outward-rectifying K^+-channel (Manis and Marx, 1991). Measurements in the chicken have shown that by activation of this channel postsynaptic potentials can be reduced in duration to about 500 μs (Reyes et al., 1996), while postsynaptic potentials in cells that lack such specialized channels, like the pyramidal cells of the mammalian cortex, have a duration of about 5 ms. Simulations show that phase locking at 5 kHz can be explained if we assume cellular mechanisms that are about twice as fast as in the chicken (Gerstner et al., 1996).

Thus, with the processes underlying phase locking, the auditory system has "invented" a means to represent time that can be used for further computations. I shall discuss one of these (coincidence detection) in the following section, but it should be kept in mind that the importance of time measurement goes far beyond this, because, for example, speech perception also depends on the precise encoding of temporal events.

Coincidence detection

If a neuron's response depends on the temporal difference in the time of arrival of its inputs, one may call it a coincidence detector, because two simultaneously arriving spikes may fire such a neuron, whereas two spikes arriving at different times might not be able to do so. Simultaneously arriving spikes elicit simultaneous excitatory postsynaptic potentials that sum up to exceed firing threshold. In this way, a neuron's response is an indicator of binding together two inputs. I shall first briefly mention the general meaning of coincidence detection and then turn to the special mechanisms found in the owl's brain.

Coincidence detection plays a role not only in the measurement of ITD for sound localization but in many other neural processes that occur in different neural substrates and on a large range of time scales: associative learning (Kandel and Schwartz, 1982), motion detection (Borst and Egelhaaf, 1989), long-term potentiation (Konnerth et al., 1996), synchronization of neural activity (Singer and Gray, 1995), range detection in bats (Suga, 1988), depth vision by spatial or temporal disparity (Wagner and Frost, 1993; Carney et al., 1989), and coordination of cerebellar activity (Heck, 1993). The computation of coincidence detection is performed by neurons having quite different morphology: from pyramidal cells in the mammalian cortex to dendrite-lacking cells in the nucleus laminaris of the owl. Likewise, several different molecular mechanisms are involved, for example, NMDA receptors in the hippocampus (Konnerth et al., 1996), outward rectification of potassium currents in the auditory system (Manis and Marx, 1991; Reyes et al., 1996), and serotonin receptors in conjunction with G protein–dependent intracellular cascades in sensitization in the snail (Kandel and Schwartz, 1982). The different computational speeds of the molecular processes together with neural gross morphology and conduction times account for the wide range in relevant time scales: from microseconds in measuring interaural time differences to seconds in associative learning. Nevertheless, the formal description, the algorithm, is always the same.

Coincidence detection in the microsecond range in the auditory system is used to represent ITDs. It depends on the high precision phase-locking described in the last section and on several further conditions. First, a special neural circuitry is necessary. Second, some regulatory mechanism has to bind together inputs with similar delays. In addition, the coincidence-detecting cells have to be similarly sensitive to time as the input cells and the cells must be able to segregate inputs from the left brain side from inputs from the right brain side.

The principal idea for the realization of an adequate neural circuit dates back some 50 years (Jeffress, 1948). According to Jeffress (1948), the cells that measure these small time differences act as coincidence detectors, and the neural network innervating the coincidence detectors is built of cables that act as delay lines. Jeffress' proposal is realized in remarkable detail in the owl (Carr and Konishi, 1990). The coincidence-detecting neurons are the neurons in the nucleus laminaris, the first station of binaural convergence in the auditory pathway. The delay lines are formed by the axon collaterals of the cells of the nucleus magnocellularis (Fig. 7.5).

A regulatory mechanism is necessary because the times that have to be measured are in the range of microseconds, while the total delay from the ear drum to the coincidence detector lies in the range of 2 to 4 ms. Gerstner et al. (1996) proposed that Hebbian mechanisms might allow the cells to select inputs with the correct delay.

Not only do the cells seem to use Hebbian mechanisms, but we also see morphological specializations in the coincidence-detecting neurons. Nerve cells can be divided into a soma, a dendritic tree, and an axon. The dendritic tree integrates incoming information. While, in principal, binding by a Hebbian mechanism may also work via axodendritic synapses and passive or active conductances in a dendritic tree, in cells of nucleus laminaris a correlation between frequency tuning and dendritic arborization exists. Cells tuned to frequencies above approximately 4 kHz do not have dendritic trees at all, but the afferent axon terminals synapse on the soma (Carr and Boudreau, 1993). Thus, the reduction of the dendritic tree is a further specialization that underlies temporal sensitivity in the microsecond range.

The issue of the separation of the inputs from the left and right sides has only partly been resolved. If a cell is trained with a constant ITD and then stimulated with varying ITDs, the cell responds with a higher spike rate to the ITD used in the training phase. Thus, the cell is able to perform the segregation under these conditions. In the natural situation, however, the cell receives inputs having many different ITDs. Additional mechanisms are necessary to explain segregation of inputs from the left and right sides (Kempter et al., unpublished).

Thus, what coincidence-detecting neurons can do is to bind two events together. This is more than just summing up many inputs for the generation of a rate code. Coincidence detection is an important computation, because it may reveal some connection between these events. In associative learning, for example, an unconditioned stimulus is paired with a conditioned stimulus. Similar binding strategies might play a role in the synchronization of brain activity that is supposed to underlie the extraction of "higher" brain function (Singer and Gray, 1995) and even consciousness (Crick, 1994). At a less speculative level, combination-sensitive neurons have been described in the bat, where they serve for range determination or for velocity measurements (Suga, 1988). There are many more examples, and one, the possible involvement of combination-sensitive neurons in speech perception (Sussman 1989; Sussman et al., 1998), is discussed below.

Across-frequency integration. A biological stimulus is often very complex, stimulating different sensory modalities and having different qualities. The brain analyzes stimuli by decomposing them. Thus, visual components are analyzed by the eye or acoustic components by the ear. Likewise, different qualities within a modality are also separated. There is, for example, an analysis within separate frequency bands in the peripheral auditory pathway; we find a time pathway and an intensity pathway (Fig. 7.5). Nevertheless, we sense only one stimulus. Thus, after decomposing a stimulus for analysis, the different components of the stimulus must again be bound together to generate behavior. Coincidence detection is a first mechanism to achieve this. However, the neural responses representing a stimulus after a first coincidence-detection computation are often ambiguous. Thus, the response shown in Figure 7.7 depends in a periodic manner on ITD. This precludes the representation of one location in space, and, thus, false targets or target attributes appear. This is one of the reasons for many illusions. A well-known example is the false-target problem in stereo vision. If we look at the popular autostereograms (Tyler and Clarke, 1990), it takes some time until we see the three-dimensional shape. What our brain does while we are looking at the picture but still not perceiving the depth is to find the correct matches between the information reaching the right eye and that reaching the left eye.

If a hunting animal wants to survive under evolutionary pressure, it must try to reduce false targets as much as possible. Thus, there should be algorithms after the stage of primary coincidence detection to remove the ambiguity in the response of the neurons performing the initial coincidence detection. These computations occur in

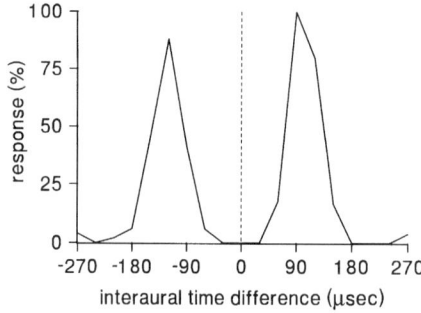

Figure 7.7. Interaural time difference curve. The cyclic response function has a period of 210 ms that is equivalent to the period belonging to the stimulating frequency (4761 Hz). The peaks thus occur at interaural phase differences of 90/270 = 0.43 and -120/270 = –0.57

hierarchically higher structures. In the following I shall describe such an algorithm that seems to play a role in removing ambiguity in the output of the coincidence-detecting neurons in the auditory system in some detail. This computation takes place three synapses after the computation of coincidence detection in the external nucleus of the inferior colliculus (Fig. 7.5). I shall first outline what the ambiguity looks like in the responses of the coincidence-detecting cells, then show how the ambiguity arises, and finally introduce a solution to the ambiguity problem.

Cells in nucleus laminaris are the first that exhibit sensitivity to ITD. ITD sensitivity might be measured by counting the number of spikes occurring in a certain time interval after stimulus onset. The spike counts for the responses to the different ITDs constitute the so-called ITD curve (Fig. 7.7). Coincidence detectors respond best when the spikes arrive together. This can be demonstrated from the period histograms (Fig. 7.6B). If we shift the period histogram obtained by stimulating the left ear by 90 ms to the right, in this simulation adapted to the real responses shown in Figure 7.7, it coincides with the period histogram obtained by stimulating the right ear. Consequently, 90 µs ITD elicited the highest response in the ITD curve (Fig. 7.7). Because ITD curves in nucleus laminaris are periodic to both small-band and broad-band stimuli, such laminaris neurons cannot represent a single ITD; they represent more than one ITD. The response shown here is very regular. Within the range of ITDs tested, the curve exhibits two response peaks and three response minima. The response changes almost follow a sinusoid.

Why are the neurons unable to detect the correct ITD? As has been mentioned before, the representation of ITD is a binaural process. Becuase there are signals to the left and right ears, the correct match of the sounds has to be determined. Thus, a false-target problem exists here just as it has been described for stereo vision above. The solution to the false-target problem is easy if the sound is broad band as indicated in the upper curves of Figure 7.8A. The correct match can always be found. For the tones shown in the lower part of Figure 7.8A, several matches are possible if the onset of the sound is not known. Then it cannot be decided which troughs on the left and right sides correspond with each other. Even if the stimulus consists of noise, narrow-band neurons receive inputs from a small-frequency range. Therefore, the ITD curves of narrow-band neurons (Figs. 7.7 and 7.9A) are periodic. The temporal difference of the response peaks in the ITD curve corresponds with one period of the stimulus tone. Because these narrow-band neurons respond maximally to more than one ITD, they cannot signal ITD unambiguously but only the phase equivalent of the ITD. In technical terms, the neuron's response shows maxima at

ITD = Interaural phase difference/frequency +k • 2 π;   k = 0, ±1, ±2,... (1)

This equation is shown graphically in Figure 7.8B for frequencies from 1 to 10 kHz and for ITDs from −300 to +300 µs. One peak occurs for all frequencies at +90 µs. For a frequency of 4800 Hz, the best frequency of the neuron with the ITD curve shown in Figure 7.7, a second peak around −120 ms is expected (Fig. 7.8B). Figure 7.7 shows a second peak at exactly this time difference. Note also that for other frequencies similar phase ambiguities occur (Fig. 7.8B).

7 Hunting in Barn Owls

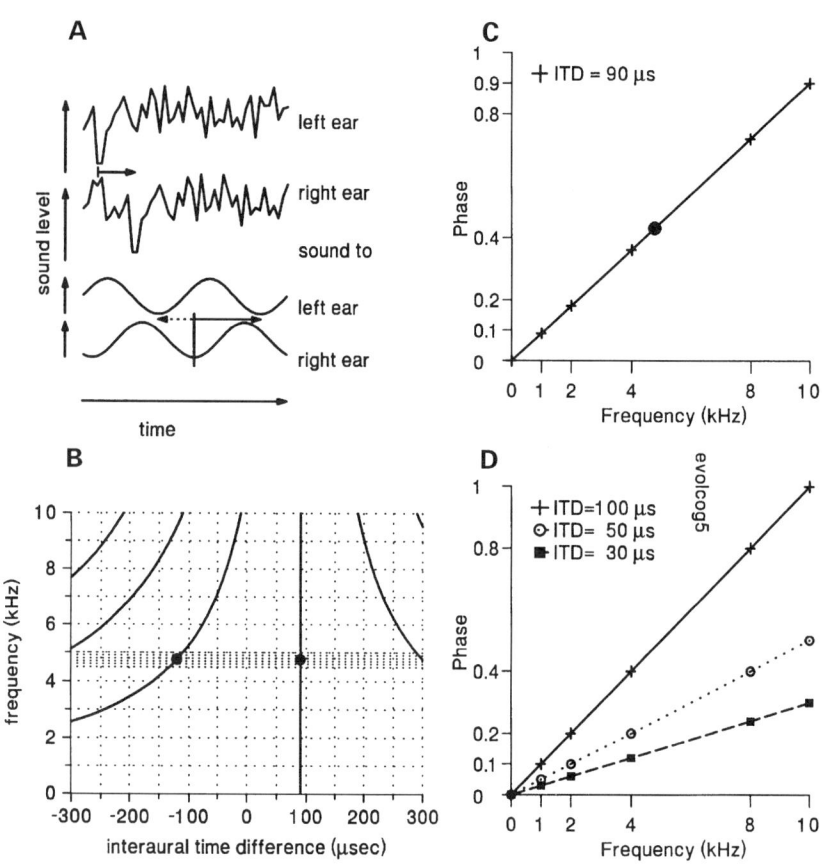

Figure 7.8. Phase ambiguity and its resolution. The schematic drawings show how phase ambiguity may arise if the stimulus is a tone (*A, bottom*). Phase ambiguity is absent if the stimulus is broad-band noise (*A, top*). (*B*) Graph showing the appearance of response peaks in ITD curves as a function of frequency. The dots and the tiny dashes show the example given in Figure 7.7. The regions marked by the tiny dashes center around 4761 Hz. The dots denote the locations of the response peaks. The thick lines show a theoretical construct under the assumption that one response peak occurs at 90 µs for all frequencies. The locations of the neighboring peaks change as functions of frequency. (*C*) The phase of the response (0.43 from the example in Fig. 7.4) is plotted as a function of frequency (4.761 kHz from the example in Fig. 7.7) (dot). The phase-frequency pairs of neurons having a common response peak at 90 µs but, being tuned to different frequencies (1, 2, 4, 8, 10 kHz), lie on a straight line. The slope of the straight line corresponds to the common response peak. (*D*) Differently sloped lines represent different interaural time differences.

Although the Jeffress model mentioned earlier explains the principle of binaural interaction by coincidence detection, this model cannot explain the representation of one sound location by the brain without further assumptions. One reason is that this model is formulated without taking the frequency dependence of the responses into account. As has just been described, narrow-frequency tuning in concert with phase-locking may create problems for sound localization because a coincidence-detecting neuron will be unable to discriminate inputs that are exactly one period apart.

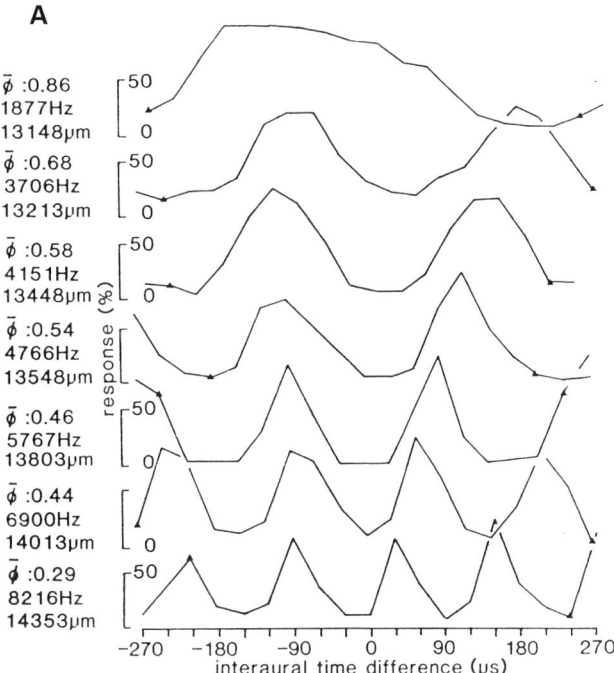
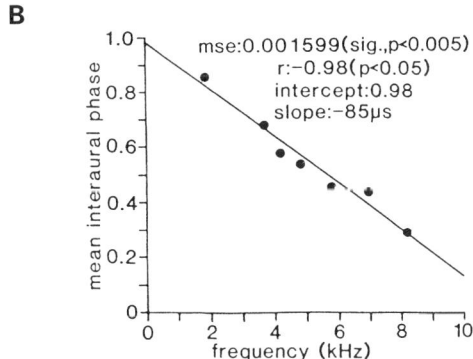

Figure 7.9. Arrays of neurons with an *array-specific* interaural time difference (ITD). (A) Recordings from seven neurons located in different depths (μm on the left) and tuned to different frequencies (Hz) and different interaural phases (ϕ, triangles on the ITD curves indicate range used for determining ϕ). Note that all curves except for the one associated with the lowest frequency tuning exhibit ambiguities in the representation of ITD. (B) If the information of all recordings is pooled in a phase-frequency plot, an unambiguous representation of ITD is achieved as indicated by the mean square error (mse) and the correlation coefficient (r).

There are two ways to solve this problem. The first one is to restrict analysis of behaviorally relevant ITDs to a range of frequencies at which the ambiguity problem does not occur. This would be 90 µs for the response shown in Figure 7.7. This might be a solution in some animals like the cat, because the ambiguity would arise only above about 1200 Hz. For humans, the limit would be about 750 Hz, and for the barn owl it lies around 3000 Hz. Thus, the barn owl cannot make use of this solution, because it has to analyze ITDs in a frequency range at which its head creates measurable ILDs. This is, as mentioned earlier, the frequency range above approximately 5 kHz. Therefore, the barn owl needs to employ a different solution to the ambiguity problem. It resolves the ambiguity occurring in the upper frequency range by integrating over several frequencies. Thus, an additional concept is necessary for the representation of auditory space. This concept is referred to as *across-frequency integration*.

Equation 1 is plotted in Figure 7.8C for an ITD of 90 µs and different frequencies. If we take an ITD of 90 µs, we have a corresponding phase of 0.09 cycles at 1 kHz (1 kHz has a period of 1000 µs), a corresponding phase difference of 0.36 cycles at 4 kHz, and of 0.9 cycles at 10 kHz. Thus, if we keep time constant, phase changes linearly with frequency. In this plot, ITD is the slope of the regression line in Figure 7.8C. If we look at the whole relation as in Figure 7.8B, we see that there is only one ITD for which the response is constant over all frequencies. This is the ITD, marked by a vertical line that connects the ITD curves at the different frequencies. If we change ITD one period to the left or right and connect responses that have the same values, we get curved lines (Fig. 7.8B). The straight line connects responses of equal relative height. Because the slope of the regression line in the phase-frequency plots indicates the ITD, different slopes represent different ITDs (Fig. 7.8D). Note that this is not the only way how across-frequency integration may take place. Neuronal responses of any equal height, not only at the maximal response as was assumed in the generation of the graphs of Figure 7.8B–D, might be combined (Yin and Kuwada, 1983).

We have seen from a theoretical analysis that across-frequency integration might solve the phase-ambiguity problem. Do mechanisms of across-frequency integration exist in the owl's brain? For across-frequency integration, cells tuned to different frequencies have to be combined in a specific way: The best combination would be in the way sketched in the mathematics of Figure 7.8B,C. Such across-frequency integration was observed (Fig. 7.9; see also Wagner et al., 1987). Neurons in the lateral shell of the central nucleus of the inferior colliculus (ICcls) are still narrowly tuned to frequency. ITD curves from seven recordings obtained at different depths (and therefore frequencies) are shown in Figure 7.9A. This array of neurons has one ITD at which the relative response is stimulus independent as shown by statistical analysis (Fig. 7.9B). This array of neurons projects to one neuron in the next higher station of the auditory pathway, the ICx. By this across-frequency integration a new property—unambiguous representation of ITD—emerges in the ICx neuron (Wagner et al., 1987). One might say that the ITD associated with the straight line is characteristic for a cell, and therefore the term "characteristic delay" was coined (Rose et al., 1966), and, indeed, ICx neurons exhibit characteristic delays (Takahashi and Konishi, 1986).

Thus, the neural algorithm for the transformation of an ambiguous code to an invariant code in the sound-localization pathway of the owl is across-frequency integration. This algorithm follows the rule that cells tuned to different frequencies but having a constant relation of phase and frequency project onto one cell in the next station. By this integration, the cell in the hierarchically higher station becomes not only broadly tuned to frequency, but becomes also endowed with the information to unambiguously represent one location in auditory space. This mechanism is similar to mechanisms of binding discussed in the visual literature (Singer and Gray, 1995), because features of a signal (object) are bound together. Thus, neurons in ICx represent a high-level extraction of an acoustic feature, ITD. Because these neurons are able to represent one location in space by also exhibiting selectivity for ILD, they have been termed *space-specific* neurons (Knudsen and Konishi, 1977).

One space-specific neuron can represent one location in auditory space. To represent the entire auditory space, many space-specific neurons, each tuned to slightly different locations, are necessary. Indeed, space-specific neurons are systematically arranged in the ICx to form a map of auditory space (Knudsen and Konishi, 1977). This map of auditory space is involved in sound-localization behavior, because small lesions in the map lead to predictable sound-localization deficits (Wagner, 1993).

In Figure 7.8 and Equation 1, I have outlined a theory that combines neurons responding to phase-frequency combinations that are linearly related. This was motivated by the good correlation between theory and observations made with stimuli presented via earphones (Figs. 7.8 and 7.9). Thus, one locus was represented by a linear phase-frequency relationship. Indeed, if the phase-frequency relationship is measured for sources at loci in frontal auditory space, linear relationships result (Brainard et al., 1992). For lateral auditory space, however, the relation is no longer linear (Brainard et al., 1992). Therefore, a linear relationship would not represent one locus in space, but many of them in a frequency-dependent way. Thus, the linear theory is a good approximation for frontal space only. For other locations in auditory space, the theory must be extended. The binding is most likely done by behavioral feedback (i.e., those phase-frequency combinations are bound together that lead to the best hunting success).

Further Brain Adaptations Subserving Sound-Localization Behavior

What I have explained thus far is how one sound locus can be represented in the brain. In addition, I have shown that the neural substrates performing these computations play a role in sound localization. The picture drawn thus far is fairly simple compared with the complexity of the hunting behavior outlined in "*Hunting as a Complex Behavior*", above. We have to explain why owls do not always react to sound stimuli, how owls remember sounds and sound loci, how information about the movement of a stimulus is combined with information about static stimuli, and how all these pieces of information are integrated with the other components of the hunting behavior. There are only partial solutions to these questions, and I shall briefly discuss several aspects now: integration of auditory and visual information, acoustic motion detection, the involvement of the telencephalon in sound localization, neural correlates of memory, and, finally, possible neural correlates of attention.

With the across-frequency integration from ICcls to ICx, the process of representation of static sound sources in the owl's brain is completed. From the ICx, this information is projected to the optic tectum (Knudsen and Knudsen, 1982). In the optic tectum sound localization information is combined with the visual information about a sound source (Knudsen and Knudsen, 1983). The optic tectum is a multilayered structure (Fig. 7.4, left pictures). Fifteen layers are distinguished in birds, which can be roughly divided into superficial and deep layers. The optic tectum contains a map of visual space that is evident in all layers. This map is represented in eye coordinates in most vertebrates. Owls are unable to move their eyes more than a few degrees; therefore, the visual tectal map in the owl is in head coordinates. Because auditory information is also mapped in head coordinates, it is easy to integrate the two maps in the tectum (Knudsen, 1982). The alignment is achieved through an instructive signal from the visual system to the auditory pathway (Knudsen and Knudsen, 1985). Alignment of visual and auditory maps in the midbrain is also found in other animals (Stein and Meredith, 1993). The specialty of the owl, however, is that auditory responses are found in both the superficial and the deep layers (Olsen et al., 1989), while in other animals, like cats and monkeys, auditory cells are sparse and only found in the deeper layers (Stein and Meredith, 1993). In the awake owl, electrical stimulation in the optic tectum causes head turns directed to the location in space that is represented by the part of the optic tectum being stimulated (duLac and Knudsen, 1990).

For effective hunting, the owl should take into account every available piece of information. Apart from static information about a sound source, there is also information about the movement of a source. Wagner and Takahashi (1990, 1992) found cells in the colliculus inferior of the owl that were sensitive to the motion direction of a sound source. The motion direction–sensitive cells were specifically arranged: Most cells on the right brain side were sensitive to clockwise motion (Wagner et al., 1994). Because the right brain side represents mainly left auditory space, these cells responded when the sound source moved leftward and thus might help the animal to focus a source in frontal space, where spatial resolution is highest.

The map of auditory space in the ICx is not the only neural representation of spatial loci. There is also a telencephalic pathway that is important for sound localization (Knudsen et al., 1993). The first station in the telencephalon is the so-called Field L. In this region, space-specific neurons were found first (Knudsen et al., 1977). However, space-specific neurons are not arranged in a map of auditory space in Field L. Neurons tuned to one location are clustered around each other, but neighboring locations in space are not represented at neighboring locations in Field L. Similar observations were made in other telencephalic areas, like the auditory part of the archistriatum (Cohen and Knudsen, 1995). Thus, the organizational principle in the telencephalon is different from that in the midbrain. There is a loop back from the telencephalon to the midbrain. In this way, the telencephalon may influence responses in the midbrain. Brainard (1994) proposed that there may be a division of labor between the two pathways: The midbrain pathway may subserve orienting responses, while the telencephalon may be required for complex localization behaviors.

Further evidence for a possible role of the telencephalon in sound-localization behavior came from experiments that investigated the involvement of memory in sound localization (Knudsen and Knudsen, 1996). In these experiments, first a visual zeroing stimulus was turned on. This stimulus elicited a head turn towards 0 azimuth and 0 elevation (Fig. 7.1D). Then the owl heard a sound from one spatial location, for example, 30° to the left. The bird turned its head to that location. Next the owl heard a second auditory stimulus, a buzz from the zero position, that elicited a second, stimulus-guided head turn. A short time after the second turn (0.1 to 2 seconds), the visual zeroing stimulus was turned off. This was the signal for the owl to make a third, memory-guided head turn toward the remembered location of the first sound and a subsequent flight to a rail in front of the loudspeaker of the first sound. Normal owls could perform this task without any problems, whereas owls with unilateral lesions in the archistriatum refused to fly in many cases when the sound came from that spatial hemifield, which had been represented by the lesioned area. Lesioned owls would still fly with little error when the sound came from that hemifield the representation of which was still intact.

The telencephalon may also be involved in the variability of the responses toward sounds described earlier that may be caused by changes in arousal or attention. How the owl's brain represents arousal or attention is still unclear. There are, however, some data available from visual motion detection that suggest possible mechanisms. When monkeys were trained to attend to a certain locus in space and at the same time the responses of cells in cortical area MT were recorded, the motion-direction sensitivity of the cells depended on the locus of attention. When attention was focused to a locus that overlapped with the spatial receptive field of the recorded cell, then motion-direction sensitivity was high, but when attention was turned to a spot outside the receptive field, motion-direction sensitivity decreased or was absent (Treue and Maunsell, 1996). Attention might influence the responses of the space-specific neurons in the same way.

What I have presented in this section is a hierarchy of computations that underlie sound-localization behavior. What we understand best thus far are the simplest computations like phase locking and coincidence detection. We have a fair understanding of across-frequency integration, auditory-visual integration and the substrates involved in memorizing sound loci and are at the beginning of understanding acoustic motion detection and the different roles of the telencephalon and the midbrain in these behaviors. Each of these aspects has been analyzed separately. These experiments have led to plausible explanations. What has not been done is to integrate the different aspects, that is, to move beyond a reductionistic analysis. This is not easy, because it requires us to formulate testable hypotheses on how this integration can happen on a neural basis.

In the following, I shall turn to two further aspects: one related to correlation between lifestyle and adaptations in owls and the other to the general meaning of the physiological algorithms discussed thus far.

Differences in the Representations of Acoustic Space in Diurnal and Nocturnal Owls

I have presented some data on adaptations of the owl's brain, and I have claimed that these specializations are a consequence of the nocturnal hunting of the barn owl. How can we know that this is true? The owl family itself offers a control for this hypothesis. Some owls are more nocturnal than others. Koch (1997) has compared feather specializations in nocturnal and diurnal owls and found fewer specializations in diurnal species. The vane of the ruff feathers was more orderly built in the nocturnal owls than in the diurnal owls: In nocturnal owls, the number of radii did not change along the the length of the rami, while in diurnal owls, a decrease in the number of radii was observed.

To obtain good two-dimensional resolution in hearing, one should use the two most reliable sound parameters, ITD and ILD, for different spatial coordinates and not as, for example, humans do, use both for the computation of azimuth. This can be achieved by an asymmetry in the ears. Ear asymmetry is more likely to occur in nocturnal owls and in those that specialize in small rodent prey (Norberg, 1987; Voous, 1989). This is an adaptation to hunting by listening. As has been mentioned above, an ear asymmetry affects mainly ILDs such that the axis along that ILD rotates out of the horizontal plane. Indeed, nocturnal owls are able to use ILDs to measure elevation, whereas diurnal owls are not. The morphological adaptations should also lead to different physiological responses. If there is no ear asymmetry, a spatial limitation of ILD tuning should not be observed, but if there is an ear asymmetry, spatial receptive fields should be limited in both azimuth and elevation. Volman and Konishi (1990) and Wise et al., (1988) analyzed spatial receptive fields of auditory cells in the ICx. In nocturnal owls, like the barn owl, the saw-whet owl, and the long-eared owl, spatial receptive fields were restricted in both azimuth and elevation. In diurnal owls, like the burrowing owl and the great-horned owl, the receptive fields were only restricted in azimuth, but not in elevation. This means that in diurnal owls we have a situation similar to other diurnal animals and humans. In conclusion, then, the comparison of diurnal and nocturnal owls demonstrates more specializations in nocturnal owls consistent with the hypothesis that these specializations have evolved with hunting in the dark.

GENERAL MEANING OF COINCIDENCE DETECTION AND ACROSS-FREQUENCY INTEGRATION

Owls are specialists for sound localization and have evolved effective neural algorithms to represent sound locations in their brain. What can we learn from these specializations about the general organization of brains and about problem solving in brains? I have already mentioned the general meaning of coincidence detection. In the following I shall discuss a possibly more general meaning of across-frequency integration and show that such an algorithm may play a role in the generation of neural information underlying cognitive behavior.

Linguists are currently trying to conceptualize the categorization of human speech sounds and they try to find representations in the brain that are neurobiologically viable and consistent with neural algorithms found in the auditory pathway. Sussman et al., (1998) argued that speech sounds that form contrastive categories in the phonological systems of languages are not too different from biologically important sounds in mammals and birds. From an evolutionary point of view, one might speculate that neural algorithms used in acoustic communication or sound localization may also be utilized in the representation of speech sounds.

An unsolved problem in speech research is the invariant mapping between the physical speech signal and the unit of message (see, e.g., Liberman and Mattingly, 1985). The speech signal is extremely variable as examples of the same phoneme are often physically different depending on the context in which they occur. For example, the [b]'s in *beat, bit, bait, bet, bat, bought, boat, boot,* and *but* are categorized as the phoneme /b/, although in every example /b/ is physically different. The question arises whether there is a possibility to map the physical signal into a meaningful speech signal, like a phoneme. Sussman (1989) tried to do this for stop consonant place of articulation (/b/,/d/,/g/) across vowel contexts. Spectrograms demonstrate that acoustic energy is concentrated in specific frequency regions or formants. Formants represent acoustic resonances of the vocal tract. Usually several formants, termed F1, F2, F3. . . . can be discriminated. During the production of isolated vowels, the formants are relatively constant. When we produce a more complex signal like a /da/, the formant frequencies change in response to the changing filter functions of the vocal tract. These frequency modulations are known as *formant transitions*. The transition of the second formant encodes best the dynamic consonant-to-vowel change (Liberman et al., 1967). The transition onset (F2-onset) and offsets (F2-vowel) can be determined and graphically displayed (Fig. 7.10A for /b/). F2-onset and F2-vowel are linearly related. In other words, the different examples mentioned above for the phoneme /b/ are linearly related in the context of F2-onset and F2-vowel (Fig. 7.10A). This holds also for /d/ and for /g/. The difference between the /b/, the /d/, and the /g/ lies in the slope of the straight line in the F2-onset–F2-vowel plot. The empirically determined relations of the speech-signal output are also known as *locus equations*. These locus equations have be validated cross-linguistically (Sussman et al., 1998).

Sussman (1989) has speculated that the linear relation between F2-onset and F2-vowel is not due to a genetic program, but is developmentally regulated and arises as a constraint due to the way the nervous system analyzes speech sounds. There are at least two steps necessary for this task. First, the F2-onset and the F2-vowel have to be bound together. This may happen in coincidence-detecting neurons. Sussman (1989) draws an analogy to the combination-sensitive neurons of the bat, which also bind together two different frequency components (Suga, 1988). Binding together F2-onset and F2-vowel, however, is not sufficient to represent a consonant unambiguously. We have the same problem as with the representation of ITD: Different F2-onset–F2-vowel components also signal the same consonant. Sussman (1989) has put forward the idea of across-frequency integration outlined earlier to postulate similar mechanisms and structures for the solution of the speech problem: functional

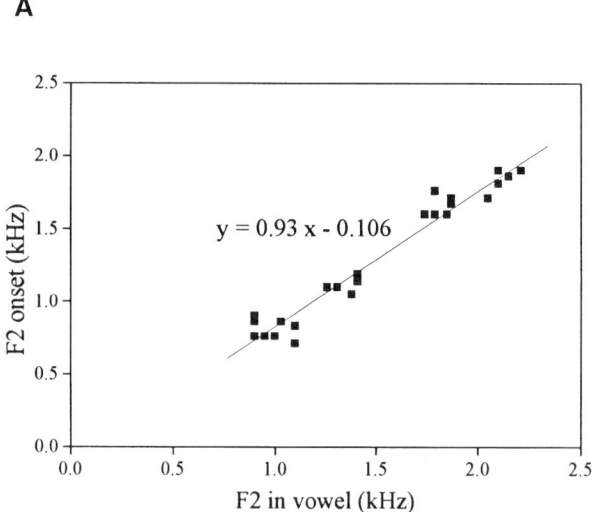

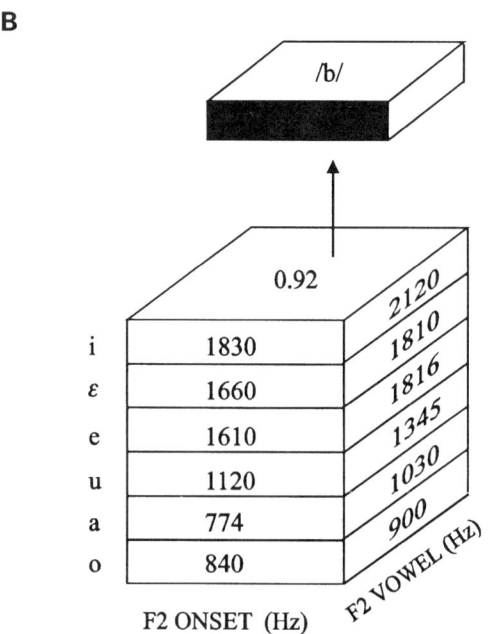

Figure 7.10. The concept of across-frequency integration in stop-consonant representation. (*A*) The locus equation for /b/. Note that F2-onset (at the transition of the consonant to the vowel) and F2 in vowel (at the time when the vowel is pronounced) are linearly related across different vowels (assembled after Sussman 1989, Fig. 7.3A). (*B*) Scheme of representation of /b/ in a two-dimensional map (assembled after Sussman 1989, Fig. 7.5). Sussman speculates that the representation of stop consonants may follow a similar rule as the representation interaural time difference in the owl (Wagner et al. 1987).

arrays with invariant properties that are absent in the individual elements of the arrays. Sussman (1989) and Sussman et al., (1991) also made an anatomical proposal for their model, and they again borrowed from the findings in the auditory system. They drew slabs in a similar way as we had done for the owl (Fig. 7.10B; see also Wagner et al., 1987). The different slabs would represent different slopes, each representing one invariant aspect, while the subslabs could not represent the consonant invariantly. These arrays would project to a hierarchically higher station. The output of the higher order neuron would represent one consonant only. What this analogy shows is that neural algorithms might have a wide application and seem not to be dedicated to a specific task in one species.

Although I regard Sussman's proposal as a good example for the general application of neural algorithms, such a statement should not be made without words of caution. Simply drawing an analogy does not suffice. A proposal about how such arrays might be generated in ontogeny is necessary, because the variation in the vocal tract is too large for genetic preprogramming of the locus equations, and there is no necessity of a linear representation. In the speech signal, the signals that should form the slabs are not present in the signal simultaneously. How, then, can they be combined? Sussman et al., (1991) made a proposal the neurobiological validity of which is not yet clear.

CONCLUSIONS

Evolution has shaped neural algorithms as it has shaped morphology and anatomy. The barn owl was used as an example to discuss adaptation for hunting when the prey is not visible to the predator. Peripheral specializations help to amplify incoming sounds and to suppress flight noises. Similar morphological specializations related to the lifestyle of an animal are often found: Penguins have a special body form that allows them to swim effectively, the wing form in vultures is optimal for soaring, and that of albatrosses and shearwaters helps them to save energy when gliding low over the waves of the oceans. Peripheral specializations suggest adaptations in sensory and/or motor pathways, and, thus, for most of the peripheral specializations we expect corresponding adaptations in the brain. What we see is an increase in brain mass in those nuclei that process the specific information. This holds for animals from very different taxa, like electric fish, lungless salamanders, owls, and bats, to name but a few. Thus, the brain is plastic enough to react to evolutionary pressure and to shape brain anatomy likewise. The brain may also invent new algorithms, and the appearance of NMDA receptors and their computational capacity in vertebrates may been seen in this context. However, invertebrates that lack NMDA receptors are also able to perform computations that bind two stimuli together. In this respect the algorithms seem to be more conservative than brain anatomy.

Neuroscientists are reductionists in that they dissect behavior and study only some aspects of it. This is necessary to obtain quantitative data. In the end, however, the behavior as a whole needs an explanation. Behavior is not monocausal; it is probably more than the sum of all its aspects studied by neuroscientists. This leaves us with a problem when trying to explain behavior from neurobiological data. Neuroethology has tried to bridge this gap by using natural stimuli for the analysis of neural representations of the world. It has been quite successful in doing so. The barn owl provides a good example for this claim (Konishi, 1993). Since the first papers by Konishi and his collaborators Knudsen and Pettigrew some 20 years ago, we have learned quite a lot about the neural mechanisms underlying sound localization. There is still a lot more to discover. The future direction will be both more integrative and more reductionist. On the integrative level, recordings from awake, behaving birds will help with understanding what is going on in the brain while the bird is behaving. On the more reductionist level, we shall try to further understand the neural and molecular mechanisms underlying behavior. Last but not least, everything has to be tied together by theory, because a mere description does not bring us forward enough. A good example is the theory of coincidence detection and across-frequency integration discussed in the text. If a theory is formulated appropriately, it may stimulate research in other fields. Due to the conservation of neural algorithms, this may contribute to an understanding of quite remote processes as demonstrated by Sussman and co-workers, who used algorithms from the owl to explain the representation of consonants in speech sounds.

REFERENCES

Andrew, R.J. (1982) Lateralisation of emotional and cognitive function in higher vertebrates, with special reference to the domestic chick. In J.P. Ewert, R. Capranica, and D.J. Ingle (eds.): *Advances in Vertebrate Neuroethology.* Academic Press, New York, pp. 477–510.
Borst, A., and M. Egelhaaf (1989) Principles of visual motion detection. *TINS* 12:297–306.
Brainard, M. (1994) Neural substrates of sound localization. *Curr. Opin. Neurobiol.* 4:557–562.
Brainard, M.S., and E.I. Knudsen (1993) Experience-dependent plasticity in the inferior colliculus: a site for visual calibration of the neural representation of auditory space in the barn owl. *J. Neurosci.* 13:4589–4608.
Brainard, M.S., and E.I. Knudsen (1995) Dynamics of visually guided auditory plasticity in the optic tectum of the barn owl. *J. Neurophysiol.* 73:595–614.
Brainard, M.S., E.I. Knudsen, and S.D. Esterly (1992) Neural derivation of sound source location: resolution of spatial ambiguities in binaural cues. *J. Acoust. Soc. Am.* 91:1015–1027.
Brandt, T., C Seebass (1994) *Die Schleiereule.* Aula-Verlag, Wiesbaden.
Bunn, D.S., A.B. Warburton, and R.D.S. Wilson (1990) *The barn owl.* T&A D Poyser, Calton.
Carney, T., M.A. Paradiso, and R.D. Freeman (1989) A physiological correlate of the Pulfrich effect in cortical neurons of the cat. *Vis. Res.* 29:155–165.
Carr, C.E. (1993) Processing of temporal information in the brain. *Annu. Rev. Neurosci.* 16:223–243.
Carr, C.E., and R.E. Boudreau (1993) Organization of the nucleus magnocellularis and the nucleus laminaris in the barn owl: encoding and measuring interaural time differences. *J. Comp. Neurol.* 334:337–355.
Carr, C.E., and M. Konishi (1990) A circuit for detection of interaural time differences in the brainstem of the barn owl. *J. Neurosci.* 10:3227–3246.
Changeux, J.-P. (1981) The acetylcholine receptor: an "allosteric" membrane protein. *Harvey Lect.* 75:85–254.
Cohen, Y.E., and E.I. Knudsen (1995) Binaural tuning of auditory units in the telencephalon archistriatal gaze fields of the barn owl: local organization but no space map. *J. Neurosci.* 15(7):5152–5168.
Coles, R.B., and A. Guppy (1988) Directional hearing in the barn owl (*Tyto alba*). *J. Comp. Physiol.* A 163:117–133.

Crick F. (1993) *The asthonishing hypothesis.* Macmillan, New York.
Du Lac, S., and E.I. Knudsen (1990) Neural maps of head movement vector and speed in the optic tectum of the barn owl. *J. Neurophysiol.* 63:131–146.
Feldman, D.E., M.S. Brainard, and E.I. Knudsen (1996) Newly learned auditory responses mediated by NMDA receptors in the owl inferior colliculus. *Science* 271:525–528.
Gerstner, W., R. Kempter, J.L. van Hemmen, and H. Wagner (1996) A neuronal learning rule for sub-millisecond temporal coding. *Nature* 383:76–78.
Heck, D. (1993) Rat cerebellar cortex in vitro responds specifically to moving stimuli. *Neurosc. Lett.* 157:95–98.
Hodgkin, A.L., and A.F. Huxley (1952) A quantitative description of membrane currents and its application to conduction and excitation in nerve. *J. Physiol. (Lond.)* 117:500–544.
Jeffress, L.A. (1948) A place theory of sound localization. *J. Comp. Physiol. Psychol.* 41:35–39.
Kandel, E.R., and J. H. Schwartz (1982) Molecular biology of learning: modulation of transmitter release. *Science* 218:433–443.
Karten, H.J., W. Hodos, W.J.H. Nauta, and A.M. Revzin (1973) Neural connections of the "visual Wulst" of the avian telencephalon. Experimental studies in the pigeon (*Columba livia*) and owl (*Speotyto cunicularia*). *J. Comp. Neurol.* 150:253–278.
Knudsen, E.I. (1982) Auditory and visual maps of space in the optic tectum of the owl. *J. Neurosci.* 2:1177–1194.
Knudsen, E.I. (1983) Subdivisions of the inferior colliculus in the barn owl (*Tyto alba*). *J. Comp. Neurol.* 218:174–186.
Knudsen, E.I. (1984) Synthesis of a neural map of auditory space in the owl. In G.M. Edelman, E.W. Gall, and M.W. Cowen (eds.): *Dynamic Aspects of Neocortical Function*, Neurosciences Research Foundation, Inc., pp. 375–396.
Knudsen, E.I., and M.S. Brainard (1995) Creating a unified representation of visual and auditory space in the brain. *Annu. Rev. Neurosci.* 18:19–43.
Knudsen, E.I., Y.E.Cohen, and T. Masino (1995) Characterization of a telencephalon gaze field in the archistriatum of the barn owl: microstimulation and anatomical connections. *J. Neurosci.* 15:5139–5151.
Knudsen, E.I., S.D. Esterly, and J.F. Olsen (1994) Adaptive plasticity of the auditory space map in the optic tectum of adult and baby barn owls in response to external ear modification. *J. Neurophysiol.* 71:79–94.
Knudsen, E.I., and P.F. Knudsen (1983) Space-mapped auditory projections from the inferior colliculus to the optic tectum in the barn owl. *J. Comp. Neurol.* 218:187–196.
Knudsen, E.I., and P.F. Knudsen (1985) Vision guides the adjustment of auditory localization in young barn owls. *Science* 230:545–548.
Knudsen, E.I., and P.F. Knudsen (1996) Disruption of auditory spatial working memory by inactivation of the telencephalon archistriatum in barn owls. *Nature* 383:428–431.
Knudsen, E.I., P.F. Knudsen, and T. Masino (1993) Parallel pathways mediating both sound localization and gaze control in the telencephalon and midbrain of the barn owl. *J. Neurosci.* 13:2837–2852.
Knudsen, E.I., and M. Konishi (1978a) A neural map of auditory space in the owl. *Science* 200:795–797.
Knudsen, E.I., and M. Konishi (1978b) Space and frequency are represented separately in auditory midbrain of the owl. *J. Neurophysiol.* 41:870–884.
Knudsen, E.I., M. Konishi, and J.D. Pettigrew (1977) Receptive fields of auditory neurons in the owl. *Science* 198:1278–1280.
Koch, U. (1997) *Morphometrische Untersuchungen an Kopffedern von Eulen im Hinblick auf die akustische Ortung.* Diplomarbeit der RWTH Aachen.
Kolb K.H. (1988) *Das Verhalten des Rauhfubkauzes (Aegolius funereus) beim Beutefang.* Diplomarbeit Universität Tübingen.
Konishi, M. (1973) How the owl tracks its prey. *Am. Sci.* 61:414–424.
Konishi, M. (1993) Listening with two ears. *Sci. Am.* April:66–73.
Konnerth, A., R.Y., Tsien, K. Mikoshiba, and Altman J. (1996) *Conicidence Detection in the Nervous System.* HSFP, Strasbourg.
Köppl, C. (1997) Phase locking to high frequencies in the auditory nerve and cochlear nucleus magnocellularis of te barn owl, *Tyto alba. J. Neurosci.* 17:3312–3321.
Köppl, C., O. Gleich, and G.A. Manley (1993) An auditory fovea in the barn owl cochlea. *J. Comp. Physiol.* A 171:695–704.
Liberman, A.M., and I. Mattingly (1985) The motor theory of speech perception revised. *Cognition* 21:1–36.

Liberman, A.M., F.S. Cooper, D.P. Shankweiler, and M. Studdert-Kennedy (1967) Perception og the speech code. *Psychol. Rev.* 74:431–461.
Manis, P.B., and S.O. Marx (1991) Outward currents in isolated ventral cochlear nucleus neurons. *J. Neurosci.* 11:2865–2880.
Masino, T., and E.I. Knudsen (1993) Orienting head movements resulting from electrical microstimulation of the brainstem tegmentum in the barn owl. *J. Neurosci.* 13:351–370.
Maunsell, J.H.R. (1995) The brain's visual world: representation of visual targets in cerebral cortex. *Science* 270:764–769.
Mebs, T. (1980) *Eulen und Käuze*. Franckh'sche Verlagshandlung, Stuttgart.
Moiseff, A. (1989a) Binaural disparity cues available to the barn owl for sound localization. *J. Comp. Physiol.* A 164:629–636.
Moiseff, A., (1989b) Bi-coordinate sound localization by the barn owl. *J. Comp. Physiol.* A164:637–644.
Moiseff, A., and M. Konishi (1981) Neuronal and behavioral sensitivity to binaural time differences in the owl. *J. Neurosci.* 1:40–48.
Moiseff, A., and M. Konishi (1983) Binaural characteristics of units in the owl's brainstem auditory pathway: precursors of restricted spatial receptive fields. *J. Neurosci.* 3:2553–2562.
Moore, B.C.J. (1994) *An Introduction to the Psychology of Hearing*, 4th ed. Academic press, London.
Neuhaus, W., H. Bretting, and B. Schweizer (1973) Morphologische und funktionelle Untersuchungen über den "lautlosen" Flug der Eulen (Strix aluco) im Vergleich zum Flug der Enten (*Anas playrhynchos*). *Biol. Zbl.* 92:495–512.
Norberg, A.R. (1987) Evolution, structure, and ecology of northern forest owls. Biology and conservation of Northern Forest Owls. Symp. Proc. 9–43.
Olsen, J.F., E.I. Knudsen, and S.D. Esterly (1989) Neural maps of interaural time and intensity differences in the optic tectum of the barn owl. *J. Neurosci.* 9:2591–2605.
Payne, R.S. (1962) How the barn owl locates prey by hearing. The Living Bird, First Annual of the Cornell Laboratory Of Ornithology, pp. 151–159.
Payne, R.S. (1971) Acoustic location of prey by barn owls (*Tyto alba*). *J. Exp. Biol.* 54:535–573.
Pettigrew, J.D., and M. Konishi (1976) Neurons selective for orientation and binocular disparity in the visual Wulst of the barn owl (*Tyto alba*). *Science* 193:675–678.
Quine, D.B., and M. Konishi (1974) Absolute frequency discrimination in the barn owl. *J. Comp. Physiol.* A 93:347–360.
Reyes, A.D., E.W. Rubel, and W.J. Spain (1996) In vitro analysis of optimal stimuli for phase-locking and time-delayed modulation of firing in avian nucleus laminaris neurons. *J. Neurosci.* 16(3):993–1007.
Rose, J.E., N.G. Grass, C.D. Geisler, and J.E. Hind (1966) Some neural mechanisms in the inferior colliculus of the cat which may be relevant to the localization of a sound source. *J. Neurophysiol.* 29:288–314.
Russell, I.J., and P.M. Sellick (1983) Low-frequency characteristics of intracellularly recorded receptor potentials in guinea-pig cochlear hair cells. *J. Physiol.* (*Lond.*) 338:179–206.
Schaeffel, F., and H. Wagner (1992) Barn owls have symmetrical accommodation in both eyes, but independent pupillary responses to light. *Vis. Res.* 32:1149–1155.
Sick, H. (1937) Morphologisch-funktionelle Untersuchungen über die Feinstruktur der Vogelfeder. *J. Ornithol.* 85:206–371.
Singer, W., and C.M. Gray (1995) Visual feature integration and the temporal correlation hypothesis. *Annu. Rev. Neurosci.* 18:555–586.
Stein, B.E., M.A. Meredith (1993) *Merging of the Senses*. MIT Press, London.
Streets, T.H. (1870) Remarks of the cranium of an owl. *Proc. Acad. Nat. Sci. Phila.* 1870:73.
Suga, N. (1988) Auditory neuroethology and speech processing: complex-sound processing by combination-sensitive neurons. In G.M. Edelman, W.E. Gall, and W.M Cowan (eds.): *Auditory Function*. John Wiley and Sons, New York, pp. 679–720.
Sussman, H.M. (1989) Neural coding of relational invariance in speech: human language analogs to the barn owl. *Psychol. Rev.* 96:631–642.
Sussman, H.M., H.A. McCaffrey, and S.A. Matthews (1991) An investigation of locus equations as a source of relational invariance for stop place. *J. Acoust. Soc. Am.* 90:1309–1325.
Sussman, H.M., D. Fruchter, J. Hilbert, and J. Sirosh (1998) Linear correlates in the speech signal: the orderly output constraint. *Behav. Brain Sci.* (in press).
Takahashi, T.T., and C.H. Keller (1992) Simulated motion enhances neuronal selectivity for a sound localization cue in background noise. *J. Neurosci.* 12:4381–4390.

Takahashi, T.T., and C.H. Keller (1994) Representation of multiple sound sources in the owl's auditory space map. *J. Neurosci.* 14.

Takahashi, T., and M. Konishi (1986) Selectivity for interaural time difference in the owl's midbrain. *J. Neurosci.* 6:3413–3422.

Takahashi, T.T., and M. Konishi (1988) Projections of the cochlear nuclei and nucleus laminaris to the inferior colliculus of the barn owl. *J. Comp. Neurol.* 274:190–211.

Takahashi, T., A. Moiseff, and M. Konishi (1984) Time and intensity cues are processed independently in the auditory system of the owl. *J. Neurosci.* 4:1781–1786.

Takahashi, T.T., H. Wagner, and M. Konishi (1989) Role of commissural projections in the representation of bilateral auditory space in the barn owl's inferior colliculus. *J. Comp. Neurol.* 281:545–554.

Taylor, I. (1994) *Barn Owls.* Cambridge University Press, Cambridge.

Treue, S., and J.H.R. Maunsell (1996) Attentional modulation of visual motion processing in cortical areas MT and MST. *Nature* 382:539–542.

Tyler, C. W., and M. B. Clarke (1990) The autostereogram. *Proc. Int. Soc. Opt. Eng.* 1256:182–197.

Volman, S.F. (1994) Directional hearing in owls: neurobiology, behaviour and evolution. In M.N.O. Davies and P.R. Green, (eds.): *Perception and Motor Control in Birds*, Springer, Berlin, pp. 293–314.

Volman, S.F., and M. Konishi (1990) Comparative physiology of sound localization in four species of owls. *Brain Behav. Evol.* 36:196–215.

Voous, K.H. (1950) *Owls of the Northern Hemisphere.* MIT Press, Cambridge.

Wagner, H. (1993) Sound-localization deficits induced by lesions in the barn owl's space map. *J. Neurosci.* 13:371–386.

Wagner, H., and B. Frost (1993) Disparity sensitive cells in the owl have a characteristic diparity. *Nature* 364:796–798.

Wagner, H., H.O. Nalbach, and I. Pappe (1993) Optokinetic responses in barn owls. *Soc. Neurosci. Abstr.* 19:345.

Wagner, H. and F. Schaeffel (1991) Barn owls (*Tyto alba*) use accommodation as a distance cue. *J. Comp. Physiol.* A169:515–521.

Wagner, H. and T. Takahashi (1990) Neurons in the midbrain of the barn owl are sensitive to the direction of apparent acoustic motion. *Naturwissenschaften* 77:439–442.

Wagner, H., and T.T. Takahashi (1992) Influence of temporal cues on acoustic motion-direction sensitivity of auditory neurons in the owl. *J. Neurophysiol.* 68:2063–2076.

Wagner, H., T. Takahashi, and M. Konishi (1987) Representation of interaural time difference in the central nucleus of the barn owl's inferior colliculus. *J. Neurosci.* 7:3105–3116.

Wagner, H., T. Trinath, and D. Kautz (1994) Influence of stimulus level on acoustic motion-direction sensitivity in barn owl midbrain neurons. *J. Neurophysiol.* 71:1907–1916.

Wallman, J., and J. Velez, (1985) Directional asymmetries of optokinetic nystagmus: developmental changes and relation to the accessory optic system and to the vestibular system. *J. Neurosci.* 5:317–329.

Warchol, M.E., and P. Dallos, (1990) Neural coding in the chick cochlear nucleus. *J. Comp. Physiol.* A166:721–734.

Willigen, v.d. R., and H. Wagner (1997) Stereopsis in the barn owl (*Tyto alba*). A behavioral demonstration. In N. Elsner and H. Wässle (eds.): *Proceedings of the 25th Göttingen Neurobiology Conference.* vol. II, p. 536.

Wink, M. (1993) Molekulare Methoden in der Greifvogelforschung. *Greifvögel Falknerei* 17–28.

Wise, L.Z., B.J. Frost, and S.W. Shaver, (1988) The representation of sound frequency and space in the midbrain of the saw-whet owl. *Soc. Neurosci. Abstr.* 14:1095.

Yin, T.C., and S. Kuwada (1983) Binaural interaction in low-frequency neurons in the inferior colliculus of the cat. III. Effects of changing frequency. *J. Neurophysiol.* 50:1020–1042.

Chapter 8

EVOLUTION AND DEVOLUTION: THE CASE OF BOLITOGLOSSINE SALAMANDERS

Gerhard Roth and David B. Wake, Brain Research Institute, University of Bremen (GR) Museum of Vertebrate Zoology, University of California, Berkeley (DBW)

INTRODUCTION

In the past, the evolution of the nervous system, including the brain, was envisioned as a near monotonic increase in size, both absolute and relative, as well as in morphological and functional complexity (Ariens-Kappers et al., 1936; Romer, 1970; Jerison, 1973; Kuhlenbeck, 1977; Northcutt, 1981; Ebbesson, 1980, 1984; Sarnat and Netsky, 1981; Starck, 1982). This process of *encephalization* was assumed to start with a simple nerve plexus (as found in current cnidarians) from which emerged central nervous systems and, subsequently, by a number of significant increases in structural and functional complexity, brains (i.e., supraesophageal [cerebral] ganglia) as in platyhelminths, nemathelminths, nemertines, molluscs, annelids, and arthropods. Encephalization was thought to continue with the vertebrates, where a series of increases in structural and functional complexity characterize the evolutionary transitions from myxinoids and petromyzontids to mammals (Ariens-Kappers et al., 1936). Such an increase was viewed as favoring sensory, motor, and cognitive functions, which, in turn, contributed directly to evolutionary success (i.e., persistence, species proliferation, and number of individuals).

Such a conception of the evolution of nervous systems as a process of essentially continuous encephalization is no longer justified (see Wullimann, this volume, Chapter 1). During phylogeny, some taxa have evolved complex brains, but at the same time others have secondarily simplified brains, giving the impression of a kind of *devolution* (i.e., secondary simplification). Examples of the latter, as revealed by cladistic analysis (Roth and Wullimann, 1996), are the following: (1) Platyhelminths (about 16,000 species) are the first group of metazoans that possess bilaterally symmetrical central nervous systems. Among the freely living platyhelminths, the "turbellarians," taxa are found (e.g., the Acoela) that have completely lost a central nervous system. Moreover, the nervous systems of trematods and cestods (several thousand species) are all secondarily simplified. (2) Among molluscs, many of the 100,000 species of gastropods and all bivalves (Lamellibranchiata, 20,000 species) have moderately to strongly simplified nervous systems. (3) Strong secondary simplification of the central nervous system is likewise found in some groups of annelids (e.g., in hirudineans [Oligochaeta] and in arthropods (e.g., in mites [Acari, Arachnida; more than 30,000 species]). (4) Tentaculates (about 5000 species) as well as hemichordates and urochordates have relatively simple central nervous systems compared with other invertebrates and either represent independent cases or one single case of secondary simplification in the last common ancestor of tentaculates and deuterostomes. In other words, among invertebrates, secondary simplification of nervous systems is at least as common as is an increase in structural and functional complexity.

Among vertebrates (Fig. 8.1A), secondary simplification of nervous systems seems a rare event. There are, however, at least three groups of vertebrates that have undergone profound simplification of the central nervous system, viz., salamanders, caecilians, and lepidosirenid lungfishes. There are cases of weaker secondary simplification of the central nervous system in other taxa as well (e.g. in frogs) and of simplification at least with respect to some traits of the nervous system (e.g., unlaminated or three-layered [as opposed to six-layered] isocortex in cetaceans and insectivores) (Nieuwenhuys et al., 1998).

Secondary simplification of nervous systems seems counterintuitive under a strict adaptionist's view. Why should reduction in brain size, nerve cell number, and morphological complexity or even the loss of sensory systems be advantageous for survival? Of course, one can find adaptive scenarios even for simplification (e.g., getting rid of developmentally or metabolically "expensive" structures or functions that are no longer needed in certain environments). This is a reasonable explanation for cases in which simplification is part of a transition to sedentary or parasitic life, as is found in many invertebrates (e.g., trematods, cestodes, bivalves, hirudineans, tentaculates, hemichordates, and urochordates). Even here, however, an important question remains to be answered: Which came first, the simplification or the changes in life style? The case of the Echinodermata remains enigmatic: Why did they give up a bilateral central nervous system? Equally unexplained are the cases of secondary simplification found among vertebrates. The most dramatic one is the case of tongue-projecting salamanders, the Bolitoglossini.

THE BOLITOGLOSSINI

The Bolitoglossini, or tongue-projecting salamanders, represent, with about 180 species described, the largest group among the family Plethodontidae (about 275 species), which, in turn, comprises more than two thirds of all extant salamanders (order Caudata, approximately 400 species) (Fig. 8.1B,C). Thus, bolitoglossines constitute about 50% of living salamander species. They are almost exclusively found in North, Central, and South America (including Brazil and Bolivia) and are the only truly tropical salamanders. The largest number of species and the highest morphological and ecological diversity within the bolitoglossines are found in Central America. Several species of the genus *Hydromantes* represent the only bolitoglossines

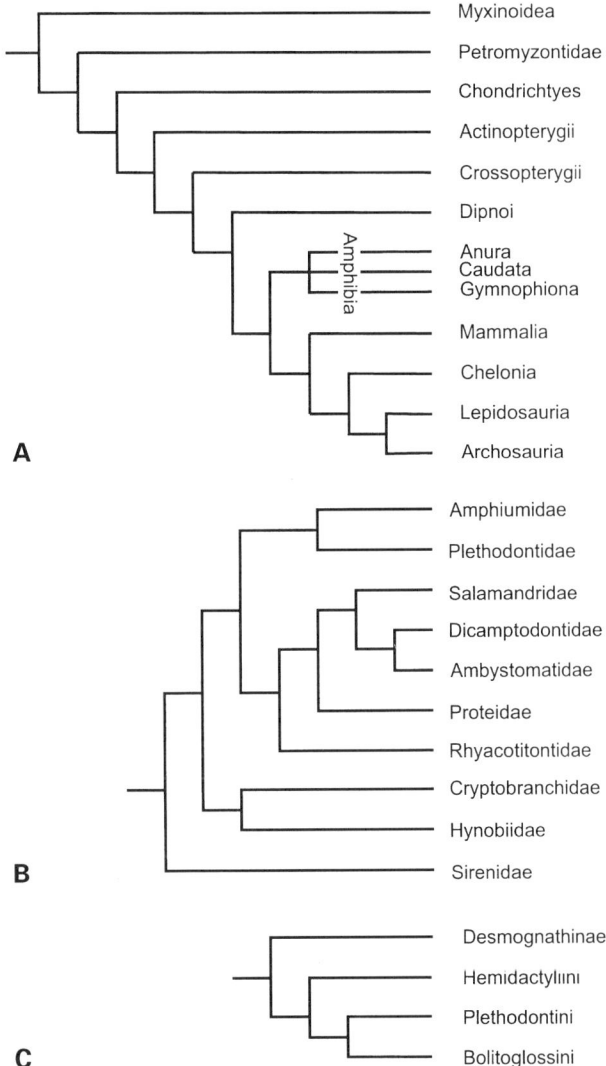

Figure 8.1. (*A*) Phylogenetic relationships of extant vertebrates. (From Roth et al., 1993.) (*B*) Phylogenetic relationships of extant taxonomic families of salamanders (Caudata). (After Larson and Dimmick, 1993.) (*C*) Phylogenetic relationships of plethodontids. (After Wake, 1966.)

living outside the New World; they are found in southern France, northern Italy, and Sardinia, although some North American species of *Hydromantes* occur in California. All nonbolitoglossine plethodontids are found exclusively in North America. The Plethodontidae are believed to have originated in eastern North America, in the Appalachian highlands, where they inhabited mountain brooks (Wilder et al., 1920; Dunn, 1926; Wake, 1966). Apparently as an adaptation to this habitat, they underwent

240   8 Evolution and Devolution: The Case of Bolitoglossine Salamanders

reduction and eventually complete loss of lungs—an event that occurred several times among salamanders other than plethodontids living in similar habitats (Beachy and Bruce, 1992). Plethodontid salamanders compensate their lunglessness by gas exchange through a highly vascularized skin and mouth cavity.

All Bolitoglossini are terrestrial. They lack aquatic larvae and have direct development (i.e., eggs are laid on land) from which tiny but adultlike salamanders hatch (Fig. 8.2.). During embryonic development, bolitoglossines do not form larval traits such as a larval hyobranchial apparatus, as do other directly developing plethodontids. The evolution of direct development and of terrestriality appears to be unrelated to lunglessness, because direct development and strict terrestriality has evolved independently many times among both lung-breathing and lungless amphibian taxa (Duellman and Trueb, 1986). The great success of plethodontid salamanders, which in some regions may exceed birds and small mammals in biomass, is certainly related to the evolution of direct development and terrestriality, because these animals are thereby freed from a biphasic life cycle and from dependence on free surface water—features that constrain other amphibians. Accordingly, terrestrial plethodontids, and bolitoglossines in particular, have invaded the most

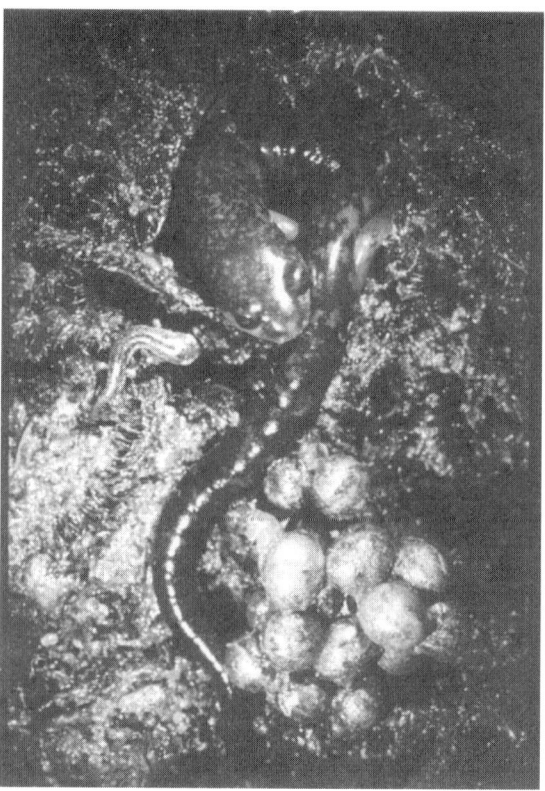

Figure 8.2. *Bolitoglossa* with eggs. (Courtesy of Dr. U. Dicke.)

diverse habitats from earthworm holes and limestone caves to bromeliads and moss mats in the trees of the tropical rain and cloud forests (Wake, 1987). Many tropical bolitoglossines are facultatively or strictly arboreal, and, not surprisingly, have diverse locomotor specializations, including acrobatic ability for life in three-dimensional environments.

Bolitoglossines are characterized by a unique feeding mechanism, i.e., a projectile tongue (Lombard and Wake, 1976, 1977, 1987; Roth, 1987). It consists of a greatly elongated hyobranchial apparatus with the tongue muscles at its anterior tip. During projection, it forms a slender projectile that is projected up to 80% of head plus body length (Deban et al., 1997) (Figs. 8.3 and 8.4). In salamanders with a biphasic life cycle, this apparatus develops from the skeleton of the hyoid and branchial arches. It consists of an unpaired median basibranchial (BB), which lies in the floor of the mouth. Two pairs of ceratobranchials (CB) articulate with the posterior end of the BB. The first and second CB on either side extend posteriorly, approaching each other, and together articulate with the epibranchial (EB). On each side of this apparatus a pair of cerytohyals lies in the floor of the mouth. In plethodontids, their anterior portion forms a flattened blade, which is attached to the lower jaw by the geniohyoideus muscle (see below), while their posterior end is cylindrical and hooked and attached to the upper jaw suspension by a ligament. The tongue pad, which contains the tongue muscles proper, is situated at the anterior end of the BB and is covered by numerous glands.

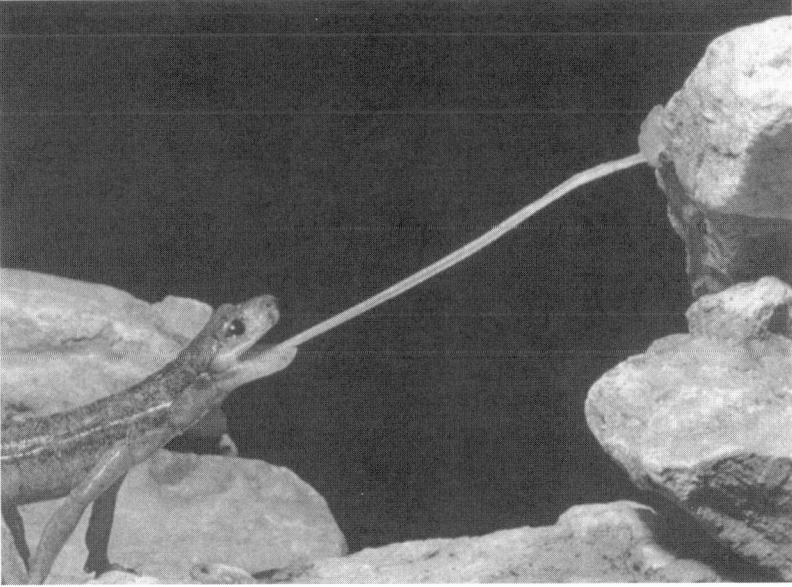

Figure 8.3. Tongue projection in *Hydromantes supramontis*. This salamander has the longest projectile tongue relative to body length. (From Deban et al., 1997.)

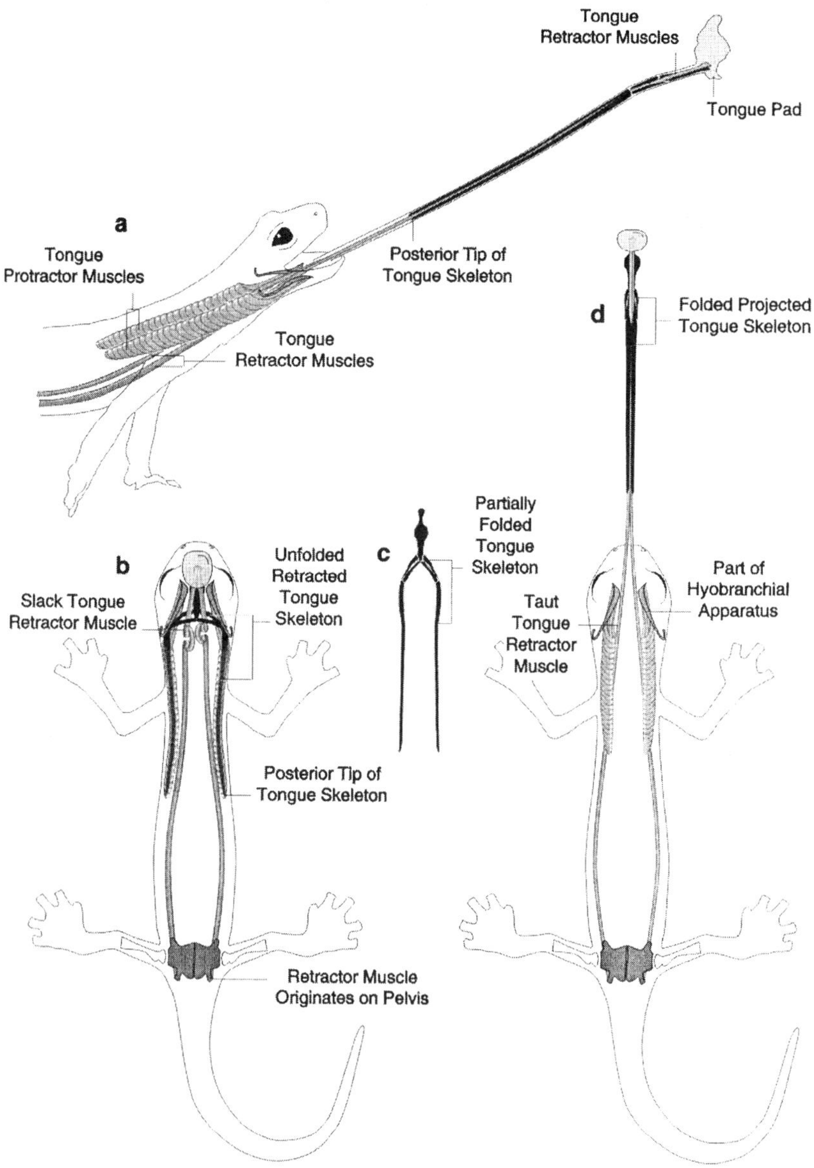

Figure 8.4. Tongue-projection system of *Hydromantes supramontis*. (*a*) Lateral view corresponding to Figure 8.3 showing the tongue skeleton (black) projected completely out of the mouth and bilaterally paired tongue protractor and retractor muscles. (*b*) Dorsal view with tongue skeleton in the unfolded retracted position, elongate posterior elements sheathed in protractor muscles, and slack, looped retractor mucles originating on the pelvis. (*c*) Tongue skeleton partially folded as in an early stage of projection. (*d*) Dorsal view showing the tongue skeleton projected entirely from the body, beyond the contracted protractor muscles, which are anchored anteriorly to the portion of the hyobranchial apparatus that remains in the mouth. The retractor muscles, now taut, run the full length of the extended tongue and body. (From Deban et al., 1997.)

The main muscles associated with this skeleton are (Fig. 8.4) (1) The subarcualis rectus I muscle, which encircles the caudal end of the EBs, forming a bulb, and extends rostrally along this element, forming a muscular sheath. It then attaches broadly to the ventral surface of the flattened anterior end of the ceratohyals. (2) The rectus cervicis profundus, which originates from the puboischium and runs along the body axis to the anterior part of the BB. (3) The geniohyoideus lateralis, which arises at the lateral edge of the ceratohyals and extends to the lower jaw. (4) The genioglossus, which—if present—extends from the ventral surface of the lower jaw on each side of the symphysis and inserts dorsally in the substance of the rostral tongue.

In all generalized salamanders (e.g., most salamandrids and ambystomatids), the hyobranchial apparatus exerts a dual function in metamorphosed animals (viz., respiration and feeding). It serves as a buccal pump for respiration in that it expands the buccal cavity. During prey capture, the tongue is pushed out of the mouth by a limited forward movement of the hyobranchial skeleton. In the Bolitoglossini, the tongue apparatus has undergone a dramatic evolution, including substantial elongation of epibranchials and loss of the genioglossus muscle, leading to free tongues in the sense that the entire hyobranchial apparatus plus retractor muscle (rectus cervicis profundus), and not only the tongue muscle proper, are projected out of the mouth (Lombard and Wake, 1976, 1977; Deban et al., 1997) (Figs. 8.3 and 8.4). The development of such a highly mobile tongue appears to be intimately connected to a reduction or loss of lungs (Wake, 1982; Roth and Wake, 1985a). This event freed the hyobranchial apparatus from the function of serving as a lung pump, giving it the chance to evolve in the direction of feeding alone. In *Bolitoglossa occidentalis*, the whole tongue reaction takes place in about 10 ms (Thexton et al., 1977); in the genus *Hydromantes*, having the longest tongue, it lasts 80 to 100 ms (Roth, 1976) (Figs. 8.3 and 8.4).

With regard to feeding strategy, many frogs and salamanders are hunters in that they actively search for prey. In contrast, Bolitoglossines are mostly ambush feeders, that is, they sit and wait (often under a cover or in a cavity) until prey comes by. The evolution of an ambush strategy probably was forced by the inability of bolitoglossines to move fast because of very low metabolic levels (see below). It may have been impossible in terrestrial environments to elude predators while hunting prey. An ambush strategy is safer and metabolically less costly, but it requires a fast and precise feeding mechanism, such as a free, projectile tongue, and very good depth perception abilities, which, in turn, require binocular, stereoscopic vision. Not surprisingly, bolitoglossine salamanders have more frontally located eyes than do other salamanders and most frogs, and therefore have a larger binocular visual field (Linke et al., 1986).

In the Bolitoglossini, we find a substantial number of retinal fibers to project to the ipsilateral optic tectum (Fig. 8.5.) in addition to the contralaterally projecting ones (Rettig and Roth, 1986). This is uncommon among other amphibians as well as among most other vertebrates except some mammals. In the bolitoglossines ipsilateral retinotectal projections may serve to enable direct comparison between information from the left and right eye in the context of stereopsis. Recent neurophysiological experiments suggest that bolitoglossines make use of the disparities between the contralateral and direct and indirect ipsilateral retinotectal projections to

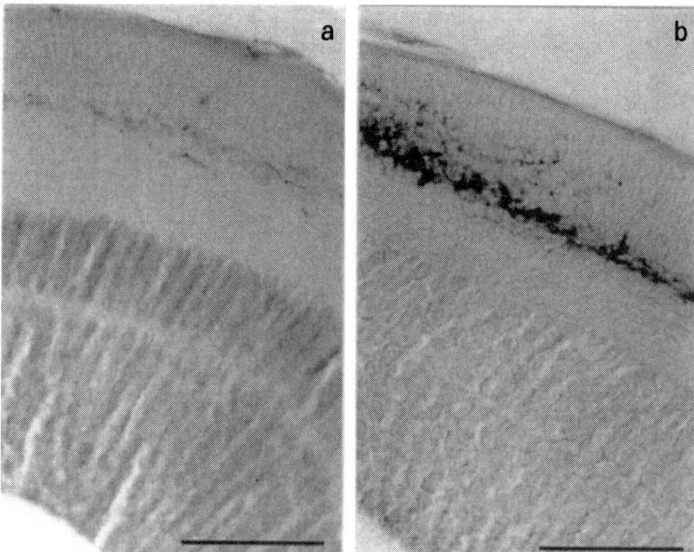

Figure 8.5. Cross section through the optic tectum of *Plethodon jordani* (*a*) and *Hydromantes italicus* (*b*) showing differences in ipsilateral retinotectal projections as revealed by retrograde biocytin labeling. Bars = 50 μm. (Courtesy of Dr. W. Wiggers.)

locate prey objects and to calculate their movement trajectories (Wiggers and Roth, 1991; Wiggers et al., 1995). Excellent stereopsis may explain why these animals almost never miss their prey and feed on prey items such as collembolans that normally escape other amphibians (Roth, 1987).

In summary, tongue-projecting salamanders are able to engage in rapid, efficient ambush feeding. Logically, one might expect these animals to possess brains at least as complex as those of frogs exhibiting comparable standards of performance in speed and precision of visually guided feeding behavior (e.g., *Rana temporaria* or *Eleutherodactylus coqui*).

THE BRAIN OF SALAMANDERS AND FROGS

The brain of salamanders—like that of other amphibians—may be divided into five major parts: (1) telencephalon; (2) diencephalon including praetectum; (3) mesencephalon; (4) cerebellum; and (5) medulla oblongata (Fig. 8.6). There is no pons in the amphibian brain.

The telencephalon (a and b in Fig. 8.6B) is composed of olfactory bulbs, pallial structures (dorsal, lateral, and medial pallium; and amygdala pars lateralis) and subpallial structures (nuclei septi, amygdala pars medialis, and striatum, including nucleus accumbens). The medial pallium represents the dorsomedial wall of the hemisphere

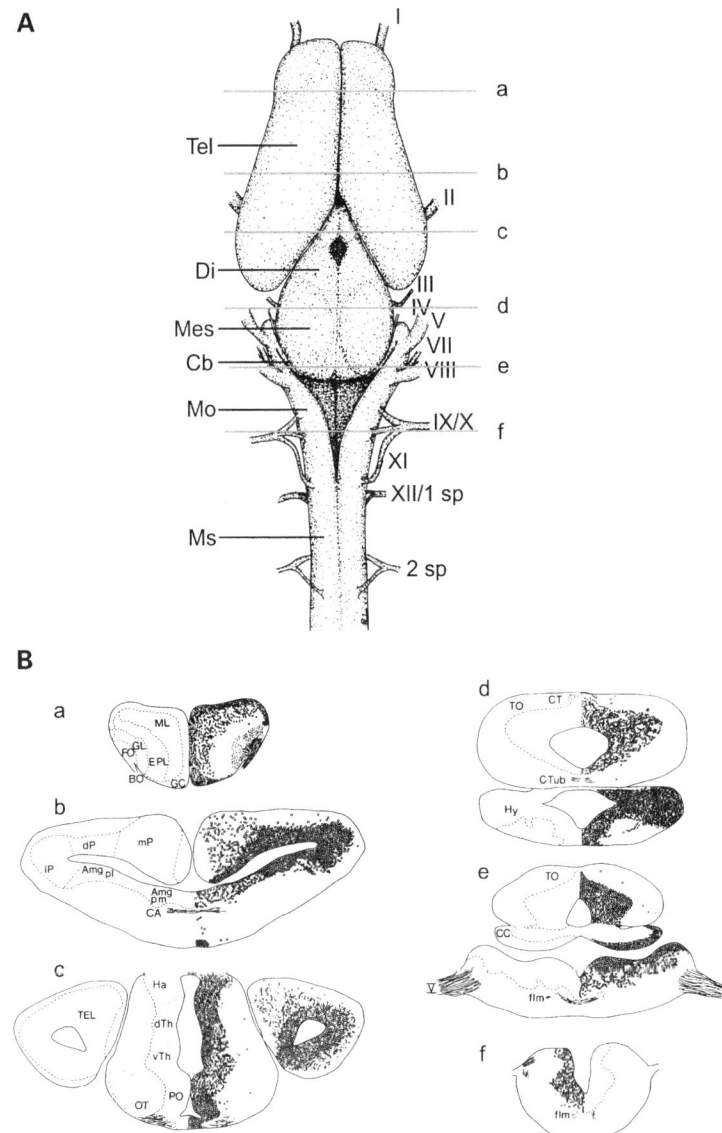

Figure 8.6. (A) Dorsal view of the brain of *Bolitoglossa subpalmata*. (B) Selected cross sections through the brain of *Bolitoglossa subpalmata* at sites indicated in A. (a) Telencephalon at the level of the olfactory bulbs. (BO) (b) Caudal telencephalon at the level of the anterior commissure. (CA) (c) Mid diencephalon (Di). (d) Mid mesencephalon (Mes). (e) Caudal mesencephalon/cerebellum/rostral medulla oblongata. (f) Mid medulla oblongata (Mo) at the entrance of the 9th nerve. Amg pl, amygdala pars lateralis; Amg pm, amygdala pars medialis; BO, bulbus olfactorius; Cb, cerebellum; CC, corpus erebelli; CT, commissura tecti; CTub, commissura tuberculi posterioris; dP, dorsal pallium; dTh, dorsal thalamus; EPL, external plexiform layer; flm, fasciculus longitudinalis medialis; GC, layer of granule cells; GL, glomerular layer; Ha, habenula; Hy, hypothalamus; lP, lateral pallium; ML, layer of mitral cells; mP, medial pallium; OT, optic tract; PO, nucleus praeopticus; TEL, telencephalon; TO, tectum opticum; vTh, ventral thalamus. (After Roth, 1987.)

and is considered to be homologous to the mammalian hippocampus, at least with regard to Ammon's horn and subiculum (Northcutt and Kaas, 1995; Roth and Westhoff, 1999). The dorsal pallium includes the pallial walls dorsal to the medial pallium and may be regarded as homologous to at least part of the mammalian isocortex (Butler and Hodos, 1996; Northcutt and Kaas, 1995). The lateral pallium is considered a homologue of the mammalian olfactory (piriform) cortex. The amygdala consists of two distinct nuclei, the pars lateralis of pallial origin, and the pars medialis of subpallial origin. The septal nuclear complex occupies the ventromedial wall of the cerebral hemispheres below the medial pallium. The striatum occupies the ventrolateral wall of the telencephalic hemisphere in a position immediately caudal to the accessory olfactory bulb.

The diencephalon (c in Fig. 8.6B) is divided into the epithalamus, dorsal thalamus, ventral thalamus, and hypothalamus. The epithalamus contains the epiphysis and the habenular nuclei, including the commissura habenularum. The dorsal thalamus is separated from the epithalamus by the sulcus dorsalis at the ventricular side. Similarly, the ventral thalamus is separated from the dorsal thalamus by the sulcus medialis and from the hypothalamus by the sulcus ventralis. The praetectum, or *synencephalon*, extends around the commissura posterior rostrally adjacent to the pars intercalaris thalami and descends ventrocaudally. Dorsally, it includes the nucleus praetectalis, ventrally and ventrocaudally, the nucleus Darkschewitsch.

The mesencephalon of amphibians (d and e in Fig. 8.6B) is divided into the tectum, a subtectal sensory zone, and the tegmentum. The tectum is treated later in greater detail in the section on the visual system. The auditory subtectal center corresponding to the anuran torus semicircularis is embedded completely in the periventricular gray matter and shows no, or very little, lamination. The tegmentum is a conglomerate of several nuclei adjacent to the rhombencephalic isthmic nucleus.

The cerebellum is small and simply organized (e in Fig. 8.6B). It consists of the corpus cerebelli, the auricula cerebelli (which are enlargements of the sensory zones of the medulla oblongata), and a nucleus cerebelli, situated ventral to the corpus cerebelli and homologized by Herrick (1948) to the deep cerebellar nuclei of mammals.

The medulla oblongata (e and f in Fig. 8.6B) is the area of termination or origin of cranial nerves IV (trochlear), V (trigeminal), VI (abducens), VII (facialis), VIII (stato-acusticus), IX (glossopharyngeus), X (vagus), and XII (hypoglossus). Its dorsal part, the alar plate of His, receives all sensory fibers from the head (except olfactory and optic fibers, which enter the forebrain), including general visceral parasympathetic sensory and gustatory fibers, as well as fibers from the trunk lateral-line system, if present. In the ventral basal plate of the medulla oblongata, the motor nuclei of nerves V to X, and partly the nucleus of nerve XII, are situated. The motor nuclei are surrounded by neurons of the reticular formation. This motor system is the coordination center of head and neck motor function, including mouth and tongue movements involved in feeding (Roth and Wake, 1985b).

In frogs as well as in most other vertebrates, many of the mentioned brain regions have a complex morphology exhibiting multiple lamination and the formation of distinct nuclei, which are often found in a migrated position. For example, the mesencephalic tectum of frogs consists of nine alternating cellular and fiber layers between the ventricle and the brain surface (Székely and Lázár, 1976), and the thalamus contains a number of morphologically distinct nuclei, some of which possess a laminar organization (Neary and Northcutt, 1983). A similar degree of histological differentiation is found in the mesencephalic tegmentum and the auditory torus semicircularis of frogs (Potter, 1965; Feng, 1983) (Fig. 8.7a–d). In contrast, the

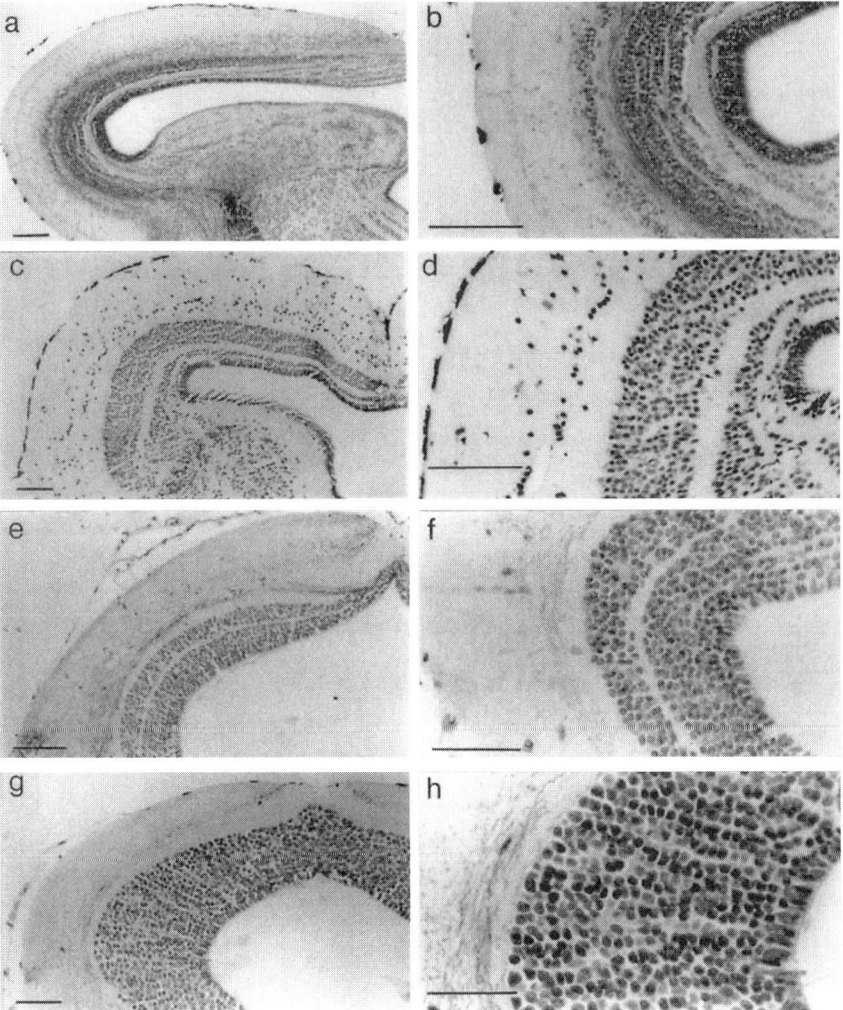

Figure 8.7. Cross sections through brains of frogs and salamanders at the level of the tectum and the dorsal tegmentum/torus semicircularis showing differences in cell size and morphological complexity. Photomicrographs are at both low (*left*) and higher (*right*) magnification (a,b). *Eleutherodactylus coqui* (cell diameter 5.8 μm); (Courtesy of Dr. Dicke, University of Bremen.) (c,d) *Bombina orientalis* (cell diameter 9.9 μm). (e,f) *Plethodon jordani* (cell diameter 11.8 μm). (g,h) *Hydromantes italicus* (cell diameter 12.5 μm). For further explanation, see text. Bars = 50 μm.

tectum, tegmentum, and thalamus of salamanders show an essentially bilayered structure, consisting of a periventricular layer of neurons (gray matter) and a superficial layer of afferent and efferent fibers and dendrites of neurons (white matter) (Fig. 8.7e–h). Only a few neurons are found in a migrated position within the white matter (Roth et al., 1990). An example is the nucleus praetectalis superficialis, which can be found in a migrated or partially migrated position. The minimum of morphological complexity among amphibians is found in the brains of bolitoglossines, which show no lamination of the tectum and no migrated nuclei at all; the spinal cord exhibits no lateral motor column present in all other limbed vertebrates (Roth and Wake, 1985b; Wake et al., 1988) (Fig. 8.8). In morphological terms, the brain of adult bolitoglossines strongly resembles that of early larvae of frogs.

This situation is just the opposite of what we would expect in the face of the specializiation of bolitoglossines toward highly efficient feeding and arboreal life and the great evolutionary success of these animals in terms of speciation, ecological diversity, and biomass. Before drawing conclusions from these data, however, we examine the visual system, the most relevant sensory system involved in feeding behavior of these animals.

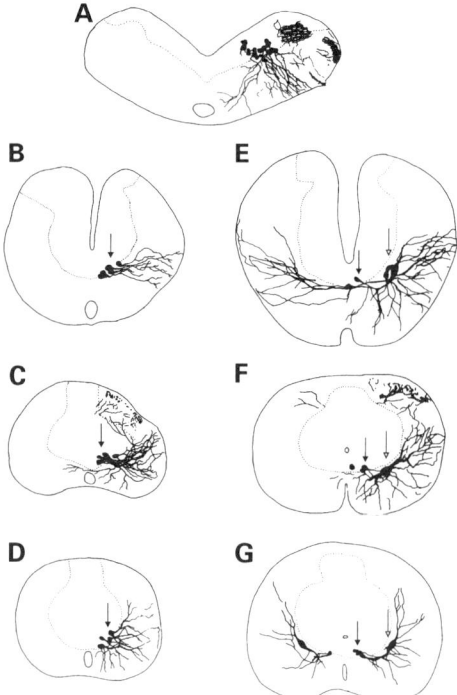

Figure 8.8. Reconstruction of transverse sections through motor nuclei related to feeding in plethodontid salamanders. A–D, *Batrachoseps attenuatus*, E–G, *Plethodon jordani*. (*A*) Motor nucleus of the facialis nerve. (*B,E*) Motor nucleus of the first spinal/hypoglossal nerve. (*C,F*) Motor nucleus of the second spinal nerve. (*D,G*) Motor nucleus of the accessory spinal nerve. While *Plethodon* possesses both a medial (arrow with solid arrowhead) and a lateral motor column (arrow with open arrowhead) in the spinal motor nuclei, *Batrachoseps* lacks a lateral motor colum. (From Roth, 1987.)

THE VISUAL SYSTEM OF BOLITOGLOSSINES

The visual system consists of the retina and its diencephalic and mesencephalic neuropils, the mesencephalic tectum, the pretectum, and the dorsal and ventral thalamus of the diencephalon, as well as the nucleus of the basal optic root and the suprachiasmatic nucleus. Another nucleus closely related to the visual system is the nucleus isthmi.

Retina and Retinofugal System

Plethodontid as well as nonplethodontid salamanders have four different morphological types of retinal ganglion cells (RGC) (Linke and Roth, 1989). In anurans, the number of types of RGC is higher, from five to seven types in *Rana pipiens* (Frank and Hollyfield, 1987). There are also differences among anurans and urodeles in the number of RGC and consequently in the number of axons of the optic nerve. Frogs have up to 470,000 optic fibers and accordingly RGC (*Rana pipiens*; Maturana, et al., 1960). In salamanders, the number of optic nerve fibers/RGC ranges from a minimum of 26,000 in the plethodontid *Batrachoseps attenuatus* (Linke and Roth, 1990) to 75,000 in the salamandrid *Notophthalmus viridescens* (Ball and Dickson, 1983). Most fibers of the optic nerve cross in the chiasma opticum to the opposite side of the brain. A certain number of the fibers, however, turn back to the ipsilateral side of the brain (see below). In salamanders and frogs, three visual terminal fields can be distinguished within the rostral thalamus, viz., the corpus geniculatum thalamicum, the neuropil Bellonci pars lateralis, and the neuropil Bellonci pars medialis. In the pretectum, retinal afferents laterally form the pretectal neuropil and more medially the uncinate field. These thalamic and pretectal projection sites are present both contralaterally and ipsilaterally, although in all amphibians—with the exception of bolitoglossines—the ipsilateral sites are much weaker than the contralateral ones (Fite and Scalia, 1976; Fritzsch, 1980; Rettig and Roth, 1986).

In the tectum of frogs, four laminas of retinofugal fibers are formed (Székely and Lázár, 1976): lamina 1 and lamina 2 are situated in layer 9 immediately below the tectal surface and consist mostly of thin, unmyelinated fibers; lamina 3 contains myelinated fibers and is situated above tectal layer 8; lamina 4, consisting of a few, thick unmyelinated fibers, is located in layer 8 and beneath it. Singman and Scalia (1990), on the basis of retrograde horseradish peroxidase tracing experiments, estimated that in *Rana pipiens* 2.3% of the overall population of ganglion cells project to the ipsilateral tectum. In the superficial white matter of the tectum of bolitoglossines as well as of other salamanders, axons of ganglion cells constitute three layers/laminas (with several sublaminas) (Wiggers, 1998). These contain direct afferents from the contralateral as well as from the ipsilateral retina, the latter amounting to 30% of the former (Rettig and Roth, 1986) (Fig. 8.5). Recent recordings in our laboratory from retinotectal afferents in the plethodontid salamanders *Plethodon jordani* and *Hydromantes italicus* suggest that RGC terminating in layer 1 tend to have relatively small receptive fields with strong inhibitory surround and respond best to changes in contrast and size of small objects. RGC in layer 2 tend to have wider receptive fields with weaker inhibitory surround and respond best to motion largely irrespective of stimulus size. Terminals in layer 3 on average again have wide receptive fields with very weak inhibitory surround. Most of these latter RGC exhibit very short latencies and are most sensitive to slow motion (Mandon and Roth, 1997). In frogs, four response types of RGC terminating in the tectum have been consistently described (Maturana et al., 1960; Grüsser and Grüsser-Cornehls, 1976), the first two of which largely correspond to layer-1 RGC of salamanders, the third to layer-2 RGC, and the fourth to layer-3 RGC of salamanders.

Thus, apart from the dramatic reduction in number of RGC and optic nerve fibers, differences in morphology and physiology between bolitoglossines and frogs are minor. Frogs may have one more morphological and physiological class of RGC judged from morphology and physiology compared with salamanders. This may be the reason for the existence of four instead of three laminas of optic nerve terminals inside the tectal white matter. The number of retinal terminal fields in the diencephalon and mesencephalon is the same in salamanders and frogs. The bolitoglossines, however, stand out among amphibians in having substantially more ipsilateral retinothalamic, retinopretectal, and retinotectal fibers than other amphibian taxa (Fig. 8.5).

Tectum

In addition to major differences in morphology of the tectum, there is a dramatic difference between anurans and urodeles in number of tectal neurons (Roth et al., 1994; 1998). Among salamanders, the lowest number of tectal neurons is found in *Batrachoseps attenuatus* (35,000) and the highest in *Salamandra salamandra* (150,000). The average number of tectal neurons in salamanders is 75,000. Among frogs, the lowest number of tectal neurons is found in *Arenophryne rotunda* (132,000) and the highest in *Eleutherodactylus coqui* (1,700,000). The average number of tectal neurons in the frogs is 720,000. Thus, frogs on average have about 10 times more tectal neurons than salamanders. Only the frog *Arenophryne rotunda* has fewer tectal neurons than any salamander. The low number of tectal neurons in salamanders compared with frogs goes along with a very low number of neurons found in migrated positions inside the white matter. In frogs, the percentage of such migrated tectal neurons ranges between 16.1 and 27.6. In salamanders, the percentage of migrated neurons ranges between 0.7 and 5, with the lowest values invariably found in the bolitoglossines (Roth et al., 1990).

Recently, comparative studies on the cytoarchitecture of the tectum were carried out in our laboratory in a number of frogs (*Discoglossus pictus*, *Eleutherodactylus coqui*) and salamanders (*Hydromantes italicus*, *Plethodon jordani*), using retrograde tracing and intracellular injection of biocytin (Dicke and Roth, 1996; Rockenhäuser and Roth, 1997; Dicke, 1999; Roth et al., 1999). In the two frog species, five types of descending projection neurons were identified (A in Figure 8.9). Type 1 neurons have a candelabra-like dendritic tree arborizing primarily in the most superficial retinorecipient lamina A or B of layer 9; the axons arborize bilaterally in the

The Visual System of Bolitoglossines 251

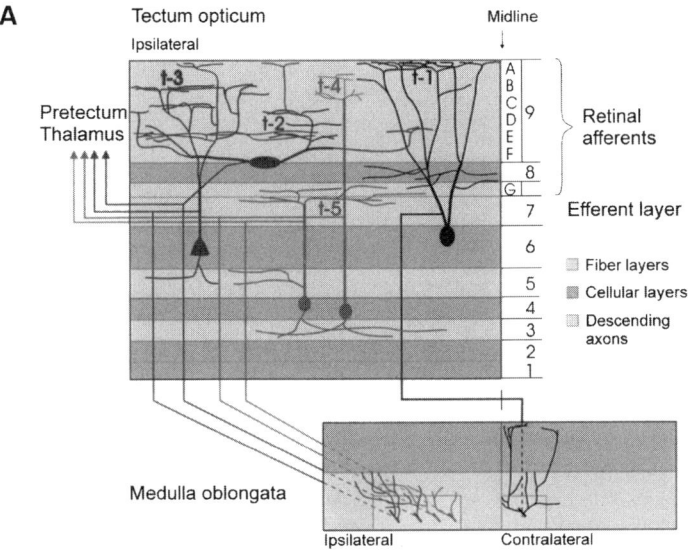

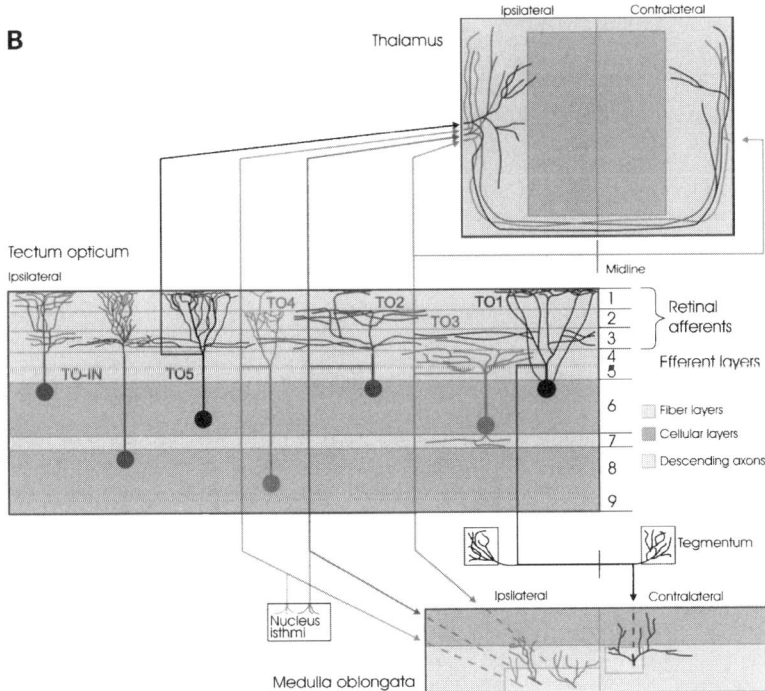

Figure 8.9. Morphological types of tectal neurons and axonal projection pattern in frogs and salamanders, as revealed by tract tracing and intracellular biocytin labeling. A: Frogs (*Discoglossus pictus*, *Eleutherodactylus coqui*). From Dicke and Roth, 1996. B: Salamanders (*Plethodon jordani*, *Hydromantes italicus*). From Roth et al., 1999. For further explanation see text.

tegmentum and descend *contralaterally*, constituting the *crossed* tecto-bulbo-spinal tract. No ascending axonal projections exist. Type 2 neurons have horizontally oriented spindle-shaped somata and a wide dendritic tree that forms up to four laminae in layer 9, the uppermost lamina overlapping with laminas A/B of retinal afferents. Type 3 neurons have pear-shaped or pyramidal somata; their dendritic tree arborizes in the deeper two laminas inside layers 9 and 8. Both types of neurons have axons ascending to the ipsilateral praetectum and thalamus, while the descending axon remains ipsilateral, constituting the *uncrossed* tecto-bulbo-spinal tract. Type 4 neurons have long and slender primary dendrites arborizing in the upper two retino-recipient laminae. They appear to have the same axonal projection pattern as types 2 and 3 neurons. Type 5 neurons have a primary dendrite that divides at the border between the periventricular gray and the white matter in a T-shaped fashion into several horizontally extending secondary and tertiary dendrites, which are mostly confined to layer 7. These neurons again have (mostly bilaterally) ascending and (exclusively ipsilaterally) descending projections. There are a number of types of tectal interneurons, (i.e., cells with no axons or axons that do not leave the tectum), that together seem to constitute about 95% of tectal cells. These five types of projection neurons are largely consistent with the types described by Székely and Lázár (1976) in *Rana esculenta* on the basis of Golgi staining and Lázár et al. (1983) and Antal et al. (1986) by retrograde labeling using cobaltic lysine as a tracer.

In the salamanders *Plethodon* and *Hydromantes*, again five types of projection neurons, called TO1 to TO5, exist (B in Fig. 8.9): TO1 neurons arborize primarily in the uppermost layer (layer 1) of retinal afferents and less intensely in layer 3. They have no ascending axons; their descending axon arborizes bilaterally in the tegmentum and constitutes the *crossed* tecto-bulbo-spinal tract. TO2 neurons arborize primarily in the intermediate and deep layers of retinal afferents (layers 2 and 3). Their ascending axon projects to the pretectum and thalamus, while their descending axon constitutes the *lateral uncrossed* tecto-bulbo-spinal tract. TO3 neurons arborize predominantly in the deep retino-recipient layer (layer 3) and in the efferent fiber layers (layers 4 and 5). They project to the pretectum and thalamus; with their descending axons they contribute to the *uncrossed* tecto-bulbo-spinal tract. TO4 neurons arborize predominantly in layers 2 and 3 and have ascending projections to the pretectum and thalamus; their ipsilaterally descending axon occupies a position lateral to the axons of TO2 neurons. TO5 neurons arborize in layers 1 and 2 or in all three layers of retinal afferents and have ascending projections; they either have no descending axons or these axons reach only the level of the nucleus isthmi. There are various subtypes of TO interneurons with respect to differences in dendritic arborization and stratification pattern, which constitute about 95% of tectal neurons.

In summary, despite the dramatic differences in overall morphology of the tectum, the cytoarchitecture and projection pattern of tectal neurons is essentially the same in frogs and salamanders. The same is true with respect to the response properties of tectal neurons. Recordings from the tectum of the toad *Bufo bufo* (Roth and Jordan, 1982) and the salamander *Hydromantes italicus* (Roth, 1982) under the same experimental conditions yielded no indication that the responses of anuran tectal cells to visual stimuli are more complex than those of salamanders.

THE FATE OF OTHER SENSORY SYSTEMS

There is no sign of reduction in the primary *olfactory* system of bolitoglossines compared with other amphibian taxa, whereas the accessory olfactory system appears to be simpler morphologically compared with salamanders with a biphasic life history, but the same "simple" appearance is found in frogs (Schmidt et al., 1988). The *somatosensory*, including the *proprioceptive*, system of plethodontid salamanders is similar to that of other salamanders and frogs as regards primary afferents, but shows remarkable differences with respect to the secondary pathways ascending to the mesencephalon and diencephalon (Dicke and Mühlenbrock-Lenter, 1998). There are more ascending tracts in *Plethodon* and bolitoglossines (*Hydromantes, Bolitoglossa*), and these tracts show substantial ipsilateral projections, whereas in the salamandrid *Pleurodeles,* ranid frogs, and *Xenopus,* projections are almost exclusively contralateral. Nothing precise is known about the *vestibular* system of salamanders.

In bolitoglossines, an *electroreceptive* and *mechanoreceptive lateral-line system* is absent, apparently because of their strict terrestriality, whereas all other salamanders possess both systems either permanently or during their aquatic stages. The *auditory system* of salamanders in general and of the Bolitoglossini in particular appears to be much simpler than in frogs. Most frogs have a well-developed auditory periphery with a tympanum and a single middle-ear bone (columella) that has a special extra-columellar extension to the tympanum. The tympanum is absent in some species of several families, and some of these species exhibit a reduction of the middle ear (e.g., *Bombina*; Stadtmüller, 1931; Smirnov, 1989). All salamanders lack an external ear (tympanum) and a middle ear cavity. One or two small middle-ear bones (operculum, columella/stapes) are fused to each other or to the otic capsule or are entirely lost (Hetherington, 1988). Most frogs have a well-developed inner ear with a papilla basilaris, the presumed homologue of the basilar lamina of amniotes, which is involved in the perception of high frequencies, and a papilla amphibiorum, a structure unique to the inner ear of amphibians and involved in the perception of low frequencies. The papilla basilaris is reduced in a number of salamander genera and is completely absent in all members of the family Plethodontidae (Lombard, 1977; Lewis and Lombard, 1988). The papilla amphibiorum is also reduced in size in plethodontids (Lombard, 1977).

In the medulla oblongata of nonbolitoglossine salamanders, the dorsal nucleus of the lateral-line sensory area receives information from the electroreceptive lateral-line system, and an intermediate nucleus receives afferents from mechanoreceptive neuromasts in its rostral portion and from the inner ear in its caudal portion, and the ventral nucleus has only vestibular functions. A dorsal and intermediate nucleus are absent in the bolitoglossines. Nonbolitoglossine salamanders have a migrated superior olive and a torus semicircularis that shows some degree of lamination; both structures are important auditory centers. In bolitoglossines, the superior olive is unmigrated and the torus semicircularis unlaminated, and both are morphologically indistinct.

In frogs, no dorsal nucleus and no rostral intermediate nucleus exist, whereas the caudal intermediate nucleus is present (Fritzsch et al., 1984; Will, 1988). In addition, there is a dorsolateral nucleus unique to anurans that receives afferents only from the papilla amphibiorum and serves as the main auditory center. The superior olive is found in a migrated position. The torus semicircularis consists of five subnuclei showing extensive cell migration and lamination. An exception is *Bombina orientalis*, in which the torus is unmigrated (Walkowiak, W., University of Köln personal communication, 1996).

In summary, in bolitoglossines some sensory systems such as the visual, somatosensory, and olfactory systems, apparently are in a structural and functional state comparable or even superior to those of other salamanders and to frogs, while other sensory systems, such as the auditory system, show strong reduction or are completely lost, such as the electro- and mechanosensory system.

CAUSES AND CONSEQUENCES OF SIMPLIFICATION IN THE CONTEXT OF PAEDOMORPHOSIS

A simple morphology characterized by the partial to complete absence of certain traits may represent a primitive (plesiomorphic) state, or it may be simplified or lost. One way in which a trait can be lost phylogenetically is secondary simplification, as, for example, may happen when an ontogenetic trajectory is truncated or when the rate of development is slowed to the point that sexual maturation occurs before morphology has attained the degree of development characteristic of ancestral and closely related forms. To determine if absence is primary or if it is a secondary loss, a phylogenetic analysis is required. For salamanders this necessitates knowledge of the ontogeny and adult morphology of relevant outgroups (viz., caecilians, anurans, amniotes, lungfishes, coelacanths, bony fishes, cartilaginous fishes, and lampreys) (cf. Fig. 8.1A). For a given character and depending on phylogenetic topology, if more than half of the outgroups for which the character state is known are more complex than salamanders, then the hypothesis that the character is secondarily simplified in salamanders is more parsimonious than the hypothesis that it is plesiomorphically simple in salamanders. In such a cladistic analysis based on 23 neural characters, Roth et al. (1993) demonstrated that salamanders are indeed secondarily simplified. Furthermore, among salamanders (Fig. 8.1B), species of the plethodontid tribe Bolitoglossini have the lowest degree of lamination and cell migration in the brain and exhibit the highest degree of secondary simplification. A parallel case of secondary simplification of the central nervous system are the American and African lungfishes (*Lepidosiren* and *Protopterus*, Dipnoi, family Lepidosirenidae). Whereas the Australian lungfish *Neoceratodus*, the coelacanth *Latimeria*, and actinopterygian fishes have more complex brains, including a multilaminated tectum mesencephali, the brain and particularly the tectum of lepidosirenids are as simple as those of salamanders (Northcutt, 1987).

Roth et al. (1993) argued that secondary simplification arises from *paedomorphosis*, a form of heterochronic evolution in which traits that characterize juveniles of ancestral taxa appear in the adult stage of descendant taxa. Paedomorphosis commonly involves different degrees of retardation, reduction, or absence of traits in adult organisms as compared with phylogenetic outgroups (Gould, 1977; McKinney and McNamara, 1991). Thus, a mosaic of fully developed (adult) traits, weakly expressed traits, and missing characters appears in adult stages of paedomorphic animals.

What are the reasons for simplicity of the salamander and particularly the bolitoglossine brain? How can the apparent paradox be solved that those salamanders showing the most sophisticated visual behavior among amphibians (i.e., the Bolitoglossini) have the simplest brain morphology among vertebrates?

The hypothesis presented here is that the observed differences in the morphology of the central nervous system between salamanders and lepidosirenid lungfishes (and to a lesser degree caecilians and a number of frogs) on the one hand and other vertebrate taxa on the other are largely a consequence of *differences in genome and cell size*. Genome size refers to the amount of DNA, here given for haploid genome (note that some authors, e.g., Olmo [1991], report *diploid* genome sizes). Differences in genome size among vertebrates are not due to polyploidy (which occurs in some populations of amphibians, but is absent in bolitoglossines), but to an increase in noncoding, mostly middle-repetitive DNA sequences (Horner and MacGregor, 1983; Olmo, 1991).

Genome size varies enormously among organisms. Among vertebrates, the smallest genome is found in teleost fishes, with less than 1 pg DNA per haploid nucleus, while lungfishes (Dipnoi) have genome sizes up to 142 pg, the largest genomes found in any animal (Olmo, 1983). Among salamanders, the smallest genome (13.7 pg) is found in the plethodontid *Desmognathus wrighti* (Hally et al., 1986; Sessions, 1984; Sessions and Larson, 1987) and the largest (83 pg) in the neotenic (perennibranchiate) *Necturus maculosus* (Olmo, 1983). The plethodontid salamander *Hydromantes italicus* (77 pg) appears to have the largest genome of any terrestrial animal, although several tropical bolitoglossine plethodontids (e.g., *Bolitoglossa subpalmata*, 64 pg) approach this value (Sessions and Larson, 1987). Species of the Bolitoglossini, on average, have larger genome sizes than other plethodontids and than other salamander families, except for the neotenic/perennibranchiate species (Olmo, 1983; Sessions and Larson, 1987).

Caecilians (Gymnophiona) also have relatively large genomes, but the largest known caecilian genome (13.2 pg per haploid nucleus; M. Wake, University of California, Berkeley, personal communication, 1998) is less than the smallest found in salamanders (13.7 pg). The smallest genome size among anurans (about 1 pg) is found in *Limnodynastes ornatus*, and the largest is found in *Arenophryne rotunda* (19 pg; Roberts, in litteris.). Although frogs generally have the smallest genome sizes among amphibians, *Bombina orientalis* has a relatively large genome (10 pg; Olmo, 1983) and shows clear signs of secondary simplification in neural as well as non-neural characters (see above). Caecilians have genome sizes intermediate between those of salamanders and anurans and have many secondarily reduced neural and non-neural characters (Schmidt and Wake, 1997). From the few characters studied in detail, the degree of simplification of caecilians appears to lie between that of anurans and salamanders.

A phylogenetic analysis reveals that an increase in genome size has occurred independently in lungfishes and amphibians as well as within the three amphibian orders Anura, Caudata, and Gymnophiona (Olmo, 1991). Furthermore, even among plethodontid salamanders (Fig. 8.1C), genome size appears to have increased several times independently (Sessions and Larson, 1987), especially in the tribes Plethodontini and Bolitoglossini. In all cases studied, the increase in genome size has the same important morphological consequences, including (1) increase in cell size; (2) decrease in cell metabolic rate; (3) decrease in cell division rate; and (4) decrease in cell differentiation rate (Van't Hof and Sparrow, 1963; Goin et al., 1968; Olmo, 1983; Sessions and Larson, 1987). These consequences lead to animals that have (1) large cells, (2) low metabolic rates, (3) few cells, (4) slow growth and slow differentiation processes, and (5) morphologies that appear to be simple, but rather are the result of *secondary simplification*.

Although the correlation between genome size and cell size is robust, that between genome size and metabolic rate in salamanders has been questioned by Licht and Lowcock (1991) on the grounds that previous studies were carried out in vitro. They used data from Gatten et al. (1991) for active animals, based on measurements of standard metabolic rates (μl O_2/g/hr) at 5°, 15°, 20° and 25°C to show a marginally significant correlation ($p < 0.02$) with genome size at 15°C and a significant correlation ($p < 0.001$) at 25°C, but not at the two other temperatures. They argue that a temperature of 25°C is unusually high for most urodeles and close to a lethal limit for amphibian development. Tropical bolitoglossines are, however, regularly active at such temperatures (e.g., *Bolitoglossa occidentalis, B. rufescens*), and Mexican ambystomatid salamanders have been recorded at temperatures in excess of 25°C on a number of occasions (Feder et al., 1982). Unfortunately, Licht and Lowcock included only three species of tropical salamanders in their study, and their data on metabolic rates of these species were incomplete.

The correlation between genome and cell size arises from the fact that large amounts of DNA lead to large nuclei and consequently to large cell volumes. Recently, Roth et al. (1994) studied the effect of genome and cell size in the brains of 22 species of salamanders and 19 species of frogs. There was a significant correlation between genome size and tectal cell diameter. In frogs, morphological complexity of the tectum was negatively correlated with cell size, while brain size was correlated with neither cell size nor morphological complexity. This means that frogs with smaller cells have more complex tecta (as well as other brain centers) independent of brain size. In salamanders, the degree of morphological complexity of the tectum was again negatively correlated with cell size, but in addition brain size was correlated with body size and with cell size (i.e., salamanders with larger brains tend to have larger cells and those with smaller brains have smaller cells).

Among anurans, the least complex morphologies of the tectum as well as of other parts of the brain were found in the species *Arenophryne rotunda* and *Bombina orientalis*—two species that have the largest and second largest genomes and cells among frogs studied thus far and are considered to be highly paedomorphic based on nonneural as well as neural characters (Smirnov, 1989; Roberts, in litteris); (Fig. 8.7c,d). Conversely, frogs with small genomes and cell sizes such as *Limnodynastes ornatus* and *Eleutherodactylus coqui* have very complex tecta (Fig. 8.7a,b). Among salamanders, small-sized species with relatively large cells but small brains such as *Batrachoseps attenuatus* and *Thorius narisovalis* have the least complex brains, but larger sized bolitoglossines with very large genomes and cells such as *Hydromantes italicus* exhibited similarly "simple" brain morphologies. On the other hand, larger sized salamanders with relatively small genome and cell sizes like *Ambystoma mexicanum* have the most complex brains among urodeles, and those with intermediate genome and cell sizes like *Plethodon jordani* exhibit intermediate degrees of morphological complexity (Fig. 8.7e,f).

It is presently unknown how increased genome size leads to retardation of brain development. There may be general effects of increased DNA replication times and, accordingly, longer cell cycle times or the effect of low metabolic rate on brain development, or more specific effects such as retarded expression of developmental genes or disturbance of epigenetic tissue interactions. Studies in our laboratory point to differences in the spatial and temporal pattern of upregulation and downregulation of cell surface and cell adhesion molecules between frogs and amniotes on the one hand and salamanders on the other (T. Becker et al., 1993; C.B. Becker et al., 1993). Not all developmental processes in the amphibian brain are retarded to the same degree. Rather, it seems that developmental processes that occur early in development are less affected than are those occurring late, which are either strongly retarded or are lacking entirely. This effect is combined with the degree of genome size increase (i.e., retardation or lack of late processes is more pronounced in species with larger genomes). The dorsal telencephalon is a late-differentiating brain structure and seems to be most affected by retardation. In all three orders of amphibians, it is very simply organized and is usually considered the morphologically least complex among gnathostome vertebrates except lepidosirenid lungfishes (Northcutt, 1987), although anurans have a somewhat more complex telencephalon than salamanders. Another late-developing brain structure is the cerebellum. Compared with most other vertebrates, it is small in anurans, even smaller in salamanders with relatively small genome sizes, and smallest in salamanders with large genomes. In contrast, the tectum and diencephalon develop relatively early, and accordingly both structures are less simplified in frogs than in salamanders (and lepidosirenid lungfishes), with caecilians ranging in between. Finally, the same holds for the medulla oblongata and spinal cord, which generally develop very early. One of the latest events occurring here is the formation of a lateral motor column due to the migration of secondary motor neurons from medial to lateral (Nishikawa et al., 1991). Accordingly, all frogs and those salamanders with small genome sizes have a well-developed lateral motor column, whereas species with large genome sizes (i.e., the Bolitoglossini) have functional "lateral" motor column neurons that fail to migrate.

Increases in genome and consequently cell size have happened many times in the animal kingdom (as well as among plants) and invariably led to increased developmental times and paedomorphic morphologies. There is no universal agreement on the origin and significance of increased genome size in vertebrates. According to the selfish DNA hypothesis (Ohno, 1972; Doolittle and Sapienza, 1980; Orgel and Crick, 1980), genome size tends to increase until this tendency is halted by countervailing selection. This would mean that an increase in genome size is a purely genomic event with no advantage or even with strong disadvantage for the organism, which has to compensate for any disadvantages in order to survive.

Attempts have been made by Szarski (1983) to view an increase in genome size in salamanders as an adaptation for survival in harsh environments ("frugal" strategy): Large genomes lead to large cells, which lead to low metabolic rates requiring less oxygen supply and less investment into nutrition. It is true that salamanders in general have very low oxygen demands (a factor that makes their cells very suitable for in vitro studies) and that they can survive for months without food intake. The latter allows them to retreat for extended periods of time into microhabitats where food is scarce (such as caves), and low demands of oxygen supply could be favorable for the lungless plethodontids, which exhibit the lowest metabolic rates among vertebrates. At the same time, such a "submergent" behavior (sensu Maiorana, 1976) minimizes exposure to predators, particularly given the fact that in the tropics predation intensity is extraordinarily high.

Another argument put forward by Szarski (1983) is that it must be more economical to build an organism from a smaller number of larger cells instead of using a large number of smaller cells. While the former arguments might be valid, the latter certainly is not, because salamanders with few and large cells develop very slowly and reach sexual maturity much later on average than other amphibians (up to 7 years in *Hydromantes italicus*). If there is a selective advantage of an increase in genome and cell size in the sense of a "frugal" strategy in salamanders in general and in bolitoglossines in particular, it is outbalanced by negative consequences such as retardation of development and simplification of the nervous system.

WHAT DO BOLITOGLOSSINES TELL US ABOUT EVOLUTION IN GENERAL AND BRAIN EVOLUTION IN PARTICULAR?

The case of bolitoglossines illustrates how a genomic, possibly nonadaptive event may deeply influence (via reproductive style and lifestyle) all levels of the life of an organism, including geographic distribution of the taxon to which it belongs. At the same time, we learn how organisms, during their "struggle for survival," developed compensatory mechanisms in order to circumvent the constraints resulting from an increase in genome size.

In the Bolitoglossini, we indeed find a unique combination of constraints resulting from an increase in genome size and its inevitable consequences for the organism as well as "tricks" that helped these animals to escape from the evolutionary trap. The first of such events was the evolution of lunglessness, which freed the hyobranchial apparatus from the constraint of serving as a lung pump, making a further evolution of the feeding function possible. The second step was the evolution of direct development and its opportunities, as explained above. Furthermore, direct development circumvents the formation of a complex larval hyobranchial apparatus. Both evolutionary steps—causally unrelated to each other—favored the formation of a specialized feeding apparatus (i.e. a free, projectile tongue). This was an important event because, due to their low metabolic rates, bolitoglossines are incapable of sustained fast locomotion in order to escape predators. Therefore, they had to become ambush feeders. In this context, increased frontality of the eyes and an increase in direct ipsilateral retinotectal projections apparently formed the basis of excellent depth perception abilities required for the use of a projectile tongue during ambush feeding. Ambush feeding and direct development facilitated arboreal life or terrestrial life in caves (it is hard to be an active hunter while climbing on trees or on the walls of caves).

What are possible compensatory processes in bolitoglossines for the observed simplicity of brain morphology and the strongly reduced number of neurons? As to simple morphology, it is to date not completely clear what functional significance the opposite situation (viz., a high degree of lamination and the formation of migrated nuclei or columnar structures) has. Separation of input and output and parallel processing of information may be facilitated by lamination, formation of nuclei, and columns, but there are numerous examples where complex information processing may happen in unlaminated nerve tissue as well (e.g., unlaminated dorsoventricular ridge in birds vs. laminated isocortex in mammals; Nieuwenhuys et al., 1998). In the amphibian tectum, the degree of lamination is strictly correlated with the number of afferent fibers and tectal neurons (see above), and it may be that tecta with a low number of afferent fibers and tectal neurons simply do not "need" a strict separation of input, output, and information processing modules. Thus, the most striking morphological difference between bolitoglossine salamanders and most other vertebrates may be a consequence of the reduction in cell proliferation rate.

Nevertheless, the fact remains that bolitoglossines have very few neurons in their brains and sensory systems—probably the fewest compared with other vertebrates with functioning sensory systems. The entire brain of most salamanders contains less than 1 million neurons (i.e., less than the brain of a honey bee). Frogs may have 5 to 10 times more neurons in their brains. Mathematical modeling and computer simulation of neuronal functions demonstrate that very smart sensory, motor, and even simple cognitive functions can be achieved by networks composed of relatively few neurons. A principle that in this context is particularly relevant in bolitoglossines is *population coding*. This principle means that certain kinds of information are not processed separately by specialized ("dedicated") neurons, but involve the joint activity of neurons with partially overlapping response properties. One great advantage of neuronal networks based on population coding is the robustness of their functions against reduction in the number of participating neurons. In plethodontid salamanders, such population coding is assumed to be present in the recognition and localization of objects (Eurich et al., 1995; Roth et al., 1998), and it has been shown by computer simulation that these functions are not dramatically reduced even when the number of neurons involved is reduced by 50% (Eurich et al., 1995). Thus, effective object recognition and localization may be accomplished by a relatively low number of neurons.

Population coding does not, however, always have the same power as networks containing many "dedicated" neurons with more specialized functions. This seems to be particularly true, when, for example, high spatial visual resolution or vision at distance is needed. Recent studies comparing *Bombina* and *Hydromantes* indeed demonstrate that the frog is better in both functions than the salamander (Göckel and Roth, 1998). A remarkable feature of the bolitoglossine visual system in this context is that it is restricted to frontal vision. Whereas many amphibians have 360° vision (some frogs even have a caudal binocular field) and eagerly respond to prey objects situated in the caudal visual field, this is not observed in bolitoglossines. Such a restriction to frontal vision was permitted only by changes in feeding strategy from hunting to ambush feeding. Inside the brain of bolitoglossines, two-thirds of tectal neurons have frontally oriented receptive fields and constitute a relatively large binocular field. This dedication of tectal neurons to frontal vision enhances the otherwise poor spatial resolution power (e.g., in the context of stereoscopic vision). The presence of an increased number of direct ipsilateral retinotectal terminals may further increase the resolution power. At the same time, the distance at which bolitoglossine salamanders reliably respond to prey items with orienting behavior is reduced from more than 1 m in most frogs to about 30 cm. In combination with the fact that visual neurons respond to angular rather than absolute size, this reduction in response distance increases visual acuity by a factor of 3 to 4.

Finally, networks being composed of large numbers of neurons seems to be required for complex and fast learning and memory formation going on in the juvenile and adult brain (i.e., beyond early imprinting processes). Students of amphibian behavior constantly noticed that the learning abilities of juvenile and adult amphibians are limited to a few domains (e.g., the distinction between palatable and noxious food items or finding their way back to their territory). Cross-modal information transfer seems to be particularly poor (e.g., from olfactory to visual). It may, thus, well be that reduction in sensory and behavioral plasticity is the price that animals with a reduced number of neurons in their brains and sense organs must pay for escaping the evolutionary trap constituted by an increase in genome size.

REFERENCES

Antal, M., N. Matsumoto, and G. Székely (1986) Tectal neurons of the frog: intracellular recording and labeling with cobalt electrodes. *J. Comp. Neurol.* 246:238–253.

Ariens-Kappers, C.U., G.C. Huber, G.C., and E.C. Crosby (1936) *The Comparative Anatomy* of the Nervous System of Vertebrates, Including Man. MacMillan, New York.

Ball, A.K., and D.H. Dickson (1983) Displaced amacrine and ganglion cells in the newt retina. *Exp. Eye Res.* 36:199–214.

Beachy, C.K., and R.C. Bruce (1992) Lunglessness in plethodontid salamanders is consistent with the hypothesis of a mountain stream origin: a response to Ruben and Boucot. *Am. Nat.* 139: 839–847.

Becker, C.G., T. Becker, and G. Roth (1993) Distribution of NCAM-180 and polysialic acid in the developing tectum mesencephali of the frog *Discoglossus pictus* and the salamander *Pleurodeles waltl*. Cell Tissue Res. 272: 289–301.

Becker, T., C.G. Becker, U. Niemann, C. Naujoks-Manteuffel, R. Gerardy-Schahn, and G. Roth (1993) Amphibian-specific regulation of polysialic acid and the neural cell adhesion molecule in development and regeneration of the retinotectal system of the salamander *Pleurodeles waltl*. *J. Comp. Neurol.* 336:532–544.

Butler, A.B., and W. Hodos (1996) *Comparative Vertebrate Neuroanatomy. Evolution and Adaptation.* Wiley-Liss, New York.

Deban, S., D.B. Wake, and Roth G. (1997) Salamander with a ballistic tongue. *Nature* 389:27–28.

Dicke, U. (1999) Morphology, axonal projection pattern and response type of tectal neurons in plethodontid salamanders. I. A tracer study of projection neurons and their pathways. *J. Comp. Neurol.* 404:473–488.

Dicke, U., and S. Mühlenbrock-Lenter (1998) Primary and secondary somatosensory projections in direct-developing plethodontid salamanders. *J. Morphol.* 238:307–326.

Dicke, U., and G. Roth (1996) Similarities and differences in the cytoarchitecture of the tectum of frogs and salamanders. *Acta Biol. Hung.* 47:41–59.

Doolittle, W.F., and C. Sapienza (1980) Selfish genes, the phenotype paradigm and genome evolution. *Nature* 284:601–603.

Duellman, W.E., and L. Trueb (1986) *Biology of Amphibians.* McGraw-Hill, New York.

Dunn, E.R. (1926) *The salamanders of the Family Plethodontidae.* Northampton, Mass.

Ebbesson, S.O.E. (1980) The parcellation theory and its relation to interspecific variability in brain organization, evolutionary and ontogenetic development, and neuronal plasticity. *Cell Tissue Res.* 213:179–212.

Ebbesson, S.O.E. (1984) Evolution and ontogeny of neural circuits. *Behav. Brain Sci.* 7:321–366.

Eurich, C., G. Roth, H. Schwegler, and W. Wiggers (1995) Simulander: a neural network model for the orientation movement of salamanders. *J. Comp. Physiol.* 176:379–389.

Feder, M.E., J.F. Lynch, H.B. Shaffer, and D.B. Wake (1982) Field body temperatures of tropical and temperate zone salamanders. *Smithsonian Herpetol. Inform. Serv.* 52:1–23.

Feng, A.S. (1983) Morphology of neurons in the torus semicircularis of the northern leopard frog, *Rana pipiens pipiens. J. Morphol.* 175:253–269.

Fite, K.V., and F. Scalia (1976) Central visual pathways in the frog. In K.V. Fite (ed.): *The Amphibian Visual System: An Interdisciplinary Approach* Academic Press, New York, pp. 87–118.

Frank, B.D., and J.G. Hollyfield (1987) Retinal ganglion cell morphology in the frog, *Rana pipiens. J. Comp. Neurol.* 266:413–434.

Fritzsch, B. (1980) *Retinal projections in European Salamandridae. Cell Tissue Res.* 213:325–341.

Fritzsch, B., A.M. Nikundiwe, and U. Will (1984) Projection patterns of lateral line afferents in anurans. A comparative HRP-study. *J. Comp. Neurol.* 229:451–469.

Gatten, R.E. Jr., K. Miller and R. Full (1991) Energetics of amphibians at rest and during locomotion. In M. Feder and W.W. Burggren (eds.): Environmental Physiology of Amphibians. Chicago, University of Chicago Press.

Göckel, M., and G. Roth (1998) *Comparative Studies on Vision at Distance in Amphibians.* Göttingen Neurobiology Report, 1998. G. Thieme, Stuttgart, p. 451.

Goin, O.B., C. J. Goin, and K. Bachmann (1968) DNA and amphibian life history. *Copeia* 1968: 532–540.

Gould, S.J. (1977) *Ontogeny and Phylogeny.* Harvard University Press, Cambridge, MA.

Grüsser, O.-J., and U. Grüsser-Cornehls (1976) Neurophysiology of the anuran visual system. In R. Llinas and W. Precht (eds.): *Frog Neurobiology.* Springer, Berlin, pp. 298–385.

Hally, M.K., E.M. Rasch, H.R. Mainwaring, and R.C. Bruce (1986) Cytophotometric evidence of variation in genome size of desmognathine salamanders. *Histochemistry* 85:185–192.

Herrick, C.J. (1948) The Brain of the Tiger Salamander *Ambystoma tigrinum.* Chicago, University of Chicago Press.

Hetherington, T.E. (1988) Metamorphic changes in the middle ear. In B. Fritzsch et al., (eds.). *The Evolution of the Amphibian Auditory System.* Wiley, New York, pp. 339–357.

Horner, H.A., and H.C. MacGregor (1983) C value and cell volume: their significance in the evolution and development of amphibians. *J. Cell Sci.* 63:135–146.

Jerison, H. (1973) *Evolution of the Brain and Intelligence.* Academic Press, New York.

Kuhlenbeck, H. (1977) *The Central Nervous System of Vertebrates, vol. V, part I: Derivatives of the Prosencephalon:Diencephalon and Telencephalon.* Karger, München.

Larson, A., and W.W. Dimmick (1993) Phylogenetic relationships of the salamander families: An analysis of congruence among morphological and molecular characters. *Herpeto. Monogr.* 7:77–93.

Lázár, G., P. Toth, E. Csank, and E. Kicliter (1983) Morphology and location of tectal projection neurons in frogs: A study with HRP and cobalt filling. *J. Comp. Neurol.* 215:108–120.

Lewis, E.R., and R.E. Lombard (1988) The amphibian inner ear. In Fritzsch et al. (eds.): *The Evolution of the Amphibian Auditory System.* Wiley, New York, pp. 93–123.

Licht, L.E., and L.A. Lowcock (1991) Genome size and metabolic rate in salamanders. *Comp. Biochem. Physiol.* 100B:83–92.

Linke, R., and G. Roth (1989) Morphology of retinal ganglion cells in lungless salamanders (Fam. Plethodontidae): an HRP and Golgi study. *J. Comp. Neurol.* 289:361–374.

Linke, R., and G. Roth (1990) Optic nerves in plethodontid salamanders (Amphibia, Urodela): neuroglia, fiber spectrum and myelination. *Anat. Embryol.* 181:37–48.

Linke, R., G. Roth, and B. Rottluff (1986) Comparative studies on the eye morphology in lungless salamanders, family Plethodontidae, and the effect of miniaturization. *J. Morphol.* 189:131–143.
Lombard, R.E. (1977) Comparative morphology of the inner ear in salamanders (Caudata: Amphibia). *Contrib. Vert. Evol.* 2:1–140.
Lombard, R.E., and D.B. Wake (1976) Tongue evolution in the lungless salamanders, family Plethodontidae. I. Introduction, theory and a general models of dynamics. *J. Morphol.* 148:265–286.
Lombard, R.E., and D.B. Wake (1977) Tongue evolution in the lungless salamanders, family Plethodontidae. II. Function and evolutionary diversity. *J. Morphol.* 153:39–80.
Lombard, R.E, and D.B. Wake (1987) Tongue evolution in the lungless salamanders, family Plethodontidae. IV: Phylogeny of plethodontid salamanders and the evolution of feeding dynamics. *Syst. Zool.* 35:532–551.
Maiorana, V.C. (1976) Predation, submergent behavior, and tropical diversity. *Evol. Theory* 1:157–177.
Mandon, S., and G. Roth (1997) *Functional classification of retinal ganglion cells in lungless salamanders (fam. Plethodontidae)*. Göttingen Neurobiology Report, 1997 G. Thieme, Stuttgart, p. 501.
Maturana, H.R., J.Y. Lettvin, W.S. McCulloch, and W.H. Pitts (1960) Anatomy and physiology of vision in the frog *(Rana pipiens)*. *J. Gen. Physiol.* 43(Suppl. 2):129–175.
McKinney, M.L., and K.J. McNamara (1991) *Heterochrony: The Evolution of Ontogeny.* New York, Plenum.
Neary, T.J., and R.G. Northcutt (1983) Nuclear organisation of the bullfrog diencephalon. *J. Comp. Neurol.* 213:262–278.
Nieuwenhuys, R., H.J. ten Donkelaar, and C. Nicholson (1998) *The Central Nervous System of Vertebrates*, vol. 3. Springer, Berlin.
Nishikawa, K., G., Roth, and U. Dicke (1991) Post-hatching development of motor neurons and motor columns in the anterior spinal cord of salamanders. *Brain Behav. Evol.* 37:368–382.
Northcutt, R.G. (1981) Evolution of the telencephalon in non-mammals. *Annu. Rev. Neurosci.* 4:301–350.
Northcutt, R.G. (1987) Lungfish neural characters and their bearing on sarcopterygian phylogeny. In: W.E. Bemis, W.W. Burggreen, and N.E. Kemp (eds.): *The Biology and Evolution of Lungfishes.* Alan R. Liss, New York, pp. 277–297.
Northcutt, R.G., and J.H. Kaas (1995) The emergence and evolution of mammalian isocortex. *Trends Neurosc.* 18:373–379.
Ohno, S. (1972) So much "junk" in our genome. In H. H. Smith (ed.): *Evolution of Genetic Systems.* Brookhaven Symposium on Bioology. Gordon and Breach, New York, pp. 366–370.
Olmo, E. (1983) Nucleotype and cell size in vertebrates: a review. *Bas. Appl. Histochem.* 27:227–256.
Olmo, E. (1991) Genome variations in the transitions from amphibians to reptiles. *J. Mol. Evol.* 33:1–25.
Orgel, L., and F. Crick (1980) Selfish DNA: the ultimate parasite. *Nature* 284:604–607.
Potter, H.D. (1965) Mesencephalic auditory region of the bullfrog. *J. Neurophysiol.* 28:1132–1154.
Rettig, G., and G. Roth (1986) Retinofugal projections in salamanders of the family Plethodontidae. *Cell Tissue. Res.* 243:385–396.
Rockenhäuser, A., and G. Roth (1997) Morphological classification of tectal cells in the frog *Discoglossus pictus*. Göttingen Neurobiology Report, 1997. G. Thieme, Stuttgart, p. 530.
Romer, A.S. (1970) *The Vertebrate Body*, 4th ed. Saunders, Philadelphia.
Roth, G. (1976) Experimental analysis of the prey catching behavior of *Hydromantes italicus* Dunn (Amphibia, Plethodontidae). *J. Comp. Physiol.* 109:47–58.
Roth, G. (1982) Responses of the optic tectum of the salamander *Hydromantes italicus* to moving prey stimuli. *Exp. Brain Res.* 45:386–392.
Roth, G. (1987) *Visual Behavior in Salamanders. Studies of Brain Function.* Springer, Berlin.
Roth, G., J. Blanke, and D.B. Wake (1994) Cell size predicts morphological complexity in the brains of frogs and salamanders. *Proc. Natl. Acad. Sci. U.S.A.* 91:4796–4800.
Roth, G., Dicke U., and W. Grunwald (1999) Morphology, axonal projection pattern and response types of tectal neurons in plethodontid salamanders. II. Intracellular recording and labeling experiments. *J. Comp. Neurol.* 404:489–504.
Roth, G., U. Dicke, and W. Wiggers (1998) Vision. In H. Heatwole (ed.): *Amphibian Biology, vol. 3: Sensory Perception.* Beatty & Sons, Surrey.
Roth, G., W. Grunwald, and C. Naujoks-Manteuffel (1990) Cytoarchitecture of the tectum mesencephali in salamanders. A Golgi and HRP study. *J. Comp. Neurol.* 291:27–42.
Roth, G., and M. Jordan (1982) Response characteristics and stratification of tectal neurons in the toad *Bufo bufo* L. *Exp. Brain Res.* 45:393–398.

Roth, G., C. Naujoks-Manteuffel, K. Nishikawa, A. Schmidt, and D.B. Wake (1993) The salamander nervous system as a secondarily simplified, paedomorphic system. *Brain Behav. Evol*. 42:137–170.
Roth, G., and D.B. Wake (1985a) Trends in the functional morphology and sensorimotor control of feeding behavior in salamanders: an example of internal dynamics in evolution. *Acta Biotheor*. 34:175–192.
Roth, G., and D.B Wake (1985b) The structure of the brainstem and cervical spinal cord in lungless salamanders (family Plethodontidae) and its relation to feeding. *J. Comp. Neurol*. 241:99–110.
Roth, G., and G. Westhoff (1999) Morphology and axonal projection pattern of neurons in the medial pallium of the frog *Discoglossus pictus. Eur. J. Morphol*. 37: 166–171.
Roth, G., and M.F. Wullimann (1996) Evolution der Nervensysteme und Sinnesorgane. In J. Dudel, R. Menzel, and R. F. Schmidt (eds.): *Neurowissenschaft. Vom Molekül zur Kognition*. Springer-Verlag, Berlin.
Sarnat, H.B., and M.G. Netsky (1974) *Evolution of the Nervous System*. Oxford, London.
Schmidt, A., C. Naujoks-Manteuffel, and G. Roth, (1988) Olfactory and vomeronasal projections and the pathways of the nervus terminalis in ten species of salamanders; a whole-mount study employing the horseradish-peroxidase technique. *Cell Tissue Res*. 251:45–50.
Schmidt, A., and Wake, M.H. (1997) Cellular migration and morphological complexity in the caecilian brain. *J. Morphol*. 231:11–27.
Sessions, S.K. (1984) *Cytogenetics and Evolution of Salamanders*. Ph.D. Dissertation, University of California, Berkeley.
Sessions, S.K., and A. Larson (1987) Developmental correlates of genome size in plethodontid salamanders and their implications for genome evolution. *Evolution* 41:1239–1251.
Singman, E.L., and F. Scalia (1990) Quantitative study of the tectally projecting retinal ganglion cells in the adult frog: I. The size of the contralateral and ipsilateral projections. *J. Comp. Neurol*. 302:792–809.
Smirnov, S.V. (1989) Postmetamorphic skull development in *Bombina orientalis* (Amphibia, Discoglossidae), with comments on neoteny. *Zool. Anz*. 223:91–99.
Stadtmuller, F. (1931) Varianten im Mittelohrgebiet bei *Bombinator* (Columella auris, Hyalbogenspanne, Tuba auditiva). *Gegenbaur's Morphol. Jahrb*. 66:196–219.
Starck, D. (1982) *Vergleichende Anatomie der Wirbeltiere*, vol. 3. Springer, Berlin.
Szarski, H. (1983) Cell size and the concept of wasteful and frugal evolutionary strategies. *J. Theor. Biol*. 105:201–209.
Székely, G., and G. Lázár (1976) Cellular and synaptic architecture of the optic tectum. In: R. Llinas, and W. Precht (eds.): *Frog neurobiology*. Springer, Berlin, pp. 407–434.
Thexton, A.J., D.B. Wake, and M.H. Wake (1977) Tongue function in the salamander *Bolitoglossa occidentalis. Arch. Oral Biol*. 22:361–366.
Van't Hof, J., and A.H. Sparrow (1963) A relationship between DNA content, nuclear volume, and minimum mitotic cycle time. *Proc. Natl. Acad. Sci.U.S.A*. 49:897–902.
Wake, D.B. (1966) Comparative osteology and evolution of the lungless salamanders, family Plethodontidae. *Mem. S. Calif. Acad. Sci*. 4:1–111.
Wake, D.B. (1982) Functional and developmental constraints and opportunities in the evolution of feeding systems in urodeles. In D. Mossakowski and G. Roth (eds.): *Environmental Adaptation and Evolution*. Fischer, Stuttgart, pp. 51–66.
Wake, D.B. (1987) Adaptive radiation of salamanders in Middle American cloud forests. *Ann. Missouri Bot. Gard*. 74:242–246.
Wake, D.B., K.C. Nishikawa, U. Dicke, and G. Roth (1988) Organization of the motor nuclei in the cervical spinal cord of salamanders. *J. Comp. Neurol*. 278:195–208
Wiggers, W. (1999) Projections of single retinal ganglion cells to the visual centers. An intracellular staining study in a plethodontid salamander. *Vis. Neurosc*. 16:1–13.
Wiggers, W., and G. Roth (1991) Anatomy, neurophysiology and functional aspects of the nucleus isthmi in salamanders of the family Plethodontidae. *J. Comp. Physiol*. 169:165–176.
Wiggers, W., G. Roth, C. Eurich, and A. Straub (1995) Binocular depth perception mechanisms in tongue-projecting salamanders. *J. Comp. Physiol*. 176:365–377.
Wilder, I.L. Whipple, and E. R. Dunn (1920) The correlation of lunglessness in salamanders with a mountain brook habitat. Copeia 84:63–68.
Will, U. (1988) Organization and projections of the area octavolateralis in amphibians. In Fritzsch, B. et al., (eds.): *The Evolution of the Amphibian Auditory System*, Wiley, New York, pp. 185–208.

Chapter 9

EVOLUTIONARY CONSTRAINTS OF LARGE TELENCEPHALA

Gerd Rehkämper, Heiko D. Frahm, and Michael D. Mann
C. and O. Vogt Institute of Brain Research, University of Düsseldorf, (G.R., H.D.F.) and Department of Physiology and Biophysics, Medical Center, University of Nebraska (M.D.)

EVOLUTION—WHAT DOES THAT MEAN?

The term *evolution* has a long tradition in natural science and was even used in pre-Darwinian times. Animaculists and ovulists used it to describe the development from a single sperm or a single egg to the adult organism. Modern usage is primarily associated with Darwin's theory of the origin of species (Darwin, 1859). Nevertheless, different research interests and strategies are subsumed under the term *evolution*. One is phylogenetic, in which investigators attempt to establish a genealogy of living species through time. Their results might be presented in a cladogram, which also defines the relatedness of living species. In Germany, Ax (1987) has referred to this as *phylogenetic systematics*. This work was originally formulated by Hennig (1966) and elaborated by many investigators (e.g., Eldredge and Cracraft, 1980).

Although these authors refer to Darwin, one might question whether they have followed the proposal of "Taking Darwin Seriously" (Ruse, 1986) in the strict sense. Bowler (1996) and Ruse (1997) have drawn attention to the fact that the perception of Darwin's ideas by his contemporary scientists, such as Thomas Henry Huxley and Ernst Haeckel, was very selective. At the same time, these authors had a strong interest in systematics, and their legacy is still identifiable in modern comparative morphology.

Rehkämper (1997) has tried to demonstrate that the innovation in Darwin's theory is the introduction of the actualistic principle into biology. This principle states that only phenomena that are amenable to investigation at the current time are suitable for formulating scientific hypotheses and explanations. As a result, the living animal becomes the focus, and the hypothesis is that the success of a species is the result of functional selection and adaptation to a species-specific ecological niche. Function depends on structure, and thus functional morphology can contribute to these endeavors. Structural information by itself is, however, useless. It is the activity of the nervous system that produces behavior and, thus, constrains evolutionary success and development.

The central nervous system itself is both structure and associated function. Examining its structure may be easy, whereas analyzing its function is often much more difficult methodologically. Comparative neuromorphology can, however, be used as a propaedeutic approach. It can help to find the key that has opened a peculiar ecological niche in which a given species has successfully survived.

To summarize, evolution is adaptation via natural selection. Neuromorphology offers a tool that can help to bring into focus what a species is adapted to and selected for physiologically and behaviorally.

BRAIN AND BRAIN PART SIZE AS A HEURISTIC TOOL

The brains of different vertebrate species are not the same. One parameter that is easily measurable is absolute brain size. This can be described using parameters of length, height, and width. These parameters, however, might be influenced by external factors (e.g., the anatomy of the skull). In contrast, brain weight seems to be more independent of such influences and is often used. It can easily be converted to brain volume using the specific weight of brain tissue (1.036 g/cm^3 in mammals; Stephan, 1960). Many of the famous brain collections have been established primarily to get information on brain size and brain composition, yielding a large amount of such data.

It is a sort of credo of neurobiology that delineating the quantitative aspects of the brain, such as size (or number of cells or amount of neuropil) would help to understand the brain, that is, to clarify its function. We share this point of view. Not everyone, however, does. Philosophers or psychologists are often willing to identify a causal relation between the brain and functions such as cognition and consciousness or even vision and hearing, but they do not find it suitable to measure the brain and its parts. Their arguments are sometimes very hard to counter. There are, however, facts that support the usefulness of investigating the brain quantitatively to understand a living species. If a brain part is found to be completely reduced in a species, then the function it normally subserves may not exist in that species or may not be accomplished in the same way as in that species having the brain part in question. The olfactory and the visual systems are cases in point. Whales, which do not possess olfactory structures, are anosmic. The mole rats (rodents), which lack eyes capable of reception of visual images, are blind. The golden mole (insectivore) is said not to possess an optic nerve (Le Gros Clark, 1932); it is blind as well. By analogy, one may conclude that an enlargement of a brain part has functional importance. In a way, this is supported by investigations outside a comparative approach. Nottebohm (1981) has noted that the size of a motor control nucleus alters in correlation with the seasonal singing behavior of the male songbird. During the season when the birds sing, the nucleus is large; in times when they do not sing, it is small. This alteration involves neurogenesis (Paton and Nottebohm, 1984) and underlines the relationship between size and functional demands of brain structures. We will later refer to other papers that support such insights. It should, however, be mentioned here that Gahr (1997) questioned these results and discussed methodical problems associated with differing delineation criteria.

Another problem has to be treated adequately. Comparing absolute brain (part) sizes may yield data that are biologically implausible (for a review, see Stephan et al., 1986). Hardly anyone argues that whales and elephants are superior to humans in central nervous capacities, such as intelligence or cognition, although their brains are absolutely larger. The problem is that their bodies are also absolutely larger. The allometric approach, taking body weight into consideration, reduces the risk of misleading interpretations. It has become a useful tool in identifying adaptive peculiarities of the species. This approach defines average correlations between brain (part) size and body weight and thus allows one to identify species that are above or below average. An index can be calculated describing the amount of deviation from this average, that is, the degree of encephalization or telencephalization or diencephalization. In a large variety of mammalian and avian species such indices correspond to ecological, ethological, or evolutionary categories (see Stephan et al. 1991; Rehkämper et al. 1991a; Boire and Baron, 1994; Baron et al., 1996).

It must be realized, however, that natural selection can act on body size alone, on brain size alone, or on both. Alternatively, brain size may change as a correlated trait even though selection is only for increased or decreased body size. This has been discussed by Towe and Mann (1995).

The impact of the evolution of body size becomes visible in secondarily miniaturized mammals, such as *Miopithecus talapoin* (Stephan et al., 1981). For this monkey, a large calculated encephalization index is not necessarily reflected in brain function, for example, in cognitive behavior. On the other hand, there are animals with unusually large body sizes. The gorilla and the orangutan are good examples (Zilles and Rehkämper, 1988). Here, the females have "normal" body weights, whereas the males have above normal weights. As a consequence the encephalization indices for the two sexes are different. Obviously, there are evolutionary pressures that lead to altered body weight.

On a related topic, Towe and Mann (1995) described a natural experiment that was unintentionally done by humans. The authors investigated brain size and body size in pocket gophers (*Thomomys bottae perpes*) whose homes were covered by alfalfa, which is an agriculturally used plant of high energy content. These animals were compared with pocket gophers from the same species occupying normal habitat (i.e., desert shrubland). In the case of the alfalfa experiment, the increased food resources can be considered to select for increased body weight alone. Brain weight would then increase only as needed to cope with the increase in body size.

The brains of the alfalfa field animals followed the same somatic scaling relations as those of animals from the desert shrubland. All differences were fully explained by the sexual dimorphism in the somatic variables. Slopes of the brain–body relations for males and females in the two sites were nearly identical and similar to those predicted from a geometric model based on the statistical characteristics of the samples. Towe and Mann (1995) argued that these slopes define the increase in brain size required to serve an increased body size with no changes in lifestyle. This being the case, some broad generalizations about the evolutionary history of some other rodents are possible.

The value of this slope, approximately 0.18, is considerably lower than the overall slope (0.69) found by Mann et al. (1988) for myomorph rodents (not including *Thomomys*), suggesting that there has been considerable selection among rodents for increased brain size. If there had not been such selection, the slope for myomorph rodents would be 0.18. This selection for increased brain size would be in addition to any selection for increased body size alone. Slopes for different genera within this group are different—some are quite high; some are near 0.18. Particular genera, such as *Peromyscus* (slope around 0.79), may have been under strong pressure to increase brain size, whereas other genera, such as *Rattus*, may have been under little or no pressure for increased brain size (Fig. 9.1). In this view, genera with intermediate slopes may have experienced intermediate pressures for increased brain size or mixed pressures to increase body size and, independently, brain size. Thus, this investigation of brain–body relationship generates new hypotheses that should be tested.

WHAT FACTORS INFLUENCE BRAIN SIZE OR BRAIN PART SIZE?

Neurobiologists have put causes of alteration in brain size into four categories: (1) There is no brain size alteration; (2) brain size alteration is an epiphenomenon; (3) brain size is influenced by individual learning; and (4) brain size and brain part size reflect adaptation.

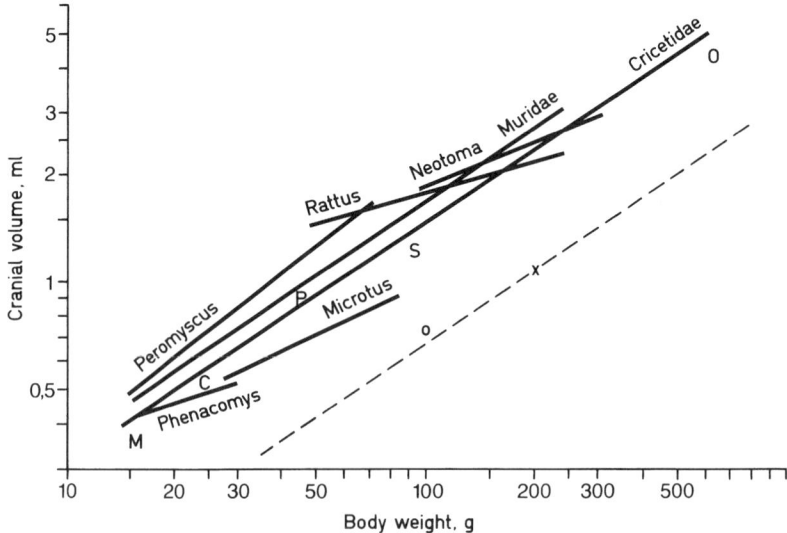

Figure 9.1. Log-log plot of mean body weight versus mean cranial volume (brain size) for various genera in the families Muridae and Cricetidae. The reduced major axes for genera with more than one subspecies are drawn. O, *Ondatra*; M, *Mus*; S, *Sigmodon*; P, *Phyllotis*; and C, *Clethrionomys*. The dashed line is plotted with a 2/3 slope through the value for *P. montanus* (x); the value for *T. mordax* (o) lies nearby. (From Mann et al., 1988, by permission of Karger, Basel.)

We would like to outline these points of views. Then we present our own data on brain diversity in birds and mammals, and, finally, we evaluate these theories on alteration in brain size with due consideration of our own data.

There Is No Brain Size Alteration

This discussion is associated with attempts to evaluate the influence of body size on brain size. Snell (1892) and Dubois (1897) drew attention to the fact that brain size does not increase with body weight isometrically but allometrically, and they estimated the exponent of the log–log relation to be about 2/3. This value has been used in many treatments; however, there has always been a debate whether body weight alone is a suitable variable for comparison. For example, using ideas from Kleiber (1961) or Jolicoeur and Heusner (1971), Martin (1981) argued that the basic metabolic rate should also be considered. Clearly, the brain operates the body, but the body has to take care of the brain's nutrition. Because the metabolic demand of the brain is large, metabolic rate may exert constraints on brain size. Armstrong (1982, 1983, 1985) made use of Stephan's data on brain size and body size in primates and corrected the body weights for basic metabolic rates as far as the data were available. She found that there was no longer a difference in relative brain size between prosimians and simians, as has been calculated by Stephan et al. (1988) using body weight alone as independent variable.

Martin (1990) worked intensively with this hypothesis, and he suggested that brain size is a function of maternal nutrition during the offspring's ontogenesis (Martin, 1995). Human evolution is thus no longer seen as primarily characterized by increasing brain size from *Australopithecus* via *Homo habilis* and *H. erectus* to *H. sapiens*. Instead, alteration in dietetic regimes is considered to be more basic, and the large brain is understood as a side effect, which might or might not be advantageous. It should be pointed out that not everyone supports Martin's ideas. Harvey and Krebs (1990), for example, were unable to confirm a number of predictions of Martin's metabolic theory. Towe and Mann (1995) have also expressed reservations about these ideas.

Brain Size Alterations Are Epiphenomena

For the argument developed in the last paragraph, alterations in brain size were regarded as a consequence of changes that have nothing to do with the brain function proper.

Alterations in brain size are presented as one of the major topics of comparative neurobiology, but Deacon (1990) suggests that some problematic assumptions prevent important insights into the evolution of the brain and alterations in brain size. "Anthropocentrism," "*scala naturae* thinking," "bigger is better concepts," and "larger brains do have more association areas" are some catchwords, the heuristic value of which is questioned by Deacon (1990). He argues for an approach that considers the intensity of information processing and proposes network allometry. Furthermore, modes of neurogenesis are seen as key to understanding brain size. He interprets evolution as primarily an historic process of development, either phylogenetically or ontogenetically. The central point of Darwin's theory, however, is not historical development but functional adaptation and corresponding selection (Rehkämper, 1997; see below).

Finlay and Darlington (1995) also drew attention to the ontogenesis of the brain. They pointed out that species showing prolonged neurogenesis do have large brains. The period of neurogenesis comes to an end with the beginning of cytogenesis (i.e., neuronal differentiation). Interestingly, Finlay and Darlington (1995) have excluded olfactory parts of the brain from their concept because these do not support their theory.

Roth et al. (1994) published a paper dealing with the brain of frogs and salamanders. They were puzzled by the fact that brains that are architectonically simple are nevertheless relatively large. They looked more carefully into brain structure and realized that the size of the nucleus of the neurons is different in different species, reflecting differences in genome size. Large genomes require large cell nuclei, and, as a consequence, perikarya and total brains are large. The evolutionary advantage of large genomes, however, is said to have nothing to do with brain function. Thus, alterations in brain size are not of primary importance. On the other hand, alterations in genome size cannot be without consequence.

Jerison (1955, 1973, 1977, 1985, 1994) identified biologically relevant alterations in brain size and defined so-called extra neurons, neurons in excess of those needed to manage a body of a given size. These Jerison sees as the substrate for intelligence. One problem with Jerison's concept is that he neglects the importance of brain composition. He argues that brain composition is all the same and that the size of the telencephalon, with the isocortex, can be predicted if the size of the total brain is known. Thus, it is not the total brain size that is an epiphenomenon in the chain of Jerison's arguments, but the size of brain parts.

Brain Size Is Influenced by Individual Learning

Krebs et al. (1989) investigated food-storing and non–food-storing tits of different species of the genus *Parus* and measured the volume of the hippocampus. They found that food storers have a relatively larger hippocampus than non–food storers do. In a second study, newly hatched food-storing tits were separated into two groups (Clayton and Krebs, 1994). The first one had a chance to perform food storing; the second did not. The enlarged hippocampus in animals that stored food suggests that individual learning might influence the size of a brain part and thus of the total brain, although there are open questions, such as how to rule out the effects of motor performance.

Another type of alteration of brain part size (i.e., some part is enlarged at the expense of another) is seen in primates. If a monkey has lost one finger, the somatosensory representation of that finger is lost. Stimulation of other fingers then drives the neurons that have served the lost finger (Merzenich et al., 1984; for review, see Kaas, 1991). Apparently, their areas of representation have been individually enlarged. Similarly in laboratory mice, Bronchti et al. (1992) saw an increase in the somatosensory cortex after neonatal eye removal.

Brain Size and Brain Part Size Reflect Adaptation

Stephan and co-workers collected the brains from more than 400 insectivore, primate, rodent, and bat species and studied brain size, brain composition, and body size in relation to the evolutionary level and ecoethological characteristics. These data are summarized in two review papers (primates, Stephan et al., 1981, 1988) and four books (insectivores, Stephan et al., 1991; and three volumes on bats, Baron et al., 1996). Stephan has not published a hypothesis or theory of brain size and its causes. However, he tried to explain most of the data in terms of evolutionary adaptation and selective advantage of alteration in brain size and brain composition. We will come back to this topic after a discussion of large telencephala.

DEFINITION OF "LARGE TELENCEPHALA"

The telencephalon is a brain part characteristic of all vertebrate brains. A small telencephalon is seen in the hemiparasitic agnatha, particularly in lampreys (petromyzontids), but in all other groups the telencephalon constitutes a major component of the brain. From the work of Ebbesson (1980a), we are aware that, in all classes of vertebrates, the telencephalon seems to be a destination of somatosensory, visual, and auditory as well as olfactory pathways. In every group the telencephalon appears to be engaged in motor coordination as well (for a review, see Ebbesson, 1980b). Nevertheless, the relative and absolute sizes of the telencephala are very different in different groups. We do not discuss here the methodological problems of determination and scaling of the size of the brain and its parts throughout all vertebrates. Instead, we define large telencephala as those that constitute half or more of the total brain.

From the abundance of data on mammalian and avian brains, we can say that the telencephalon in most representatives of both classes is large according to our definition (Stephan et al., 1981, 1988, 1991; Rehkämper et al., 1991a; Boire and Baron, 1994). The degree of enlargement, however, is very different, and we will deal with both classes in turn. Doing that, an allometric approach is preferred, taking body weight into consideration. Two aspects will be demonstrated: First, the large size of the telencephalon in both classes is caused by an enlargement of very different functional subunits (e.g., isocortex or its equivalent, hippocampus, olfactory bulb) in different members of the class; second, parallel evolution in mammalian and avian brains is obvious (Rehkämper and Zilles, 1991). Finally, attention is drawn to domesticated animals, particularly to their cognitive abilities.

MAMMALS

The proportion of the mammalian brain that is telencephalon varies from 49% in the insectivore *Geogale*, which has allometrically the smallest brain of all mammals, to 85% in humans (Rehkämper et al., 1986; Stephan et al., 1991), who has allometrically the largest brain among mammals. Thus, a remarkable variability is obvious. A functional interpretation of such data is difficult, however, because the telencephalon consists of several subunits, each of which serves a different function. These are the subcortical striate body and septal areas, which are not dealt with in this chapter, the hippocampal complex of the limbic system, the olfactory cortices, and the multifunctional isocortex*. Thus, we need a detailed analysis of the composition of the telencephalon to understand the biological advantage of large telencephala. It is quite obvious that telencephalic composition is not uniform but has species-specific alterations. Several trends are identifiable.

Telencephala Enlarged Because of Dominance of Olfactory Orientation

In *Geogale, Echinops,* and other Madagassian tenrecs (Tenrecidae, Insectivora), the telencephalon is dominated by olfactory cortices, according to Stephan (1975) (olfactory bulb, prepiriform region, retrobulbar region, olfactory tubercle; Figs. 9.2 and 9.3). The olfactory bulb alone is 29 times larger than in humans (allometrically), whereas the rest of telencephalon is only 1/50 of that in humans. These animals are nocturnal insect hunters, and their sensory equipment reflects their peculiar biology. Thus, it can be said that the process of their telencephalization is associated with a specialization of a specific sensory system, the olfactory system.

Telencephala Enlarged Because of Superior Spatial Cognition

A curious group of mammals are the elephant shrews, the Macroscelididae, which include the genera *Elephantulus, Macroscelides, Nasilio, Petrodromus,* and *Rhynchocyon* (Fig. 9.4). Allometrically, they have larger telencephala than those found in *Geogale, Echinops* or *Tenrec*. This size is heavily influenced by an extraordinary expansion of the hippocampus (Fig. 9.5), as shown by Stephan et al. (1981, 1991). It is 4.5 times larger than that in tenrecs and thus nearly as large as in humans (that in humans is 4.9 times larger).

The hippocampus is part of the limbic system, which is associated with affective behavior as well as with learning and memory. Recently, attention has been drawn to the role of the hippocampus in spatial orientation, and it has been argued that spatial

---

* It should be noted that we try to avoid the terms *archicortex*, *palaeocortex*, and *neocortex* (except in referring to other authors) because they are burdened with a concept of sequential appearance of such cortices during phylogeny. There is no evidence from comparative anatomy that this is true.

Definition of "Large Telencephala" 273

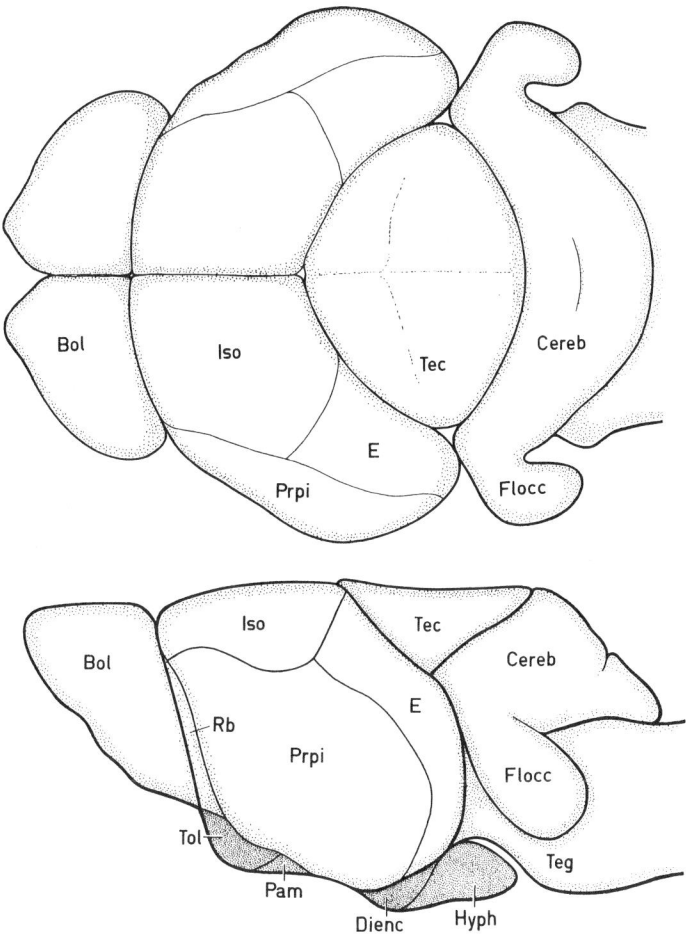

Figure 9.2. Brain of the Madagassian insectivore *Geogale aurita* in dorsal (above) and lateral (below) views. This species has one of the smallest telencephala (Bol + Iso + E + Prpi + Tol + Rb + Pam) found among mammals. Bol, olfactory bulb; Cereb, cerebellum, Dienc, diencephalon; E, entorhinal region; Flocc, flocculus; Hyph, hypophysis; Iso, isocortex; Pam, periamygdalar region; Prpi, prepiriform cortex; Rb, retrobulbar region; Tec, tectum; Teg, tegmentum; Tol, olfactory tuberculum. (Modified from Rehkämper et al., 1986.)

mapping is a specialized cognitive ability ("spatial cognition") and one of the major functions of the hippocampus (Nadel, 1991; Lipp et al., 1989; Schwegler et al., 1981). This argument is supported by neuroethological field and laboratory studies in rodents. Jacobs and Spencer (1994) studied kangaroo rats that live in large territories. The food-storing behavior of Merriam's kangaroo rat (*Dipodomys merriami*) suggests the necessity of better spatial abilities than those of the bannertail kangaroo rat (*Dipodomys spectabilis*), which does not store food. Measurements of the hippocampus have revealed that in fact Merriam's kangaroo rats exhibit significantly larger hippocampi than bannertail kangaroo rats (Jacobs and Spencer, 1994).

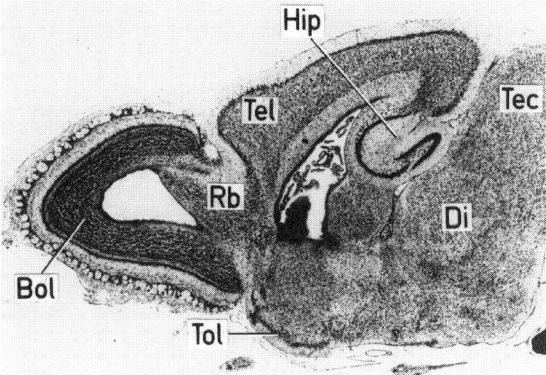

Figure 9.3. Sagittal section through the brain of the Madagassian insectivore *Echinops telfairi*; note the extremely well-devoloped olfactory bulb. Bol, olfactory bulb; Di, diencephalon; Hip, hippocampus; Rb, retrobulbar region; Tec, tectum; Tel, telencephalon; Tol, olfactory tuberculum.

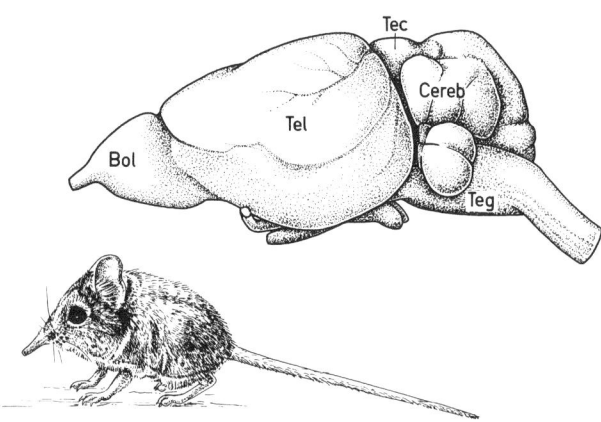

Figure 9.4. The elephant shrew *Elephantulus* and its brain. Bol, olfactory bulb; Cereb, cerebellum; Tec, tectum; Teg, tegmentum; Tel, telencephalon.

Elephant shrews have been investigated in the wild (Sauer, 1973). From these observations we know that they live in large territories, which have many shelters at different places. If an elephant shrew is threatened by a predator, it quickly runs to the nearest shelter. In this way, their biology is similar to kangaroo rats in that they, too, require a superior spatial ability. Thus, it can be said that the process of telencephalization in elephant shrews is heavily influenced by an increase in hippocampal size, perhaps reflecting a specialization for spatial cognition.

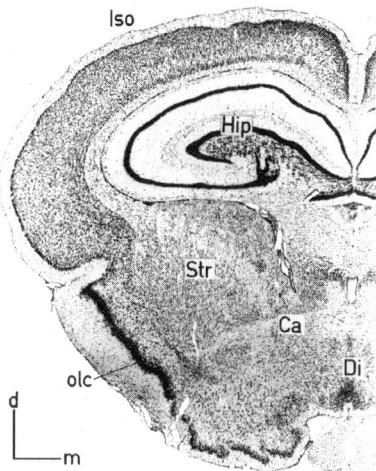

Figure 9.5. Cross section through the telencephalon of *Elephantulus*; note the large hippocampus (Hip). Ca, anterior commissure; d, dorsal; Di, diencephalon; Iso, isocortex; m, medial; olc, olfactory cortex; Str, striate body.

Telencephala Enlarged Because of a Voluminous Isocortex

We have mentioned two (olfactory cortex and hippocampus) of three cortical parts of the telencephalon in mammals. The third one is the isocortex. In most groups of mammals, the process of telencephalization is associated with an enlargement of the isocortex. Examples can be found among carnivores (Röhrs, 1985a,b, 1986a,b), ungulates (Oboussier, 1972; Ebinger, 1974; Kruska, 1970; 1973), and others. The most reliable data are available from the work of Stephan and collaborators for insectivores, rodents, and particularly primates and bats (Stephan et al., 1981, 1991; Baron et al., 1996).

The term *isocortex*, coined by Brodmann (1909), means cortex of equal structure. The equality, however, refers to the ontogenetic development of the different parts of the isocortex. It does not refer to a functional homogeny. Like the telencephalon, the adult isocortex as a whole is functionally and structurally too heterogenous to allow any evolutionary, thus adaptive, interpretation of differences in its total size. We must instead look carefully to determine which parts of the isocortex seem to be enlarged. That is not without problems.

Morphological criteria as used in cyto-, myelo-, or other architectonics do not reveal the functions of different parts of the isocortex, but the morphologist may surmount methodological limitations by integrating physiological methods into his work. Tracing is a technique between morphology and physiology. If pathways can be followed back to sensory organs, a functional interpretation is possible. From use of such techniques, a sort of a *bauplan* of the isocortex identifies an occipitally situated visual cortex, a laterocaudally situated auditory cortex, a postcentrally situated somatosensory cortex, and a precentrally located motor cortex. Such a *bauplan* could hardly be identified in very small isocortices, although various authors proposed a similar organization (e.g., in insectivores) (Brodmann, 1909; Rehkämper, 1981; Valverde and Lopez-Mascaraque, 1981; Künzle and Rehkämper, 1992; for review, see also Stephan et al., 1991); in every case, physiological proof is lacking. In larger isocortices, as found in rodents, tree shrews (*Tupaia*), and prosimians, such a *bauplan* seems to be stable, but there are species that apparently have greatly altered this *bauplan*. Such a species is the subterranean rodent *Spalax*.

Isocortex (and Therefore, Telencephalon) Enlarged Because of Elaborated Somatosensory Areas Together with a Necessity of Motor Coordination in a Subterranean Life

With electrophysiological techniques, it has been demonstrated that *Spalax* has no cortical visual representation (Necker et al., 1992). Thus, an important landmark is missing. Because the architectonic structure of the occipital cortex in *Spalax* seems hardly different from that in other rodents (e.g., the laboratory rat), anatomy alone cannot help to reveal the function of this peculiar isocortex. At the same time, we know that the isocortex of *Spalax* is relatively large and contributes disproportionately to the size of the telencephalon (encephalization index 2.7, isocorticalization index 8.4; Frahm et al., 1997). Therefore, attempts were made to investigate the isocortex of *Spalax* with methods that are relevant to both structure and function (Mann et al., 1997).

Single-unit and multiunit recordings were used to delineate the borders of the somatosensory cortex as mechanical stimulation was applied to the entire body surface (Fig. 9.6). Small injections of pontamine sky blue were used to mark the outlines of this cortical region as determined from such recordings. With these labels and with a number of paraffin series, the fresh volume of the somatosensory cortex could be calculated and compared with that for the laboratory rat. From such comparisons, it was clear that the somatosensory cortex of *Spalax* is of an unusually large size and appears to be twice as large as in the laboratory rat, which is used for comparison because suitable data on the size of the somatosensory cortex for other species, including rodents, are not available (Fig. 9.7).

Motor cortices are characterized by relatively high concentrations of α-adrenergic receptors. These can be demonstrated autoradiographically using the tritiated ligand prazosin. With this technique, we calculated the size of the motor cortex within the isocortex of *Spalax* (Rehkämper et al., 1991b). The unusual enlargement of the motor cortex even surpasses the enlargement of the somatosensory cortex (Rehkämper et al., 1995). The motor cortex in *Spalax*, in comparison with that in the laboratory rat, is more than three times larger. These data fit the biology of *Spalax*. Underground, vision is limited, and the somatosensory system is the better system for environmental monitoring in this ecological niche. At the same time, *Spalax* builds a large tunnel system with the aid of teeth, head, and neck (Nevo, 1991). This is associated with hypertrophic chewing and neck musculature and probably requires elaborated

Definition of "Large Telencephala" 277

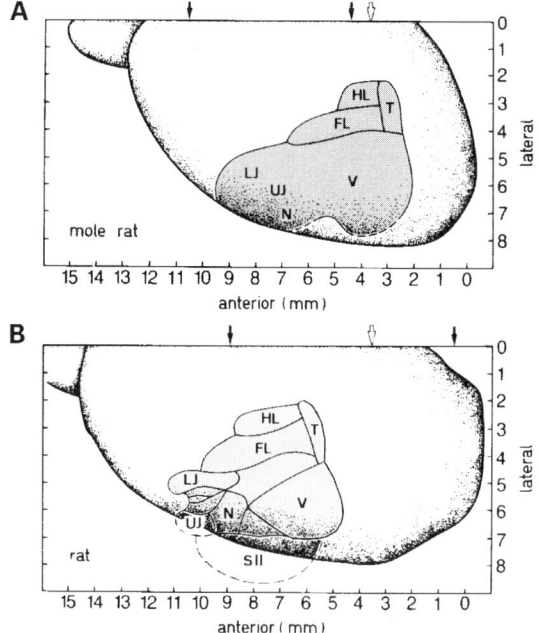

Figure 9.6. Dorsal view of the telencephalic hemispheres in the mole rat *Spalax* (modified from Necker et al., 1992) and the laboratory rat *Rattus* (modified from Chapin and Lin, 1984). The somatosensory cortex is delineated; note that it is situated much more caudally in the mole rat than in the laboratory rat. FL, forelimb; HL, hind limb; LJ, lower jaw; N, nose; T, trunc; UJ, upper jaw; V, vibrissae; SII, somatosensory cortex II; closed arrows show bregma and lambda; open arrow shows caudal end of the corpus callosum.

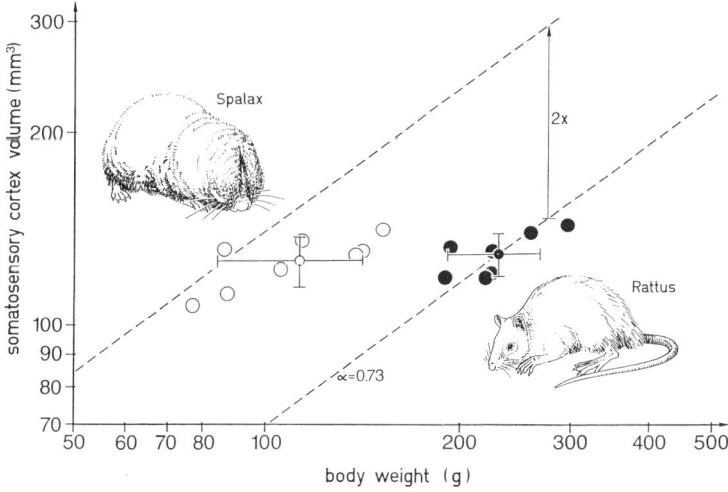

Figure 9.7. The volume of the somatosensory cortex in the mole rat and the laboratory rat related to body weight in a log-log system. Large open (mole rat) and filled (laboratory rat) circles are individual data. Small circles indicate the average values, with bars indicating the standard deviations. (From Mann et al., 1997, by permission of Verlag für Wissenschaft und Bildung, Berlin.)

motor control. Correspondingly, motor control areas outside the cortex are found to be unusually large (e.g., cerebellum, striatum, and particularly the motor nuclei of the trigeminal nerve, which innervate the chewing muscles) (Frahm et al., 1997). As far as we know, such differentiations are regularly reflected in telencephalic size, because, for example, the cerebellum is closely associated with the telencephalon by a corticopontocerebellar tract. Thus, telencephalization and isocorticalization in *Spalax* are heavily influenced by sensory specialization as well as special problems of motor coordination.

Telencephala Enlarged Because of Multimodal Integration

The catch words "telencephalization" and "isocorticalization" imply for many people the idea that these brain areas are multimodal integration centers. This function is difficult to associate with circumscribed areas of the isocortex, but it seems reasonable to assume that isocortical regions outside the primary representation areas are involved. Although quantitative data are completely lacking, it is accepted by many that the enlarged isocortices in monkeys, apes and humans have integration as a primary function (Passingham and Ettlinger, 1974; Nieuwenhuys, this volume, Chapter 6). Actually, the positron emission tomography data from neurological clinics also support such concepts. When patients are asked to solve complex problems that require multimodal integration, blood flow (and presumably also neuronal activity) is increased in areas outside sensory or motor cortices *sensu stricto* (see, e.g., Roland and Friberg, 1985). We do not, however, want to discuss this phenomenon in the mammalian context in greater detail here.

BIRDS

The proportion of the avian brain composed of telencephalon varies from 50% in galliform birds to 80% in passeriform species (Fig. 9.8), covering a range similar to that in mammals (Rehkämper et al., 1991a; Boire and Baron, 1994). One may reasonably question whether this parallelism is reflected in parallel trends in progressive telencephalization in various bird groups. An answer is made difficult because the analysis of the avian brain is not yet as advanced as that of the mammalian brain. There is, however, some evidence.

Telencephala Enlarged Because of Olfaction

Anseriform birds have relatively large telencephala (66% of the total brain in geese, Ebinger and Löhmer, 1987; 70% in ducks, Boire and Baron, 1994). At the same time, this group has a well-developed olfactory bulb (Bang and Cobb, 1968). Recently it was demonstrated that this large olfactory bulb projects to various telencephalic target

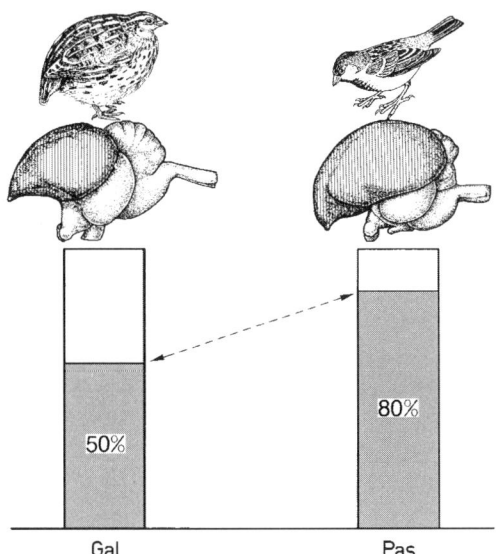

Figure 9.8. Variability of telencephalic size in relation to brain size in birds. Gal, galliform birds; *Coturnix* as an example; Pas, passeriform birds, *Passer* as an example.

areas (Fig. 9.9; Ebinger et al., 1992). A projection area is found on the mediobasal aspect of the telencephalon, which, only in anseriform birds, expands into the interhemispheric fissure and occupies a large part of the medial hemispheric surface. In fact, the olfactory structures in anseriform birds are twice as large as they are, for example, in the rock dove *Columba livia* (Ebinger et al., 1992). Quantitatively, these olfactory structures do not constitute one fourth of the telencephalon as is the case in *Geogale* and other insectivores, but the tendency is obvious. Telencephalization in this avian brain is accompanied by an expansion of olfactory structures.

Telencephala Enlarged Because of Spatial Cognition

The hippocampus likewise demonstrates a remarkable variability in avian brains. Recently, we became aware of the fact that the hippocampus of food-storing birds is larger than of nonstorers (Krebs et al., 1989; Clayton and Krebs, 1994; Sherry et al., 1992; Shettleworth, 1990). In fact, the data parallel the hippocampal data from food-storing rodents and elephant shrews (see above). Thus, a superior capacity of spatial cognition is also needed in food-storing birds. This could explain the large size of the hippocampus provided that the hippocampus has a similar function in birds.

Additional support for this hypothesis comes from homing pigeon research. These animals have a superior spatial cognition (Papi, 1995; Bingman et al., 1995). We demonstrated that the hippocampus in this breed contributes disproportionately to the larger telencephalon in comparison to nonhoming breeds (Rehkämper et al., 1988).

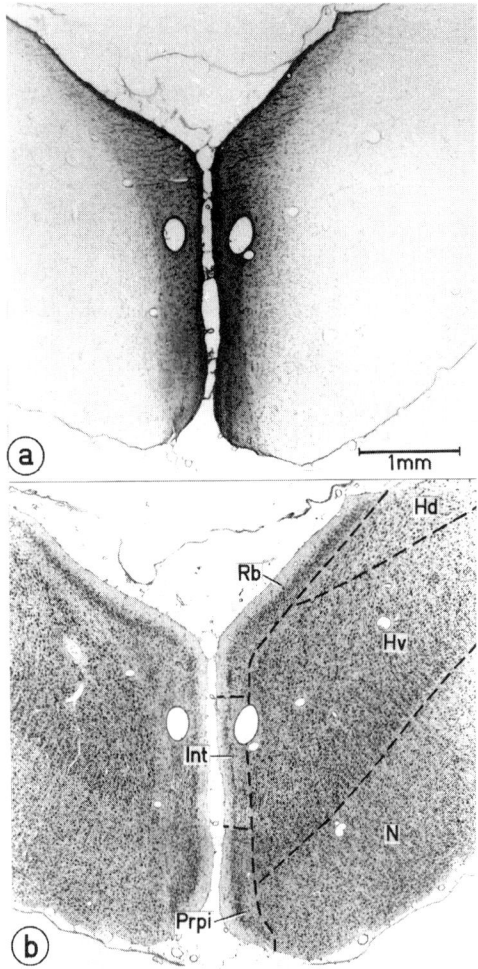

Figure 9.9. Coronal section showing olfactory structures (Rb, retrobulbar area; Int, intermediate zone; Prpi, prepiriform cortex) in the telencephalon of *Anas platyrhynchos*. (*a*) After injection of tritiated leucin into the olfactory bulb, projection areas in the ventral, medial, and dorsal part of the telencephalon are visible. (*b*) Corresponding section stained with cresyl fast violet to illustrate architectonics. Note that olfactory structures are not restricted to mediobasal parts of the telencephalon as usual but are expanded. Hd, dorsal hyperstriatum; Hv, ventral hyperstriatum; N, neostriatum. (From Ebinger et al., 1992, by permission of Springer, Berlin.)

Telencephala Enlarged Because of Isocortical Equivalents

An identification of the avian brain equivalent of mammalian "isocorticalization" is crucial. Pivotal to this identification is the definition of the mammalian isocortex and its counterpart in birds. It is true that the mammalian isocortex bears primary areas as well as secondary and associative regions. Starting from the pioneering work of Wallenberg (1898, 1903), Karten (1965, 1968, 1969, 1979, 1991), Karten and

Dubbeldam (1973), and Karten and Hodos (1970) demonstrated that the neostriatum of birds (pigeons) bears representation areas of the main sensory pathways. Additionally, the archistriatum has been identified as a motor region, and the same is true for paleostriatal areas (Zeier and Karten, 1971). These observations led to the concept that the avian neostriatum *sensu lato* was equivalent to the mammalian isocortex or at least a part of it (Nauta and Karten, 1970). This concept, which is in agreement with the results of Källen (1951,1962), is in opposition to some traditional views (e.g., Kuhlenbeck, 1967–1978), but has been increasingly substantiated (see Ulinski, 1983; Veenman et al., 1995).

We started a complete revision of the architecture of the ventral hyperstriatum and neostriatum (Rehkämper et al., 1984, 1985). It was the aim to determine whether the architecture of the avian neostriatum–hyperstriatum ventrale complex has something in common with the mammalian isocortex. The architectonic findings reveal three areas of sensory representation that correspond with the nucleus basalis, the ectostriatum, and the Field L in the terminology of previous investigations (Rehkämper et al., 1984, 1985; Rehkämper and Zilles, 1991). These areas occupy only a small part of the whole complex. In every case, it could be demonstrated that the primary areas are accompanied by small, more or less surrounding fields that are topographically similar to Brodmann's secondary areas 5 and 7, area 42, and area 18 (V2) in mammalian brains (Brodmann, 1909). Large parts of the caudal neostriatum and dorsal ventral hyperstriatum, however, lie apart from these primary and secondary areas. This again is similar to the organization of the mammalian isocortex, particularly if it is large. There, too, primary and adjoining areas are embedded in large regions that could not be classified like this.

Tracing studies revealed the connectivity of these areas. Because of its size, the caudal neostriatum* is of special interest. It accounts for approximately half of the neostriatum (53% in a domestic chicken breed, Chabo)—Field L excluded—and receives afferent fibers from all secondary areas and from the ventral hyperstriatum (Rehkämper and Zilles, 1991). Such a large number of intracortical fibers is also typical of the mammalian isocortex. At the same time, the caudal neostriatum sends fibers to the archistriatum and the paleostriatum. Both areas have been shown to be major sources of telencephalic efferent fibers forming a telencephalic control of motor systems similar to that of isocortex and striatum in mammals. We argued that in birds the whole complex of hyperstriatal and neostriatal areas corresponds to the mammalian isocortex despite its lack of a cortical organization. Topographical organization, connectivity, and function seem to be nearly identical. The largest part of these areas is composed of fields that do have the infrastructure for multimodal processes, including learning. In the chicken brain, for example, it has been demonstrated that medial parts of the neostriatum and ventral hyperstriatum play a crucial role in one-trial learning (imprinting; Stewart et al., 1984). Güntürkün (1997) has demonstrated that a dorsocaudal part of the pigeon's neostriatum is engaged in delayed alternation tasks, which in mammals are associated with the prefrontal cortex. The latter is a multimodal association area as well.

---

* In consequence of what is said in footnote 1, the terms neo-, archi- and paleostriatum must be seen problematical as well. However, in contrast to the situation in mammals there are no alternative terms which are in common use. Thus, we will not change anything in the frame of this paper.

282 9 Evolutionary Constraints of Large Telencephala

We have seen that large mammalian telencephala gained their size by an enlargement of the isocortex. The question now is whether the same is true for birds. This seems to be the case. For several reasons, we compared the brains of small-brained galliforms with large-brained passeriforms, such as songbirds and crows. The passeriforms have large telencephala, and the investigation of telencephalic composition confirms that this is due to disproportionately enlarged neostriata and hyperstriata (Fig. 9.10) (Rehkämper et al., 1991a; Rehkämper and Zilles, 1991). The data of Boire and Baron (1994) also support this view.

In mammals and especially primates, we have argued that isocorticalization is due, at least in part, to an increase in the capacity for multimodal integration. For the sake of simplicity, we propose that multimodal integration is a prerequisite for cognitive abilities that include constituting abstract categories and deductive reasoning, as well as learning and remembering (Strube, 1996). Thus, one can argue that the primate isocortex with its large nonprimary areas provides the structural basis for superior cognitive ability. This corresponds with the available psychological data (Meador et al., 1987).

A similar situation may exist in passeriform birds as well, although there is a severe lack of data, particularly from experimental psychology. Brain size and brain composition in domestic pigeons is similar to what is seen in galliform birds. Delius and collaborators have shown that, even with such small brains, cognitive tasks can be performed that are usually not associated with an avian brain (for review, see Delius,

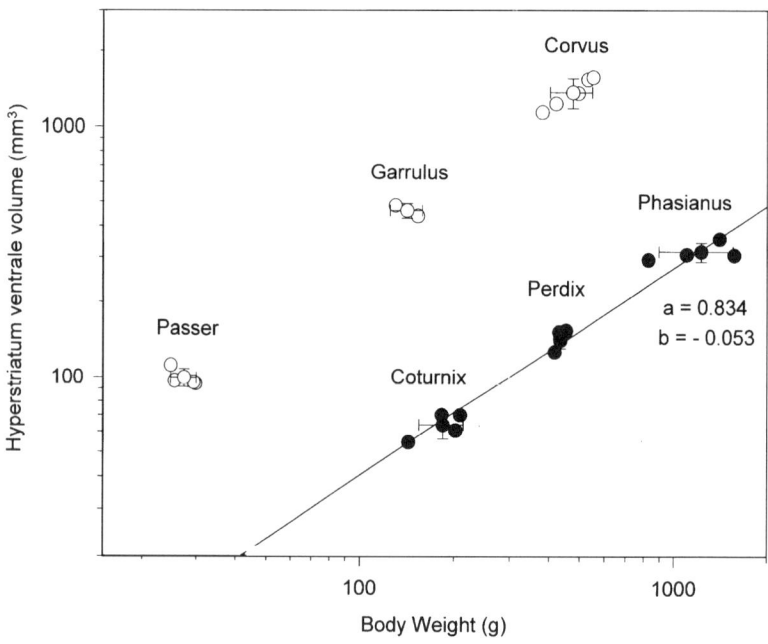

Figure 9.10. Volume of ventral hyperstriatum related to body weight in a double logarithmic system. Note that the volume of passeriform birds is much larger allometrically than in galliform birds.

1992). It is important to note that many of the tests applied to the pigeons do not ask for species-specific abilities.

If small brains and telencephala as are seen in pigeons are able to perform such remarkable cognitive tasks, one might ask: "Of what are birds with large telencephala, e.g., songbirds and crows, capable?" Even though there are a paucity of data in this regard, we do not hesitate to hypothesize that these avian species should be grouped in a cognitive ability category close to or equal to that of primates. This is supported by investigations of Benjamini (1983) on ravens and Wilson et al. (1985) on jackdaws, jays, and rooks.

DOMESTICATED ANIMALS

Comparative neurobiology of many species in the wild has pointed out a remarkable variability in size and composition of the telencephalon. In fact, no other brain part seems to respond equally to selective pressures and adaptive necessities. This view is corroborated when the telencephalon is studied in domestic animals.

Domestication research is a special branch of evolutionary research, dealing with alterations below the species level under well-defined constraints. It has been shown that the telencephalon is particularly affected by the general phenomenon of brain size reduction that characterizes the domestication process (Herre and Röhrs, 1990; Kruska, 1988). The greater the size of telencephalon of the wild form, the greater is the decrease in the domesticated form (Herre and Röhrs, 1990). Again, it is obvious that different parts of the telencephalon change their size differently under domestication.

The slope of the allometric axis describing the intraspecific relationship of brain weight and body weight is low in domestic animals, in contrast with the result of a cross-species comparison. Thus, body weight should have a lesser effect. This allows one to compare the percentage contribution of single brain parts directly within breeds of one species. In domesticated mammals we have data on olfactory cortices and the hippocampal complex. We also have many data on the isocortex as a whole.

Data on isocortical subdivisions, however, are rare. In domesticated mammals the striate area is smaller than in wild forms: 11.3% in rats, 39.9% in pigs (Herre and Röhrs, 1990), and 30.2% in sheep (Ebinger, 1975b). Plogmann and Kruska (1990) delineated the auditory cortex of domestic pigs for comparison with that in wild boars. A reduction of 32% was calculated. A single paper reported a reduction of the motor cortex in domesticated as compared with the wild sheep (Ebinger, 1975a). There are no comparable data on mammalian somatosensory areas or on isocortical areas that serve multimodal integration (i.e., those with a presumed relevance for cognition).

Because of Ebinger's work on domesticated birds (pigeons, ducks, geese, and turkeys), we have a solid database to demonstrate that at least sensory systems and their telencephalic representation areas undergo a disproportionate decrease in size (Fig. 9.11) (for review, see Ebinger, 1996). This is true for the visual ectostriatum in turkeys (25%; Ebinger and Röhrs, 1995) or the somatosensory basal nucleus in geese and mallards (7% in geese, Ebinger and Löhmer, 1987; 24% in mallards, Ebinger, 1995).

284   9   Evolutionary Constraints of Large Telencephala

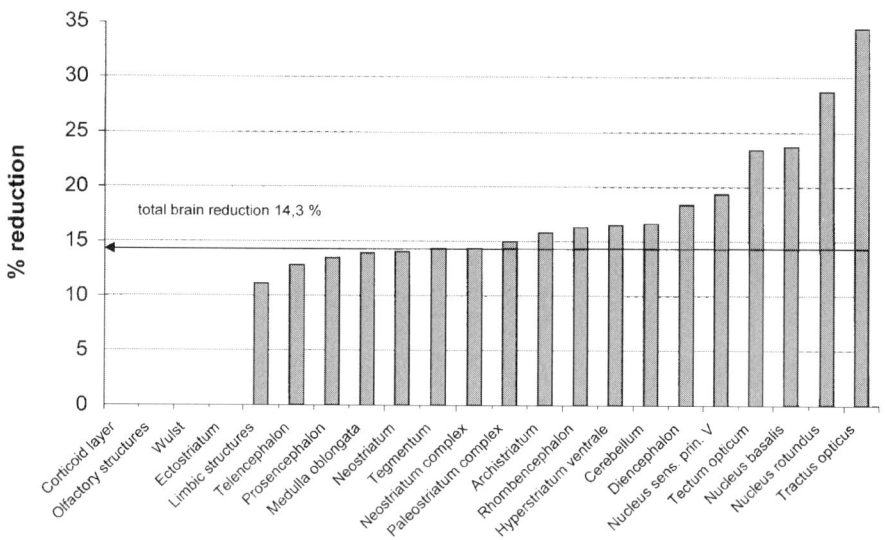

Figure 9.11. Diagram illustrating the percent reduction of brain subdivision volumes in domesticated mallard compared with the wild form. Arrow line indicates the percent decrease in total brain volume. (Modified from Ebinger, 1995.)

Measurements of multimodal integration centers (i.e., neostriatum and ventral hyperstriatum), demonstrate a reduction as well. There is evidence, however, that this depends on the breed studied. Interestingly, in homing pigeons, these areas do not seem to be reduced as much as in other breeds. The homing ability of homing pigeons is a multimodal cognitive phenomenon (Papi, 1991, 1995; Bingman et al., 1994, 1995). One would expect multimodal areas to be particularly large in homing pigeons. Our data on brain composition in this breed compared with nonhoming breeds show that neostriatum with its large multimodal integration centers contributes to a larger degree to the telencephalon in homing than in the nonhoming breeds.

Similar values have been calculated in chickens of the breed Japanese Chabos (Rehkämper et al., 1995). Here, too, a larger neostriatum is found compared with chickens of the breed Silky hens. For these chickens, behavioral data are not yet available, but the first Skinner-box experiments point to remarkable cognitive capacities of Chabos, including categorical or conceptual behavior.

Cognitive capacities of domestic animals deserve more attention. Generally, the brains of domesticated animals are smaller than those of the wild forms. This, however, does not necessarily mean that all brain parts undergo a reduction. Klatt (1921) has suggested that brain parts engaged in associative learning might be larger in domesticated species than in their wild ancestors. It is probable that domesticated animals need special cognitive abilities to live together with humans, because association with a different species may require different communication skills. This may well be the central point of the domestication problem. There are data that support this idea. Some breeds of dogs (e.g., poodles) that live closely with humans are unable to organize social systems among themselves. When a human is integrated, however, the situation changes, and an effective system is built up that includes the human (Feddersen-Petersen, 1994). This could be viewed as a problem of cognition, which has been solved by the domesticated animal through superior learning capacities. Thus, it might be that reduction of telencephalic size in the course of domestication is accompanied by progressive development of cognitive abilities. On the other hand, it could be that humans impose the organization, and the poodles no longer need their own abilities. Clearly, this idea needs to be further tested.

AGAIN: THEORIES OF BRAIN SIZE AND BRAIN COMPOSITION

We presented our data in a way that they support the adaptationist hypothesis. The reduction of the visual cortex in *Spalax* together with an enlargement of the somatosensory representation areas could be explained in this way. The data on domesticated animals also offer support for this hypothesis. Selection pressures that led to the current configurations for wild animals are largely unknown; those that selected domesticated animals are known. Thus, they can be seen as a sort of experiment to visualize brain plasticity and the selective pressures that can change brain shape. We now would like to come back to the initially presented hypotheses of brain size alteration and discuss them against the background of our own data and thoughts.

The arguments of Roth et al. (1994) that genome size can determine brain size and complexity independent of functional considerations and of Clayton and Krebs (1994) that experience plays a role in determining the size of brain parts cannot be discussed adequately within the framework of our approach, because we do not have appropriate data. Particularly, the impact of individual learning processes on the morphometry of the brain would be very interesting to investigate further. Homing pigeons, for example, would be a good model to test their hypotheses.

The variation seen in brain composition is not in agreement with the isometry hypothesis (all brain parts increase to the same degree) as formulated by Jerison (see above). This theory could not predict the reduction of visual cortex in *Spalax*, and it does not come to grips with what is seen in pigeon or chicken breeds. Previously, Fox and Wilczynski (1986) showed that somatic brain regions, which are necessary "to maintain vegetative, sensorimotor, and related behavior," for example, the spinal cord and the brain stem, scale by a different exponent of body weight than nonsomatic brain regions, for example, forebrain and cerebellum. Frequently, individual parts of the brain are found to scale against body weight with different slopes (Stephan et al., 1991; Rehkämper et al., 1991a). All these data do not support Jerison's chain of arguments. In addition, Holloway (1979) points out that it is not neural mass alone that is important, but the internal organization of the brain, which he calls "wiring." This would also be true for functional subparts of the brain as measured in Stephan's studies or in the present Chapter. Unfortunately, the wiring is much more difficult to study in living animals and impossible in fossils, which play an important role in Jerison's work.

Jerison (1985) seems to be aware of such problems, but he points out that focusing on the isocortex alone (i.e., on an isolated brain part), might underevaluate the olfactory-guided "intelligence," one type among many that he recognizes. These different types of intelligence, however, need to be defined more clearly. Otherwise, every activity of the nervous system would be, in a way, intelligent, and the term would lose any heuristic value.

The data of Armstrong (1985; see above) on brain size in prosimians, in comparison with monkeys, are difficult to understand in biological terms. To us, it seems unreasonable to assume that prosimians and monkeys are neurobiologically identical. The same can be said for passerine and nonpasserine birds, which have been compared by Armstrong and Bergeron (1985). In neither case is there any behavioral and psychological data to support that equality.

Deacon (1990; see above) proposed a displacement theory that seems to integrate some other concepts (e.g., Ebbesson's parcellation theory). It is assumed that competitive axonal interaction during ontogenesis leads to a loss of connections, or acquisition of additional connections, or replacement of one class of connections by another. As a consequence, morphometric alterations occur. Deacon's introduction to his theory (1990) included a demand for functional analysis. The living animal in its environment is not, however, a part of his theory. This is illustrated clearly when he argues, "Multiplication of cortical areas might be accounted for, not as augmentation of function, but as response to a growing size differential. This must certainly be a rich source for 'preadaptation'." (Deacon, 1990, p. 685).

For us, the crucial point in evolutionary biology is not only to ask how brains acquired their typical size and shape, but, even more important, to ask what an animal can do with such a brain to survive. This is where selection comes in. Problems of phylogeny, as discussed by Deacon (1990), are not in the center of interest of evolutionary neurobiology. It is illuminating when Gould (1975) states that interspecific comparison in neuromorphometry "is by far the worst to consult for information about evolutionary *mechanisms*. It represents the static scaling of contemporary adults within a group; it is not the result of ancestral–descendant sequences among the forms constituting it. It provides scaling criteria for the functional morphologist, but it does not represent the path traveled by an organism towards that adaptation" (p. 277). For us, evolutionary research in the post-Darwinian era is much closer to functional morphology than to phylogeny. This has to do with the actualistic strategy of Darwin (Rehkämper, 1997), as it must be. Functional morphology is observable in the present time, phylogeny only in the past.

Deacon and others criticized Stephan and collaborators for being trapped in *scala naturae* thinking. We regard that as a superficial interpretation. This argument seems to be made automatically whenever scaling is an obvious method of analysis. Scaling is, however, nothing more than a simple approach to sorting morphometric data in an objective and reproducible manner. It enables us to find species that deviate from some predicted values. Such species are "hot spots" that might be examined in greater detail. There is no hidden philosophy in such calculations, except the conviction that there is an underlying relationship in the various measurements of brain and body size. Hot spots are of interest for the evolutionary neurobiologist because they might indicate particularly strong selective pressures and stimulate fruitful research on the biology of an identified species.

The position of Deacon (1990) is not necessarily contradictory to the points of view of Finlay and Darlington (1995; see above) as far as the influence of ontogenesis is concerned. These authors argue that (1) the length of neurogenesis defines the size of the brain and that (2) in the end, the sizes of brain parts in different brains can be predicted if the size of the total brain is known. Whereas the condition of the adult brain may well be influenced by the mode of development, we can hardly imagine that this developmental factor is neutral to adaptation and selection. It should also be noted that their first assertion is true only if the "rate" of neurogenesis is constant across species.

Finlay and Darlington's second point (1995) is not immune from two methodological problems shared by many scaling studies. First, there is no doubt that their calculations are correct. One might ask, however, if it is biologically acceptable to calculate "mouse to elephant" curves. When the body weight range is large, it is expedient to use double logarithmic plots, making it look as if the data points (brain size, brain part size) are very near the line. This gives the impression that no differences (or at least only small differences) exist. Because in such calculations many species are represented by a limited number of individuals, there is an insufficient database to test differences statistically. This, however, is not a proof of uniformity. One example helps visualize this point. Finlay and Darlington (1995, their Fig.1) stress the point that there is a linearity in the relation of iso(neo)cortical size and brain size in insectivores, prosimians, simians, and bats. At first glance it looks as if the isocortex of the largest insectivore, *Solenodon*, is similar in size to that in the small simian *Cebuella*. Because in these two species brain size is nearly identical, they may be compared directly. The isocortex of *Solenodon* measures 661 mm^3 and that of *Cebuella* 2.535 mm^3. Thus, the *Cebuella* brain, which is similar in size to that of *Solenodon*, bears an isocortex approximately four times larger. We think this difference is biologically important.

Second, the slopes of subgroups might be significantly different from the overall slope. Harvey (1988) and Healy and Harvey (1990) have calculated such slopes for different groups that are defined as systematic entities or nutritional groups. They clearly demonstrated that such groups do have different slopes. Mann et al. (1988) have described the same phenomenon. Following the ideas of Rempe (1962), Rempe and Weber (1972), and Hofmann (1982), Rehkämper et al. (1991c) demonstrated a mathematical method for dealing with this problem. They compared brain and body sizes in hummingbirds and galliform birds. Hummingbirds are extremely small, whereas galliform birds may reach remarkable sizes. Shifting the data to a common origin and standardizing the variances allows one to calculate a slope that adequately describes brain size–body size relationships in both groups. This slope can be used for comparison after the data have been transferred back to the original position before variances were standardized.

CONCLUSIONS

Evolution is understood as functional adaptation. This concept has been used to deal with large telencephala found in some species of both mammals and birds. It emphasizes the necessity of considering the functional heterogeneity of the telencephalon in attempting to understand its size from a biological point of view.

Methodologically, an allometric approach that takes body weight into consideration is favored. This helps to identify the impact of the body on the brain and, thus, to differentiate brain evolution from independent evolution of body size as is seen sometimes.

In mammals, large telencephala may be associated either with voluminous olfactory cortices or with expanded hippocampi. Large isocortices are generally found in animals with large telencephala. Again, biologically relevant specializations such as large somatosensory systems or large motor systems have been evolved. Often, parts of the isocortex associated with cognitive functions have been enlarged disproportionately.

Variability in telencephalic size typical of mammalian brains is likewise found in avian brains, although birds have not been studied to the same extent. Many data support the hypothesis that, in the avian brain, the neostriatum and hyperstriatum complex plays the role of the mammalian isocortex. Within this complex, large areas have the infrastructure for cognitive capacities, and there is strong evidence that birds likewise exhibit a trend toward a volumetric increase in the size of structures that serve cognition. Among the birds, passeriform species occupy a leading position.

Thus, birds and mammals show a parallelism in evolutionary trends that leads to analogies (or homoplasies and convergences) in brain organization. In Darwinian terms of evolution, such analogies are probable. If one group has found a strategy that appears to be of biological advantage, it is likely that other groups will use this advantage as well. Examples are glossophagine bats and hummingbirds. Both groups make use of nectar, and the key to this biology is hovering flight. To this end, extrapyramidal motor areas such as cerebellum, nucleus ruber, and inferior olive are allometrically enlarged (Stiefken, 1993; Kinkel, 1994).

Domestication is evolution under man-made constraints. In this special case, cognitive abilities might play a crucial role. However, we are far from having satisfying data about either cognitive capacities or the brain structures associated with cognition.

ACKNOWLEDGMENTS

We thank Reinhold Necker (Bochum), Peter Ebinger (Hannover), and Christian Werner (Düsseldorf) for helpful discussions on earlier drafts of this Chapter. The skillful work of Christine Opfermann-Rüngeler (graphics and artwork) and Claudia Stolze (histology and photography) is kindly acknowledged.

REFERENCES

Armstrong, E. (1982) A look at relative brain size in mammals. *Neurosci. Lett.* 34:101–104.
Armstrong, E. (1983) Metabolism and relative brain size. *Science* 220:1302–1304.
Armstrong, E. (1985) Relative brain size in monkeys and prosimians. *Am. J. Phys. Anthropol.* 66:263–273.
Armstrong, E., and R. Bergeron, (1985) Relative brain size and metabolism in birds. *Brain Behav. Evol.* 26:141–153.
Ax, P. (1987) *The Phylogenetic System. The Systematization of Organisms on the Basis of Their Phylogenesis.* J. Wiley & Sons, New York.
Bang, B.G. and S. Cobb (1968) The size of the olfactory bulb in 108 species of birds. *Auk* 85:55–61.
Baron, G., H. Stephan, and H.D. Frahm, (1996) *Comparative neurobiology in chiroptera*, vols. 1–3. Birkhäuser, Basel.
Benjamini, L. (1983) Studies in the learning abilities of brown necked ravens and herring gulls. I. Oddity learning. *Behaviour* 84:173–194.
Bingman, V., G. Casini, C. Nocjar, and T.-J. Jones, (1994) Connections of the piriform cortex in homing pigeons (*Columba livia*) studied with fast blue and WGA-HRP. *Brain Behav. Evol.* 43:206–218.
Bingman, V.P., T.-J. Jones, R. Strasser, A. Gagliardo, and P. Ioalé (1995) Homing pigeons, hippocampus and spatial cognition. In E. Alleva, A. Fasolo, H.P. Lipp, L. Nadel, and L. Ricceri, (eds.): *Behavioural Brain Research in Naturalistic and Semi-Naturalistic Settings: Possibilities and Perspectives.* Kluwer, Dordrecht, pp. 207–224.
Boire, D., and G. Baron, (1994) Allometric comparison of brain and main brain subdivisions in birds. *J. Brain Res.* 35:49–66.
Bowler, P. (1996) *Life's Splendid Drama.* University of Chicago Press, Chicago.
Brodmann, K. (1909) *Vergleichende Lokalisationslehre der Großhirnrinde.* Ambrosius Barth, Leipzig.
Bronchti, G., N. Schönenberger, E. Welker, and H. van der Loos, (1992) Barrel field expansion after neonatal eye removal in mice. *Neuroreport* 3:489–492.
Chapin, J.K., and C.S. Lin, (1984) Mapping the body representation in the SI cortex of unanesthetized and awake rats. *J. Comp. Neurol.* 229:199–231.
Clayton, N., and J. Krebs, (1994) Hippocampal growth and attrition in birds affected by experience. *Proc. Natl. Acad. Sci. U.S.A.* 91:7410–7414.
Darwin, C. (1859) *On the Origin of Species by Means of Natural Selection.* Murray, London.
Deacon, T. (1990) Rethinking mammalian brain evolution. *Am. Zool.* 30:629–705.
Delius, J.D. (1992) Comparative cognition of identity. In P. Bertelson, P. Eelen, and G. d'Ydewalle, (eds.): *International Perspectives on Psychological Science, vol., Leading Themes.* Lawrence Erlbaum, Hillsdale, NJ, pp. 25–40.
Dubois, E. (1897) Über die Abhängigkeit des Hirngewichts von der Körpermasse bei den Säugethieren. *Arch. Anthropol.* 25:1–28.
Ebbesson, S.O.E. (1980a) The parcellation theory and its relation to interspecific variability in brain organization, evolutionary and ontogenetic development and neuronal plasticity. *Cell Tissue Res.* 213:179–212.
Ebbesson, S.O.E. (ed.) (1980b) *Comparative Neurology of the Telencephalon.* Plenum, New York.
Ebinger, P. (1974) A cytoarchitectonic volumetric comparison of brains in wild and domestic sheep. *Z. Anat. Entwickl. Gesch.* 144:267–302.
Ebinger, P. (1975a) A cytoarchitectonic volumetric comparison of the area gigantopyramidalis in wild and domestic sheep. *Anat. Embryol.* 147:167–175.
Ebinger, P. (1975b) Quantitative investigations of visual brain structures in wild and domestic sheep. *Anat. Embryol.* 146:313–323.
Ebinger, P. (1995) Domestication and plasticity of brain organization in mallards *(Anas platyrhynchos). Brain Behav. Evol.* 45:286–300.
Ebinger, P. (1996) Domestikationsbedingte Änderungen von Hirn und Verhalten beim Hausgeflügel. In G. Rehkämper, and H. Greven, (eds.): *Beiträge zur Biologie der Haus- und Nutztiere. Acta biol. benrodis*, Suppl. 3, Verlag Natur & Wissenschaft, Solingen pp. 37–52
Ebinger, P., and R. Löhmer, (1987) A volumetric comparison of brains between greylag geese (*Anser anser* L.) and domestic geese. *J. Hirnforsch.* 28:291–299.
Ebinger, P., G. Rehkämper, and H. Schröder, (1992) Forebrain specialisation and the olfactory system in anseriform birds. *Cell Tissue Res.* 268:81–90.

9 Evolutionary Constraints of Large Telencephala

Ebinger, P., and M. Röhrs, (1995) Volumetric analysis of brain structures, especially of the visual system in wild and domestic turkeys (*Meleagris gallopavo*). *J. Brain Res.* 36:219–228.

Eldredge, N., and J. Cracraft, (1980) *Phylogenetic Patterns and the Evolutionary Process.* Columbia University Press, New York.

Feddersen-Petersen, D. (1994) Ethologische Untersuchungen zu Fragen des Normalverhaltens, zur Ermittlung sozialer Umweltansprüche und zur Präzisierung des Begriffes der "tiergerechten Haltung" von Haushunden. *Kleintierpraxis* 39:669–684.

Finlay, B.L., and R.B. Darlington, (1995) Linked regularities in the development and evolution of mammalian brains. *Science* 268:1578–1584.

Fox, J.H., and W. Wilczynski, (1986) Allometry of major CNS divisions: towards a reevaluation of somatic brain–body scaling. *Brain Behav. Evol.* 28:157–169.

Frahm, H.D., G. Rehkämper, and E. Nevo, (1997) Brain structure volumes in the mole rat, *Spalax ehrenbergi* (Spalacidae, Rodentia) in comparison to the rat and subterrestrial insectivores. *J. Brain Res.* 38:209–222.

Gahr, M. (1997) How should brain nuclei be delineated? Consequences for developmental mechanisms and for correlations of area size, neuron numbers and functions of brain nuclei. *TINS* 20:58–62.

Gould, St. J. (1975) Allometry in primates, with emphasis on scaling and the evolution of the brain. In F. S. Szalay (ed.): *Approaches to Primate Paleobiology.* Karger, Basel, pp. 244–292.

Güntürkün, O. (1997) Cognitive impairments after lesions of the neostriatum caudolaterale and its thalamic afferents in pigeons: functional similarities to the mammalian prefrontal system? *J. Brain Res.* 38:133–143.

Harvey, P. (1988) Allometric analysis and brain size. In H.J., Jerison and I. Jerison (eds.): *Intelligence and Evolutionary Biology.* NATO ASI Series G 17. Springer, Berlin, pp. 199–210.

Harvey, P., and J.R. Krebs (1990) Comparing brains. *Science* 249:140–146.

Healy, S. D., and P. Harvey (1990) Comparative studies of the brain and its components. *Neth. J. Zool.* 40:203–214.

Hennig, W. (1966) *Phylogenetic Systematics.* University of Illinois Press, Urbana.

Herre, W., and M. Röhrs (1990) *Haustiere—zoologisch gesehen. 2. Auflage.* Fischer, Stuttgart.

Hofman, M.A. (1982) Encephalization in mammals in relation to the size of the cerebral cortex. *Brain Behav. Evol.* 20:84–96.

Holloway, R.L. (1979) Brain size, allometry, and reorganization: towards a synthesis. In M.E. Hahn, et al. (eds.): *Development and Evolution of Brain Size: Behavioral Implications.* Academic Press, New York, pp. 59–88.

Jacobs, L.F., and W.D. Spencer, (1994) Natural space-use patterns and hippocampal size in kangaroo rats. *Brain Behav. Evol.* 44,125–132.

Jerison, H.J. (1955) Brain to body ratios and the evolution of intelligence. *Science* 121:447–449.

Jerison, H.J. (1973) *Evolution of the Brain and Intelligence.* Academic Press, New York.

Jerison, H.J. (1977) The theory of encephalization. *Ann. N.Y. Acad. Sci.* 299:146–160.

Jerison, H.J. (1985) Animal intelligence as encephalization. *Philos. Trans. R. Soc. Lond. Biol.* 308:21–35.

Jerison, H.J. (1994) Evolution of the brain. In D.W. Zaidel, (ed.): *Neuropsychology, Handbook of Perception and Cognition.* Academic Press, San Diego, pp. 53–82.

Jolicoeur, P., and A.A. Heusner, (1971) The allometry equation in the analysis of the standard oxygen consumption and body weight of the white rat. *Biometrics* 27:841–855.

Kaas, J.H. (1991) Plasticity of sensory and motor maps in adult mammals. *Annu. Rev. Neurosci.* 14:137–167.

Källén, B. (1951) Embryological studies on the nuclei and their homologization in the vertebrate forebrain. *Kgl. fysiogr. Sällsk. Lund Handl. N.F.* 62, 5:1–36.

Källén, B. (1962) II. Embryogenesis of brain nuclei in the chick telencephalon. *Erg. Anat. Entwickl.* 36:62–82.

Karten, H.J. (1965) Projections of the optic tectum of the pigeon (*Columba livia*). *Anat. Rec.* 151:369.

Karten, H.J. (1968) The ascending auditory pathway in the pigeon (*Columba livia*). II. Telencephalic projections of the nucleus ovoidalis thalami. *Brain Res.* 11:134–153.

Karten, H.J. (1969) The organization of the avian telencephalon and some speculations on the phylogeny of the amniote telencephalon. *Ann. N.Y. Acad. Sci.* 167:164–179.

Karten, H.J. (1979): Visual lemniscal pathways in birds. In A.M. Granda, and J.H. Maxwell (eds.) *Neural Mechanism of Behavior in the Pigeon.* Academic Press, New York, pp. 409–430.

Karten, H.J. (1991) Homology and evolutionary origins of the neocortex. *Brain Behav. Evol.* 38:264–272.

Karten, H.J., and J.L. Dubbeldam, (1973) The organization and projections of the palaeostriatal complex in the pigeon *(Columba livia). J. Comp. Neurol.* 148:61–90.
Karten, H.J., and Hodos, W. (1970) Telencephalic projections of the nucleus rotundus in the pigeon *(Columba livia). J. Comp. Neurol.* 140:35–52.
Kinkel, H. (1994) *Vergleichend-allometrische Untersuchungen zur Volumenentfaltung von Kerngebieten im Hirnstamm von Hühnervögeln (Galliformes), Singvögeln (Passeriformes) und Kolibris (Trochilidae).* Dissertation, Med. Fakultät, Universität Köln.
Klatt, B. (1921) *Studien zum Domestikationsproblem. Untersuchungen am Hirn. Bibliotheca genetica,* Band II. Borntraeger, Leipzig.
Kleiber, M. (1961) *The Fire of Life.* Wiley, New York
Krebs, J., D.F. Sherry, S.D. Healy, V.H. Perry, and A.L. Vaccarino (1989) Hippocampal specialisation in food storing birds. *Proc. Natl. Acad. Sci. U.S.A.* 86:1388–1392.
Kruska, D. (1970) Über die Evolution des Gehirns in der Ordnung Artiodactyla Owen 1848, insbesondere der Teilordnung Suina Gray 1868. *Z. Säugetierkde* 35:214–238.
Kruska, D. (1973) Cerebralisation, Hirnevolution und domestikationsbedingte Hirngrößenänderungen innerhalb der Ordnung Perissodactyla Owen 1848, und ein Vergleich mit der Ordnung Artiodactyla Owen 1848. *Z. Zool. Syst. Evol. Forsch.* 11:81–103.
Kruska, D. (1988) Mammalian domestication and its effect on brain structure and behavior. In H.J. Jerison and I. Jerison (eds.): *Intelligence and evolutionary biology.* NATO ASI Series, Vol. G17. Springer, Berlin, pp. 211–250.
Kuhlenbeck, H. (1967–1978) *The Central Nervous System of Vertebrates,* 5 vols. Karger, Basel.
Künzle, H., and G. Rehkämper, (1992) Distribution of cortical neurons projecting to dorsal column nuclear complex and spinal cord in the hedgehog-tenrec, *Echinops telfairi. Somatosens. Motor Res.* 9: 185–197.
Le Gros Clark, W.E. (1932) The brain of the insectivora. *Proc. Zool. Soc. Lond.* 4:975–1013.
Lipp, H.P., H. Schwegler, W.E. Crusio, D.P. Wolfer, M.-C. Leisinger-Trigona, B. Heimrich, and P. Driscoll (1989) Using genetically-defined rodent strains for the identification of hippocampal traits relevant for two way avoidance behavior: a non invasive approach. *Experientia* 45:845–859.
Mann, M.D., S.E. Glickman, and A.L. Towe (1988) Brain/body relations among myomorph rodents. *Brain Behav. Evol.* 31:111–124.
Mann, M.D., G. Rehkämper, H. Reinke, H.D. Frahm, R. Necker, and E. Nevo, (1997) Size of somatosensory cortex and of somatosensory thalamic nuclei of the naturally blind mole rat, *Spalax ehrenbergi. J. Brain Res.* 38:47–59.
Martin, R.D. (1981) Relative brain size and basal metabolic rate in terrestrial vertebrates. *Nature (Lond.)* 293:57–60.
Martin, R.D. (1990) *Primate Origins and Evolution: A Phylogenetic Reconstruction.* Chapman and Hall, London.
Martin, R.D. (1995) Hirngröße und menschliche Evolution *Spektrum Wissenschaft September,* pp. 48–55.
Meador, D.M., D.M. Rumbaugh, J.L. Pate, and K.A. Bard (1987) Learning, problem solving, cognition, and intelligence. In G. Mitchell, and J. Erwin (eds.): *Behavior, Cognition, and Motivation. Comparative Primate Biology,* Vol. 2, Part B. Liss, New York, pp. 17–83.
Merzenich, M.M., R.J. Nelson, M.P. Stryker, M.S. Cynader, A. Schoppmann, and J.M. Zook (1984) Somatosensory cortical map changes following digit amputation in adult monkeys. *J. Comp. Neurol.* 224:591–605.
Nadel, L. (1991) The hippocampus and space revisited. *Hippocampus* 1:221–229.
Nauta, W.J.H., and H.J. Karten, (1970) A general profile of the vertebrate brain, with sidelights on the ancestry of cerebral cortex. In F.O. Schmitt, (ed.): *The Neurosciences.* Second Study Program, Rockefeller University Press, New York, pp. 7–26.
Necker, R., G. Rehkämper, and E. Nevo (1992) Cortical representation of the somatosensory system in the blind mole rat, *Spalax ehrenbergi:* an electrophysiological investigation. *Neuroreport* 3:505–508.
Nevo, E. (1991) Evolutionary theory and processes of active speciation and adaptive radiation in subterranean mole rats, *Spalax ehrenbergi* superspecies, in Israel. *Evol. Biol.* 25:1–125.
Nottebohm, F. (1981) A brain for all seasons: cyclical anatomical changes in sensory control nuclei of the canary brain. *Science* 214:1368–1370.

Oboussier, H. (1972) Evolution of the mammalian brain. Some evidence on the phylogeny of the antilope species. *Acta Anat.* 83:70–80.
Papi, F. (1991) Olfactory navigation. In P. Berthold (ed.): *Orientation in Birds.* Birkhäuser, Basel, pp. 52–85.
Papi, F. (1995) Recent experiments on pigeon navigation. In E. Alleva, A. Fasolo, H.P. Lipp, L. Nadel, and L. Ricceri, (eds.): *Behavioural Brain Research in Naturalistic and Semi-Naturalistic Settings: Possibilities and Perspectives.* Kluwer, Dordrecht, pp. 225–238.
Passingham, R.E., and G. Ettlinger, (1974) A comparison of cortical functions in man and the other primates. *Int. Rev. Neurobiol.* 16:233–299.
Paton, J.A., and F. Nottebohm (1984) Neurons generated in the adult brain are recruited into functional circuits. *Science* 225:1046–1048.
Plogmann, D., and D. Kruska, (1990) Volumetric comparison of auditory structures in the brains of european wild boars *(Sus scrofa)* and domestic pigs *(Sus scrofa f. dom.) Brain Behav. Evol.* 35:146–155.
Rehkämper, G. (1981) Vergleichende Architektonik des Neocortex der Insectivora. *Z. Zool. Syst. Evol. Forsch.* 19:233–263.
Rehkämper, G. (1997) Zur frühen Rezeption von Darwins Selektionstheorie und deren Folgen für die vergleichende Morphologie heute. *Sudhoffs Arch.* 81:171–192.
Rehkämper, G., H.D. Frahm, and M. Mann (1995) Brain composition and ecological niches in the wild or under man-made conditions (Domestication). In E. Alleva, et al. (eds.): *Behavioral Brain Research in Naturalistic and Seminaturalistic Settings: Possibilities and Perspectives.* Kluwer, Dordrecht, pp. 83–103.
Rehkämper, G., H.D. Frahm, and K. Zilles (1991a) Quantitative development of brain and brain structures in birds (Galliformes and Passeriformes) compared to that in mammals (Insectivores and Primates). *Brain, Behav. Evol.* 37:125–143.
Rehkämper, G., H.D. Frahm, K. Zilles, and E. Nevo (1991b) *Spalax*—Zentralnervöse Anpassungen eines blinden Tieres. Arbeitstagung Würzburg 1990. *Anat. Anz.* 172:67.
Rehkämper, G., E. Haase, and H.D. Frahm (1988) Allometric comparison of brain weight and brain structure volumes in different breeds of the domestic pigeon, *Columba livia f.d.* (Fantails, Homing pigeons, Strassers). *Brain Behav. Evol.* 31:141–149.
Rehkämper, G., K.-L. Schuchmann, A. Schleicher, and Zilles, K. (1991c) Enzephalisation in Humming birds (*Trochilidae*). *Brain Behav. Evol.* 37:85–91.
Rehkämper, G., H. Stephan, and W. Poduschka (1986) The brain of *Geogale aurita* Milne-Edwards and Grandidier 1872 (Tenrecidae, Insectivora). *J. Hirnforsch.* 27:391–399.
Rehkämper, G., and K. Zilles (1991) Parallel evolution in mammalian and avian brains: cytoarchitectonical and cytochemical analysis. *Cell Tissue Res.* 263:3–28.
Rehkämper, G., K. Zilles, and A. Schleicher (1984) A quantitative approach to cytoarchitectonics. IX. The areal pattern of the hyperstriatum ventrale in the domestic pigeon, *Columba livia f.d. Anat. Embryol.* 169:319–327.
Rehkämper, G., K. Zilles, and A. Schleicher (1985) A quantitative approach to cytoarchitectonics. X. The areal pattern of the neostriatum in the domestic pigeon, *Columba livia f.d. Anat. Embryol.* 171:345–355.
Rempe, U. (1962) Über einige statistische Hilfsmittel moderner zoologisch-systematischer Untersuchungen. *Zool. Anz.* 169:93–140.
Rempe, U., and E.E. Weber (1972) An illustration of the principal ideas of MANOVA. *Biometrics* 28:235–238.
Röhrs, M. (1985a) Cephalisation bei Feliden. *Z. Säugetierkde.* 50:234–240.
Röhrs, M. (1985b) Cephalization, neocorticalization and the effect of domestication on brains of mammals. In H.R. Duncker, and G. Fleischer (eds.): *Functional Morphology in Vertebrates.* Fischer, Stuttgart, pp. 545–547.
Röhrs, M. (1986a) Cephalisation, Telencephalisation und Neocorticalisation bei Mustelidae. *Z. Zool. Syst. Evol. Forsch.* 24:157–166.
Röhrs, M. (1986b) Cephalisation bei Caniden. *Z. Zool. Syst. Evol. Forsch.* 24:300–307.
Roland, P., and L. Friberg (1985) Localization of cortical areas activated by thinking. *J. Neuropsychol.* 53:1219–1243.
Roth, G., J. Blanke, and D.B. Wake (1994) Cell size predicts morphological complexity in the brains of frogs and salamanders. *Proc. Natl. Acad. Sci. U.S.A.* 91:4796–4800.

Ruse, M. (1986) *Taking Darwin Seriously.* Basil Blackwell, Oxford.
Ruse, M. (1997) *Monad to Man. The Concept of Progress in Evolutionary Biology.* Harvard University Press, Cambridge, MA.
Sauer, E.G.F. (1973) Zum Sozialverhalten der kurzohrigen Elefantenspitzmaus, *Macroscelides proboscideus. Z. Säugetierkde* 38:67–97.
Schwegler, H., H.-P. Lipp, H. Van der Loos, and W. Buselmaier (1981) Individual hippocampal mossy fiber distribution in mice correlates with two way avoidance performance. *Science* 214:817–819.
Sherry, D.F., L.F. Jacobs, and S.J.C. Gaulin (1992) Spatial memory and adaptive specialization of the hippocampus. *TINS* 15:298–303.
Shettleworth, S.J. (1990) Spatial memory in food-storing birds. *Philos. Trans. R. Soc. Lond. Biol.* 329:143–151.
Snell, O. (1892) Die Abhängigkeit des Hirngewichts von dem Körpergewicht und den geistigen Fähigkeiten. *Arch. Psychiat. Nervenkrankh.* 23:436–446.
Stephan, H. (1960) Methodische Studien über den quantitativen Vergleich architektonischer Struktureinheiten des Gehirns. *Z. Wiss. Zool.* 164:143–172.
Stephan, H. (1975) Allocortex. In W. Bargmann (ed.): *Handbuch der mikroskopischen Anatomie des Menschen.* Band IV, Teil 9. Springer, Berlines.
Stephan, H., G. Baron, and H.D. Frahm (1988) Comparative size of brains and brain components. In H.D. Steklis, and J. Erwin (eds.): *Comparative primate biology, vol. 4. Neurosciences.* Liss, New York, pp. 1–38.
Stephan, H., G. Baron, and H.D. Frahm (1991) *Comparative Brain Research in Mammals, vol.1, Insectivora* Springer, New York
Stephan, H., G. Baron, H.D. Frahm, and M. Stephan (1986) Größenvergleiche an Gehirnen und Hirnstrukturen von Säugern. *Z. mikrosc. Anat. Forsch. Leipzig* 100:189–212.
Stephan, H., H.D. Frahm, and G. Baron (1981) New and revised data on volumes of brain structures in insectivores and primates. *Folia Primatol.* 35:1–29.
Stewart, M., S.P.R. Rose, T.S. King, P.L.A. Gabbott, and R. Bourne (1984) Hemispheric asymmetry of synapses in chick medial hyperstriatum ventrale following passive avoidance training: a stereological investigation. *Dev. Brain Res.* 12:261–269.
Stiefken, V. (1993) *Vergleichende Untersuchungen zur Größe von motorischen Zentren in Cerebellum und Hirnstamm der Fledermäuse.* Dissertation, Med. Fakultät, Universität Köln.
Strube, G. (1996) Kognition. In G. Strube, B. Becker, C. Frecksa, U. Hahn, K. Opwis, and G. Palm (eds.): *Wörterbuch der Kognitionswissenschaft.* Stuttgart, Klett-Cotta, pp. 303–317.
Towe, A.L., and M.D. Mann (1995) Habitat-related variations in brain and body size in pocket gophers. *J. Brain Res.* 36:195–201.
Ulinski, P.S. (1983) Dorsal ventricular ridge: a treatise on forebrain organization in reptiles and birds. In R.G. Northcutt (ed.): *Wiley Series in Neurobiology.* John Wiley and Son, New York, pp. 1–265.
Valverde, F., and L. Lopez-Mascaraque (1981) Neocortical endeavor: basic neuronal organization in the cortex of the hedgehog. 11th Int. Cong. Anat. In *Glial and Neuronal Cell Biology.* Liss, New York, pp. 281–290.
Veenman, C.L., J.M. Wild, and A. Reiner (1995) Organization of the avian "cortico-striatal" projection system: a retrograde and anterograde pathway tracing study in pigeons. *J. Comp. Neurol.* 354:87–126.
Wallenberg, A. (1898) Eine Verbindung caudaler Hirnteile der Taube mit dem Striatum. *Neurol. Zentralbl.* 17:300–302.
Wallenberg, A. (1903) Der Ursprung des Tractus isthmo-striaticus oder bulbo-striaticus der Taube. *Neurol. Zentralbl.* 22:98–101.
Wilson, B., N.J. Mackintosh, and R.A. Boakes (1985) Transfer of relational rules in matching and oddity learning by pigeons and corvids. *Q. J. Exp. Psychol.* 37B:313–332.
Zeier, H., and H.J. Karten (1971) The archistriatum of the pigeon: organization of afferent and efferent connections. *Brain Res.* 31:313–326.
Zilles, K., and G. Rehkämper (1988) The brain of the Orang-utan, *Pongo satyrus*, with special reference to its telencephalon. In J. Schwartz (ed.): *Biology of the Orang-Utan.* Oxford University Press, New York, pp. 157–176.

PART II

Cognition: From Neural Basis to Behaviour

Chapter 10

BRAIN AND COGNITIVE FUNCTION IN TELEOST FISHES

Leo S. Demski and Joel A. Beaver, Division of Natural Sciences and Pritzker Marine Biology Laboratory, New College of the University of South Florida

INTRODUCTION

Studies concerning neural correlates of cognitive behaviors, particularly learning, memory, spatial orientation, and communication, have primarily used mammalian and avian subjects (see papers in Kesner and Olton, 1990; and most other contributions to this volume) and as such represent information on only two of the seven major vertebrate classes. This is understandable considering the great brain differentiation and complex behavior attributed to the two groups. Of the remaining vertebrates, the bony fishes present special opportunities because they are the dominant vertebrate radiation with a great diversity of brain and behavioral complexity. Indeed, bony fishes have also attracted considerable interest as models for behavioral analysis (Tinbergen, 1951; Lorenz, 1963; Heiligenberg, 1975; Barlow, 1993) as well as for understanding the function and evolution of neurobehavioral systems (Ingle, 1968; Aronson, 1970; Bullock, 1983; Davis and Northcutt, 1983; Northcutt and Davis, 1983a; papers in Atema et al., 1988; Wullimann, 1998; for a discussion of systems in the cartilaginous fishes, see Demski and Northcutt, 1996).

Analysis of neural substrates of spatial representation has perhaps been the most fruitful area of the study of neural correlates of cognition in mammals and birds. Several useful models of hippocampal involvement in spatial representation have emerged to explain results in both laboratory tests and natural behavior (e.g., food storage memory in song birds). Fishes are an exemplary group of vertebrates with behaviors readily amenable to such studies (Braithwaite, 1998). Thus, similar investigations in fishes could yield useful comparisons with tetrapod groups and thereby provide a more comprehensive database for understanding neural/behavioral mechanisms for spatial analysis and representation. To this end, we emphasize spatial mapping in the following discussion.

In this chapter, we review and synthesize the available information on bony fish cognitive behavior and brain systems thought to subserve the functions. Hopefully, this information will be useful in providing starting points for future research. The first section reviews examples of presumed cognitive functions involved in teleost behavior both in the laboratory and under natural conditions. The next three sections each represent a different approach to identifying potential neural substrates for teleost cognition: analysis of the effects of brain lesions on cognitive functions; identification of correlations among brain development, behavioral capacity, and sensory ecology; and elucidation of neural pathways and mechanisms in species with hypertrophy of brain areas likely to be involved in navigation and orientation in spatially complex environments.

STUDIES ON COGNITION IN FISHES

Formal analysis of cognitive function has only recently been applied to fishes and specifically to only a few members of the largest and most diverse group, the modern bony fishes or teleosts (approximately 24,000 species) (Grande, 1995). Many laboratory studies have indicated that some fishes possess the ability to learn in situations ranging from habituation to complex instrumental conditioning, including reversal learning and use of secondary reinforcers (see reviews by MacPhail, 1982; Overmier and Hollis, 1990). The studies have to some extent been considered in a framework of animal cognitive theory (e.g., constructs for working memory components have been postulated). Several authors have demonstrated that the methods of cognitive ethology can be used to provide new insights into aspects of fish behavior such as partner choice, foraging patterns, and space utilization (for reviews of general features of cognitive ethology, see Wyers, 1985; Dugatkin and Wilson, 1993; Beckoff, 1996).

More information is available on the cognitive aspects of orientation and navigation in the three-dimensional space characteristic of most aquatic environments. Considerable observational and experimental data suggest that many teleost species retain a detailed working knowledge of their immediate surroundings and, in some cases, much wider areas such as foraging sites across large areas of coral reefs (Helfman et al., 1982; Dodson, 1988: Wilson and Wilson, 1992; Burke, 1995; Braithwaite, 1998). Even exploration in an open aquarium by goldfish is spatially organized (Kleerkoper el al., 1974). Of particular note is the seminal work by Aronson (1951, 1971) on the orientation in the gobiid fish *Bathygobius soporator*. The fish will jump from tide pool to tide pool when prodded. They are usually successful at landing in a safe (i.e., wet) area even though they cannot see the target zone. Using artificial tide pools that permitted manipulation of zones and landmarks, Aronson demonstrated that the gobies swim over the area of the flooded pools at the artificial "high tide" and form spatial maps based on various landmarks. They use the maps to later orient jumps to adjacent pools at "low tide" when the landmarks are not in view. Similarly, Markel (1994) reported that spatial learning and memory were used by blackeye gobies (*Coryphopterus nicholsi*) in escaping to their burrows in response to prodding by the investigator.

Experimental studies on goldfish have demonstrated that visual landmarks and size constancy are used in food acquisition (Pitcher and Magurran, 1983; Douglas et al., 1988; Warburton, 1990; Braithwaite et al., 1996; Douglas, 1996) and that they are capable of solving spatial tasks using allocentric frames of reference that seemingly require development of complex spatial representations of their immediate surroundings (Rodriguez et al., 1994). Probable use of spatial memory has also been reported for the behavior of Siamese fighting fish (*Betta splendens*) tested in a radial arm maze (Roitblat et al., 1982) and the feeding activities of coral reef damselfishes (Noda et al., 1994) and butterflyfishes (Reese, 1989).

The above cited examples are mostly cases where vision plays an important, and probably dominant, role in spatial mapping. Spatial mapping based primarily on other senses has been described for certain fishes that occupy dimly lighted environments. African elephantnose fish (*Gnathonemus petersii*) can detect objects in their environment by sensing disturbances in weak electric fields produced by discharges from their electric organs. Using an apparatus in which fish were rewarded for finding an aperture in a partition, Cain (1995) demonstrated that the fish use electroreception to form a sensory image of their immediate environment. This information is coupled with hydrostatic sensing (probably via pressure receptors located at the prootic bulla and swim bladder) to give a depth profile to the image. Later the fish locate the aperture without electric organ discharge, indicating that they can integrate information from other senses into a cognitive map based essentially, or at least initially, on electrosensory information.

Blind cave fish (*Anoptichtys jordani*, now recognized as a blind form of *Astyanax mexicanus*; see further below) are able to establish an internal representation of their environment using the lateral-line sense. The fish swim over and thereby explore their immediate surroundings at a speed that maximally stimulates the lateral-line organ (Teyke, 1989). During this time, a spatial representation of the environment is developed. Afterwards, the fish move within the area at speeds that are suboptimal for such stimulation. Thus, they are probably using other cues in concert with the environmental map to navigate successfully in the cave area. Once again, the map seems to be used in guiding behavior via feedback from senses other than those primarily used for map development.

Examples of spatial maps with other senses are not available; however, ictalurid catfish experimentally deprived of vision and olfaction can locate food with their hypertrophied taste system (Bardach et al., 1967; Atema, 1971), and it is likely they might utilize gustation to at least augment mapping images based earlier on other senses. The finding of a gustatory projection to the central and dorsomedial areas of the telencephalon in this group (Kanwal et al., 1988; Lamb and Caprio, 1993) supports the idea. Recent observations of descending projections from those telencephalic areas to the inferior lobe and torus lateralis, structures with connections to gustatory nuclei, in the goldfish (Rink and Wullimann, 1998), and of afferents from the preglomerular tertiary gustatory nucleus to the dorsomedial region of the telencephalon and efferents from the later to the inferior lobe in the distantly related cichlid *Oreochromis (Tilapia) niloticus* (Yoshimoto et al., 1998) suggest that gustatory mapping in the telencephalon and diencephalon may be fairly universal among euteleosts. Tavolga (1971) has postulated that the sea catfish (*Arius felis*) may locate objects and navigate using reflected sounds produced by swim bladder contractions. If substantiated, the observations suggest the possibility of an acoustically based spatial map.

These studies on nonlesioned fish suggest that various sensory systems are used by teleosts to create long-lasting neural representations of environmental maps. The currently available neuroanatomical evidence indicates that all sensory systems are represented in the telencephalon and, perhaps with the exception of chemoreception, in the cerebellum and tectum as well (Wullimann, 1998). Thus, reports of the effects of lesions in these structures will be considered next.

BRAIN LESIONS AND COGNITIVE BEHAVIOR IN FISHES

Telencephalon: Nonspatial Learning

There have been numerous studies in teleosts concerning the effects of bilateral telencephalic hemisphere removal on nonspatial learning ranging from habituation, classical conditioning, and appetitive instrumental conditioning to active and passive avoidance (Kaplan and Aronson, 1967, 1969; Savage, 1980; Overmier and Hollis, 1983; 1990; Ohnishi, 1997). The vast majority of these experiments have used goldfish as subjects. Exceptions are studies by Kaplan and Aronson (1967, 1969) on cichlids and by Warren (1961) and Davis and Kassel (1983) on paradise fish. Goldfish do not have the largest and most differentiated telencephalon among teleosts, and, for this reason, caution must be exercised in generalizing these findings to fishes with large telencephala such as various coral-reef teleosts (see further below). To summarize, Overmeir and Hollis (1983, 1990) indicate the following as results of bilateral telencephalic ablation in fishes.

Effects not directly related to learning: (1) loss of olfaction (as expected); (2) reduction in response variability; (3) decrease in spontaneous locomotion; (4) decrease in general activity levels in nonschooling fishes; and (5) increase in general activity levels in schooling fishes

Habituation: some impairment of long-term or short-term habituation, depending on tests

Pavlovian conditioning: no substantial effects over a wide range of parameters, including higher order conditioning

Instrumental conditioning: no deleterious effect when reward is delivered promptly on completion of response

Choice-dependent learning: is impaired when the learned response and reward are separated either spatially or temporally (see Ohnishi, 1997)

Avoidance learning: avoidance responding is not blocked but responses are unstable, slow to develop, and extinguish rapidly—deficits occur both in the learning process and retention of the response

Long-term memory of learned entities before ablation: no effect in instrumental responding when fish are preoperatively trained and tested 8 days after the ablation

Reversal learning: marked impairment is observed with telencephalic lesions

The losses of function have been interpreted as resulting from the disruption of telencephalic systems that mediate responses to secondary reinforcements (Overmier and Hollis, 1983, 1990) or that involve short-term memory consolidation in extra-telencephalic areas (Ohnishi, 1997). The results indicate that the teleostean telencephalon functions in several types of learning, probably through more than one neural process, and that the structure does so via interactions with more caudal brain centers, possibly the cerebellum (see below).

Telencephalon: Spatial Learning

Salas et al. (1996a,b) have carried out two studies that indicate that the telencephalon of goldfish is involved in place learning. They employed a test apparatus patterned after one used to demonstrate that goldfish could perform a test requiring space constancy (Ingle and Sahagian, 1973). Salas et al. (1996a) reported that telencephalic lesions disrupted performance in a choice paradigm based on space constancy, but not in a cue-directed choice. Similarly, in tests with a four-arm maze, telencephalic ablation led to problem-solving deficits when fish were forced to use a place-learning strategy but not when they could employ an egocentric turning strategy (Salas et al., 1996b). The results of both studies strongly suggest that the telencephalon is involved in the formation of cognitive maps with relational representation of aspects of the environment. Loss of the telencephalon leads to a shift to learning via discrimination of cues alone. The authors compare the findings to studies of hippocampal damage in mammals and birds but do not make direct comparisons of telencephalic structures between the goldfish and tetrapods because, as they point out, differences in development of the telencephalon (evagination in tetrapods, eversion in bony fishes; see Northcutt and Braford, 1980; Nieuwenhuys and Meek, 1990) have confused the issue of homology between the groups. Unfortunately, fish with more restricted lesions in the telencephalon have not been tested within this design. Thus, the experimental evidence clearly indicates that goldfish employ cognitive mapping in their behavior and that the telencephalon utilizes such in spatial learning.

Observations in salmon possibly also relate to telencephalic analysis of spatial information. Hofmann and Meyer (1993) report that visually evoked activity in the telencephalon changes noticeably during the metamorphic smolt transformation, in contrast to tectal activity, which remains at the presmolt level. This is a period in which fish prepare for their seaward migration and imprint to their natal freshwater streams. Although the imprinting is most likely based primarily on olfaction (Hasler and Scholz, 1983), a role for visual stimuli cannot be ruled out. Alternately, the enhanced visual function could relate to increased ability to orient and navigate with respect to objects in the stream and ocean environments or perhaps to sun direction.

To date, there is no experimental data on telencephalic involvement in spatial learning in species with the greatest development of the nonchemosensory processing areas of the telencephalon; such fishes include many coral reef fishes and the freshwater mormyrids. The former inhabit the spatially most complex environments where vision is clearly useful for orientation and navigation, whereas the latter "see" an elaborate electrical image of their season-dependent turbid surroundings. It seems likely that some of the telencephalic enhancements are involved in cognitive mapping and that lesion studies in these fishes would provide significant results. An anatomical analysis of some pathways likely involved in spatial orientation and navigation is being carried out presently in our laboratory with several coral reef species (see below).

Cerebellum

Several studies have implicated the teleost cerebellum in learning. Karamian (1956) reported that conditioned reflexes to either a light- or sound-conditioned stimulus (CS) disappeared and could not be reinstated in goldfish and carp in which the total cerebellum (the corpus or main part and valvula, a portion that extends into the midbrain ventricle below the tectum) had been ablated. This was in contradiction to the effects of telencephalon removal, where the conditioned responses were readily attainable. The effects of ablating the corpus alone were studied in two fish, one tested with light as the CS and the other with sound as the CS. In the former, positive responses did not occur until the test of the fourth day, and then no stable conditioned response developed even after a month of testing. With the latter, no conditioned responses occurred for the first 10 days of testing, but within 1 month a normal response had been established. The author states that the differences may be correlated to the observation that the corpus is more involved in visual function as opposed to the valvula, which receives a greater acoustic input (see further below). The author cites work by G.A. Malyukina (1954) on conditioned reflexes to a lateral-line–mediated CS. Extirpation of the telencephalon or optic tectum did not affect the rate of establishment or the stability of the responses, whereas total removal of the cerebellum prevented the development of responses or resulted in a loss of preoperative conditioning. The results suggest a role of the cerebellum in the establishment and retention of conditioned responses; however, caution must be applied to these conclusions because histological verification of the brain damage is not given.

Aronson and his co-workers (Aronson and Herberman 1960; Kaplan and Aronson, 1969; Aronson, personal communication) continued the study of telencephalic and cerebellum involvement in learning in fishes. They used cichlids (a member of the Perciformes, the most diversified order of fishes and indeed the largest order of vertebrates; see further below and Nelson, 1984) with fairly well-developed visual pathways and telencephalic hemispheres (see further below) in both operant and avoidance conditioning paradigms.

Removal of either the telencephalon or the corpus of the cerebellum (with complete histological documentation) in *Tilapia macrocephla* (now *Oreochromis*) did not result in loss of a food-rewarded operant response (hitting a target for a food pellet), but in both cases response latencies and variability were increased. The latencies for the fish with cerebellar lesions were somewhat greater than for those with telencephalic ablation.

Kaplan and Aronson (1969) studied the effects of telencephalon and corpus removal on light-conditioned avoidance responding. Their results indicated that cerebellar extirpation caused far more severe learning deficits than did telencephalon removal. Some cerebellar cases never learned to avoid even after the conditioned stimulus–unconditioned stimulus interval was increased fourfold. Some made intermittent avoidances, but none reached the criterion for stabilization of the avoidance response. Indeed, the subjects only responded to the CS in 80% of the tests. Qualitative observations indicated that cerebellar ablates did not use preparatory reactions such as waiting at the escape hole as did the sham-operated animals. The deficits were not caused by motor disturbances because, within 24 hours of surgery, minor disturbances of equilibrium disappeared and "the cerebellar-ablated subjects could not be distinguished from the sham-operated subjects on the basis of posture, locomotion, or feeding behavior."

Thus, it seems that the corpus and possibly valvula of the cerebellum are involved in the conditioning process, perhaps at a more fundamental level than the telencephalon. Although there is no direct information on the role of the cerebellum in spatial mapping, examples below indicate that some fishes with large telencephala and complex spatial behavior also have highly developed cerebella. The mormyrid elephantnose fish have an exceptionally well-developed corpus of four large lobes and an even larger valvula that covers most of the dorsal aspect of the remainder of the brain (Nieuwenhuys and Nicholson, 1969). The structure is thought to be involved in processing electrosensory information (see review by Meek, 1992). As pointed out in the first section, such information can be used to form spatial maps. Tangs and surgeonfishes (Acanthuridae) form large schools each morning which then proceed to graze over wide areas of coral reefs in organized movement patterns (Barlow, 1974a,b; Montgomery et al., 1989). These teleosts have a greatly enlarged corpus compared with other reef fishes with more restricted home ranges (Aronson, 1963; Demski, unpublished data). Thus, one can postulate that development of elaborate spatial mapping capabilities likely involves interrelated cerebellar and telencephalic neural machinery.

Tectum

Although there are considerable data on tectal anatomy and electrophysiology in a variety of teleosts (Meek, 1983; Vanegas, 1983; Vanegas and Ito, 1983), we found limited information on potential cognitive functions of the structure. Sanders (1940) carried out a study in goldfish in which lesions of the dorsal tectum or its presumed telencephalic connections interfered with retention of second-order olfactory learning with visual stimulation as a "reward"; however, confirmation of this work is lacking. It appears that most studies on brain mechanisms and learning have employed tasks probably incompatible with the possible "blindness" resulting from tectal lesions. Springer and co-workers (1977) describe the effects of tectal ablation on five visually mediated behaviors in goldfish, but the observed losses in function can be attributable to primary sensory deficits (see further below). Observations from a variety of sources provide indirect support for tectal involement in teleost spatial behavior.

The tectum has well-defined connections with both the dorsal telencephalon and cerebellum (see above). Its development is positively correlated with the differentiation of these structures, which have been implicated in teleost cognition (see above and details in following sections). In certain species, the tectum appears to integrate information from more than one modality (e.g., visual and electrosensory cues) to map the position of objects in the environment (Bastian, 1982; Meek, 1983). Repetitive tetanic electrical stimulation (1 to 5 Hz) of the optic nerve can produce long-term potentiation (LTP) of synaptic activity in the isolated goldfish tectum (Lewis and Teyler, 1986). The LTP could repesent mechanisms involved in spatial learning and memory.

Tectal stimulation in several teleosts has elicited coordinated eye movements and complex swimming, postural, and other behavior patterns in a variety of teleosts (Akert, 1949; Meyer et al., 1970; Demski, 1983; Vanegas, 1983; Al-Akel et al., 1986; Herrero et al., 1998). The results suggest that the tectum regulates organized movements that, in certain cases, may relate to stimulus-generated spatial maps. In this regard, Springer and co-workers (1977) report that tectal ablation in goldfish eliminates the normal optomotor swimming in response to rotating stripes in a rotating drum but not the optokinetic nystagmus or eye tracking movements associated with the moving stripes. The authors suggest that "the tectum serves a premotor function in addition to its sensory role." Observations (Fiebig et el., 1985) that eye movements have been evoked by stimulation of the telencephalon in piranhas (*Serrasalmus nattereri*) are consistent with the suggested importance of telencephalic-tectal-cerebellar interconnections in controlling spatially related behaviors (see further details below).

RELATIVE BRAIN SIZE AND DEVELOPMENT: IMPLICATIONS FOR COGNITIVE FUNCTION IN FISHES

A number of brain–body size studies have been carried out in bony fishes (see below), and some of these include measurements of specific regions. The following deals with such information in the broad context of relating morphological differences with probable differences in cognitive abilities and as such, possible neural substrates for sensory and sensorimotor processing involved in cognition in bony fishes. We comment only on the most recent studies in which standardized procedures have been employed. A similar discussion for the elasmobranch fishes (sharks, skates, rays) has recently been put forth and is not considered here (Demski and Northcutt, 1996).

Studies in Minnows (Cypriniformes)

The minnows are the most diverse group of freshwater teleosts, comprising approximately 2000 species with major radiations in North America and Eurasia (Banister,

1995). They live in water ranging from clear to highly turbid. Some have chin barbels with elaborate chemosensory capabilities. The group, along with catfishes, make up the majority of the Otophysi, fishes that have superior hearing in part because of a series of small bones that form the Weberian apparatus. The device conducts acoustic vibrations from the swim bladder to the inner ear much as the middle ear ossicles do in tetrapods (Lauder and Liem, 1983). Indeed, in Schellart's analysis (1992) of the relative development of vision, hearing, and lateral-line capabilities, the cyprinids have the highest hearing index and vary greatly within the lower to middle range in the vision index.

The results of studies on several European minnows (Kotrschal and Junger, 1988; Kotrschal and Palzenberger, 1992) indicate correlations between habitat, especially level of turbidity, and brain structure type. Species living in turbid waters are primarily bottom feeders that extract prey from the substrate; these forms have well-developed gustatory systems. Other aquatic environments include a greater number of feeding generalists, hunters, as well as planktivores, with better visual systems at the expense of the chemosensory systems. Generalists and other vision-orientated fishes tend to have better developed octavolateralis systems. It is notable that higher "integrative" centers show little association with any particular morphotype in all these studies. It is apparent from the data, however, that the gustatory specialists that have the largest vagal lobes do not exhibit enhancement of the telencephalon or the corpus of the cerebellum. In contrast, associations of vision and acousticolateralis systems seem to be associated with increases in these two central nervous system structures.

Cambray (1994) studied brain diversity in two sister species of South African minnows. *Pseudobarbus afer* lives in a clear perennial mountain stream while *Pseudobarbus asper* is found in a turbid intermittent river. *Pseudobarbus afer* has a significantly larger eye, telencephalon, optic tectum, and corpus of the cerebellum. The facial and vagal lobes did not differ between the species. The author suggests that selection for visual function in a clear environment has resulted in the differences between the brains of the two species. Thus, the coordinated development of the telencephalon, optic tectum, and cerebellum appears linked to selection for mechanisms of cognitive mapping in the visually richer environment.

Huber and Rylander (1991) compared tectal differentiation—as measured by the thickness of its individual layers—and growth measures of telencephalon and cerebellum in related species of two genera of minnows (*Notropis* and *Cyprinella*) living in turbid versus clear water. As predicted, they found that the thickness of tectal layers as well as the overall tectum was greater in the latter. Of particular interest to cognitive functions were the incidental findings that enlargement of the cerebellum was positively correlated with the thickness of one of the most complex tectal layers, the stratum fibrosum et griseum superficiale, and that increased growth of the telencephalon was positively correlated with that of the corpus of the cerebellum. The results are consistent with the above suggestion that the telencephalon and cerebellum are both integration centers for higher complex behavior often of a visual orientation.

Blind and Sighted Characins

Peters and co-workers (1993) measured brain area sizes in a characin species, *Astyanax mexicanus*, in which some subtypes live in or near caves while others retain the ancestral condition of living in well-lighted rivers. The authors demonstrated that the optic lobes were greatly reduced in the cave types with nonfunctional eyes and the longest history as a troglobiont form compared with the surface types and two of the other cave dwelling forms with somewhat reduced but functional eyes and a more recent history of surface living. This was expected; however, the telencephalon was significantly larger (estimated about 40% by volume) in the former than the others. The cerebellum was approximately the same size in all four subtypes studied. The results indicate that development of the sensory capacities other than vision in the extremely specialized cave species may be responsible for the telencephalic enhancement. This recalls the results of Telye (1989; see above), who found that cave fishes use the lateral-line system to form a spatial map of their surroundings. Perhaps loss of vision resulted in an increased capacity for such a mapping function and this function required an enhanced telencephalon. With vision intact, the mapping may have been more associated with the tectum.

The Cichlids of the African Great Lakes

The cichlid fishes (Cichlidae) are percomorph teleosts with many derived characteristics, including an enlarged pretectum and other distinct features indicating dominance of vision among senses (Fernald and Shelton, 1985; Presson et al., 1985; Wullimann and Meyer, 1990; Wullimann and Roth, 1992). Cichlids are widely distributed in most fresh waters in South and Central America and Africa. The greatest cichlid radiation is in the Great Lakes of Africa, where each lake supports a unique assemblage of several hundred distinct species exhibiting great behavioral and morphological diversity. Staaden and co-workers (1994/1995) provide a principle factor analysis of data on whole brain measurements of 189 species from the Great Lakes yielding correlations of relative brain area development with behavioral and morphological specialties. They measured seven brain size parameters and used several statistical procedures to identify correlated factors that account for variation in the data set. The most significant correlation was that between telencephalon measurements and those of the cerebellum and the optic tectum. The telencephalon size was less strongly positively correlated with that of the hypothalamus. Cerebellum and optic tectum measurements were also very strongly positively correlated. For these cichlids, the most significant principle component (accounting for 31% of the variation) concerned differences in telencephalon size; "indicating that evolutionary changes in brain morphology of cichlids in the East African lakes relate primarily to the development of this complex association center" (Staaden et al., 1994/1995). The other components concerned development of special sensory modalities, with differences in structures involved in lateral-line mechanoreception accounting for 13.8% of the variation, olfactory-related structures 9.9%, and visual structures 6.2%.

The overall greater variation in telencephalic structures suggests that they relate to increases in complexity of sensory and behavioral systems in one or more modality. The positive correlation between the telencephalic and tectal development suggests that vision may have a more profound effect on the telencephalic enlargement than either the lateral-line or olfactory senses. It is noteworthy that the corpus of the cerebellum development was also strongly correlated with that of the tectum and telencephalon. The findings support the previous suggestion (see above) that, at least in percomorphs, telencephalic-tectal-cerebellar neural associations form functional units that have been selected for specific behavioral capabilities most likely involving cognitive functions.

Coral Reef Percomorphs

As mentioned above, many coral reef percomorphs have elaborate behavior, including complex spatial and social learning (see Introduction). This makes them particularly interesting subjects for the comparative analysis of total and regional brain development, especially concerning areas potentially involved in cognitive functions (see Fig. 10.1 for a cladistic analysis of percomorph fishes). Ridet, Bauchot, and their co-workers have carried out an extensive series of studies comparing whole brains among a variety of teleosts covering most of the major phyletic groups with the prime exception of the Osteoglossomorpha. The majority of fishes catalogued were coral reef species (Bauchot et al., 1977, 1989; Ridet and Bauchot, 1990a,b, 1991). Adjusting for body weight, the authors computed an encephalization index. This demonstrated, for the most part, that reef percomorphs have the largest brains. Of this group, the squirrelfishes and soldierfishes (Beryciformes, Holocentridae), the filefishes and triggerfishes (Tetraodontiformes, Balistidae), and the perchlike fishes (Perciformes—surgeonfishes, Acanthuridae; wrasses, Labridae; damselfishes, Pomacentridae; hawkfishes, Cirrhitidae; snappers, Lutjanidae; seabasses, Serranidae; jacks, Carangidae; emperors, Lethrinidae; cardinals, Apogonidae; and others) have the highest encephalization indexes (Fig. 10.2). They conclude that brains are enlarged in the more derived groups and especially the visually dominated percomorphs associated with reefs.

Wullimann (1997) has recently formulated a hypothesis that supports the idea that the ancestors of these fishes evolved elaborate novel visual pathways associated with the pretectal area, in particular the nucleus glomerulosus. He provides compelling evidence for the rapid evolution of this visual pathway in fishes occupying the newly generated, visually complex scleractinian coral and hippuritacean bivalve reefs. The work of Bauchot, Ridet, and colleagues also supports this hypothesis. Hypertrophy of visual systems in these fishes is also indicated by high densities of photoreceptors in the retina, especially in areas of visual streaks (Ali and Anctil, 1976; Ito and Murakami, 1984; Collin and Pettigrew, 1988a,b, 1989; Collin, 1989), a foveate retina in seabass (Schwassmann, 1968; Ali and Antil, 1976), and enlarged optic lobes with thickening of several layers (Kishida, 1979). Indeed, when several parameters are used to develop a visual index, these fishes and closely related freshwater and temperate fishes consistently are rated the highest (Schellart, 1992; Schellart and Prins, 1993).

308 10 Brain and Cognitive Function in Teleost Fishes

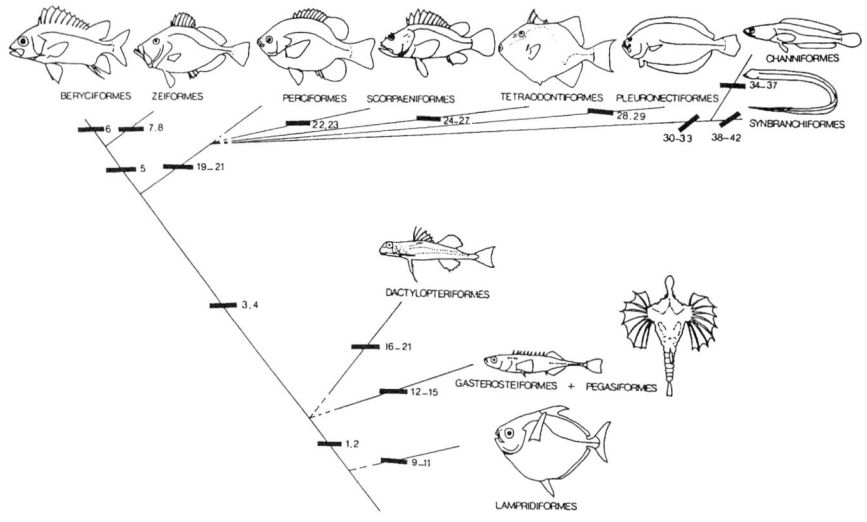

Figure 10.1. Cladogram of the Percomorpha. Coral reef species are primarily in two lineages, one that leads to the Beryciformes (squirrelfishes and soldierfishes) and the other that includes Perciformes (basslike fishes) and Tetraodontiformes (triggerfishes and filefishes). See Lauder and Liem (1983) for list of characters represented by numbers on bars. (From Lauder and Liem, 1983, by permission of Harvard University Press, Cambridge.)

There has been less work dealing with the relative regional differentiation and development of the brain in coral reef percomorphs. Aronson (1963) called attention to the enlarged telencephalon of squirrelfishes (Beryciformes) and surgeonfishes (Perciformes). In the former, he demonstrated histologically that the nonolfactory pallium was primarily responsible for the enlargement. Observations of whole brains (Tuge et al., 1968; Schroeder, 1980; Demski, 1995a,b, 1998; Chin, 1996) are consistent with Aronson's report and extend the group of coral reef percomorphs with enlarged telencephala to include members of the Tetraodontiformes (primarily the Balistidae) and other species of Beryciformes and Perciformes.

Ridet and Bauchot (1990b) measured the relative volumes of a number of brain areas in 72 teleosts, including coral reef percomorphs of the orders Beryciformes, Perciformes, and Tetraodontiformes. They used photographs of brain sections to quantitatively estimate relative brain volumes (method in Ridet and Bauchot, 1990a) The authors measured the "non-olfactory areas of the telencephalon" separately as the telencephalic hemispheres minus the zone of primary olfactory projection and the olfactory bulbs. The nonolfactory region had the greatest variability among species studied. The variation in the nonolfactory areas of the telencephalon to spinal cord ratio was especially diagnostic in separating species with the greatest relative development of telencephalic areas most likely involved in cognitive functions (Fig. 10.3). The orders scoring highest in this regard were the Beryciformes (soldierfishes) Tetraodontiformes (filefishes, triggerfishes, and puffers), and Perciformes (including many reef and other types, e.g., snappers, damselfishes, and grunts), a finding

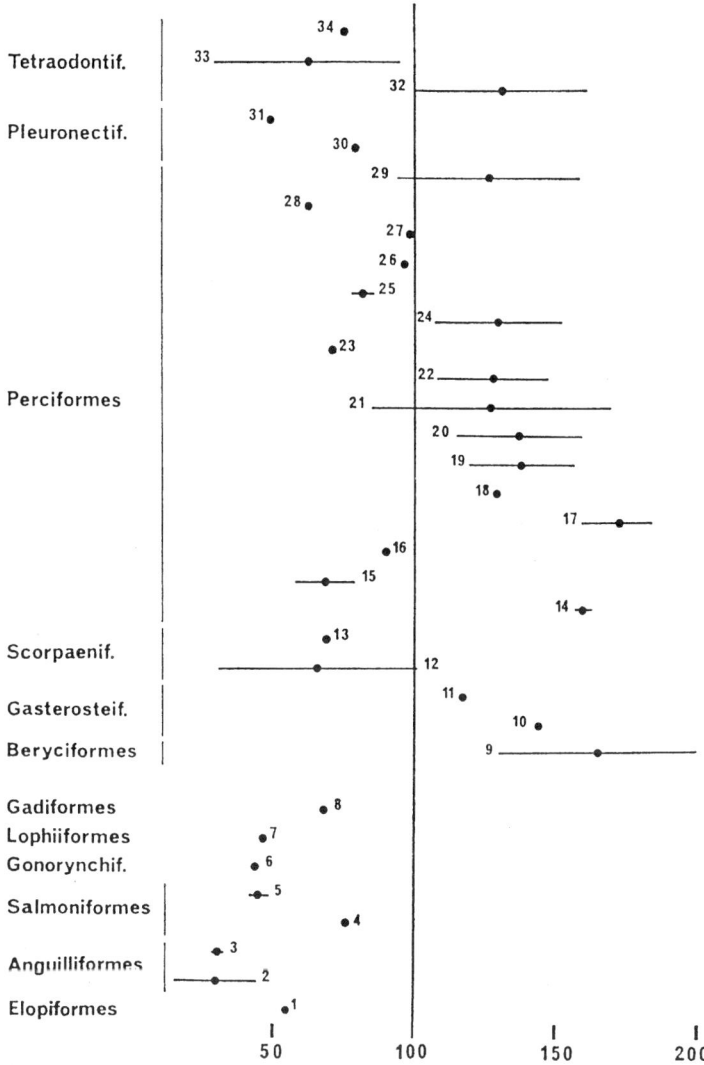

Figure 10.2. Encephalization indices (brain weight/body weight ratios) for 113 Hawaiian teleosts. The orders are listed to the left, and the numbers indicate families as listed below. Of particular interest for cognitive studies are the fishes with the largest brains. They belong to three orders (i.e., Beryciformes [squirrelfishes and soldierfishes], Perciformes [basslike fishes], and Tetraodontiformes [triggerfishes and filefishes]). Families illustrated: 1, Elopidae; 2, Muraenidae; 3, Congridae; 4, Aulopidae; 5, Synodidae; 6, Chanidae; 7, Antennariidae; 8, Brotulidae; 9, Holocentridae; 10, Aulostomidae; 11, Fistularidae; 12, Scorpaenidae; 13, Hoplichtyidae; 14, Serranidae; 15, Pseudochromidae; 16, Kuhlidae; 17, Apogonidae; 18, Lutjanidae; 19, Mullidae; 20, Chaetodontidae; 21, Pomacentridae; 22, Cirrhitidae; 23, Mugilidae; 24, Labridae; 25, Scaridae; 26, Parapericidae; 27, Xiphasiidae; 28, Eleotridae; 29, Acanthuridae; 30, Bothidae; 31, Pleuronectidae; 32, Balistidae; 33, Tetraodontidae; 34, Diodontidae. (From Bauchot et al., 1977.)

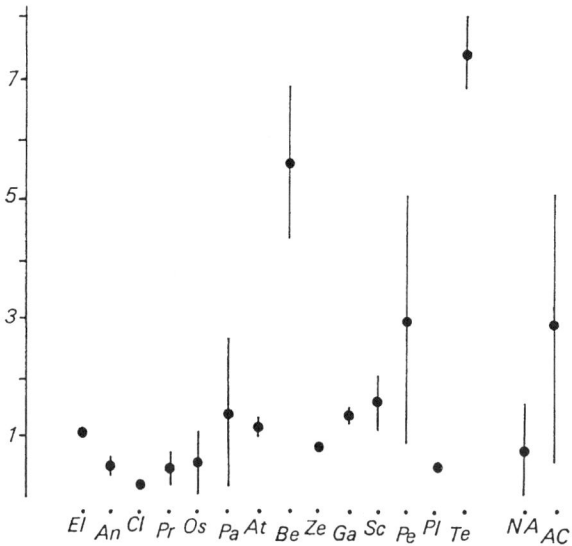

Figure 10.3. Indices of the ratio of size of the nonolfactory telencephalon to the medulla in 72 teleost species. The Acanthopteryii (AC), which include the percomorphs, have generally higher scores than the non-Acanthopteryii (NA), which include members of the following systematically more basal groups: An, Anguilliformes; At, Atheriniformes; Cl, Clupeiformes; El, Elopiformes; Os, Ostariophysi; Pa, Paracanthopterygii; Pr, Protoacanthopterygii. The fishes with the highest ratios are in the same percomorph orders as are those with the largest whole brains (see Fig.10.1), that is, members of the Beryciformes (Be; squirrelfishes and soldierfishes), Perciformes (Pe; basslike fishes), and Tetraodontiformes (Te; triggerfishes and filefishes). The somewhat greater variation within the Perciformes is probably a result of the great diversity within the group, which has a number of freshwater as well as reef species. Other percomorph orders measured were Ga, Gasterosteiformes; Pl, Pleuronectiformes; Sc, Scorpaeniformes; and Ze, Zeiformes. (From Ridet and Bauchot, 1990b, by permission of Academic Verlag, Berlin.)

comparable to the above-mentioned observations of the whole brains. Ratios of the tectum to the olfactory bulb development suggest that these fishes are primary microsmatic, vision specialists. The areas for acousticolateralis functions were not measured separately. Thus, the extent of importance of these senses is not revealed in this study.

Several tentative conclusions can be drawn from the comparative brain size studies. Enlargements of the telencephalon are usually associated with animals living in a strong photic environment and are highly positively correlated with increases in differentiation of both the tectum and the cerebellum. It seems reasonable to assume that such multiregional enhancements represent selection for integrated higher level visual processing mechanisms. In some special cases, (e.g., blind cave fishes or electric fishes), the acousticolateralis systems may be the primary sense responsible for the telencephalic size increases. Electrophysiological studies underline the potential importance of integrated telencephalic-tectal-cerebellar systems in teleosts. Friedlander (1983) demonstrated that telencephalic electrical stimulation caused significant changes in unit activity in the tectum in largemouth black bass (*Micropterus salmoides*). Lee and Bullock used discrete electrical stimulation in the central area of the telencephalon (area dorsalis telencephali pars centralis) in catfish (*Ictalurus nebulosus*) to profoundly influence field potentials and unit activity in both the tectum (Lee and Bullock, 1990a) and the corpus of the cerebellum (Lee, 1984; Lee and Bullock, 1990b,c). Anatomical studies concerning these pathways are considered in some detail in the next section.

MICROCIRCUITRY OF TELENCEPHALIC ENHANCEMENTS IN SELECTED PERCOMORPHS

Demski and co-workers have begun a more detailed investigation of the neural architecture of the hypertrophied telencephalon of representatives of the Beryciformes, Perciformes, and Tetraodontiformes (see Fig. 10.1 for the systematic relationships of these groups). Based on a preliminary survey (Chin, 1996), the following representative species were chosen for study: Beryciformes—squirrelfishes, *Holocentrus ascensionis* and *Holocentrus rufus* (Holocentridae); Perciformes—pinfish, *Lagodon rhomboides* (Sparidae); bluegill sunfish, *Lepomis macrochirus* (Centrarchidae); Texas cichlid, *Cichlasoma cyanoguttatum* (Cichlidae); white grunt, *Haemulon plumieri* (Haemulidae); graysby, *Epinephelus cruentatus*; coney, *Epinephelus fulvus* (Serranidae); ocean surgeonfish, *Acanthurus bahianus*; blue tang, *Acanthurus coeruleus* (Acanthuridae); cardinal or flamefishes, *Apogon* sp. (Apogonidae); the popeye catalufa *Pristigenys serula* (Priacanthidae); several damselfishes of the genus *Pomacentrus*, (Pomacentridae); and Tetraodontiformes—queen triggerfish, *Balistes vetula* (Balistidae). Within the Perciformes, the pinfish, bluegills, and Texas cichlids were included as they have less well-developed telencephala and as such provide a more generalized percomorph baseline for comparison to the more highly developed reef fishes. Indeed, Northcutt and co-workers (Northcutt and Braford, 1980; Northcutt and Davis, 1983b) used sunfish (Lepomis) (Fig. 10.4) as their representative percomorph in papers often used as the starting point for comparison of nuclear areas within the telencephalon of bony fishes (Figs. 10.5 and 10.6).

Representative sections of the study species brains were stained with cresyl violet and in some cases with the rapid Golgi method. The results indicate that the reef fishes exhibit a particularly striking development in three areas of the pallial nonolfactory telencephalon, the dorsal part of the area dorsalis telencephali pars lateralis (Dld), the area dorsalis telencephali pars medialis (Dm), and the area dorsalis telencephali pars centralis (Dc) (Demski and Beaver, 1996, 1997). More recently (Demski, 1998; Demski et al., 1998), the connections of the areas have been studied using the neural tracer biotinylated dextran amine (BDA). The experimental work has been primarily on squirrelfishes and secondarily on pinfish, Texas cichlids, bluegills, white grunts, popeye catalufas, and ocean surgeonfishes. A general appreciation for the telencephalic enhancements typical of the reef fishes can be gained by comparing the whole brain diagram (Fig. 10.5) and Nissl-stained transverse sections (Fig. 10.6) provided for the sunfish (*Lepomis*) with those from our work on squirrelfishes (Figs. 10.7 to 10.9).

312   10 Brain and Cognitive Function in Teleost Fishes

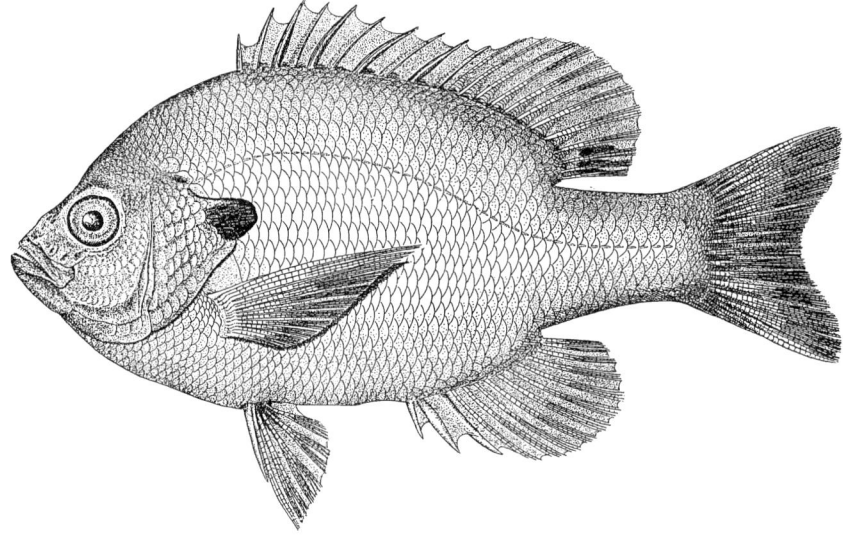

Figure 10.4. Drawing of the freshwater bluegill sunfish *Lepomis macrochirus*. Sunfish have been used as the benchmark percomorph for brain studies (see Fig. 10.5, 10.6 and text for details). (From Goode, 1884, by permission of United States Government Printing Office, Washington.)

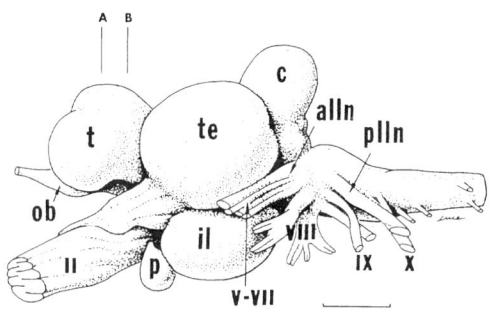

Figure 10.5. Lateral view of the *Lepomis* brain. The lines indicated by A and B represent the levels of the transverse sections shown in Figure 10.6. alln, Anterior lateral-line nerve; c, corpus of the cerebellum; il, inferior lobe of hypothalamus; ob, olfactory bulb; p, pituitary gland; plln, posterior lateral-line nerve; t, telencephalon; te, optic tectum; II, optic nerve; V–VII, trigeminofacial complex; VIII, octaval nerve; IX, glossopharyngeal nerve; X, vagal nerve. Bar = 2mm. (From Northcutt and Braford, 1980, by permission of Plenum Press, New York.)

It should be noted that Ito and co-workers (see Murakami et al., 1983; Yamane et al., 1996) carried out detailed studies on telencephalic connections of the enlarged telencephalon in a scorpaeniform rockfish, *Sebastiscus marmoratus*. The findings provide significant information on a sister group of both the Perciformes and Tetraodontiformes (Fig. 10.1). Comparisons with brains we have studied indicate that *Sebastiscus marmoratus* has a telencephalon most similar to some of the basslike Perciforms (e.g., the seabasses [Serranidae], cichlids [Cichlidae], and sunfishes [Centrarchidae]).

Microcircuitary of Telencephalic Enhancements in Selected Percomorphs 313

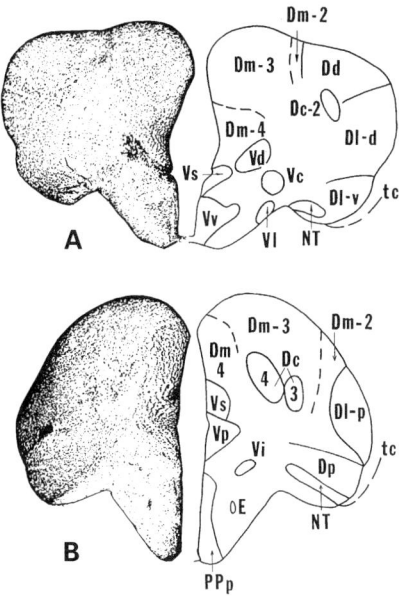

Figure 10.6. Transverse Nissl-stained sections of the *Lepomis* telencephalon. The levels of the sections are indicated in Figure 10.5. Note the radial cords of cells in Dl-d in A. The Dc area No. 4 in B projects to the tectum in bluegills (see text for details). Dc-2, -3, -4, parts of the central zone of area dorsalis telencephali; Dl-d, dorsal part of lateral zone of area dorsalis telencephali; Dl-p, posterior part of area dorsalis telencephali; Dl-v, ventral part of lateral zone of area dorsalis telencephali; Dm-2, -3, -4, parts of medial zone of area dorsalis telencephali; Dp, posterior zone of area dorsalis telencephali; E, entopeduncular nucleus; NT, nucleus taenia; PPp, parvocellular part of periventricular preoptic nucleus; tc, tela choroidea; Vc, commissural nucleus of area ventralis telencephali; Vd, dorsal nucleus of area ventralis telencephali; Vi, intermediate nucleus of area ventralis telencephali; Vl, lateral nucleus of area ventralis telencephali; Vp, postcommissural nucleus of area ventralis telencephali; Vs, supracommissural nucleus of area ventralis telencephali; Vv, ventral nucleus of area ventralis telencephali. (From Northcutt and Braford, 1980, by permission of Plenum Press, New York).

Area Dorsalis Telencephali Pars Lateralis (Dorsal Part)

The area dorsalis telencephali pars lateralis is a pallial region on the lateral aspect of the telencephalon (Figs. 10.5, 10.6, 10.8 and 10.9) that receives input from a tectal recipient nucleus in the diencephalon (see further below and Murakami et al., 1983; Northcutt and Wullimann, 1988; Braford, 1995; Yamane et al., 1996; Wullimann, 1998). This pallial zone is especially well developed in squirrelfishes (Figs. 10.8 and 10.9), damselfishes, and surgeonfishes. In all cases, the small cells of the area form a "cortexlike" outer zone separated from large cells of Dc by a complex capsule of mostly myelinated axons (Figs. 10.9 to 10.11). In squirrelfishes, the area receives an ipsilateral projection from the tectal recipient nucleus prethalamicus (Ebbesson, 1980; Ito et al., 1980; Ito and Vanegas, 1983; Vanegas and Ito, 1983; Ito and Vanegas, 1984), which is located in the rostral diencephalon.

314   10 Brain and Cognitive Function in Teleost Fishes

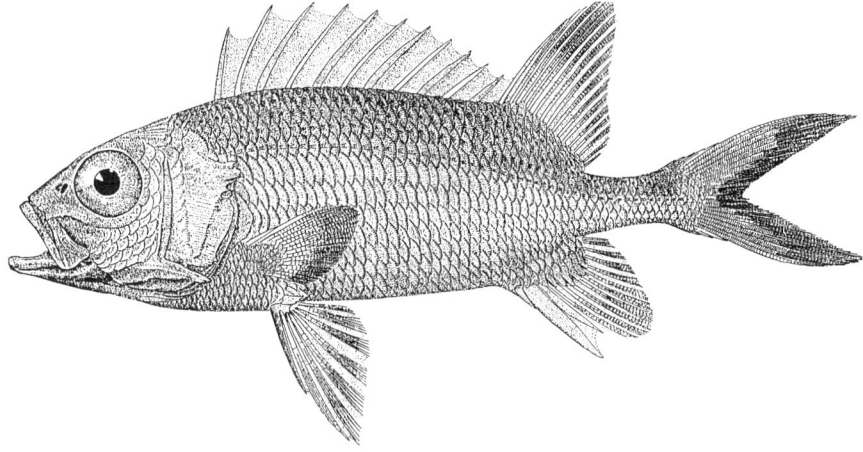

Figure 10.7. Drawing of the squirrelfish *Holocentrus ascensionis*. These Atlantic coral reef fish are most active at night. Their large eyes are indicative of enhanced visual pathways that extend to the telencephalon (see text for details). (From Goode, 1884, by permission of United States Government Printing Office, Washington).

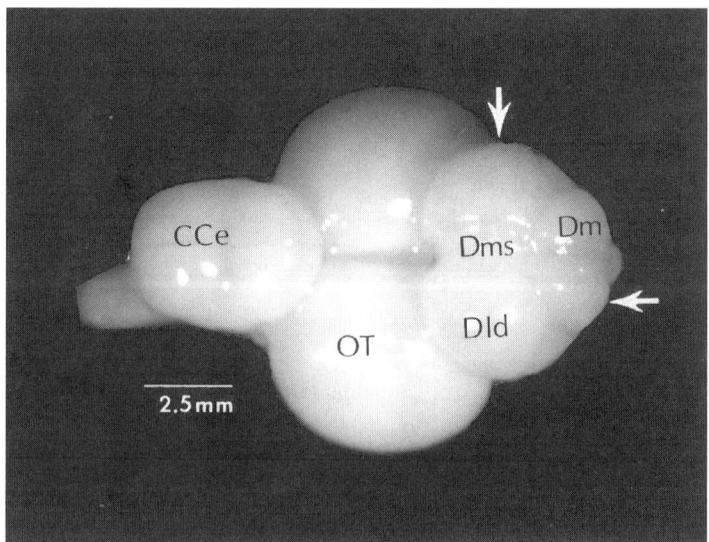

Figure 10.8. Photograph of the dorsal surface of a squirrelfish brain, illustrating some of the enlarged areas of the dorsal telencephalon. The area dorsalis telencephali pars medialis has a more "typical" ventral portion (Dm), which forms a separate lobe, and a more "specialized" portion, which is seen as a thin superficial band (Dms) medial to the dorsal portion of the area dorsalis telencephali pars lateralis (Dld) of the dorsal lobe. The Dld is the primary target for a topographic projection from the diencephalic nucleus prethalamicus, which receives a strong tectal input (see text for details). The arrows indicate the level of the transverse section in Figure 10.9 and the plane of section of the parasagittal section in Fig. 10.11. OT, optic tectum; CCe, corpus or body of the cerebellum.

Microcircuitary of Telencephalic Enhancements in Selected Percomorphs 315

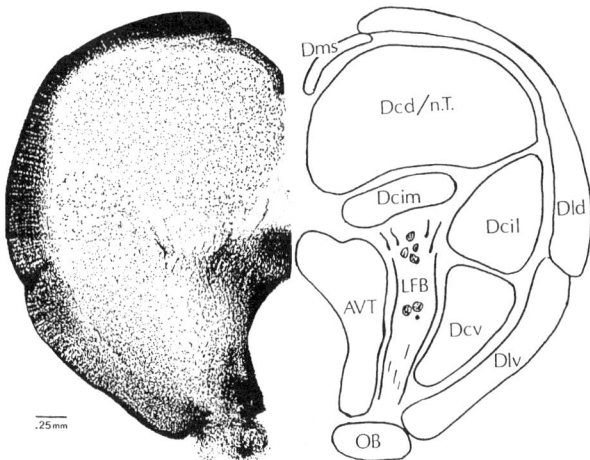

Figure 10.9. Transverse section through the squirrelfish telencephalon (see arrow in Fig. 10.8 for level). Nissl-stained cell bodies are shown on the left side in a high contrast photomicrograph; outlines of the major brain nuclei and fiber tracts are given on the right. Note the dense cell packing and radially directed cords in the "cortexlike" Dld and the cell-sparse fiber capsule that separates the area from the Dcd/n.T. The regions form part of a proposed loop between the telencephalon and the tectum (see text for details). AVT, area ventralis telencephali; Dcil, intermediolateral part of area dorsalis telencephali pars centralis; Dcd/n.T, dorsal part of area dorsalis telencephali pars centralis, renamed *nucleus tectalis* because of its tectal projection; Dcim, intermediomedial part of area dorsalis telencephali pars centralis; Dcv, ventral part of area dorsalis telencephali pars centralis; Dld, dorsal part of area dorsalis telencephali pars lateralis; Dlv, ventral part of area dorsalis telencephali pars lateralis; Dms, superficial part of area dorsalis telencephali pars medialis; LFB, lateral forebrain bundle; OB, olfactory bulb.

Our recent studies indicate that the projection is topographically organized, most likely retaining the retinotopic pattern of the tectum (Demski and Beaver, 1996, 1997) Fig. 10.10). The position and connections of the nucleus prethalamicus suggest that it is homologous to the rostral preglomerular nucleus (see Northcutt and Wullimann, 1988; Wullimann, 1998). The latter is part of the posterior tubercle complex, a group of nuclei most likely homologous to portions of the subthalamus (Northcutt and Wullimann, 1988; Braford, 1995) or to basal plate portions of the dorsal and ventral thalamus of tetrapods (Wullimann and Puelles, 1999). Dld implants of BDA in pinfish, Texas cichlids, and popeye catalufas retrogradely label cells in the rostral preglomerular nucleus, whereas the area receives labeled afferents following tectal implants in these fishes. The comparative observations confirm the tectal–telencephalic connection. Nissl-stained sections reveal a similar rostral preglomerular nucleus in the other fishes in our study group. The nucleus is especially prominent in the surgeonfishes and tangs, where it strongly resembles the nucleus prethalamicus of squirrelfishes. The preglomerular complex has reciprocal connections with widespread areas of the telencephalon, including pathways related to nonvisual sensory input (e.g., from the acousticolateralis and gustatory systems).

In squirrelfishes, the Dld has connections with the other two hypertrophied pallial areas (Demski et al., 1998), that is, it receives afferents from a specialized portion of

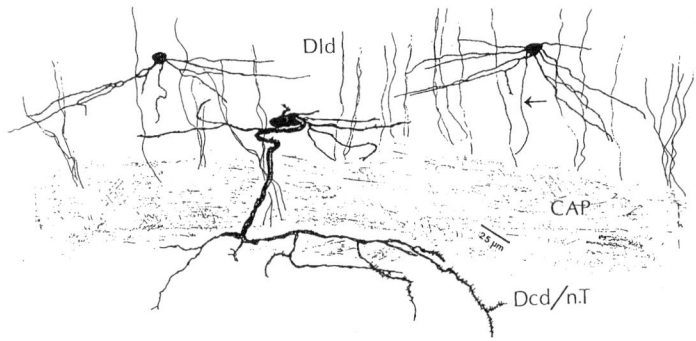

Figure 10.10. Camera lucida diagram of a rapid Golgi-stained section of a squirrelfish brain. The section is centered on the fiber capsule (CAP) separating the tectal-related areas Dld (dorsal part of area dorsalis telencephali pars lateralis) and Dcd/n.T (dorsal part of area dorsalis telencephali pars centralis, renamed *nucleus tectalis* because of its tectal projection). The smaller cells in Dld are the typical type found in great number in the area. Their spiny dendrites fan out in a rough semicircle directed toward the capsule. Their axons originate from the soma or basal potion of a dendrite (arrow) and move toward the capsule without branching. They branch in the capsule and continue to do so as they spread out, covering the large spiny dendrites of the Dcd/n.T cells. Axons from a number of these cells, which are out of the plane of section, are illustrated as a parallel array. The large cell in the center is referred to as a *bridge cell*, as it has dendritic processes in both zones. It appears to give off an axon that branches within the Dld (not shown). The newly described cell type may be involved in a short feedback system if it receives contacts from the small Dld cell axons in Dcd and projects its axonal terminals onto the dendrites of the cells in Dld (see text for additional details).

the Dm (Dms, see explanation below and Fig. 10.9 and 10.10) and has reciprocal connections with the tectofugal part of Dc (Dcd or nucleus tectalis, see below and Figs. 10.9 to 10.11). Regarding the latter, the main projection of the small "cortical" cells of Dld is into the Dcd, where their axons fan out over the large spiny dendrites of the Dcd cells. Relatively large, specialized cells (bridge cells) are scattered throughout the Dld in a layer just superficial to the fiber capsule that separates the Dld from the underlying Dcd (Fig. 10.10). The bridge cells usually have one to two long thick processes that resemble dendrites. The processes pass into the capsule where they may extend for some distance and are likely to receive axonal contacts from the fibers therein. They leave the capsule to enter the adjacent Dcd, where they branch repeatedly, ending as fine processes with long spines. In the Dld, the bridge cells have smaller branched "dendrites" emanating from the soma or the abovementioned large processes and a straight unbranched process that appears to give rise to a multibranching axonal system. The "axonal" processes run parallel to the surface as they course through the radially directed cords of the small "cortical" cells. Thus, the bridge cells literally bridge the capsule to interconnect the Dld and Dcd.

The system may function as a short feedback loop, if—as seems likely—the bridge cell dendrites in Dcd are contacted by the diverging axons of the "cortical" cells (see Fig. 10.11 for a summary diagram). Dcd projects topographically to several layers of the tectum. It also projects to the nucleus prethalamicus; however, a topographical representation has not been demonstrated in this case (see further below and Fig. 10.11). The possibility that retinotopic maps are maintained

Microcircuitary of Telencephalic Enhancements in Selected Percomorphs 317

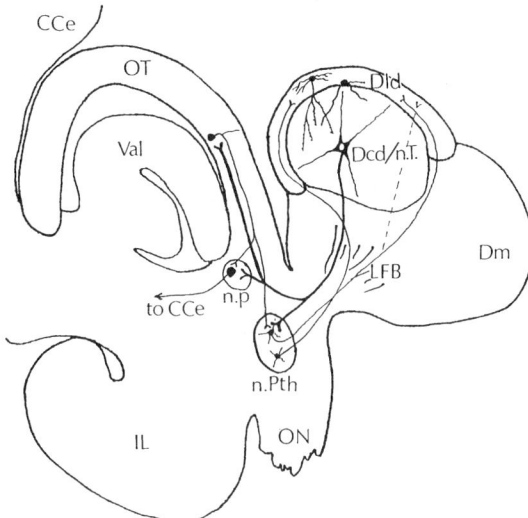

Figure 10.11. A drawing of a parasagittal section through the telencephalon, diencephalon and midbrain of a squirrelfish (see arrow in Fig. 10.8 for the level). Illustrated are connections of the hypertrophied dorsal telencephalon thought to be involved in visual functions, including spatial mapping, probably in relation to diurnal, crepuscular, and nocturnal orientation and navigation in the coral reef environment. Small "cortical-like" neurons and larger bridge cells are illustrated in the Dld (dorsal part of area dorsalis telencephali pars lateralis); they relate the area to the underlying Dcd/n.T (dorsal part of area dorsalis telencephali pars centralis, renamed *nucleus tectalis* because of its tectal projection), which in turn projects to the tectum and two diencephalic areas, the nucleus prethalamicus (n.Pth) and the precerebellar nucleus paracommissuralis (n.p). The optic tectum (OT) also projects to both diencephalic nuclei. Nucleus prethalamicus appears to send topographically arranged afferents to the Dld. Thus closed loops are formed that potentially interconnect the visual telencephalon (Dld and Dcd/n.T), the tectum, and the corpus or body of the cerebellum (CCe). See Figures 10.9 and 10.10 and text for additional information. Dm, area dorsalis telencephali pars medialis; IL, inferior lobe of the hypothalamus; LFB, lateral forebrain bundle; ON, optic nerve; Val, valvula of the cerebellum.

throughout the connections of nucleus prethalamicus to Dld, Dld to/from Dcd, Dcd back to the tectum and nucleus prethalamicus is unresolved because the detailed organization of tectal projections to nucleus prethalamicus has not yet been determined. Regarding the latter, preliminary observations suggest at least a gross topographical projection. Thus, it seems likely that the Dld/Dcd interacts with the tectum in the processing of visually based spatial information.

Area Dorsalis Telencephali Pars Centralis

In the three percomorph orders discussed here, the area dorsalis telencephali pars centralis contains several nuclei consisting of large multipolar cells with spiny dendrites and axons that for the most part appear to enter the lateral forebrain bundles or the fiber capsules surrounding the cell groups (Figs. 10.5, 10.6, and 10.8 to 10.11). Tectal tracer injections in squirrelfishes, pinfish, white grunts, Texas cichlids, popeye catalufas, and bluegills have resulted in retrograde labeling in one of the largest nuclei of the Dc (Dcd in Figs. 10.9 to 10.11, squirrelfish brains). The cell group is characterized by medium to large evenly spaced cells surrounded by a heavy fiber capsule.

The tectal connection has been confirmed by anterograde transport following implants of horseradish peroxidase into the nucleus in squirrelfishes (Ito et al., 1982) and the rockfish *Sebastiscus* (Murakami et al., 1983) or BDA into the Dc area in squirrelfishes (Demski and Beaver, 1997) and pinfish (Demski et al., 1999). In addition, lesions in Dc result in degeneration of afferents to the tectum in *Sebastiscus* (Murakami et al., 1983) and the sea bass *Serranus scriba* (Lazarevic et al., 1989). In squirrelfishes the nucleus is the largest within Dc and forms most of the dorsal aspect of the telencephalon as it fuses across the midline (Fig. 10.9). The cell group in the bluegill is Dc group No. 4 as defined for sunfish by Northcutt and co-workers (1980, 1983a) (Fig. 10.6). In both squirrelfishes and pinfish, the area receives a heavy projection of fine beaded axons from the adjacent Dld as revealed by anterograde transport from Dld cells filled by local BDA implants (see also above) and confirmed by Golgi studies in squirrelfishes. Based on cell type, topography, and connections to the tectum, the Dcd is considered homologous among the species studied and is hereafter referred to as the *nucleus tectalis* (n.T) of Dc (Figs. 10.9 to 10.11).

Although tracer studies have not been carried out in surgeonfishes[1], damselfishes, and sea basses, observations of Nissl-stained sections indicate considerable enlargement of an encapsulated portion of Dc. The areas have multipolar neurons of similar configuration and even spacing as those of the n.T. They also demonstrate large oval cells with one or two large processes, and their somata are located immediately superficial to the capsule. Thus, in Nissl material, they closely resemble the bridge cells of squirrelfishes. We tentatively conclude that these areas represent the n.T and the overlying Dld. Tracer and Golgi studies are being performed to test the suppositions. The comparative findings suggest that at least portions of the Dld and the n.T of Dc have evolved in concert, probably as a result of selective pressure for circuits that enhance visual processing in the most complex aquatic environment, the coral reefs.

The n.T is probably a primitive character for actinopterygian fishes as a similar, albeit less well-developed, tectal projecting nucleus has been reported for the telencephalon of nonpercomorph teleosts, including the osteoglossomorph knifefishes (Braford, 1995), the cypriniform carp (Luiten, 1981; Ito and Kishida, 1977) and goldfish (Grover and Sharma, 1981; Wullimann and Meyer, 1993), the characiform piranha (Fiebig et al., 1983), the siluriform channel catfish (Bass, 1981; Schlussman et al., 1990), and probably even the nonteleostean gar *Lepisosteus* (Northcutt, 1982).

In squirrelfishes anterograde transport from n.T implants of horseradish peroxidase (Ito et al., 1982) or BDA (Demski and Beaver, 1997) also revealed a projection to the nucleus paracommissuralis (Fig. 10.11). The latter provides afferents to the body (corpus) of the cerebellum in squirrelfishes (Ito et al., 1982: Demski and Beaver, unpublished observations) and other euteleosts (Wullimann and Meyer, 1993). The projection from the n.T to the nucleus paracommissuralis has also been identified by anterograde transport of BDA in pinfish (Demski et al., 1999). Thus, in at least two species, the n.T has connections with the potential to distribute information in parallel

---

1   Tectal BDA implants in a surgeonfish fill Dcd cells (L. Demski, unpublished observations)

to both the tectum (directly) and via nucleus paracommissuralis to the body of the cerebellum. Based on anterograde transport from tectal implants in squirrelfishes, pinfish, and Texas cichlids, the tectum also projects to nucleus paracommissuralis (Demski, 1998; Demski et al., 1999); the pathway provides yet another loop for a putative distributed processing system for analyzing and perhaps modulating spatial information (Fig. 10.11).

In squirrelfishes, BDA implants or injections (Demski and Beaver, 1997; unpublished observations) or horseradish peroxidase injections (Ito et al., 1982) into the n.T retrogradely label cells in most of the telencephalic regions, in the nucleus prethalamicus and other nuclei of the preglomerular complex, the locus coeruleus, and the raphe. Until confirmed via anterograde transport studies, the results must be interpreted with caution because the tracer placements probably caused damage to fibers of the lateral forebrain bundle as well as the capsule surrounding the nucleus. The results strongly suggest that the area has complex connections indicative of a probable substrate for higher integrative functions. As mentioned previously, electrical stimulation in the Dc in catfish has a profound effect on both tectal (Lee and Bullock, 1990a) and cerebellar (Lee, 1984; Lee and Bullock, 1990b,c) electrical activity. The findings are consistent with the above hypothesis.

Area Dorsalis Telencephali Pars Medialis

The third region that is enlarged in the reef species is the area dorsalis pars medialis (Dm). It is particularly prominent in triggerfishes and squirrelfishes (Figs. 10.8 and 10.11) where it separates into a large individual lobe. The cytoarchitecture of Dm is more uniform than in the pars lateralis. The "cortical-like" cells are larger, less spiny, and not arranged in rough columns as in Dld. The position and connections of Dm have prompted tentative homologies with the dorsal striatum (caudatoputamen) (Northcutt and Braford, 1980; Northcutt and Davis, 1983b), pallial amygdala (Braford, 1995), or medial pallium (hippocampus) (Murakami et al., 1983) of tetrapods. In a variety of fishes the Dm receives input from the preglomerular complex of the diencephalon and projects to the inferior lobe of the hypothalamus; the preglomerular afferents have been variously associated with taste and octavolateralis functions (Echteler and Saidel, 1981; Murakami et al., 1983, 1986; Striedter, 1991; Braford, 1995; Rink and Wullimann, 1998; Wullimann, 1998; Yoshimoto et al., 1998). It is also reported to receive input from the ventromedial nucleus of the thalamus, a connection thought to represent multimodal input (Ito et al., 1986). In our own recent studies, microimplants or injections of BDA into the Dm of squirrelfishes, pinfish, and Texas cichlids retrogradely labeled the small "granule" cells in the posteromedial or commissural portion of the preglomerular nuclear complex. In the above species and the ocean surgeonfish, such tracer implants anterogradely labeled fibers in the inferior lobe (Demski, Beaver, Barlow and Teelucksingh, unpublished observations).

Physiological studies of Dm are consistent with the indications of multisensory function based on the anatomically defined connections described above. Prechtl and co-workers (1998) have recorded evoked potentials in Dm to acoustic, electrosensory, and visual stimulation in mormyrid electric fish, and Kanwal et al. (1988) have recorded single unit activity in the area in response to gustatory stimulation in catfish. Thus, the Dm is a prime candidate for a locus for multimodal sensory integration, perhaps involved in memory and/or response initiation in a manner suggestive of limbic function in tetrapods.

Behavioral studies are also consistent with this hypothesis. Small lesions in Dm disrupt the normal balance among aggressive, reproductive, and parental behaviors in sticklebacks (Segaar and Nieuwenhuys,1963) and, depending on position, can increase or decrease aggression in Siamese fighting fish (Bruin, 1983). Electrical stimulation in the area in free-swimming bluegills evoked arousal, defensive behavior, and, at increased intensity, rapid escape responses (Demski, 1969). Similar results have been obtained in studies on goldfish (Savage, 1971; Quick and Laming, 1988), where such stimulation was also demonstrated to be negatively reinforcing (Boyd and Gardner, 1962; Savage, 1971). Savage's description (1971) of the response of a goldfish to Dm stimulation is particularly relevant, as it suggests that the fish was reacting to mental images. "At increased current values (40–60 µA) there was a greater tendency for the animal to react to 'non-existent' objects. Thus instead of merely erecting its fins whilst swimming, the animal would stop and hang motionless, in some cases even swimming slowly backwards."

It should also be noted that in the percomorphs the size of the inferior lobe (see Fig. 10.5 for dimensions and location), especially its largest area, the nucleus diffusus, appears positively correlated with the development of the Dm (Demski, unpublished observations; see also examples in Tuge et al., 1968). The association is most likely related to the interconnections of the areas (see above). The triggerfishes have these lobes enlarged to an extent not encountered in any other group (see Wullimann et al., 1984; Wullimann, 1987; Demski unpublished observations). The differentiation of the percomorph inferior lobe is most likely related to the development of the complex pretectum in species inhabiting the newly evolved scleractinian/hippuritacean reefs (Wullimann, 1997) because the nucleus glomerulosus, the largest portion of the complex, has its exclusive output to the inferior lobe. The nucleus glomerulosus receives input from visually related pretectal nuclei (Sakamoto and Ito, 1982; Wullimann and Meyer, 1990; Wullimann, 1998). Thus, the Dm and inferior lobe elaborations may be part of the "new" visual circuitry developed in response to the reef environment. Multisensory integration is also likely, however, because the inferior lobe in certain species, like the Dm, is known to receive inputs from taste pathways (Demski, 1981; Finger, 1983; Morita et al., 1980, 1983; Kanwal et al., 1988; Lamb and Caprio, 1993; see review by Wullimann, 1998).

It is also of interest that the major cell type in nucleus diffusus is very similar to the "cortical cells" of Dm and Dld as is the radial nature of the organization of the nucleus (Demski et al., 1975; Demski, unpublished observations). The common cytoarchitecture of the areas suggests similarity of basic neuronal functions. In this regard, electrical stimulation in the nucleus diffusus in bluegills evokes responses similar to those obtained from Dm or Dld (i.e., arousal, defensive display, swimming, and escape) rather than the feeding and aggressive activity elicited in other nearby hypothalamic regions. Tests of the effects of inferior lobe lesions on learning, memory, or visual functions have not been carried out.

It is noteworthy that, in squirrelfishes, a specialized portion of the Dm forms a thin, superficial band of tightly packed medium-sized cells situated above the fiber capsule between the Dld and the midline (Demski and Beaver, 1996) (see Fig. 10.8 and 10.9). We refer to the nucleus as the *area dorsalis telencephali pars medialis superficialis* (Dms). Retrograde transport studies indicate that the Dms provides a dense innervation of the Dld through a network of fine beaded axons and that it may also project to the torus longitudinalis (Demski et al., 1998). Verification of the latter connection via retrograde filling from toral injections has not, however, been done. The longitudinal torus is a part of the tectum with input from the cerebellar afferent nucleus lateralis valvulae (Wullimann, 1994; Wullimann and Roth, 1994) and possibly the valvula of the cerebellum (Muñoz-Cueto et al., 1998). Physiological studies indicate toral involvement in eye movement and responses to dimming light (see details in Northmore et al., 1983; Gibbs and Northmore, 1996). It appears to have timing functions similar to those of the cerebellar parallel fiber system (Meek, 1992; Bell et al., 1997). The putative relationship of the Dms with the torus suggests a loop between the visual telencephalon and tectum that perhaps operates in parallel to the Dc projection to the tectum proper (Demski, and Beaver, unpublished observations).

Behavioral Studies on the Enlarged Telencephalon of Percomorphs

From the foregoing, in squirrelfishes and most likely some other reef teleosts, the hypertrophied dorsal telencephalon has several pathways for interaction with the tectum and probably the cerebellum. The connections may well be substrates for controlling behavior utilizing visually based spatial maps (Fig. 10.11). Behavioral studies are consistent with the suggestion.

Laming (1987) demonstrated that habituation to visual illumination in one eye in the squirrelfish *Holocentrus rufus* would transfer to tests in the other eye and that transection of the anterior commissure, the largest connection between the hemispheres, blocked the transfer. Laming combined the anterior commissure transection with lesions in one hemisphere to test for disruption of the habituation on the lesioned side. Because the transfer pathway was blocked, he could use stimulation of the non-lesioned side as a control for the lesion effects. He found that lesions of the Dl did not change the habituation significantly, whereas large lesions in the posterior-dorsal portion of Dc (what appears from his figures to be part of n.T) seriously disrupted the response (e.g., one animal required 53 trials to habituate to stimulation in the eye contralateral to the lesion, i.e., the one connected to the lesioned Dc, compared with only 7 for stimulation in the other eye). A similar effect on habituation to the onset of illumination was also reported for goldfish (Rooney and Laming, 1986).

Laming's results support the anatomical findings (see above) that the visual pathway to the telencephalon is from retina to the contralateral tectum and telecephalon. They are also consistent with results from degeneration studies that suggested pathways for interconnection of the two hemispheres in squirrelfishes (Vanegas and Ebbesson, 1976; Vanegas and Ebbesson, 1980). The lack of effect of Dl lesions was interpreted to mean that the telencephalic visual processing was not involved in the habituation responses, whereas the disruptive effect of the Dc damage was thought to result from loss of its function as a multisensory integrative center.

We have carried out some preliminary behavioral studies on squirrelfishes at the Institute for Marine Science in Roatan, Honduras (Demski and Beaver, unpublished observations). The dorsal portion of the telencephalon, including large parts of Dld, Dms, and part of the n.T of Dc but not Dm, was ablated with suction in two animals. As opposed to normal and sham-operated fish, the telencephalon ablates did not attempt to re-enter the rocky shelters provided in their tanks but rather swam in large circles in the center of the tank, typically with their dorsum partly out of the water. The fish were sacrificed within 1 week because of time constraints but showed little change in their behavior throughout the postoperative period. More elaborate studies are planned based on the results.

Although it is difficult to interpret the behavioral results in squirrelfishes without knowing the precise location and extent of the lesions, the findings clearly indicate involvement of at least part of the telencephalic–tectal loop in mediating behavioral responses to visual stimuli (see further below).

Certain teleosts exhibit a response in which they orient their ventral aspect toward the substrate. This ventral substrate response (VSR) can be a dominant factor in the position assumed by the fish (Meyer et al., 1976; 1977). It is particularly well-developed in fishes that live under ledges, such as the black croaker *Cheilotrema saturnum*, a percomorph in the family Sciaenidae. Meyer and co-workers (1976) demonstrated that the VSR is visually guided in this species and that a vertical substrate could induce tilts as great as 64° away from the vertical when illumination was from above. They also reported that such responses were no longer observed following bilateral ablation of the telencephalon. The visually less complicated dorsal light response was independent of the VSR and was still present following loss of the telencephalon. The results suggest that, in the VSR, the telencephalon is responsible for computation of the average plane of often complex substrates. Such information would most likely be integrated with that associated with the fish's orientation to gravity and the direction of illumination to determine a final position of the fish. Connections between the telencephalon and cerebellum, for example, via the projection of Dc to nucleus paracommissuralis (see above), might be instrumental in carrying out such computations.

It is interesting to note that the VSR can be primarily guided by electrosensory information in the weakly electric fish *Eigenmannia* (Meyer et al., 1976). Unfortunately, telencephalic lesions were not performed on these animals. Evidence presented in other portions of this chapter suggests that specialized electrosensory functions may relate to telencephalic enlargements similar to those associated primarily with vision (see Introduction and Summary and Conclusions). Based on this, we predict that removal of the telencephalon in these electric fishes would also result in a loss of the VSR.

SUMMARY AND CONCLUSIONS

Teleost fishes exhibit cognitive functions ranging from classical conditioning to reversal learning in instrumental conditioning. Spatial learning and memory have been well-documented both in the laboratory and under natural conditions. Most examples of spatial mapping are associated with vision as the primary sense (e.g., navigation within the complex coral reef environment). Examples of maps based on mechanoreceptive and electroreceptive lateral-line input have, however, been reported. In certain instances, maps generated with one sensory modality can be accessed by others.

Brain lesion studies implicate both the telencephalon and the cerebellum in the mediation of learned behaviors. In studies where lesions to both structures were compared directly, those of the cerebellum were more disruptive. Loss of the telencephalon in goldfish results in deficits in spatial learning, whereas more cue-dependent responses are relatively unaffected. Cerebellum abated fish have not been tested in these situations. Evidence from a number of sources suggests that tectal lesions might also affect spatial and perhaps nonspatial memory and learning; however, to our knowledge, the appropriate studies have not been carried out.

Comparative studies on brain development in closely related species inhabiting diverse environments indicate that tectal development is greatest in species living in clear water and that telencephalic and cerebellar differentiation is positively correlated with that of the tectum. In a large number of cichlid fishes of the African Great Lakes, the telencephalon had the greatest variation of the brain areas measured. The findings suggest that telencephalic pathways may be largely responsible for the behavioral differences seen among the cichlid species. The lesion and comparative results support the idea that telencephalic-tectal-cerebellar pathways may be substrates from which new behaviors are molded and that, in many instances, the behaviors involve higher level processes, including learned responses to the special environmental features.

Both qualitative and quantitative observations on whole brains and brain regions in an extensive series of fishes reveal that three orders of coral reef percomorph teleosts (Beryciformes, the squirrelfishes; Perciformes, the basslike fishes; and Tetraodontiformes, the triggerfishes) have not only the largest brains but also the greatest relative development of the nonolfactory portions of the telencephalon. Many of the fishes appear to be vision specialists that demonstrate exceptional development of three pallial regions of the dorsal telencephalon (Dld—the dorsal part of the dorsolateral area; Dc—the dorsocentral zone; Dm—the dorsomedial region). The enhancements are probably linked with development of special features in the optically related pretectum (see Wullimann, 1997) that arose in a common ancestor in response to the invasion of the newly evolved scleractinian/hippuritacean reef environment. Given the telencephalic involvement in spatial learning in goldfish, in which the area is rather undifferentiated, it seems reasonable to assume that the telencephalic enhancements in the reef fishes, which inhabit the optically richest of aquatic environments, represent to some extent adaptive specializations involved in spatial orientation and navigation.

Results of more detailed neuroanatomical studies on representatives of the three orders strengthen the argument. Most of the work has been on squirrelfishes in which the visual system from eye to tectum is particularly well-developed. Following earlier work in several laboratories, our recent studies indicate that Dld is highly developed in representatives of all three of the groups. The area receives input from a tectal recipient rostral preglomerular nucleus, which has been referred to as the *nucleus prethalamicus* in squirrelfishes. The projection is topographically organized in the squirrelfishes. Among the species we have studied, the tectal recipient preglomerular nucleus is most highly differentiated in certain of the coral reef fishes (e.g., surgeonfishes and squirrelfishes). Dld is characterized by development of a cortexlike columnar association of small neurons that project axons into the adjacent portion of Dc. The two areas are also coupled by specialized bridge cells that have processes in both areas. The Dc zone is particularly well developed in squirrelfishes, where it enlarges and fuses across the midline to cover most of the dorsal aspect of the telencephalon. The area (referred to as the *nucleus tectalis*) has a topographical projection to several layers of the tectum. It also projects back to the nucleus prethalamicus. The connections establish a potential topographically organized closed loop between the dorsal telencephalon and the tectum. Physiological studies in nonpercomorphs confirm the visual involvement of the areas.

In squirrelfishes and some other percomorphs, the nucleus tectalis also projects to the nucleus paracommissuralis, which in turn projects to the corpus of the cerebellum. The nucleus paracommissuralis also receives input from the tectum in squirrelfishes and other percomorphs. The nucleus paracommissuralis-associated pathway could widen the telencephalon–tectal loop to include the corpus of the cerebellum. Thus, the connections provide putative substrates for visually related spatial orientation and movement. Results of preliminary brain lesion studies are consistent with the hypothesis. The pathways considered are not unique to percomorphs but rather represent enhancements to patterns common to the euteleosts, which is a much wider group including many systematically more basal taxa.

The Dm is also greatly enlarged in certain reef percomorphs (e.g., in squirrelfishes and triggerfishes), where it forms a large separate lobe. Anatomical and physiological studies in nonpercomorphs indicate that the area receives input from several major senses. Its connections and elaborate development in animals like triggerfishes that demonstrate some of the most complex behavior among teleosts (see references in the Introduction; personal observations) suggest that it may be involved in memory and organization of behavior in relation to multiple environmental factors.

In squirrelfishes a specialized superficial portion of Dm (Dms) projects to Dld and possibly to the torus longitudinalis of the tectum. Physiological studies in squirrelfishes indicate that toral cells respond to saccadic eye movements and dimming illumination. The torus is known to receive input from the nucleus lateralis valvulae (which provides afferents to the cerebellum) and to project to the marginal zone of the tectum. The Dms connections could potentially associate the tectal–telencephalon visual loop with eye movements and other cerebellar or vestibular mediated responses. It might thus be involved in realignment of spatial maps with changes in eye and body position. The Dms could also be involved in behavior changes associated with the nocturnal habits of squirrelfishes. The putative pathway provides another possible loop among the visual telencephalon, tectum, and cerebellum.

The material presented in this chapter supports the hypothesis that complex visual environments lead to differentiation of areas in the teleostean telencephalon, especially those connected with the tectum and cerebellum. Although the processes described herein pertain mostly to vision, some evidence indicates that dominance of other senses in certain environments may also result in telencephalic enhancement, for example, two of the telencephalic areas hypertrophied in percomorphs (i.e., Dld and the associated part of Dc) are also enlarged in the remotely related, systematically more basal osteoglossomorph elephantnose and African knifefishes. Here, elaboration of electrosensory function rather than vision may be the primary force responsible for this development (see Introduction and Braford [1995], for additional details). Similarly, in the weakly electric South American gymnotid knifefishes, which are only remotely related to either of the abovementioned groups, an enlarged Dc projects to a hypertrophied torus semicircularis of the midbrain (Lopes Corrêa et al., 1998). In these fishes the torus semicircularis is a primary center for processing complex electrosensory information (Bastian and Heiligenberg, 1980; Carr et al., 1981).

Continued study of the telencephalic-tectal-cerebellar pathways in the hypertrophied condition (e.g., in coral reef fishes or certain electric fishes) seems to be a good strategy to gain understanding of the basic mechanisms underlying the most complex of fish behaviors and the processes controlling their evolution.

ACKNOWLEDGMENTS

The authors acknowledge the contributions made to our studies by the following students: Paul E. Barlow, Xiomara Chin, Mark I. Coffino, James W. Custis, Jason T. Deignan, Mandy J. Funderburk, Debra M. Herbstman, Claudia L. Lukas, and Keith H.Teelucksingh. We also thank Mario Wullimann for his valuable suggestions on the manuscript. The use of the facilities and the help of the staff at the Institute of Marine Science in Roatan Honduras, the collecting privileges extended to us by the Honduran Department of Fisheries, and the financial support provided in part by National Science Foundation grant IBN9724144RUI and the Leonard S. Florsheim Sr. endowment to the New College Foundation are also gratefully acknowledged. In special appreciation, this chapter is dedicated to the memory of Lester R. Aronson, who, as no one else, encouraged the first author to continue the study of teleost forebrains, including those that are hypertrophied in coral reef species.

REFERENCES

Akert, K. (1949) Der visuelle Greifreflex. *Helv. Physiol. Acta* 7:112–134.
Al-Akel, A.S., D.M. Guthrie, and JR. Banks (1986) Motor responses to localized electrical stimulation of the tectum in the freshwater perch (*Perca fluviatilis*). *Neurosciences* 4:1381–1391.
Ali, M.A., and M. Anctil (1976) *Retinas of Fishes: An Atlas*. Springer-Verlag, Berlin, 284 pp.

Aronson, L.R. (1951) Orientation and jumping behavior in the gobiid fish *Bathygobius soporator*. *Am. Mus. Novitates* 1486:1–22.
Aronson, L.R. (1963) The central nervous system of sharks and bony fishes with special reference to sensory and integrative mechanisms. In P.W. Gilbert (ed.): *Sharks and Survival*. D.C. Heath and Co., Boston, pp. 165–241.
Aronson, L.R. (1970) Functional evolution of the forebrain in lower vertebrates. In L.R. Aronson, E. Tobach, D.S. Lehrman, and J.S. Rosenblatt (eds.): *Development and Evolution of Behavior*. W.H. Freeman and Co., San Francisco, pp. 75–107.
Aronson, L.R. (1971) Further studies on orientation and jumping behavior in the gobiid fish, *Bathygobius soporator*. *Ann. N.Y. Acad. Sci.* 188:378–392.
Aronson, L.R., and R. Herberman (1960) Persistence of a conditioned response in the cichlid fish, *Tilapia macrocephala* after forebrain and cerebellar ablations. *Anat. Rec.* 138:332.
Aronson, L.R., and H. Kaplan (1968) Function of the teleostean forebrain. In D. Ingle (ed.): *The Central Nervous System and Fish Behavior*. University of Chicago Press, Chicago, pp. 107–125.
Atema, J. (1971) Structures and functions of the sense of taste in the catfish (*Ictalurus natalis*). *Brain Behav. Evol.* 4:273–294.
Atema, J., R.R. Fay, A.N. Popper, and W.N. Tavolga (1988) *Sensory Biology of Aquatic Animals*. Springer-Verlag, New York, 936 pp.
Bannister, K.E. (1995) Carps and their allies. In J.R. Paxton and W.N. Eschmeyer (eds.): *Encyclopedia of Fishes*. Academic Press, San Diego, pp. 96–100.
Bardach, J.E., J. H. Todd, and R. Crickmer (1967) Orientation by taste in fish of the genus *Ictalurus*. *Science* 155:1276–1278.
Barlow, G.W. (1974a) Extraspecific imposition of social grouping among surgeonfishes (Pisces: Acanthuridae). *J. Zool. Lond.* 174:333–340.
Barlow, G.W. (1974b) Contrasts in social behavior between Central American cichlid fishes and coral-reef surgeon fishes. *Am. Zool.* 14:9–34.
Barlow, G.W. (1993) Fish behavioral ecology: pros, cons and opportunities. *Mar. Behav. Physiol.* 23:7–27.
Bass, A.H. (1981) Telencephalic efferents in the channel catfish, *Ictalurus punctatus*: projections to the olfactory bulb and optic tectum. *Brain Behav. Evol.* 19:1–16.
Bastian, J. (1982) Vision and electroreception: integration of sensory information in the optic tectum of the weakly electric fish *Apteronotus albifrons*. *J. Comp. Physiol.* 147:287–297.
Bastian, J., and W. Heiligenberg (1980) Phase-sensitive midbrain neurons in *Eigenmannia*: neural correlates of the jamming avoidance response. *Science* 209:828–831.
Bauchot, R., M.L. Bauchot, R. Platel, and J.M. Ridet (1977) Brains of Hawaiian tropical fishes; brain size and evolution. *Copeia* 1:42–46.
Bauchot, R., J.E. Randall, J.-M. Ridet, and M.-L. Bauchot (1989) Encephalization in tropical teleost fishes and comparison with their mode of life. *J. Hirnforsch*. 30:645–669.
Bekoff, M. (1996) Cognitive ethology, vigilance, information gathering, and representation: who might know what and why? *Behav. Proc.* 35:225–237.
Bell, C., D. Bodznick, J. Montgomery, J. Bastian (1997) The generation and subtraction of sensory expectations within cerebellum-like structures. *Brain Behav. Evol.* 50 (suppl. 1):17–31.
Boyd, E.S., and L.C. Gardner (1962) Positive and negative reinforcement from intracranial stimulation of a teleost. *Science* 136:648–649.
Braford, M. R. Jr. (1995) Comparative aspects of forebrain organization in the ray-finned fishes: touchstone or not? *Brain Behav. Evol.* 46:259–274.
Braithwaite, V.A. (1998) Spatial memory, landmark use and orientation in fish. In S. Healy (ed.): *Spatial Representation in Animals*. Oxford University Press, pp. 86–102.
Braithwaite, V.A., J.D. Armstrong, H.M. McAdam, and F.A. Huntingford (1996) Can juvenile Atlantic salmon use multiple cue systems in spatial learning? *Anim. Behav.* 51:1409–1415.
Bruin, J.P.C. de (1983) Neural correlates of motivated behavior in fish. In J.-P. Ewert, R.R. Capranica and D.J. Ingle (eds.): *Advances in Vertebrate Neuroethology*. Plenum Press, New York, pp. 969–995.
Bullock, T.H. (1983) Why study fish brains? Some aims of comparative neurology today. In R.E. Davis and R.G. Northcutt (eds.): *Fish Neurobiology, vol. 2: Higher Brain Areas and Functions*. University of Michigan Press, Ann Arbor, pp. 361–368.
Burke, N.C. (1995) Nocturnal foraging habits of French and bluestriped grunts, *Haemulon flavolineatum* and *H. sciurus*, at Tobacco Caye, Belize. *Environ. Biol. Fish.* 42:365–374.

Cain, P. (1995) Navigation in familiar environments by the weakly electric elephantnose fish, *Gnathonemus petersii* L. (Mormyriformes, Teleostei). *Ethology* 99:332–349.
Cambray, J.A. (1994) Effects of turbidity on the neural structures of two closely related redfin minnows, *Pseudobarbus afer* and *P. asper*, in the Gamtoos River system, South Africa. *S. Afr.Tydskr. Dierk.* 29:126–131.
Carr, C.E., L. Maler, W. Heiligenberg, and E. Sas (1981) Laminar organization of the afferent and efferent systems of the torus semicircularis of gymnotiform fish: morphological substrates for parallel processing in the electrosensory system. *J. Comp. Neurol.* 203:649–670.
Chin, X. (1996) A photographic atlas of brains of common Caribbean reef fishes. Baccalaureate Thesis, New College of University of South Florida, Sarasota, Florida, 62 pp.
Collin, S.P. (1989) Topography and morphology of retinal ganglion cells in the coral trout *Plectropoma leopardus* (Serranidae): a retrograde cobaltous-lysine study. *J. Comp. Neurol.* 281:143–158.
Collin, S.P., and J.D. Pettigrew (1988a) Retinal topography in reef teleosts I. Some species with well-developed areae but poorly-developed streaks. *Brain Behav. Evol.* 31:269–282.
Collin, S.P., and J.D. Pettigrew (1988b) Retinal topography in reef teleosts II. Some species with prominent horizontal streaks and high-density areae. *Brain Behav. Evol.* 31:283–295.
Collin, S.P., and J.D. Pettigrew (1989) Quantitative comparison of the limits on visual spatial resolution set by the ganglion cell layer in twelve species of reef teleosts. *Brain Behav. Evol.* 34:184–192.
Davis, R.E., and J. Kassel (1983) Behavioral functions of the teleostean telencephalon. In R.E. Davis and R.G. Northcutt (eds.): *Fish Neurobiology vol. 2: Higher Brain Areas and Functions*.University of Michigan Press, Ann Arbor, pp. 237–263.
Davis, R.E., and R.G. Northcutt (1983) *Fish Neurobiology, vol. 2: Higher Brain Areas and Functions*. University of Michigan Press, Ann Arbor, 414 pp.
Demski, L.S. (1969) Behavioral effects of electrical stimulation of the brain in free-swimming bluegills (*Lepomis macrochirus*). Ph.D. Dissertation, University of Rochester, Rochester, New York, 403 pp.
Demski, L.S. (1981) Hypothalamic mechanisms of feeding in fishes. In P.R. Laming (ed.): *Brain Mechanisms of Behavior in Lower Vertebrates*. Cambridge University Press, Cambridge, pp. 225–237.
Demski, L.S. (1983) Behavioral effects of electrical stimulation of the brain. In R.E. Davis and R.G. Northcutt (eds.): *Fish Neurobiology, vol. 2: Higher Brain Areas and Functions*. University of Michigan Press, Ann Arbor, pp. 317–359.
Demski, L.S. (1995a) Forebrain enlargement in bony fishes: a preliminary analysis of phyletic trends and ecomorphological considerations. Abstract for J.B. Johnston Club at Society for Neuroscience Annual Meeting.
Demski, L.S. (1995b) Brain behavior systems in coral reef fishes: possible models for patterns and evolutionary econeurobiology. Abstract for workshop on Evolution, Neurobiology and Behavior, Krasnow Institute for Advanced Study, George Mason University, May 31–June 4.
Demski, L.S. (1998) Patterns in the evolution of the visual telencephalon of actinopterygians: cognitive mapping in a "fishy cortex." Abstract for J.B. Johnston Club at Society for Neuroscience Annual Meeting.
Demski, L.S., and J.A. Beaver (1996) Evolution of cognition in teleosts: the hypertrophied dorsal telencephalon of squirrelfish. Society for Neuroscience Annual Meeting, Abstract 60.6.
Demski, L.S., and J.A. Beaver (1997) Visually-related pathways of the hypertrophied dorsal telencephalon of squirrelfish. Society for Neuroscience Annual Meeting, Abstract 927.7.
Demski, L.S., J.A. Beaver, P. Barlow, M.J. Funderburk, and K. H. Teelucksingh (1999) The visual telencephalon of percomorph fishes: tectal and cerebellar associations. Society for Neuroscience Annual Meeting Abstract (in press).
Demski, L.S., J.A. Beaver, J.T. Deignan, and C.L. Lukas (1998) Intrinsic connections of the visually-related dorsal telencephalon of squirrelfish. Society for Neuroscience Annual Meeting, Abstract 64.3.
Demski, L.S., A.P. Evan, and L.C. Saland (1975) The structure of the inferior lobe of the teleost hypothalamus. *J. Comp. Neurol.* 161:483–498.
Demski, L.S., and R.G. Northcutt (1996) The brain and cranial nerves of the white shark: an evolutionary perspective. In A.P. Klimley and D.G. Ainley (eds.): *Great White Sharks: The Biology of Carcharodon carcharias*. Academic Press, San Diego, pp. 121–130.
Dodson, J.J. (1988) The nature and role of learning in the orientation and migratory behavior of fishes. *Environ. Biol. Fish* 23:161–182.
Douglas, R.H. (1996) Goldfish use the visual angle of a familiar landmark to locate a food source. *J. Fish Biol.* 49:532–536.

Douglas, R.H., J. Eva, and N. Guttridge (1988) Size constancy in goldfish (*Carassius auratus*). *Behav. Brain Res.* 30:37–42.

Dugatkin, L.A., and D.S. Wilson (1993) Fish behavior, partner choice experiments and cognitive ethology. *Rev. Fish Biol. Fisher.* 3:368–372.

Ebbesson, S.O.E. (1980) A visual thalamo-telencephalic pathway in a teleost fish (*Holocentrus rufus*). *Cell Tissue Res.* 213:505–508.

Echteler, S.M., and W.M. Saidel (1981) Forebrain connections in the goldfish support telencephalic homologies with land vertebrates. *Science* 212:683–685.

Fernald, R.D., and L.C. Shelton (1985) The organization of the diencephalon and the pretectum in the cichlid fish, *Haplochromis burtoni*. *J. Comp. Neurol.* 238:202–217.

Fiebig, E., S.O.E. Ebbesson, and D.L. Meyer (1983) Afferent connections of the optic tectum in the piranha (*Serrasalmus nattereri*). *Cell Tissue Res.* 231:55–72.

Fiebig, E., D.L. Meyer, and S.O.E. Ebbesson (1985) Eye movements evoked from telencephalic stimulations in the piranha (*Serrasalmus nattereri*). *Comp. Biochem. Physiol.* 81A:67–70.

Finger, T.E. (1983) The gustatory system in teleost fish. In R.G. Northcutt and R.E. Davis (eds.): *Fish Neurobiology, vol. 1: Brain Stem and Sense Organs*. University of Michigan Press, Ann Arbor, pp. 285–309.

Friedlander, M.J. (1983) The visual prosencephalon of teleosts. In R.E. Davis and R. Glenn Northcutt (eds.): *Fish Neurobiology, vol. 2: Higher Brain Areas and Functions*. University of Michigan Press, Ann Arbor, pp. 91–115.

Gibbs, M.A., and D.P.M. Northmore (1996) The role of torus longitudinalis in equilibrium orientation measured with the dorsal light reflex. *Brain Behav. Evol.* 48:115–120.

Goode, G.B. (1884) *The Fisheries and Fishery Industries of the United States: Section I Natural History of Useful Aquatic Animals with an Atlas of Two Hundred and Seventy-Seven Plates*, The United States Commisson of Fish and Fisheries, United States Government Printing Office, Washington, D.C., 297 pp.

Grande, L. (1995) Fishes through the ages. In J.R. Paxton and W.N. Eschmeyer (eds.): *Encyclopedia of Fishes*. Academic Press, San Diego, pp. 27–31.

Grover, B.G., and S.C. Sharma (1981) Organization of extrinsic tectal connections in goldfish (*Carassius auratus*). *J. Comp. Neurol.* 196:471–488.

Hasler, A.D., and A.T. Scholz (1983) Olfactory imprinting and homing in salmon. *Zoophysiology*. 14:1–134.

Heiligenberg, W. (1975) Processes controlling aggressive behavior in cichlid fish. In D.J. Ingle and H.M. Shein (eds.): *Model Systems in Biological Psychiatry*. MIT Press, Cambridge, pp. 132–148.

Helfman, G.S., J. L. Meyer, and W.N. McFarland (1982) The ontogeny of twilight migration patterns in grunts (Pieces: Haemulidae). *Anim. Behav.* 30:317–326.

Herrero, L., F. Rodríguez, C. Salas, and B. Torres (1998) Tail and eye movements evoked by electrical stimulation of the optic tectum in goldfish. *Exp. Brain Res.* 120:291–305.

Hofmann, M.H., and D.L. Meyer (1993) Visual-evoked responses in the salmon telencephalon change during smolt transformation. *Neurosci. Lett.* 155:234–236.

Huber, R., and M. K. Rylander (1991) Quantitative histological studies of the optic tectum in six species of *Notropis* and *Cyprinella* (Cyprinidae, Teleostei). *J. Hirnforsch.* 32:309–316.

Ingle, D. (1968) *The Central Nervous System and Fish Behavior*. University of Chicago Press, Chicago, 272 pp.

Ingle, D., and D. Sahagian (1973) Solution of a spatial constancy problem by goldfish. *Physiol. Psychol.* 1:83–84

Ito, H., and R. Kishida (1977) Tectal afferent neurons identified by the retrograde HRP method in the carp telencephalon. *Brain Res.* 130:142–145.

Ito, H., Y. Morita, N. Sakamoto, and S. Ueda (1980) Possibility of telencephalic visual projection in teleosts, Holocentridae. *Brain Res.* 197:219–222.

Ito, H., and T. Murakami (1984) Retinal ganglion cells in two teleost species, *Sebastiscus marmoratus* and *Navodon modestus*. *J. Comp. Neurol.* 229:80–96.

Ito, H., T. Murakami, and Y. Morita (1982) An indirect telencephalo-cerebellar pathway and its relay nucleus in teleosts. *Brain Res.* 249:1–13.

Ito, H., and H. Vanegas (1983) Cytoarchitecture and ultrastructure of nucleus prethalamicus, with special reference to degenerating afferents from optic tectum and telencephalon, in a teleost (*Holocentrus ascensionis*). *J. Comp. Neurol.* 221:401–415.

Ito, H., And H. Vanegas (1984) Visual receptive thalamopetal neurons in the optic tectum of teleosts (Holocentridae). *Brain Res.* 290:201–210.
Kanwal, J.S., T.E. Finger, and J. Caprio (1988) Forebrain connections of the gustatory system in ictalurid catfishes. *J. Comp. Neurol.* 278:353–376.
Kaplan, H., and L.R. Aronson (1967) Effect of forebrain ablation on the performance of a conditioned avoidance response in the teleost fish, *Tilapia h. macrocephala. Anim. Behav.* 15:438–448.
Kaplan, H., and L.R. Aronson (1969) Function of forebrain and cerebellum in learning in the teleost *Tilapia heudelotii macrocephala. Bull. Am. Mus. Nat. Hist.* 142:141–208.
Karamian, A.I. (1956) Evolution of the function of the cerebellum and cerebral hemispheres. *Fiziol. Zh. S.S.S.R.* 25:15–109. [Translation from Russian for the National Science Foundation (USA) by Israel Program for Scientific Translation, Jerusalem, 1962.]
Kesner, R.P., and D.S. Olton (1990) *Neurobiology of Comparative Cognition.* Lawrence Erlbaum Associates, Hillsdale, New Jersey, 476 pp.
Kishida, R. (1979) Comparative study on the teleostean optic tectum. Lamination and cytoarchitecture. *J. Hirnforsch.* 20:57–67.
Kleerekoper, H., J. Matis, P. Gensler, and P. Maynard (1974) Exploratory behavior of goldfish *Carassius auratus. Anim. Behav.* 22:124–132.
Kotrschal, K., and H. Junger (1988) Patterns of brain morphology in mid-European Cyprinidae (Pisces, Teleostei): a quantitative histological study. *J. Hirnforsch.* 29:341–352.
Kotrschal, K., and M. Palzenberger (1992) Neuroecology of cyprinids: comparative, quantitative histology reveals diverse brain patterns. *Environ. Biol. Fish.* 33:135–152.
Lamb, C.F., and J. Caprio (1993) Diencephalic gustatory connections in the channel catfish. *J. Comp. Neurol.* 377:400–418.
Laming, P.R. (1987) Behavioural arousal and its habituation in the squirrel fish, *Holocentrus rufus*: the role of the telencephalon. *Behav. Neural Biol.* 47:80–104.
Lauder, G.V., and K.F. Liem (1983) The evolution and interrelationships of the actinopterygian fishes. *Bull. Mus. Comp. Zool.*, 150:95–197.
Lazarevic, L., L. Rakic, M. Gojkovic and Z. Draškovic (1989) Striatal projections in the teleost *Serranus scriba. Iugoslav. Physiol. Pharmcol. Acta* 25:53–63.
Lee, L.T. (1984) Response of the cerebellum to stimulation of telencephalon in the catfish (*Ictalurus nebulosus*). *J. Neurophysiol.* 51:1394–1408.
Lee, L.T., and T.H. Bullock (1990a) Cerebellar units show several types of early responses to telencephalic stimulation in catfish. *Brain Behav. Evol.* 35:278–290.
Lee, L.T., and T.H. Bullock (1990b) Cerebellar units show several types of long-lasting posttetanic responses to telencephalic stimulation in catfish. *Brain Behav. Evol.* 35:291–301.
Lee, L.T., and T.H. Bullock (1990c) Responses of the optic tectum to telencephalic stimulation in catfish. *Brain Behav. Evol.* 35:313–324.
Lewis, D. and T.J. Teyler (1986) Long-term potentiation in the goldfish optic tectum. *Brain Res.* 375:246–250.
Lopes Corrêa, S.A., K. Grant, and A. Hoffmann (1998) Afferent and efferent connections of the dorsocentral telencephalon in an electrosensory teleost, *Gymnotus carapo. Brain Behav. Evol.* 52:81–98.
Lorenz, K., (1963) *On Aggression.* Harcourt, Brace and World, New York, 306 pp.
Luiten, P.G.M. (1981) Afferent and efferent connections of the optic tectum in the carp (*Cyprinus carpio* L.) *Brain Res.* 220:51–65.
Macphail, E.M. (1982) *Brain and Intelligence in Vertebrates.* Oxford University Press, New York, 423 pp.
Malyukina, G.A. (1954) Cited in Karamian, 1956, pp 33.
Markel, R.W. (1994) An adaptive value of spatial learning and memory in the blackeye goby, *Coryphopterus nicholsi. Anim. Behav.* 47:1462–1464.
Meek, J. (1983) Functional anatomy of the tectum mesencephali of the goldfish. An explorative analysis of the functional implications of the laminar structural organization of the tectum. *Brain Res. Rev.* 6:247–2197.
Meek, J. (1992) Why run parallel fibers parallel? Teleostean Purkinje cells as possible coincidence detectors, in a timing device subserving spatial coding of temporal differences. *Neuroscience* 48:249–283.
Meyer, D.L., R. Becker, and W.Graf (1977) The ventral substrate response. Comparative investigation of the VSR about the roll and the pitch axis. *J. Comp. Physiol.* 117:209–217.

Meyer, D.L., W. Heiligenberg, and T.H. Bullock (1976) The ventral substrate response. A new postural control mechanism in fishes. *J. Comp. Physiol.* 109:59–68.

Meyer, D.L., D. Schott, and K.-P. Schaefer (1970) Reizversuche im Tectum opticum freischwimmender Kabeljaue bzw. Dorsche (*Gadus morrhua* L.). *Pflugers Arch. Ges. Physiol.* 314:240–252.

Montgomery, W.L., A.A. Myrberg, Jr., and L. Fishelson (1989) Feeding ecology of surgeonfishes (Acanthuridae) in the northern Red Sea, with particular reference to *Acanthurus nigrofuscus* (Forsskål). *J. Exp. Mar. Biol. Ecol.* 132:179–207.

Morita, Y., H. Ito., and H. Masai (1980) Central gustatory paths in the crussian carp, *Carassius carassius*. *J. Comp. Neurol.* 191:119–132.

Morita, Y., T. Murakami, and H. Ito (1983) Cytoarchitecture and topographic projections of the gustatory center in a teleost, *Carassius carassius*. *J. Comp. Neurol.* 218:378–394.

Muñoz-Cueto, J.A., C. Sarasquete, and O. Kah (1998) The torus longitudinalis in the gilthead seabream: an undescribed fiber tract link with the valvula cerebelli. *Histol. Histopathol.* 13:391–394.

Murakami, T., T. Fukuoka, and H. Ito (1986) Telencephalic ascending acousticolateral system in a teleost (*Sebastiscus marmoratus*), with special reference to the fiber connections of the nucleus preglomerulosus. *J. Comp. Neurol.* 247:383–397.

Murakami, T., Y. Morita, and H. Ito (1983) Extrinsic and intrinsic fiber connections of the telencephalon in a teleost, *Sebastiscus marmoratus*. *J. Comp. Neurol.* 216:115–131.

Nelson, J.S. (1984) *Fishes of the World, 2nd ed*. John Wiley and Sons Inc., New York, 523 pp.

Nieuwenhuys, R., and J. Meek (1990) The telencephalon of actinopterygian fishes. In E.G. Jones and A. Peters (eds.): *Cerebral Cortex, vol. 8A, Comparative Structure and Evolution of Cerebral Cortex, part I*. Plenum Press, New York, pp. 31–73.

Nieuwenhuys, R., and C. Nicholson (1969) A survey of the general morphology, the fiber connections, and the possible functional significance of the gigantocerebellum of mormyrid fishes. In R. Llinás, (ed.): *Neurobiology of Cerebellar Evolution and Development*. American Medical Association, Chicago, pp.107–134.

Noda, M., K. Gushima, and S. Kakuda (1994) Local prey search based on spatial memory and expectation in the planktivorous reef fish, *Chromis chrysurus* (Pomacenridae). *Anim. Behav.* 47:1413–1422.

Northcutt, R.G. (1982) Localization of neurons afferent to the optic tectum in longnose gars. *J. Comp. Neurol.* 204:325–335.

Northcutt, R.G., and M.R. Braford, Jr. (1980) New observations on the organization and evolution of the telencephalon of actinopterygian fishes. In *Comparative Neurology of the Telencephalon*. S.O.E. Ebbesson (ed.): Plenum Press, New York, pp. 41–98.

Northcutt, R.G., and R.E. Davis (1983a) *Fish Neurobiology, vol. 1: Brain Stem and Sense Organs*. University of Michigan Press, Ann Arbor, 414 pp.

Northcutt, R.G., and R.E. Davis (1983b) Telencephalic organization in ray-finned fishes. In R.E. Davis and R.G. Northcutt (eds.): *Fish Neurobiology, vol. 2: Higher Brain Areas and Functions*. University of Michigan Press, Ann Arbor, pp. 203–236.

Northcutt, R.G., and M.F. Wullimann (1988) The visual system in teleost fishes: morphological patterns and trends. In J. Atema, R.R. Fay, A.N. Popper, and W.N. Tavolga (eds.): *Sensory Biology of Aquatic Animals*. Springer-Verlag, New York, pp. 515–552.

Northmore, D.P.M., B. Williams, and H. Vanegas (1983) The teleostean torus longitudinalis: responses related to eye movements, visuotopic mapping, and functional relations with the optic tectum. *J. Comp. Physiol.* 150:39–50.

Ohnishi, K. (1997) Effects of telencephalic ablation on short-term memory and attention in goldfish. *Behav. Brain Res*. 86:191–199.

Overmier, J.B., and K.L. Hollis (1983) The teleostean telencephalon in learning. In R.E. Davis and R.G. Northcutt (eds.): *Fish Neurobiology, vol. 2: Higher Brain Areas and Functions*. University of Michigan Press, Ann Arbor, pp. 265–284.

Overmier, J.B., and K.L. Hollis (1990) Fish in the think tank: learning, memory, and integrated behavior. In R.P. Kesner and D.S. Olton (eds.): *Neurobiology of Comparative Cognition*. Lawrence Erlbaum Associates, Hillsdale, NJ, pp. 205–236.

Peters, N., V. Schacht, W. Schmidt, and H. Wilkens (1993) Gehirnproportionen und Ausprägungsgrad der Sinnesorgane von *Astyanax mexicanus* (Pisces, Characinidae). *Z. Zool. Syst. Evol. Forsch.* 31:144–159.

Pitcher, T.J., and A.E. Magurran (1983) Shoal size, patch profitability and information exchange in foraging goldfish. *Anim. Behav.* 31:546–555.

Prechtl, J.C., G. von der Emde, J. Wolfart, S. Karamursel, G.N. Akoev, Y.N. Andrianov, and T.H. Bullock (1998) Sensory processing in the pallium of a mormyrid fish. *J. Neurosci.* 18:7381–7393.

Presson, J., R.D. Fernald, and M. Max (1985) The organization of retinal projections to the diencephalon and pretectum in the cichlid fish, *Haplochromis burtoni*. *J. Comp. Neurol.* 235:360–374.

Quick, I.A., and P.R. Laming (1988) Cardiac, ventilatory and behavioural arousal responses evoked by electrical brain stimulation in the goldfish (*Carassius auratus*). *Physiol. Behav.* 43:715–727.

Reese, E.S. (1989) Orientation behavior of butterflyfishes (family Chaetodontidae) on coral reefs: spatial learning of route specific landmarks and cognitive maps. *Environ. Biol. Fish* 25:79–86.

Ridet, J.-M., and R. Bauchot (1990a) Analyse quantitative de l'encéphale des téléostéens: Caractères evolutifs et adaptatifs de l'encéphalisation. I. Généralitiés et analyse globale. *J. Hirnforsch.* 31:51–63.

Ridet, J.-M., and R. Bauchot (1990b) Analyse quantitative de l'encéphale des téléostéens: Caractères evolutifs et adaptatifs de l'encéphalisation. II. Les grandes subdivisions encéphaliques. *J. Hirnforsch.* 31:433–458.

Ridet, J.-M., and R. Bauchot (1991) Analyse quantitative de l'encéphale des téléostéens: Caractères evolutifs et adaptatifs de l'encéphalisation. III. Analyse multivariée des indices encéphaliques. *J. Hirnforsch.* 32:439–449.

Rink, E., and M.F. Wullimann (1998) Some forebrain connections of the gustatory system in the goldfish *Carassius auratus* visualized by separate DiI application to the hypothalamic inferior lobe and the torus lateralis. *J. Comp. Neurol.* 394:152–170.

Rodríguez, F., E. Durán, J.P. Vargas, B. Torres, and C. Salas (1994) Performance of goldfish trained in allocentric and egocentric maze procedures suggests the presence of a cognitive mapping system in fishes. *Anim. Learn. Behav.* 22:409–420.

Roitblat, H.L., W. Tham, and L. Golub (1982) Performance of *Betta splendens* in a radial arm maze. *Anim. Learn. Behav.* 10:108–114.

Rooney, D.J., and P.R. Laming (1986) Localization of telencephalic regions concerned with habituation of cardiac and ventilatory responses associated with arousal in the goldfish (*Carassius auratus*). *Behav. Neurosci.* 100:45–50.

Sakamoto, N., and H. Ito (1982) Fiber connections of the corpus glomerulosum in a teleost, *Navodon modestus*. *J. Comp. Neurol.* 205:291–298.

Salas, C., C. Broglio, F. Rodríguez, J.C. López, M. Portavella, and B. Torres (1996a) Telencephalic ablation in goldfish impairs performance in a "spatial constancy" problem but not in a cued one. *Behav. Brain Res.* 79:193–200.

Salas, C., F. Rodríguez, J.P. Vargas, E. Durán, and B. Torres (1996b) Spatial learning and memory deficits after telencephalic ablation in goldfish trained in place and turn maze procedures. *Behav. Neurosci.* 110:965–980.

Sanders, F.K. (1940) Second-order olfactory and visual learning in the optic tectum of the goldfish. *J. Exp. Biol.* 17:416–434.

Savage, G.E. (1971) Behavioural effects of electrical stimulation of the telencephalon of the goldfish, *Carassius auratus*. *Anim. Behav.* 19:661–668.

Savage, G.E. (1980) The fish telencephalon and its relation to learning. In S.O.E. Ebbesson (ed.): *Comparative Neurology of the Telencephalon*. Plenum Press, New York, pp. 129–174.

Schellart, N.A.M. (1992) Interrelations between the auditory, the visual and the lateral line systems of teleosts; a mini-review of modeling sensory capabilities. *Neth. J. Zool.* 42:459–477.

Schellart, N.A.M., and M. Prins (1993) Interspecific allometry of the teleost visual system; a new approach. *Neth. J. Zool.* 43:274–295.

Schlussman, S.D., M.A. Kobylack, A.A. Dunn-Meynell, and S.C. Sharma (1990) Afferent connections of the optic tectum in channel catfish *Ictalurus punctatus*. *Cell Tissue Res.* 262:531–541.

Schroeder, D.M. (1980) The telencephalon of teleosts. In *Comparative Neurology of the Telencephalon*. S.O.E. Ebbesson (ed): Plenum Press, New York, pp. 99–115.

Schwassmann, H.O. (1968) Visual projection upon the optic tectum in foveate marine teleosts. *Vis. Res.* 8:1337–1348.

Segaar, J., and R. Nieuwenhhuys (1963) New etho-physiological experiments with male *Gasterosteus aculeatus*, with anatomical comment. *Anim. Behav.* 11:331–344.

Springer, A.D., S.S. Easter, Jr., and B.W. Agranoff (1977) The role of the optic tectum in various visually mediated behaviors of goldfish. *Brain Res.* 128:393–404.

Staaden, M.J. van, R. Huber, L.S. Kaufman, and K.F. Liem (1994/95) Brain evolution in cichlids of the African Great Lakes: brain and body size, general patterns, and evolutionary trends. *Zoology* 98:165–178.
Striedter, G.F. (1991) Auditory, electrosensory, and mechanosensory lateral line pathways through the forebrain in channel catfishes. *J. Comp. Neurol.* 312:311–331.
Tavolga, W.N. (1971) Acoustic orientation in the sea catfish, *Galeichthys felis*. *Ann. N.Y. Acad. Sci.* 188:80–97.
Teyke, T. (1989) Learning and remembering the environment in the blind cave fish *Anoptichthys jordani*. *J. Comp. Physiol. A.* 164:655–662.
Tinbergen, N. (1951) *The Study of Instinct*. Oxford University Press, London, 228 pp.
Tuge, H., K. Uchihashi, and H. Shimamura (1968) *An Atlas of the Brains of Fishes of Japan*. Tsukiji Shokan, Tokyo, 240 pp.
Vanegas, H., and H. Ito (1983) Morphological aspects of the teleostean visual system: a review. *Brain Res. Rev.* 6:117–137.
Vanegas, H., and S.O.E. Ebbesson (1976) Telencephalic projections in two teleost species. *J. Comp. Neurol.* 165:181–196.
Vanegas, H., and S.O.E. Ebbesson (1980) Projections of the teleostean telencephalon. In S.O.E. Ebbesson (ed.): *Comparative Neurology of the Telencephalon*. Plenum Press, New York, pp. 117–127.
Vanegas, H. (1983) Organization and physiology of the teleostean optic tectum. In R.E. Davis and R.G. Northcutt (eds.): *Fish Neurobiology, vol. 2: Higher Brain Areas and Functions*. University of Michigan Press, Ann Arbor, pp. 43–90.
Warburton, K. (1990) The use of local landmarks by foraging goldfish. *Anim. Behav.* 40:500–505.
Warren, J.M. (1961) The effect of telencephalic injuries on learning by paradise fish, *Macropodus opercularis*. *J. Comp. Physiol. Psychol.* 54:130–132.
Wilson, R., and J.Q. Wilson (1985) *Pisces Guide to Watching Fishes: Understanding Coral Reef Fish Behavior*. Pisces Books, Houston, 275 pp.
Wullimann, M.F. (1987) The hypothalamic, ventricular channel-system and its phylogenetic distribution among fishes. *Proc. V Congr. Europ. Ichthyol. Stockholm.* pp. 65–72.
Wullimann, M.F. (1994) The teleostean torus longitudinalis: a short review on its structure, histochemistry, connectivity, possible function and phylogeny. *Eur. J. Morphol.* 32:235–242.
Wullimann, M.F. (1997) Major patterns of visual brain organization in teleosts and their relation to prehistoric events and the paleontological record. *J. Paleobiol.* 23:101–114.
Wullimann, M.F. (1998) The central nervous system. In D.H. Evans (ed.): *The Physiology of Fishes, 2nd ed*. CRC Press, Boca Raton, pp. 245–282.
Wullimann, M., W. Finck, and D.G. Senn (1984) A hypothalamic channel-system in the inferior lobes of a triggerfish (*Rhinecanthus aculeatus*, Balistidae). *Experientia* 40:725–727.
Wullimann, M.F., and D.L. Meyer (1990) Phylogeny of putative cholinergic visual pathways through the pretectum to the hypothalamus in teleost fish. *Brain Behav. Evol.* 36:14–29.
Wullimann, M.F., and D.L. Meyer (1993) Possible multiple evolution of indirect telencephalo-cerebellar pathways in teleosts: studies in *Carassius auratus* and *Pantodon buchholzi*. *Cell Tissue Res.* 274:447–455.
Wullimann, M.F,. and L. Puelles (1999) Postembryonic neural proliferation in the zebrafish forebrain and its relationship to prosomeric domains. *Anat. Embryol.* 329:329–348.
Wullimann, M.F., and G. Roth (1992) Is the nucleus corticalis of teleosts a new cholinergic central nervous system for vertebrates? *NeuroReport* 3:33–35.
Wullimann, M.F., and G. Roth (1994) Descending telencephalic information reaches longitudinal torus and cerebellum via the dorsal preglomerular nucleus in the teleost fish, *Pantodon buchholzi*: a case of neural preaptation? *Brain Behav. Evol.* 44:338–352.
Wyers, E.J. (1985) Cognitive behavior and sticklebacks. *Behavior* 95:1–10.
Yamane, Y., M. Yoshimoto, and H. Ito (1996) Area dorsalis pars lateralis of the telencephalon in a teleost (*Sebastiscus marmoratus*) can be divided into dorsal and ventral regions. *Brain Behav. Evol.* 48:338–349.
Yoshimoto, M., J.S. Albert, N. Sawai, M. Shimizu, N. Yamamoto, and H. Ito (1998) Telencephalic ascending gustatory system in a cichlid fish, *Oreochromis (Tilapia) niloticus*. *J. Comp. Neurol.* 392:209–226.

Chapter 11

COGNITION IN INSECTS: THE HONEYBEE AS A STUDY CASE*

Randolf Menzel, Martin Giurfa, Bertram Gerber, and Frank Hellstern, Institut für Neurobiologie, Freie Universität Berlin

INTRODUCTION: BRAIN, BEHAVIOR, AND BIOLOGY OF HONEYBEES

Behavior and Biology of Honeybees

Insects are small animals and therefore have small brains. Intuitively, small brains might be thought to provide the animal with less computational power, and, thus, insects might be expected to be less complex in their behavior than vertebrates. On a normalized scale, however, the brain size of honeybees is in the range of that of anamniote vertebrates. The cephalization index (Jerison's cephalization index: [brain weight/body weight] 2/3) equals 0.012 in the honeybee ([1 mg/85 mg] 2/3). In vertebrates, this index ranges between 0.007 (anamniotes) and 0.07 (birds, mammals) (Jerison, 1969; Russel, 1979). Still, the small absolute number of neurons (960,000 neurons in a volume of 1 mm3, Witthöft, 1967) might impose rigid constraints on brain function and limit behavioral flexibility, and in this respect insect brains share anatomical properties with salamanders (see Roth and Wake, this volume, Chapter 8). It might be, however, that it is not the total number of neurons but the relative temporal organization of excitation that is critical for brain function (Singer and Gray, 1995; Rieke et al., 1997) Furthermore, the computational power of single neurons might be far more important than current opinion suggests (Yuste and Tank, 1996), and the relatively large size of neurons of invertebrate brains may even provide additional units of function.

Is such a design more prone to stereotyped function, and are there additional major differences in the cognitive capacities of small brains with large neurons? Such a question can be addressed only by studying the output of the brain (i.e., the behavior of the animal) and its behavioral flexibility. Paradigms developed to analyze behavioral flexibility in vertebrates may be used for this purpose. Then it becomes possible to address questions such as which kinds of behavioral flexibility occur in insects, and are cognition-like concepts, such as *expectation, attention, prediction,* and *concept*

---

* This chapter is dedicated to the memory of Dr. Martin Hammer, who substantially contributed to the concepts presented here.

formation needed to describe behavioral flexibilities in insects. Moreover, it is worth asking how an insect brain supports such behavioral flexibility in order to search for possible mechanistic explanations of cognitive functions.

The multitude of flexible behaviors produced by the small number of peripheral and central neurons of a particular insect, the honeybee *Apis mellifera*, is most impressive. Honeybees are fast and elegant flyers, they quickly learn to manipulate a large range of differently constructed flowers for extracting pollen and nectar, and they do this in an effective way (Heinrich, 1984). They care for the brood, feed and clean their larvae according to their age and needs, and flexibly organize the distribution of tasks in their society (Frisch, 1967; Seeley, 1995). They communicate about the needs of the colony (nectar, pollen, water, propolis), and, with the aid of a ritualized body movement (waggle dance), they inform each other about the location and quality of a distant food source or a potential new nest site (Frisch, 1967).

Honeybees perceive colors in a trichromatic fashion over a spectral range that extends into ultraviolet and is shortened in the red (Menzel and Backhaus, 1991), and they discriminate patterns (Wehner, 1981; Srinivasan, 1994). These visual cues can be learned as signals for food or for the hive entrance (Menzel, 1985). Honeybees use the pattern of polarized light in the sky to navigate according to a time–compensated celestial compass (Wehner and Rossel, 1985). Compass directions between the hive and feeding sites are learned for each new feeding site and are related to the surrounding landmarks in such a way that compass directions can be inferred from them when the sky is overcast (Frisch and Lindauer, 1954; Dyer and Gould, 1981). The flight direction relative to the sun compass is converted into an angle of the body length axis relative to gravity during the waggle dance on the vertical comb. Flight distances are measured visually (Esch and Burns, 1995, 1996; Srinivasan et al., 1996) and transposed into the frequency of body movements during the communicative waggle dance. The precise localization of the hive entrance or a feeding site is learned relative to its associated landmarks (Cartwright and Collett, 1983), and landmarks en route are learned in a sequential order (Chittka and Geiger, 1995). A sense of the earth's magnetic field is used to facilitate learning the relative position of a food source (Collett and Baron, 1994) and performing the waggle dance more accurately (Lindauer and Martin, 1972).

The choice between food sources is not random but depends very much on experience at the various food sources (Greggers and Menzel, 1993). The effort invested in obtaining the food and its caloric value allow the bees to build specific memories of the food sources and guide foraging decisions (Waddington, 1985; Menzel et al., 1993). Odors also play an important role in the organization of the community and as learned signals of food sources. They are learned particularly quickly and are very well discriminated (Bitterman et al., 1983). The number of odors honeybees can discriminate appears to be nearly unlimited (Vareschi, 1971).

Thus, honeybees are able to retain information and recall it later in relevant occasions and appropriate contexts. New information is integrated into information already acquired and stored in discrete units. It can only be concluded that such a rich perceptual and behavioral repertoire and such a wide range of adaptive processes cannot be the product of an inflexible form of information processing, but must result from well-developed modes of learning and memory. The next step is to ask how complex such a memory is, whether memory leads to internal representations, and whether some form of operation on internal representations does occur during memory retrieval and formation. Can such an operation lead to an expectation about the future as a consequence of earlier learning? How rich are these representations, and what might be meant by "expectation" in an insect? How are those operations performed by the brain of a honeybee?

As in all studies on cognition in animals, we face the problem that assumptions about the existence of representations and operating on them can often be refuted by seemingly simpler assumptions that should be preferred over more complex ones, (e.g., by explaining behavioral flexibility in associative terms). Because applying Occam's razor and Morgan's canon (Morgan, 1894) is critical for interpreting results on cognitive capabilities of animals, it will be our special concern to focus on paradigms testing predictions that cannot be met by assumptions on associative activity.

To address the problem of cognition in the honeybee as a case study, we first give a short overview of the design of this insect's brain. Then we look into simple forms of associative learning and briefly outline experimental evidence that allows us to raise the question whether the establishment of *elementary* associations might involve cognition-like processes of attention or expectation and prediction. We then move on to forms of associative learning that involve relational dependencies. We shall call the latter *configural* forms of learning (Rudy and Sutherland, 1992). Examples are drawn from olfactory conditioning, visual learning in a natural setting, and navigation. We demonstrate that honeybees evince the capacity of building not only elementary but also configural associations, and thus we shall conclude that the learning performance of an insect like the honeybee can, at least qualitatively, be comparable with that of vertebrates. This indicates that, even if vertebrate and invertebrate structures differ at the neural and sensory levels, similar neuronal mechanisms of solving problems posed by the environment may have been implemented through natural selection.

Design of an Insect Brain

The arthropod brain differs from that of the vertebrate brain in several basic features. It is subdivided into neuropils that are formed by well-structured arrangements of synaptically connected dendrites and axodendrons (Fig. 11.1). The neural tissue is compact and does not include ventricles or internal fluid-filled spaces. Neurons communicate via their dendrites and their axodendrons, but somata are usually excluded from the processing of electrical signals. Most of the somata lie in the epithelial layer surrounding the brain (supra- and subesophageal ganglion) and the ventral ganglia of the body segments. Although the number of neurons in the insect brain is rather small, some neurons may be large in comparison to the size of the brain (Fig. 11.1). Several neurons have been identified structurally, and two of these neurons have also been functionally identified at the level of the individual neuron, the VUMmx1 with its soma in the subesophageal ganglion and its axodendrons in the supraoesophageal ganglion, and the Pe–1, a mushroom body extrinsic neuron, which

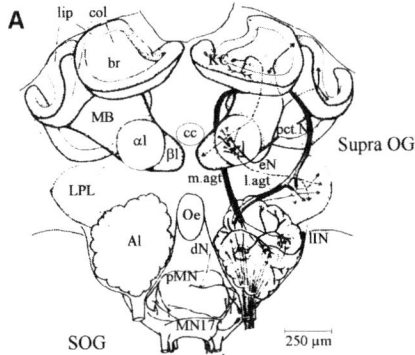

Figure 11.1. (A) The brain of the honeybee consists of the subesophageal ganglion (SOG) and the supraoesophageal ganglion (Supra OG). The supraoesophageal ganglion receives input from the compound eyes via the visual ganglia (to the right and left, not shown) and the chemo– and mechanosensory receptors on the antennae and other parts of the head. Several highly organized structures are embedded in a diffuse neuropil. These structures are the antennal lobes (Al), the mushroom bodies (MB), and the central complex (cc). The figure highlights the structures and neurons involved in olfactory coding and learning. The Al receives input from 60,000 chemosensory receptor neurons that project to 160 spherical glomerular compartments in the Al. The 160 glomeruli are interconnected by local interneurons (lIN) and give rise to projection neurons, which connect Al the with the MB and a lateral brain region, the lateral protocerebral lobe (LPL). The projection neurons run in three distinct fiber tracks (m.agt, l.agt, and ml.agt, the latter not shown). The MB is a higher order multisensory integration center consisting of 160,000 densely packed neurons, the Kenyon cells (KC). The input of the MB is separated according to sensory modalities; the lip (which receives olfactory input), the collar (col) (receiving visual input), and the basal ring (br), whose input is uncertain. The MBs are connected to all other brain regions via extrinsic neurons (eN) leaving the MB in the alpha and beta lobes (αl, βl). One of these neurons is the PE1, an identified neuron projecting from the αl to the LPL. Descending neurons (dN) originating in the LPL connect the Supra OG and the SOG and drive the premotor and motor neurons (pMN, MN) in the SOG. *contd on opposite page.*

connects the mushroom body with the premotor output region of the brain (Fig.11.1). It is quite possible that there are many such individually recognizable neurons. The VUMmx1 neuron (Fig. 11.1B), for example, extends throughout the supraesophageal ganglion and connects it to the subesophageal ganglion, which is associated with those three body segments serving the mouth parts behind the frontal head segments. Other neurons interconnect neuropils, (e.g., the antennal lobes [Al]) with the mushroom bodies (MBs) and the MBs with the lateral protocerebrum. Each of these neurons belongs to a rather small group of neurons (from 2 to 2000 neurons per group) of similar structure and function and can easily be identified as a member of this group. For example, the neurons connecting the Al with the MBs do so via three tracts, each of which is composed of only a few hundred axons (Fig. 11.1A). Thus, uniqueness and small number of neurons appear to be a general design feature of the insect brain.

We do not yet understand whether such a design leads to basically different computational processes compared with brains that are less constrained in their absolute size and cell number, as in most vertebrate brains, but we recognize that each neuron

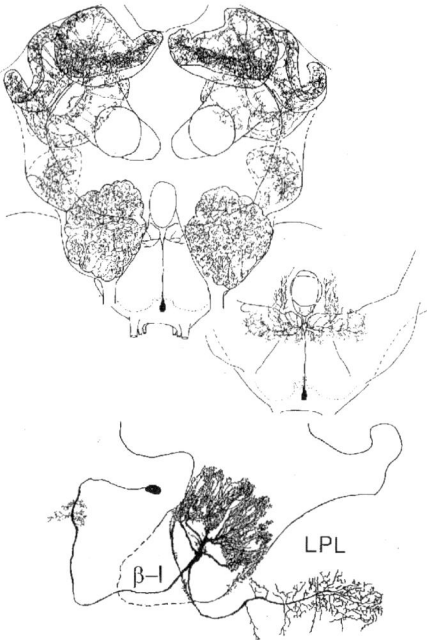

Figure 11.1. contd.
(B) A few of the 960,000 neurons in the honeybee brain have been identified at the individual cell level. Two examples are shown: the PE1 (lower panel) and the VUMmx1 (upper pannel). The latter neuron belongs to a group of ventral unpaired median neurons (six in each of the three SOG neuromeres), whose somata are located in the ventral midline of the SOG. These neurons receive input from sucrose receptors in the proboscis and probably on the antenna, and other neurons in the SOG. VUMmx1 is one of these neurons and projects to the paired Al, MB , and LPL structures in the Supra OG. It converges with neurons of the olfactory pathway. The VUMmx1 was found to instruct the brain about the reinforcing component of sucrose stimulation during appetitive olfactory learning (see text). (from Hammer and Menzel, 1995, by permission of Society for NeuroScience, Washington).

addresses a much larger relative portion of other brain neurons than is the case in vertebrates. Are such neurons capable of implementing higher computational power in the sense that they in themselves are sufficient to produce or modulate units of behavior? A positive answer to this question may be provided by studying the neuron VUMmx1 (Hammer, 1993). This neuron converges with the olfactory pathway in the honeybee brain at three sites, the Al, the lip and basal ring region of the input area (calyx) of the MB, and the lateral protocerebral lobe (LPL), an output region of the brain (Fig. 11.1B). Sucrose stimulation triggers the extension of the proboscis as a reflex response (see below) and leads to excitation of VUMmx1. Although stimulation of VUMmx1 itself does not lead to reflexive proboscis extension, this neuron mediates the reinforcing function of reward during appetitive olfactory learning: its depolarization substitutes the reward in olfactory conditioning (Hammer, 1993). Thus, a single neuron is sufficient to instruct the honeybee brain about the reinforcing value of a stimulus and to implement, already at a single-cell level, some characteristic properties postulated for reinforcement in associative learning (Hammer and Menzel, 1995; Hammer, 1997).

The visual ganglia (lamina, medulla, lobula), the primary chemosensory processing neuropil (the Al), and a few smaller neuropils (dorsal lobe, the mechanosensory and motor center of the antennae; the unpaired central complex with the protocerebral bridge and the central body, which are thought to be involved in higher order motor processing) are well separated from the more diffuse neuropils (Fig. 11.1A). The most obvious and voluminous structures in the insect brain are the two MBs. In the case of the honeybee, each MB consists of two calyces of identical substructure, each with 160,000 tightly packed neurons, the Kenyon cells. Such neurons receive their input in the calyx region and send two collaterals to the alpha and bete lobe, the output regions of the MB (Mobbs, 1982). The calyx region of honeybees is subdivided into three major input areas (i.e., lip, collar, and basal ring) that receive input from different sensory systems. Olfactory projection neurons connecting the antennal lobe with the MBs project to the lip but not to the collar (Mobbs, 1982, 1984; Homberg, 1984). Visual projection neurons from the medulla and the lobula project to the MBs in a complementary way (viz., to the collar but not to the lip) (Mobbs, 1982, 1984; Gronenberg, 1986; Bicker et al., 1993). Thus, the compartmentalization of the MB inputs suggests separate central systems for processing visual and olfactory signals. The connectivity of the basal ring is uncertain: Initial reports of visual (Gronenberg, 1986) and olfactory (Mobbs, 1982) input could not be substantiated (Mobbs, 1984, 1985; Bicker et al., l993). An interaction between visual and olfactory processing might, thus, occur downstream of the input region of the MBs. This suggestion is in line with the observation that, although the MB input is clearly separated in modality, its output neurons are typically multimodal (Erber, 1978; see also Maronde, 1991) for additional convergence points of visual and olfactory processing).

The multisensory convergence in the MBs suits them well for highe order multimodal computations, in particular for relational, context-dependent neural plasticities. Indeed, the MBs are known to be intimately related to olfactory learning and memory (Hammer and Menzel, 1995; Menzel and Müller, 1996). So far, however, there is no evidence allowing us to implicate the MBs directly in either visual or cross -modality learning processes in the bee.

ELEMENTARY AND CONFIGURAL FORMS OF LEARNING IN CLASSICAL CONDITIONING

The Preparation: Classical Conditioning of the Proboscis Extension Reflex

Honeybees can be conditioned to olfactory stimuli. The experimental situation as shown in Figure 11.2 allows the free movement of the bee's antennae and mouth parts. The antennae are the main chemosensory organs. When they are touched with sucrose solution, the honeybee reflexively extends its proboscis to reach and suck the sucrose.

Elementary and Configural Forms of Learning in Classical Conditioning

Unlike sucrose solution, odorants do not release such a reflex in naive animals. If, however, an odorant is presented immediately before the sucrose solution (forward pairing), an association is formed that enables the odorant to release the proboscis extension response (PER) in a following test. This effect is clearly associative and involves classic, but not operant, conditioning (Bitterman et al., 1983). Thus, the odorant can be viewed as the conditioned stimulus and the sucrose solution as the reinforcing, unconditioned stimulus. PER conditioning shows most of the basic characteristics of classic conditioning, namely, acquisition (Fig. 11.2B) and extinction, differential conditioning and reversal learning (Fig. 11.2C), stimulus specificity and generalization, dependence on odorant as well as on reinforcement intensity, dependence on the temporal interval between stimulus and reinforcement, and dependence on the temporal interval between learning trials (Menzel, 1990). Physiological correlates of such behavioral phenomena can be found at different levels, ranging from molecular biology and biochemistry to single identified neurons and optical imaging of neuronal ensembles using $Ca^{2+}-$ as well as voltage-sensitive dyes (Hammer and Menzel, 1995; Menzel and Müller, 1996).

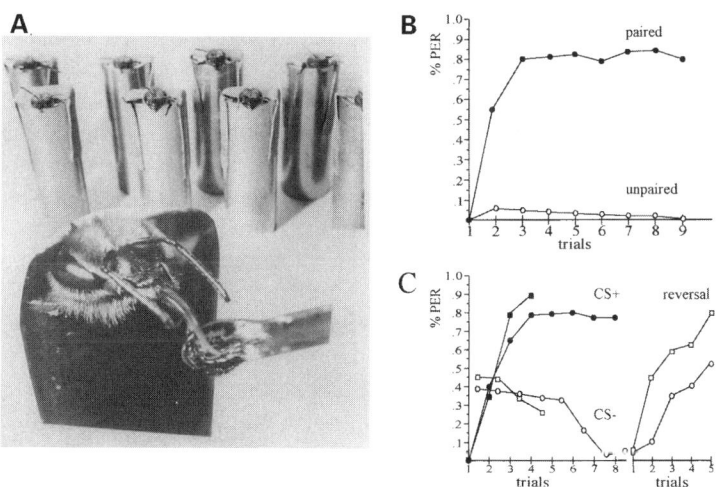

Figure 11.2. (A) The proboscis extension response (PER) paradigm. Honeybees are harnessed in little metal tubes in such a way that they are free to move their antennae and mouthparts. Touching the antennae with a drop of sucrose solution releases the PER in hungry bees. The PER can be conditioned to an olfactory stimulus by forward pairing of the odor with sucrose. The bees will respond with the PER later when the odor is given alone. (B) Acquisition of the PER by bees trained by either multiple forward pairing trials of conditioned stimulus (CS) and unconditioned stimulus (US) (paired) or by unpaired presentations of CS and US (unpaired). During training with forward pairings, the CS preceded the US by 2 seconds during a trial; therefore, each forward conditioning trial also includes a test situation, the 2 seconds of CS presentation before the onset of the US. An extension of the proboscis during this period is evaluated as a conditioned response and expressed as probability of PER in a group of bees (ordinate). (C) Differential conditioning with four (squares) or eight (circles) trials (left graph). During differential conditioning, one odor is paired with sucrose (CS+); the other odor is presented unpaired (CS–) between the CS+ trials. The interval between CS+ and CS– trials was 5 minutes. During reversal training (30 minutes after differential conditioning), the former CS– is now paired with the sucrose stimulus and, thus, becomes the CS+ (right graph) (see text).

A Cognitive Approach to Memory Dynamics

Memory is the capacity to retain acquired information and to use it for future behavior. In the context of association theory, memory is nothing but the potential of a conditioned stimulus to bring an established associative link into action. Learning, however, might be viewed as a process of acquiring information rather than responses (Tolman, 1932). Support for such a cognitive interpretation of memory and learning in the honeybee comes from the fact that memory formation is not identical with the process of acquisition. Memory needs time to develop and proceeds through phases of qualitative differences with respect to its susceptibility to interfering events and its content. Memory phases may also differ regarding retrievability and interaction with newly learned tasks. All these aspects of memory have been proved to exist in the honeybee (Menzel, 1990).

The fact that memory formation needs time to develop (Fig. 11.3A) and shows the typical U–shaped time course with a "dip" around 3 minutes (the "Kamin effect"; Kamin, 1957) may be indicative of a consolidation process and/or a time-dependent retrieval effect. Evidence for both mechanisms exists in honeybees (Menzel, 1990). The two stages of memory apparent in Figure. 11.3A can be viewed as unavoidable consequences of the neural and cellular machinery underlying the formation of long-term memory because strengthening an existing memory trace may take time. There is strong experimental support for this interpretation in many animals, including the honeybee (Menzel and Müller, 1996). Additionally, it may also reflect processes that integrate different attributes of the learning event (e.g., its novelty, its configuration with other stimuli; see below) into an existing memory in such a way that the initial memory contains the elementary associations and the processed memory the constructed configural forms (Rudy, 1996). There are some hints in favor of this interpretation in honeybees as well. The specificity of stimulus memory rises over time (Fig. 11.3B), and generalization between stimuli of the same modality (olfaction) is different shortly after olfactory conditioning and at longer intervals (Menzel, 1990; Smith, 1991). Thus, the memory content is, indeed, different at different times after conditioning, but the mechanistic basis for these differences is not yet understood.

The hypothesis that the "dip" function reflects memory consolidation is mainly based on a number of studies suggesting that around 3 minutes after a single learning trial memory shows a time window of high susceptibility to interference (Menzel, 1990; Hammer and Menzel, 1995). To investigate how the consolidation status affects long–term retention, we tested intertrial intervals (ITIs) of 30 seconds, 1 minutes, 3 minutes and 20 minutes that cover the "dip" function (Fig. 11.3C). Interestingly, long–term retention (LTR) depends nonmonotonously on the ITI (Fig. 11.3A); this contrasts with the monotonous increase of LTR usually observed in mammals with increasing ITIs (Hintzman, 1974). To explain the low LTR levels for 3 minutes ITIs, we suggest that memories established on consecutive trials interfere with each other's consolidation during the previously mentioned window of high interference susceptibility and are consolidated at each other's expense (Hintzman, 1974). This may be due to two memories competing for a limited neural capacity for consolidation. Low LTR levels for 30 seconds ITIs could be explained by two

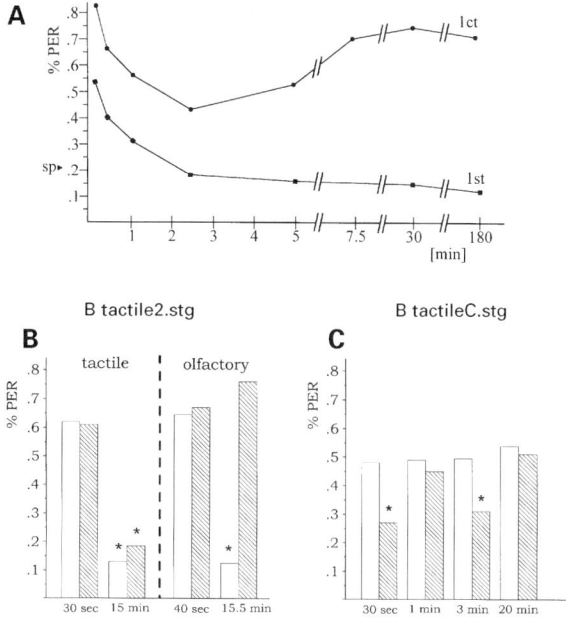

Figure 11.3. Memory dynamics. (A) A single conditioning trial in the proboscis extension response (PER) paradigm (1ct) induces a highly dynamic retention. Retention is high immediately after the conditioning trial and then loses strength, but increases again afterward (consolidation). A single trial with the unconditioned stimulus alone (one sensitization trial, 1st) leads to an increased response (to an olfactory stimulus), which relaxes to spontaneous level (sp) within a few seconds. Thus retention at short intervals (<3 minutes) is highly dominated by nonspecific arousal. (After Menzel, 1990.) (B) The early and the late memory phases differ with respect to their contents. If, for example, a tactile stimulus to the antennae is used to test stimulus specificity of the memory after an olfactory conditioning trial, one finds that PER to both olfactory (dark bars) and tactile (light bars) stimulation is high during the early phase (30 seconds after one trial conditioning), but is low for tactile and high for olfactory stimuli during the late phase (15 minutes after conditioning). Thus, consolidation leads to more specific memory over time. (C) Memory dynamics during acquisition is also reflected in long–term memory. Changing the inter trial interval (abscissa) between multiple (five) learning trials induces memories of various strengths in the long–term range (4 days, dark bars) but not in the intermediate–term range (1 day, light bars). The intertrial interval has a nonmonotonous effect on long–term retention (LTR) in that response levels for very short (30 seconds) and intermediate (3 minute) intertrial interval decrease from day 1 to day 4, whereas training with 1 or 20 minute intertrial intervals results in stable long–term retention.

mechanisms: (1) habituation could impair the capacity of reward to induce LTR (Hintzman, 1974). However, the number of sucrose stimulations leading to habituation is much higher (>200 trials, Braun and Bicker, 1992), than the number of conditioning trials used in our case (five). Thus, habituation may not completely account for our results with 30 seconds ITIs. (2) Backward inhibitory learning (for honeybees, see below) could play an additional role (Ewing et al., 1985; but see Barnet et al., 1995). A sucrose reward on the first trial could exert both an excitatory effect on the preceding and, with short ITIs, an inhibitory effect on the following odorant presentation. For honeybees, the time course of inhibitory backward learning (see below) is consistent with such a role, at least for very short ITIs.

The Elementary-Configural Distinction

In the field of associative learning, it has become increasingly clear that there might be two forms of associations: elementary and configural associations (Rudy and Sutherland, 1992; Pearce, 1994). To illustrate this distinction, consider the following two discrimination problems: The first problem involves reinforced presentations of a stimulus A and unreinforced presentations of a stimulus B (A+/B–). This discrimination can be solved by forming associations to each single (elementary) stimulus with its respective outcome. The second problem involves reinforced presentations of two stimulus compounds (AB+ and CD+) and unreinforced presentations of two other compounds made up from other combinations of the same elements (AC– and BD–). To solve this discrimination task, subjects cannot rely on single components but have to respond to specific stimulus configurations (i.e., to A only if it occurs in the context of B, but not in the context of C, and to D only if it occurs in the context of C but not in the context of B). Thus, the learned configuration is unique and can be discriminated from its components.

Cognitive Aspects of Elementary Forms of Conditioning?

Traditionally, classic conditioning has been viewed as an automatized, passive process in the sense that whenever a neutral stimulus (A) and a reinforcing stimulus (+) occur together, they are associated. In other words, a joint occurrence of A and reinforcement (A+) was thought to be both necessary and sufficient to induce associative learning. Associative processing of internal representations of stimuli in the brain would, then, be a simple, one–to–one function of these stimuli in the external world. This is not, however, an adequate conceptualization, as the next paragraph will make clear.

Backward inhibitory learning. Learning psychologists recognized that a stimulus A that precedes reinforcement (forward pairing, A+) subsequently leads to conditioned responses. When the sequence of stimuli is reversed (backward pairing, +A), however, no or weaker conditioning occurs. Recent research has revealed that backward pairing does not result in an absence of learning, but often in inhibitory learning (Moscovitch and Lolordo, 1968; Wagner and Larew, 1985). In other words, whether an excitatory or inhibitory association will be formed can be regulated by the nervous system according to the temporal relation between the stimuli involved (Rescorla and Wagner, 1972).

Backward inhibitory conditioning has recently been demonstrated in honeybees by both retardation of acquisition and summation assays (Hellstern et al., 1997) (Fig. 11.4). The extent of inhibition depends nonmonotonously on the interval between reinforcement and A: Maximal inhibition is observed with a 15 second interval between reinforcement and A, whereas shorter (6 second) as well as longer (30 to 600 second) intervals result in less or no inhibition. This is qualitatively in line with experiments on the rabbit nictitating membrane reflex (Wagner and Larew, 1985) and, thus, confirms for an invertebrate predictions of some of the most widely accepted formal associative learning theories developed for mammals (Sutton and Barto, 1981; Wagner, 1981; Klopf, 1989).

Blocking. Is the predictive value of a stimulus for reinforcement sufficient for an association to be established? An experiment by Kamin (1968) showed that this is not the case: Training a compound stimulus AX after a pretraining phase with one of its elements (A) produces less conditioned responding to X during a final test than in a control group that did not experience pretraining with A. Thus, pretraining of A has somehow *blocked* the development of conditioned responses to X. Such a phenomenon has, therefore, been called *blocking*. In other words, whether or not an association is formed between X and reinforcement can be regulated by the nervous system according to whether or not an association between A and reinforcement already exists. This finding was instrumental for most current formal theories on associative learning, and two basic approaches have been used to try to explain its mechanistic basis. Although both are formally very similar, they differ in the processes thought to underlie blocking. The first approach (Rescorla and Wagner, 1972; Sutton and Barto, 1981) holds that reinforcing stimuli can only support associations when they occur in an unpredictable way. Because during training with AX reinforcement is already predicted by A, that predicted reinforcement is no longer effective in supporting an association with X. Thus, the effectiveness of reinforcement processing is suggested to be regulated according to its predictedness. The second approach (e.g., Mackintosh, 1975) holds that during training with AX, subjects do not devote attention to X because it is embedded in an already well–known event. Thus, it is suggested that processing of X is regulated by an attentional process.

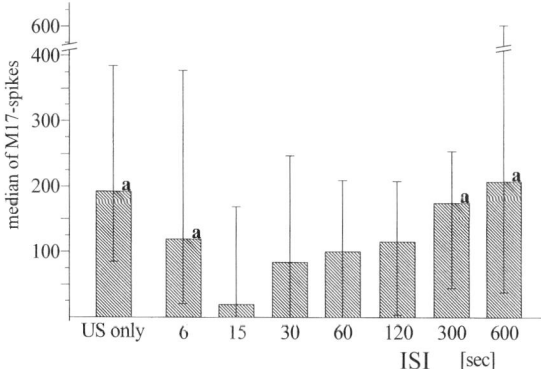

Figure 11.4. Conditioned inhibition. A single backward–pairing trail of an olfactory conditioned stimulus (CS) and a sucrose unconditioned stimulus (US) produces conditioned inhibition with a nonmonotonous interstimulus interval (ISI) dependency. Eight groups of bees are first conditioned with one backward trial. The groups differ by the interstimulus interval (6, 15, 30, 60, 120, 300, 600 seconds; US only: no CS). Half an hour later, the bees receive one CS/US forward trial with an optimal interstimulus interval of 2 seconds. Again half an hour later the strength of the conditioned response is tested in an extinction trial. The strength of the response is evaluated by the number of muscle potentials of a muscle (M17) involved in proboscis extension (ordinate). The response strengths between the groups differ according to their experimental history (df = 7, T = 14.93, p < 0.05, H test). Groups that significantly differ from the group with a 15 second ISI are marked by an a. (after Hellstern et al., 1997).

In the behavioral literature on vertebrates, it is not yet clear which of these two models is more appropriate. The two models differ with respect to processing of either reinforcement or X (and these differences are especially important for a physiological analysis), because different neural pathways are involved. Both approaches have stimulated physiological investigations that have either implicated midbrain dopamine neurons in variations of reinforcement processing (Schultz et al., 1997) or the amygdala in variations of X processing (Holland, 1993). Taken together, associative stimulus processing can be regulated in a flexible fashion to suppress processing of already predicted reinforcing stimuli and/or to focus attention on novel events and away from known ones.

Blocking within binary odorant mixtures has been demonstrated in bees by Smith and Cobey for PER conditioning and has been considerably elaborated (Smith, 1996, 1997). We were not successful, however, in reproducing these results (Gerber, 1998). Thus, the question whether blocking occurs in olfactory PER conditioning is still partially open, particularly in terms of which control procedures need to be used. In free–flying honeybees, substantial efforts to find blocking have failed (reviewed by Bitterman, 1996). Those efforts involved cross–modality compounds (vision and olfaction), and the results suggested that compound processing within one modality might follow different rules compared with cross–modality compounds (Bitterman, 1996). Recently, Couvillon et al. (1997) did find blocking in free–flying honeybees within both the visual and the olfactory modalities, but not across modalities. These results were taken as supporting the "independence" assumption (Bitterman, 1996), which holds that elements of cross–modality compounds change associative strength independently of each other. This would be a fundamental difference in honeybee learning compared with vertebrate learning. Taken together, the generality of blocking across stimulus modalities and between learning paradigms is still uncertain.

Second–order conditioning. The presence of reinforcement is not necessary in all cases of conditioning. Such evidence comes from "second-order conditioning" in mammals (Rescorla, 1980). If a stimulus A is paired with reinforcement in a first experimental phase (A+) and then paired with a second stimulus X in the absence of reinforcement (AX–) in a second phase, conditioned responses to X typically develop as well. Subsequent research has revolved around the question whether responses to X are based on chain–like associations (X associated with A, associated with reinforcement) or whether X is associated with an internal representation of reinforcement triggered by A (Holland, 1990). Regardless of these considerations, the physical presence of reinforcement apparently is not a necessary condition for an excitatory association to be formed.

Thus far, second–order conditioning has not been convincingly demonstrated in honeybee classic conditioning. Earlier reports (Takeda, 1961; Bitterman et al., 1983) might be regarded as preliminary due to a lack of thorough control procedures.

Taken together, elementary associative learning is more complex than often thought (Rescorla, 1988; Holland, 1993), and at least some of these complex aspects likewise apply to honeybee olfactory conditioning. Reinforcement that is present may not be associated with preceding stimuli (blocking) but the absence of reinforcement might (second-order conditioning). Furthermore, the kind of associations formed depends on the predictive relation of stimuli to reinforcement (the forward–backward distinction). To account for these findings, association theories had to incorporate cognition–like processes of attention (Mackintosh, 1975) and/or of expectation and prediction (Rescorla and Wagner, 1972; Sutton and Barto, 1981). With respect to brain physiology, these models suggest highly flexible associative processing of stimuli that is far beyond an automatic, one–to–one function of events occurring in the external world. In this sense, cognition–like processes seem to govern to some extent the establishment of elementary associations in the honeybee as well.

Configural Forms of Conditioning

Biconditional discrimination. In their natural environments, animals are confronted not with single stimuli indicating certain events but with a large number of stimuli at any moment of their lives. They need to be able to integrate these stimuli in such a way that they can select those combinations that are reliable predictors for important events such as the emergence of food, predators, or conspecifics. In this situation, elementary associations alone are often insufficient to solve the problem; therefore, configural associations have to be assumed. Depending on the nature of co–occurring stimuli, a single stimulus might be indicative of different behaviors. Accordingly, the question of how this integration works has always been of great interest for the analysis of stimulus processing and learning. Saavedra (1975) showed that rabbits are able to solve a biconditional discrimination task in which four different stimuli (A, B, C, D) are presented in binary combinations. For example, combinations AB and CD are followed by reinforcement (+), whereas the combinations AC and BD are not. Rabbits learn that a stimulus A presented in the context of a stimulus B is different from the same stimulus A when presented in the context of a stimulus C. As a consequence, rabbits respond less to nonreinforced than to reinforced compounds. Elementary theories based on the assumption that the response to a stimulus compound depends solely on the summed associative strengths of single elements cannot explain such an outcome.

In the case of the honeybee, recent studies have shown that honeybees are capable of solving such configural problems in the PER -paradigm (Hellstern et al., 1995). In an olfactory biconditional discrimination task with binary compounds composed of two odorants, honeybees responded more strongly to the reinforced compounds (AB+, CD+) than to the unreinforced compounds (AC−, BD−). Only five presentations of each compound, regardless of being reinforced or unreinforced, were sufficient to obtain these results—a fact that underlines the remarkable learning capacities of this insect. Additional test trials revealed that the responses to the compound cannot be predicted on the basis of the responses to the single elements.

Negative and positive patterning. Furthermore, another class of patterning problems is used to investigate whether elementary or configural associations are formed (Woodbury, 1943; Bellingham et al., 1985; Lachnit and Kimmel, 1993). Here, either two single stimuli are followed by reinforcement (A+, B+) while a binary compound of the same stimuli is not (AB–, negative patterning), or the single elements are nonreinforced (A–, B–) but the compound is followed by reinforcement (AB+, positive patterning). The fact that less responses occur to the single elements than to the compound in positive patterning can be explained by elementary theories like the Rescorla–Wagner model (Rescorla and Wagner, 1972). Simple summation of the associative strengths of the two elements is sufficient to obtain higher associative strength and, consequently, higher responsiveness to the compound. Negative patterning (where the responses to the compound are less than those to each of the two single elements), however, can only be explained if configural associations are taken into account. Only theories including considerations of a unique cue (Whitlow and Wagner, 1972), a configural cue (Rudy and Sutherland, 1992) or a configural unit (Pearce, 1994) can explain such an outcome. In negative patterning, the compound can, via a configural association, gain or lose associative strength more or less independently of the single elements.

PER conditioning can also be used to test whether honeybees are able to solve patterning problems. Positive patterning has been found (Hellstern, unpublished data, 1998). The responses to the compound exceeded by far those to single elements. Preliminary data on negative patterning suggest that under certain conditions bees are also able to solve this problem (i.e., to respond less to the compound than to the single elements). The ability to respond to one stimulus in two different ways depending on the context in which the stimulus occurs has also been shown under natural conditions (see below).

LEARNING IN THE NATURAL CONTEXT

Context–Dependent Learning and Retrieval

Are elementary associations sufficient to explain learning behavior of honeybees under natural conditions? Karl von Frisch's classic training experiments (Frisch, 1914, 1967) showed elementary associations to be critical for guiding learning of natural stimuli (colors, odors, and shapes of flowers; locations of foraging places and nest sites). Cues closely attached to food and nest sites are so easily and quickly learned (Menzel, 1985) that one may ask whether relational conditions between cues and their configuration with other memories into unique forms of more complex memories might be a strategy applied by such a small brain. For example, honeybees trained to forage on a blue target at place A in the morning and on a yellow target at place B in the afternoon subsequently search for blue at A and for yellow at B at any time of the day (Menzel, unpublished data) (Fig. 11.5). Furthermore, they choose blue and yellow equally often at a place half way between A and B.

Additional evidence for context–dependent learning and memory retrieval comes from the analysis of the waggle dance (Frisch, 1967) and from navigation experiments (Menzel et al., 1996). Consider the following situation (see Fig. 11.7A, below): Honeybees are trained to forage at two feeding sites: at S_m (630 m from the hive toward 115° from north) in the morning and at S_a (790 m, 40°) in the afternoon. If these bees are captured when leaving the hive and are released at S_a in the morning and at S_m in the afternoon, they will fly straight back to the hive along a route that they use to fly from the respective feeding site (S_a or S_m) to the hive. In such a situation, the bees have retrieved the memory for the correct flight path toward the hive from long–term memory storage. In addition, they have changed their motivation, because they were captured at the moment of leaving the hive heading toward S_m in the morning and S_a in the afternoon. Thus, landmarks characterizing S_m and S_a act as retrieval cues, activate a memory for the return flight path associated with these cues, repress a memory, which would have guided bees to the other feeding place along a flight path originating at the hive, and induce a change in the bees' motivation, from departing from the hive to returning to the hive.

This interpretation is supported by the following observation. The replacement of active memory by a newly recruited working memory is not possible in all motivational states. Honeybees just arriving at the feeding site or leaving it after feeding choose the compass flight directions they would have taken had they not been transported and released at the unexpected site. Thus, bees at the food source have such a strong active memory of the vectors between hive and feeding site, or are so much less attentive to the learned local cues they are experiencing at the unexpected release site, that the active memory cannot be replaced by a newly recruited working memory (Menzel et al., 1998). We conclude from this kind of experiment that in both the spatial and temporal domains multiple forms of memory exist. The connections between these memories can be viewed as strings of associations between separate

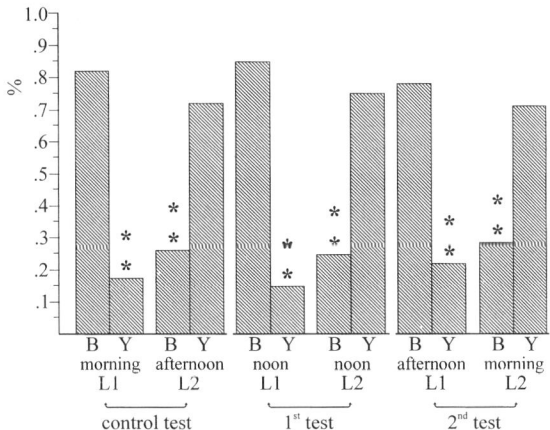

Figure 11.5. Context–specific memory retrieval in free–flying honeybees. Groups of bees are trained in a dual choice color discrimination task to a blue target (B) at location L1 in the morning (10 to 11 am) and to yellow (Y) at location L2 in the afternoon (2 to 3 pm). L1 is located 35 m to the west, L2 45 m to the north of the hive. The local landmarks at L1 and L2 are very different (walls of a building at L1; bushes and lawn at L2). The control test shows that bees choose the colors connected with the two locations. In a first test, bees are tested at midday (12 noon to 1 pm) simultaneously at both locations. The bees, which come to the two locations outside of their training time, choose correctly for the respective location. In a second test, bees are tested at L1 in the afternoon and at L2 in the morning. Again they choose correctly for the respective location and not for the time of the day. Number of choices: control test: morning L1 1260, afternoon L2 1090; first test: noon L1 584, noon L2 614; second test: afternoon L1 372, morning L2 402; c2– test, **: $p < 0.01$.

memories or as aspects of a unique spatial representation. Below, we present experiments that test these interpretations. In particular, we want to emphasize the richness of these spatiotemporal memories and their mutual dependencies, as well as the transfer of traces between two stages of long–term memory—an active form and a remote form—that provides a reference and can be retrieved by appropriate cues. The transfer between these two forms depends not only on external cues but also on the bee's internal status (i.e., its motivation). The internal status appears to define the attentiveness toward stimuli and/or the strength of the active memory.

Serial Order in a Spatiotemporal Domain

The structure of the active memory is accessible by experiments that test the sequence of behavioral units. The question is, does the animal "expect" a particular signal or outcome in a stepwise fashion when passing through a learned sequence of events, or are the cues of each event associatively connected just to the next event in such a way that a chain of simple associations lead the animal from one event to the next? Foraging honeybees experience such sequences on two scales (viz., on a large scale, when passing landmarks on the way toward the goal, and on a small scale, when making the final approach flight and choosing between a number of potential food sources).

On a large scale, honeybees visually estimate the distance to and from a feeding place by estimating the speed of the flow field and the time flown (Esch and Burns, 1996; Srinivasan et al., 1996). In addition, they learn the sequence and number of landmarks in such a way that they search for the food source at the correct relative position according to the sequence and number of landmarks passed on the way toward the food source (Chittka and Geiger, 1995; Chittka et al., 1995). Bees are trained to fly a fixed distance between the hive and the feeding site along a flight path marked by a succession of landmarks, likewise separated by fixed distances. When the distance between such an array of successive, equal landmarks of equal distance is stretched, honeybees shift their search frequencies to distances larger than the trained one. When the array is compressed, honeybees search at closer distances. Therefore, honeybees are not only guided by the actual distance between hive and feeder, but also navigate according to the relationship between the sequential arrangement of landmarks. This result is compatible with the idea that honeybees establish a memory of the number of landmarks to be passed before reaching the goal. The behavior of the honeybees is more than simple judgment of inequality, such as many versus few (Gelman and Gallistel, 1978; Davis and Memmott 1982). In the sense of Davis and Memmott (1982), the observed behavior of the honeybees fulfills the criteria of counting. Gelman and Gallistel (1978) and Davis and Perusse (1988), however, incorporate another requirement into their definition of time counting, the "abstraction principle". This principle purports that after having learned to perform a given behavioral unit assigned to a certain number of objects counted, the subject should be able to transfer this knowledge onto a set of objects of a different quality. This was not yet tested in honeybees but appears unlikely. According to Davis and

Perusse (1988), if the basic criteria of counting are fulfilled, but a transfer of the counting performance has not been shown, the respective animal's behavior should be referred to as "protocounting".

Such a strategy appears to be a feature of memory for sequences on a large as well as on a smaller scale. In the latter case, honeybees are trained to sequentially visit five food sources arranged in a particular geometric order (Kratzsch et al., 1998). Bees were able to learn some feeder arrangements with high precision, particularly those in which directionality of flight is maintained. Such behavior resembles that known as traplining in foraging Hymenoptera (Heinrich, 1976, 1979; Thomson, 1996) and, accordingly, plays an important role in natural behavior. The memory underlying this behavior must represent the overall spatial arrangement of landmarks. Again, one may argue that a chain of simple associations may account for the bees' behavior. In the case of the landmark arrangements learned by the bees, it would have to be quite an impressive chain of associations, both between landmarks (i.e., beacons at the food sources) and between landmarks that are passed by, during related flight turns on the way toward the food source. Alternatively, one may favor the cognitive view that interprets the spatial memory as a unique representation of the elements in their relative sequential positions and their specific meaning for the animal.

The cognitive interpretation is supported by the following results. Honeybees foraging in a patch of four artificial feeders with different flow rates of sucrose solution adjust their choice of feeders according to their flow rate. In other words, they match their choice frequency with each feeder's average reward rate, although the actual reward at each feeder depends not only on its flow rate but also on the time interval between visits (Greggers and Menzel, 1993). Such a matching performance is only possible if bees recognize each feeder as a unique food source, store the time elapsed since the last visit separately for each feeder, and establish a memory trace that integrates a measure of the reward strength (e.g., licking time) over a longer period of time. Closer inspection of the signals used to distinguish each feeder within the patch shows that the bees use two strategies: (1) simple associations between locally restricted olfactory cues perceived only in immediate contact with the feeder and its reward rate and (2) learning the spatial location of the four feeders (Greggers and Mauelshagen, 1997) (Fig. 11. 6). Spatial localization can be achieved by using two different kinds of information (viz., relative position with respect to landmarks without any local cues [as shown in Fig 11.6A), and local visual cues [colors], that need to be large enough to allow a simultaneous view of the three alternative feeders when leaving any one of the four feeders [not shown in Fig. 11.6]. The results are consistent with the interpretation that two fundamentally different memories control the choice process in feeding. In the first case, the honeybees form simple associations between an olfactory cue and the amount of reward in multiple trials. In the second case, matching is based on some kind of configural learning. The different reward rates are memorized indirectly by learning the location of the feeder. The conditioned stimulus "location" has only a vaguely defined relationship to the reward rate. Although the presence of landmarks and the spatial relationship of the arrangement of the color marks precisely define the location, these cues do not predict, for example, how long it takes to get there or how much food will be there.

Thus, recognition of a location should activate a retrieval system in which the feeders are compared simultaneously, and reward rates experienced at any one feeder are associated with this feeder in a spatial context with the others.

The Representation of Space in Navigation

The ability of animals to create a novel shortcut has been taken as an indication of a maplike organization of spatial memory, often referred to as a *cognitive map* (Tolman, 1948; O'Keefe and Nadel, 1978; Thinus–Blanc, 1987; however, see Bennett, 1996). There is no evidence thus far that honeybees store spatial arrangements of landmarks and scenes in such a manner (Wehner and Menzel, 1990; Wehner, 1992; Collett, 1996; Dyer, 1996; Menzel et al., 1996), because simpler navigation mechanisms (route following and landmark piloting) may exist and were found to explain the use of novel shortcuts (Menzel, 1989; Dyer, 1991; Geiger et al., 1995). This lack of evidence may well, however, result from the methods applied in the experiments on honeybee navigation, namely, the intense training to a particular feeding place along a defined route. Even if honeybees had acquired some geometric representation of landmarks through exploratory flights at the beginning of their foraging career or during initial training to other places (Menzel et al., 1990; Wehner et al., 1990; Dyer, 1991), intense training along one route could lead to an elimination of information about spatial arrangements of landmarks outside the route. Honeybees heading out for a food site S_m in the morning and finding themselves at S_a (because they were transported and released there by the experimentalist) should fly directly to S_m, if they consult a spatial memory of the relevant locations (hive, two feeding sites S_m and S_a) in the form of a geometric map (Fig. 11.7A). This is not, however, what honeybees do. Instead, they fly straight back to the hive or continue along their compass bearing depending on their motivational state (see above). Again, we have to be cautious about concluding from the negative outcome of this experiment that honeybees lack a maplike spatial representation. Because new routes are more risky, they might be overridden by "safety programs" such as flying back to the hive for reorientation or continuing to fly according to the current active memory (compass direction).

Given these possible constraints, we therefore asked whether honeybees trained to two locations (S_m in the morning, S_a in the afternoon) fly novel short cuts when released at two unexpected new sites, either a fully unfamiliar site (S_4; see Fig. 11.7A) or a site halfway between the two trained feeding sites that partially resembles features of the surrounding landscape of the two known feeding sites (S_3; Fig. 11.7A). At the fully unfamiliar place (site S_4), honeybees always choose the direction corresponding to the current state of their vector memory. If site S_3 were equally unfamiliar to them as site S_4 is, we would expect them to behave similarly, that is, to choose only the compass directions. If, however, site S_3 can be located as being between the two familiar sites, then the honeybees might be able to fly straight back to the hive along a novel route. This is indeed the case for about 50% of the bees released at S_3: They are able to fly the novel direct route toward the hive. The same bees released at S_a or S_m fly their corresponding hiveward direction (S_a Hive or S_m Hive, respectively) according to their motivational state (hive departing and hive arriving bees)

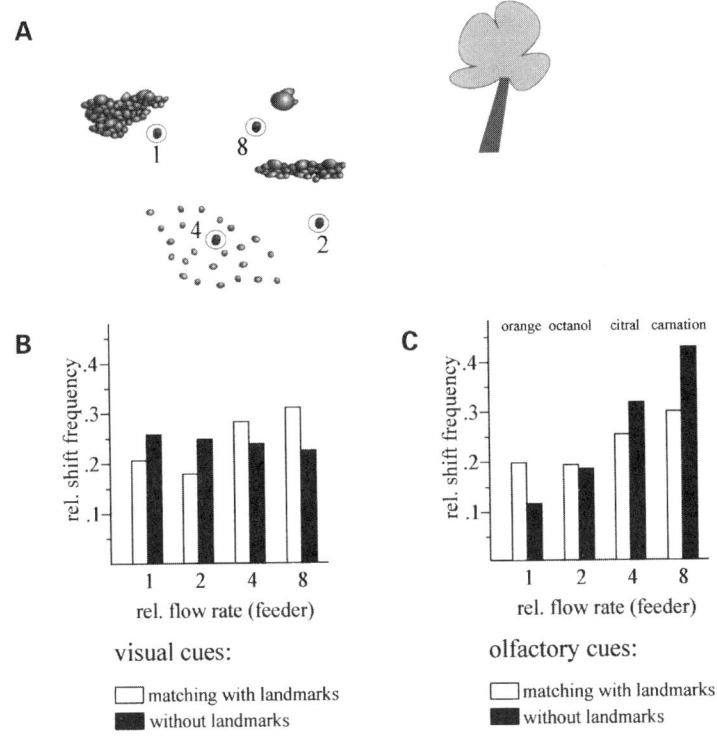

Figure 11.6. (A) Single honeybees forage in a patch of four electronic feeders. The feeders differ with respect to the flow rate of sucrose solution (the numbers, 1, 2, 4, and 8 give the relative flow rates of the four feeders). (B) In a natural setting with landmarks and different small color marks at the entrance to the feeders, bees choose the feeders with the higher flow rate over those with the lower flow rate (relative shift frequency, ordinate). If the landmarks are not visible and the color marks are so small that they cannot be seen by the bee from a distance, matching behavior collapses, indicating that the relative position of the feeders to landmarks is used to associate flow rate with feeder. (C) In a second experiment, the feeders are marked with different odors. Now choice frequency is matched with flow rate (in absence of landmarks, as well), indicating that feeder odor can also be associated with flow rate. Interestingly, matching behavior is better in the absence of landmarks and is better than in the case of local color marks both with and without landmarks. This effect is interpreted as a learning strategy in which information is transferred between feeders if landmarks are available. In other words, if they can be related to the same landmarks, the four feeders are configured into a patch, but are learned by elementary associations if local olfactory cues alone are used to identified them. (After Greggers and Mauelshagen, 1997.)

(Fig. 11.7B). The other 50% flew according to the compass memory currently residing in active memory. All bees in the motivational state of arriving or departing from either food source chose the compass direction. Control experiments excluded the possibility of orientation toward a beacon close to the hive (Menzel et al., 1998).

How do honeybees manage to fly straight to the hive from site S_3? Three hypotheses come to mind.

1. Bees may indeed integrate the spatial arrangement of landmarks into a maplike geometrical representation and locate sites S_m, S_a, S_3, and the hive

352   11 Cognition in Insects: The Honeybee as a Study Case

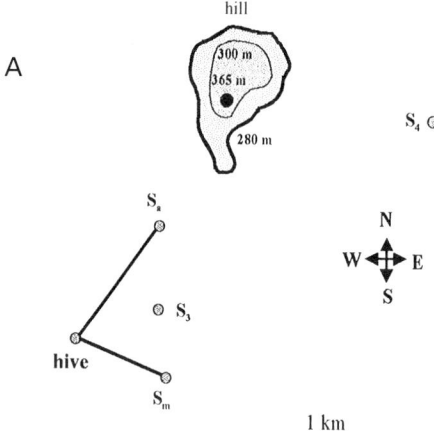

Figure 11.7. Flying novel routes in honeybees. (A) A group of bees is trained to collect sugar solution at location S_m in the morning and at S_a in the afternoon. The distances and directions of the feeding site from the hive are 115° and 630 m for S_m and 40° and 790 m for S_a. A prominent distant landmark is a cone–shaped mountain standing 150 m above the wide and flat agricultural area surrounding it. S_3 and S_4 are the novel release sites. S_3 is half way between S_m and S_a, whereas S_4 is far away (3 km) from both. *continued on opposite side.*

accordingly. In this case, they would spot the unfamiliar release site S_3 on the map and steer along the shortest route toward the hive.

2. Bees may have stored only the compass directions between the two feeding sites and the hive. Landmarks at the feeding sites serve as retrieval cues for the respective compass directions. When released at site S_3, they recognize the partial resemblance of landmark cues that characterize both feeding sites and retrieve both compass memories. Having both in their working memory, they may apply a vector-averaging process (Collett et al., 1996) similar to that working automatically during path integration (Wehner et al., 1996) and fly in the resulting direction.

3. Bees may not perform any kind of processing between the two memory contents associated with sites S_m and S_a and retrieved by the partial resemblance of landmark constellations at site S_3, but may simply refer sequentially to one memory for a while or to the other when guiding their flight path. In this case, isolated associations are sufficient to explain the behavior, and one would expect the bees to fly along a zigzag course indicating the sequential activation of sensorimotor routines to two different memories.

We never observed this kind of zigzag flight; in fact, bees flying in different directions at site S_3 or those of the control groups (i.e., bees that only had experience with site S_m or S_a and, thus, did not fly along the novel shortcut) did not differ from bees flying directly to the hive. Thus, the third hypothesis appears to be unsupported (Menzel et al., 1998).

Although these findings meet the basic requirements for the presence of a cognitive map (hypothesis 1), hypothesis 2 cannot be rejected and appears to be a more

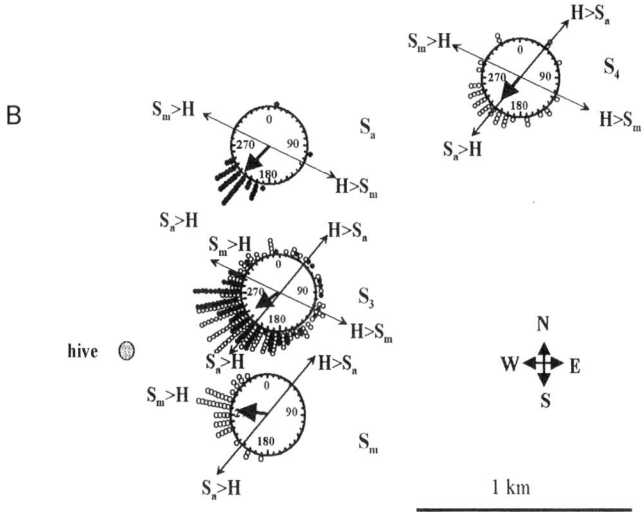

Figure 11.7. contd.
(B) The four big circles depict the distribution of vanishing bearings of the bees caught on arrival at the hive (H) from S_m in the morning (filled circles) and from S_a in the afternoon (open circles) and then displaced to different release sites. The thick black arrows represent the mean angles of the distribution of vanishing bearings as the center of mass of the data on a polar histogram (in the case of S_3, the two arrows corresponding to the two groups of bees released there are coincident and, therefore, indistinguishable). The number of animals released at each place (n) and the vector length (r) for each release site are S_a (n = 33, r = 0 86); S_3 (n = 81, r = 0.58); S_m (n = 39, r = 0.83); S_4 (n = 37, r = 0.61). The long thin arrows extending from each circle indicate the directions the bees might have taken. Bees arriving from S_m were displaced to S_a; they fly back to the hive along the S_a Hive vector. Bees arriving from S_a were displaced to S_m; they also fly back along the correct vector (i.e., S_m Hive). In both cases, the bees referred to the compass direction toward the hive that they had associated with the landmarks characterizing S_a and S_m. At the new release site S_3, half way between S_m and S_a, both the morning (S_m) and the afternoon (S_a) bees depart toward the hive, choosing a novel flight path that they had never flown before. The distribution of vanishing bearings for bees released in the morning (filled circles) and in the afternoon (open circles) lead to two mean vectors. These two vectors lie so close that they overlap, giving the impression of only one vector in the center of the circle S_3. However, S_a bees displaced to S_4 (a distant release site) fly along the compass vector that they would have flown if they had not been transported and released at a new site. These bees are thus unable to refer to any learned landmarks and thus continue along a compass direction residing in their current memory (From Menzel et al., 1998, by permission of Academic Press, London.).

parsimonious explanation (see below). Whether such a memory organization is classified as a cognitive map, however, depends on how the limitation to homeward–directed flights is interpreted and how rich the map is. A cognitive map should allow the honeybee to take shortcuts toward any intended location within the represented area and in any motivational state. This, however, is not the case. In contrast to the finding by Gould (1986), honeybees, for instance, never flew novel shortcuts between feeding sources (i.e., from S_3 to S_m or from S_3 to S_a). Such a limitation may exclude the possibility of a maplike organization of spatial memory, but it could also result from a secondary effect, namely, a safety program forcing the honeybee to continue according to the content of its working memory or to fly back first to the hive for reorientation, ignoring any other potential options.

The richness of spatial memory may allow for the possibility that honeybees heading out for a destination "expect" to pass particular landmarks (Chittka and Geiger, 1995; see above) and to experience a certain location of the goal relative to those landmarks. Honeybees trained to fly along a sequence of boxes in which the exit hole was marked by different visual cues (e.g., colors, patterns) show that they expect the right stimulus at the right place in the sequence (Collett et al., 1993). More experiments to test the idea of "expectation" at a larger scale, however, need to be performed.

A blocking phenomenon in the spatial domain may be indicative of expectation. In an experiment performed by Chittka and Kunze (1996), bees were trained to collect food in the neighborhood of a large landmark within an otherwise landmark–free area. They learned a new flight direction back to the hive only if the food source was experienced at an unexpected location relative to the large landmark. When they experienced the landmark at the "expected" place, learning the new flight direction was blocked.

In any case, honeybees apparently activate separately acquired memories and apply them in a novel, adaptive sense. Such a capacity may be interpreted as being indicative of basic forms of cognition (Markl, 1985). Retrieval of more than one memory by the associated cues, generalization between the cues, expectancy–driven learning at a low level of complexity, and context–dependent learning have been demonstrated in honeybee navigation. It is necessary to emphasize, however, that on the basis of existing data it is not justified to conclude that honeybees construct a spatial memory in the form of a mental map comparable with the one accessible to our own introspection. Attempts to demonstrate that honeybees, for example, refuse to fly to a place located in an "impossible" area (e.g., in the middle of a lake) indicated by a dancing honeybee (Gould and Gould, 1982) are not convincingly supported by data. The claim that honeybees extract computational rules from regular stepwise movements of the feeding place and "foresee" the next step (Gould and Gould, 1982) could not be reproduced (Menzel, unpublished data). Thus it appears that the navigational capabilities of honeybees cannot be explained by referring, on the one hand, only to elementary associations or chains of such associations; on the other hand, they might also not be as complex as they should be if a single unifying spatial representation (in the form of a cognitive map) is assumed.

Visual Discrimination Learning in Honeybees: Generalization, Categorization, and Concept Formation

Beyond large-scale navigation, foraging honeybees exhibit sophisticated strategies for recognizing their targets in a close–up approach. Learning colors, odors, patterns, and even textures is well documented in such an appetitive context (Wehner, 1981; Kevan and Lane, 1985; Menzel, 1985, 1993; Srinivasan, 1994). Handling the learned information is highly flexible, and generalizing to novel stimuli is possible (Giurfa, 1991; Giurfa et al., 1994). Such an adaptive capability is advantageous for an organism that needs to cope with a changing environment and, thus, with possible variations of the sensory cues learned before. Among others, some changes may be due to different viewpoints adopted when approaching the target or to changes in the physical nature of the stimuli.

Generalization depends on the perceptual distance among stimuli (Spence, 1937) and is stronger for stimuli that lie close to each other in a perceptual space. For example, honeybees trained to a vertical flower pattern and presented with different angular orientations of the same pattern discriminate and choose preferentially the trained orientation, but their choice of the alternative ones is strictly associated with their degree of overlapping with the trained shape in the lower visual field (Giurfa et al., 1995). In this case, discrimination follows a simple matching rule in which the degree of coincidence between a memorized and an actually perceived image is calculated, and stimuli are ranked accordingly (Collett and Cartwright, 1983; Gould, 1985).

Generalization for colors (Giurfa, 1991) and odors (Vareschi, 1971) has also been demonstrated. The problem in such generalization tasks, however, is to identify the dimensions defining the perceptual space in which stimuli are evaluated and ranked as being similar or different. This has been achieved in the case of honeybee color vision (Backhaus, 1991; Menzel and Backhaus, 1991). Here, the color space has been shown to be defined by two opponent neural processes that code (in an antagonistic manner) the signals from the three photoreceptor types, the short–wave, the middle–wave, and the long–wave type (ultraviolet, blue, and green, respectively). Perceptual distance between pairs of stimuli may be calculated in this bidimensional color space by means of a city block metric, a metric in which the relevant parameter for discrimination refers to the algebraic sum of the distances between the two perceptual loci along the two dimensions (Backhaus, 1991). A distance like this constitutes a good measure of the discrimination and generalization abilities of honeybees for pairs of color stimuli (Giurfa et al., 1994). Things are more problematic for odor and pattern perception because of the difficulty in finding perceptual measures of stimuli similarity. For these sensory modalities more studies are required to understand the basis of stimuli generalization.

Generalization of a reinforced feature may occur using simple matching rules. Honeybees may generalize and choose novel patterns on the basis of a reinforced common feature. For instance, they may easily learn the orientation of patterns (Hateren et al., 1990; Giger and Srinivasan, 1995), and, once trained to discriminate vertical from horizontal stripes, they can transfer the information learned to different kinds of patterns sharing the features vertical versus horizontal (Hateren et al., 1990). In this case, the degree of overlap with a memorized feature was not a reliable cue, able to perform the discrimination task. Thus one should conclude that bees learned the orientation as a cue itself and transferred it to novel stimuli. This task may be easily achieved by selective activation of orientation detectors present in the medulla, a visual neuropil of the honeybee brain (Yang and Maddess, 1997). In this case, it suffices that the orientation of the novel patterns falls within the tuning field of the neuronal detectors for the novel pattern being recognized as the same as, or as similar to, the one previously reinforced (Srinivasan et al., 1994). Thus generalization may be achieved by a neuronal mechanism that focuses exclusively on the orientation of pattern elements, and thus follows a simple matching rule.

A cognitive interpretation of the same results, however, would state that honeybees evinced a primary level of categorization. Categorization implies that not only is a collection of stimuli partitioned into groups but also that knowledge of the category to which an object belongs tells us something about its properties (Estes, 1994). Therefore, categorization involves an implicit knowledge of the stimulus properties. Typically, a categorization experiment involves discrimination in which reward is not signaled by a single stimulus, but, instead, by a variety of stimuli that share some common characteristics. This was, indeed, the case in the experiment cited above. Moreover, the requirement of a transfer to novel instances having these common characteristics is also satisfied. In that sense, honeybees do not seem to be very different from mammals, which assign individual stimuli to categories on the basis of the features of which they are composed (Pearce, 1994). Feature analysis is one of the mechanistic explanations provided for categorization (Lea, 1984). The essence of this explanation is that features that are reliably present on reinforced trials gain considerably more associative strength than the irrelevant features. Once this has occurred, then the discrimination is solved, and even novel stimuli are classified correctly.

It is tempting to say that animals are able to categorize because they possess a concept. Concepts are mental representations of classes, and their most salient function is to promote cognitive economy (Estes, 1994). Although the terms category and concept are often used interchangeably, the latter involves a higher level of abstraction. For instance, the interpretation of concepts like "elegant" or "irregular" involves aspects of memory beyond those essential for the interpretation of categorization in terms of a reinforced feature. In other words, categorization may be the basis for concept formation, but may not be identical with it. It is relatively easy to talk about *concepts* when they are used by humans, but rather difficult to specify what the term means when applied to animals and even more difficult in the case of an insect such as the honeybee. Can honeybees form concepts, and , if so (in the case of an insect), what does *concept* mean?

Recent evidence indicates that honeybees may develop a concept of bilateral symmetry (Giurfa et al., 1996). Symmetry is a rather abstract property of a wide variety of objects. It is not specifically encoded in particular features of a pattern, but exists independently of the global or local properties of the shape (i.e., in the fact that half of the figure is identical to the other half when reflected across its vertical midline). Single individually marked honeybees are trained with a succession of eight triads. A group of bees is trained for symmetry and another for asymmetry. The triads of the former group each consists of a rewarded symmetrical stimulus and two different nonrewarded asymmetrical stimuli presented simultaneously. Each triad of the asymmetrical group consists of a rewarded, asymmetrical stimulus and two different nonrewarded symmetrical stimuli (Fig.11.8). Training with each triad is interspersed with multiple-choice, and generalization tests where novel stimuli, symmetrical and asymmetrical, are presented. The patterns tested are chosen such that only symmetry but no other parameter (area, contour length, overall orientation, and so forth) can account for stimulus discrimination. By randomizing pattern parameters other than symmetry and by changing the patterns from one triad to the other, bees are prevented from building a template for a particular reinforced pattern. They should, instead, extract from the succession of extremely different, reinforced patterns the fact that symmetry (or asymmetry) is the rewarded cue (Fig. 11.8).

From test seven onward, bees extracted the symmetry or asymmetry feature and transferred it to the novel stimuli. The results indicate that bees are indeed able to detect and abstract symmetry or asymmetry (Giurfa et al., 1996). Honeybees showed a slight predisposition for learning and abstracting symmetry, because, when trained for it, they chose somewhat more frequently, came closer to, and hovered longer in front of the novel symmetrical stimuli than the bees trained for asymmetry did for the novel asymmetrical stimuli. Therefore, a bias, either innate or resulting from the insects' experience with symmetrical flowers in the field, seems to be overimposed on the performance inculcated by the training procedure.

Although these results demonstrate that honeybees may categorize stimuli on the basis of their symmetry (including a transfer to novel instances), they may not be convincing enough to speak of the formation of a symmetry concept. For instance, assuming that bees possess symmetry detectors in their visual neuropils, a fact that still needs to be elucidated, the results could be explained on the basis of selective activation (or inhibition) of such feature detectors throughout the training procedure. In that sense, performance would not be as different as that observed for the generalization of pattern orientation (see above). Further experiments are necessary to establish whether symmetry learning involves the use of a concept of symmetry. As suggested by Lea (1984), reversal experiments are critical to detect whether animals handle the whole set of information as an unique concept. In a reversal experiment, the alternative information for the formerly reinforced concept is now rewarded. Because both categories belong to the same concept, animals should not have problems in performing as well as with the feature rewarded earlier. Such experiments have been recently performed on symmetry abstraction by bees. Bees that learned to transfer to novel symmetrical or asymmetrical stimuli are subsequently trained in a reversal schedule (Giurfa et al., 1998). Once a performance plateau is reached, the alternative feature is rewarded: asymmetry, if previously rewarded for symmetry, and vice versa. Bees immediately switch to the previously unrewarded stimuli, thus showing that symmetry and asymmetry need not be learned separately but constitute complementary aspects of the same information. In control experiments, honeybees are trained in a first phase to solve a task different from symmetry categorization and are then subjected to a reversal schedule where they are trained to categorize stimuli on the basis of their symmetry. These latter experiments did not show rapid learning of the symmetry/asymmetry information in the second phase of the experiment. Thus, the immediate switch toward the alternative information observed in the reversal symmetry–asymmetry schedule is a mere consequence of having learned one of these items of information in the first phase of the experiment. We conclude from this that symmetry can be learned as a perceptual category by honeybees because it can be extracted as an independent visual pattern feature and that symmetry learning in honeybees fulfills the requirements of concept formation in the sense that honeybees transfer the abstracted information to novel items and learn symmetry as a complement of asymmetry and vice versa.

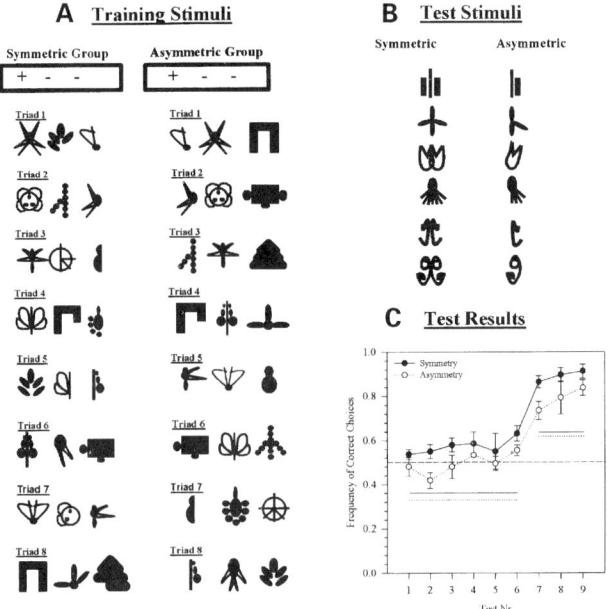

Figure 11.8. Honeybees are able to form generalized representations of symmetry versus asymmetry. Single individually marked, free–flying honeybees are trained with eight successive triads of stimuli (A) for either symmetry or asymmetry. Triads of the symmetrical group consist of a rewarded (+) symmetrical stimulus and two different nonrewarded (–) asymmetrical stimuli each, presented simultaneously. Triads of the asymmetrical group consist each of a rewarded (+) asymmetrical stimulus and two different nonrewarded (–) symmetrical stimuli. Reward is provided by sugar solution. Stimuli are very diverse, except for their symmetrical or asymmetrical outline. Training with each triad is interspersed with multiple–choice, generalization tests. (B) During tests, novel stimuli (symmetrical and asymmetrical) are presented. None is rewarded. (C) For each test stimulus, the number of choices by the bee and the intensity and duration of each choice is recorded by means of microphones behind the test stimuli. From test seven onward, bees trained to discriminate bilaterally symmetrical from nonsymmetrical patterns learn the task and appropriately transfer it to the novel stimuli, thus demonstrating an ability to detect and abstract symmetry or asymmetry as an independent visual pattern feature (after Giurfa et al., 1996).

A question that remains unanswered is whether our training procedure allows a concept of symmetry to develop or triggers an already existing concept of symmetry based namely on the fact that symmetry is a natural indicator of phenotypic and genotypic quality (Moller, 1990, 1992, 1993). If so, such a concept may be innate or result from the experience honeybees have with symmetrical flowers in the field. At the present time, it is impossible to answer these questions. Experiments with naive honeybees in their first foraging flights may indicate whether such a capability is related to the level of foraging experience of the insects. In any case, it is worth mentioning that at the beginning of the training procedure insects do not show a particular bias toward symmetry or asymmetry. They choose randomly between both stimuli categories (see test 1, Fig. 11.8). This shows that the formation of a concept of symmetry observed in our experiments is basically inculcated by our training procedure.

Therefore it is tempting to suggest that insects, with their rather simple nervous systems, may exhibit basic forms of cognitive capabilities, such as categorization and concept formation. The formation of a concept in an insect may reflect a capability to flexibly handle information pertaining to relevant objects in its environment. In that sense, concept formation, although possible, may be constrained by the characteristics of the animal's ecological niche. In other words, honeybees may abstract symmetry from a set of different stimuli and transfer it to novel stimuli because of the adaptive value that such a cue has in nature, because it signals more rewarding flowers. We would not expect honeybees to be able to develop other kinds of concepts without an ecological correlate; however, this hypothesis needs to be tested.

CONCLUSION

Basic Cognition with a Small Brain

A number of research programs (up to the present mainly including vertebrates) strongly suggest that simple forms of associative learning lead to richer behavioral plasticities than are usually acknowledged. To account for these behavioral findings, theories of simple associative learning had to incorporate cognition–like concepts of attention and/or of expectation and prediction. Evidence for a contribution of such cognitive processes in invertebrates is relatively scarce. In the honeybee, the PER preparation is a promising behavioral model in which these issues have begun to be addressed. Although a rich body of data exists, the question is still unanswered whether or not simple olfactory PER conditioning involves cognition–like processes such as attention and/or expectation and prediction.

However, elementary forms of associative learning are not sufficient to explain all facets of conditioning present in the honeybee. Honeybees are capable of solving problems that require the use of configural associations (e.g., biconditional discrimination). Thus, the ability to build configural associations shows that learning performance of an insect (with its small brain) can, in part, and at least qualitatively, be compared with that of vertebrates. This indicates that—even if vertebrates and invertebrates differ at the structural neural level—similar functional ways of solving problems posed by the environment were implemented and, therefore, the same theoretical approaches can be taken for the analysis of such forms of learning. Furthermore, testing basic cognitive properties with the olfactory PER conditioning paradigm provides the potential to combine behavioral and physiological analyses at the level of single identified neurons and small volumes of neuropils. It might, thus, be possible to address the question of how behavioral complexity relates to neural complexity.

In a natural context, navigation constitutes a plastic behavior in which paths flown by honeybees over distances of kilometers represent thousands of times the size of an individual. They can efficiently return to memorized places: the nest and/or the feeding site. In both the spatial and temporal domains, multiple forms of memory exist and are connected associatively. Context dependencies induce chains of associations between separated memories, and external cues and motivational state define which memories are brought into an active form. Results from different experiments are consistent with the idea that honeybees have specific expectancies for stimuli in space, thus suggesting that their spatial memory is based on a unique representation of the elements in their relative positions. Novel routes can be established in long–range navigation, but a cognitive map is not required for explaining them: A process that averages memory contents for different navigation vectors may already account for such a behavioral performance. Thus, navigational capacities of honeybees cannot be explained by referring only to elementary associations or chains of such associations and are, therefore, more complex than previously thought.

Honeybees can categorize objects on the basis of common features. Multiple sequential learning sets are necessary for such a performance. Such categorization may be the basis for a behavior such as concept formation. Therefore, although close–up pattern recognition has properties of stereotyped image matching, it is not bound to these simple forms of visual processing. Further learning may lead to the extraction of particular visual features such as symmetry, which is then applied in a concept–like way to new images.

The Ecological Niche and Basic Cognition

Different species adapted to different ecological niches may have rather little in common regarding their cognitive capacities, because evolutionary pressure should have selected them for specific adaptations. Alternatively, different environments may pose similar demands, and, thus, convergent evolution may have led to similar cognitive processes. All animals extract information about the external and internal world from the temporal contingencies of events and gain from them the ability to respond in advance to expected events. Nonassociative and associative forms of learning, therefore, are properties of all animals with a nervous system (Thorpe, 1963). Many animals need to return to a particular place for safety reasons or for the care of offspring and rely on observatory or incentive learning. Accordingly, such kinds of learning are common properties of many species, even those with a rather simple nervous system such as annelids and snails.

The basic rules of nonassociative and associative learning can be found in all animals with a nervous system. The obvious differences between animals in their wide range of behaviors is related to the complexity of their sensory and motor world, and this is also the primary factor in brain size. A richer sensory input provides the potential to gain more specific information about the intricacies of stimulus relationships and confounding properties. More differentiated memories are based on such information, but, in addition, need a memory–organizing process that extracts information from multiple experiences. The logical structure of the world is embedded in the configuration of stimuli and actions of the animal. Thus, similar stimuli may signal different meanings in different contexts, multiple learning signals may share a common feature that can be extracted only by integrating multiple learning events, and redundant information may become important when certain stimuli are lacking.

The brain of the honeybee appears to be capable of extracting the logical structure of the world to an impressive extent. What are its specific limitations compared with those of bigger brains, and what may be the structural/functional basis for them? To address such a question, one would need to know more about the deficiencies of small brains, an approach that has not yet been considered very much. Future research may refer to the following arguments.

A brain that is able not only to process the rich inputs from the sense organs but also to form memories across modalities implementing the logic structure of these inputs may need additional brain volume to support additional neuronal cross–talk and more widespread synaptic plasticities. The picture emerging from studies on the neural basis of adaptive behaviors is one in which these additional properties of the brain do not replace the basic functions but rather are built on top of them (Squire, 1987; Kandel and Squire, 1992; LeDoux, 1992). Such additional faculties may lead to new pathways connecting separate sensory centers, additional computational properties of existing neural tissue, and, possibly, to additional mechanisms of neural plasticity necessary to implement multifactorial dependencies. This view is as yet only vaguely supported by experimental evidence. The main problem appears to be that these additional cognitive capacities are difficult to identify. A further problem is that the additional neural structures may be hard to depict. Are they incorporated into existing neural nets and intimately entangled with them, or are they added to the existing ones? If existing neural structures are re–structured to serve new functions, does this need to correspond to major changes in the neural connectivity, the number of neurons, and the volume of the structure?

Insect brains may provide particularly suitable cases for examining such questions. Sensory and motor integration centers are compartmentalized and well separated. In particular, the mushroom bodies of the arthropod brain are thought to be related to additional demands resulting from highly developed olfactory communication systems in social insects and from multisensory integration underlying brood care and navigation in Hymenoptera (Alten, 1910; Howse, 1974, 1975; Erber et al., 1987). The mushroom bodies increase in volume when honeybees start their foraging life, that is, when new multisensory learning is demanded (Withers et al., 1993; Durst et al., 1994; Fahrbach et al., 1995). Because the involvement of mushroom bodies in olfactory learning of insects is well documented (Balling et al., 1987; Menzel, 1990; Davis, 1993; de Belle and Heisenberg, 1994; Hammer and Menzel, 1995; Rybak and Menzel, 1998), and its multisensory input is proven both neuroanatomically and neurophysiologically (Mobbs, 1982; Erber et al., 1987; Rybak and Menzel, 1993), they provide an ideal structure for studying the questions posed above. In the honeybee, one might be able to clarify whether elementary associations are formed without the contribution of the mushroom bodies, whether the mushroom bodies are necessary to organize memory formation at other sites, and whether the structural complexity of mushroom bodies rises with the demands on configural learning. Also, comparing mushroom bodies in different insects with different abilities to show configural forms of learning, and/or manipulating the contribution of the mushroom bodies during such forms of learning, may be a valid approach to finding answers to these questions.

ACKNOWLEDGMENTS

Continuous support from the Deutsche Forschungsgemeinschaft is gratefully acknowledged. We are also grateful for support from the A.v. Humboldt–Stiftung (to M.G.), die Studienstiftung des Deutschen Volkes (to B.G.), and the Berlin–Brandenburgische Akademie der Wissenschaften.

REFERENCES

Alten, H.V. (1910) Zur Phylogenie des Hymenopterengehirns. *Z. Naturwiss.* 46:511–590.
Backhaus, W. (1991) Color opponent coding in the visual system of the honeybee. *Vis. Res.* 31:1381–1397.
Balling, A., G.M. Technau, and M. Heisenberg (1987) Are the structural changes in adult *Drosophila* mushroom bodies memory traces? Studies on biochemical learning mutants. *J. Neurogenet.* 4:65–73.
Barnet, R.C., N.J. Grahame, and R.R. Miller (1995) Trial spacing effects in pavlovian conditioning: a role for local context. *Anim. Learn. Behav.* 23:340–348.
Bellingham, W.P., K. Gillette–Bellingham, and E.J. Kehoe (1985) Summation and configuration in patterning schedules with the rat and rabbit. *Anim. Learn. Behav.* 13:152–164.
Bennett, A.T.D. (1996) Do animals have cognitive maps? *J. Exp. Biol.* 199:219–224.
Bicker, G., S. Kreissl, and A. Hofbauer (1993) Monoclonal antibody labels olfactory and visual pathways in *Drosophila* and *Apis* brains. *J. Comp. Neurol.* 335:413–424.
Bitterman, M.E. (1996) Comparative analysis of learning in honeybees. *Anim. Learn. Behav.* 24:123–141.
Bitterman, M.E., R. Menzel, A. Fietz, and S. Schäfer (1983) Classical conditioning of proboscis extension in honeybees (*Apis mellifera*). *J. Comp. Psychol.* 97:107–119.
Braun, G., and G. Bicker (1992) Habituation of an appetitive reflex in the honeybee. *J. Neurophysiol.* 67:588–598.
Cartwright, B.A., and T.S. Collett (1983) Landmark learning in bees—experiments and models. *J. Comp. Physiol.* 151:521–543.
Chittka, L. and K. Geiger (1995) Can honeybees count landmarks? *Anim. Behav.* 49:159–164.
Chittka, L., K. Geiger, and J. Kunze (1995) The influences of landmarks on distance estimation of honey bees. *Anim. Behav.* 50:23–31.
Chittka, L., and J. Kunze (1996) The significance of landmarks for path integration in homing honeybee foragers. Naturwissenschaffen. 82:341–343.
Collett, T.S., (1996) Insect navigation *en route* to the goal: multiple strategies for the use of landmarks. *J. Exp. Biol.* 199:227–235.
Collett, T.S., and J. Baron (1994) Biological compasses and the coordinate frame of landmark memories in honeybees. *Nature* 368:137–140.
Collett, T.S., J. Baron, and K. Sellen (1996) On the encoding of movement vectors by honeybees. Are distance and direction represented independently? *J. Comp. Physiol. [A]* 179:395–406.
Collett, T.S., and B.A. Cartwright (1983) Eidetic images in insects: their role in navigation. *TINS* 6:101–105.
Collett, T.S., S.N. Fry, and R. Wehner (1993) Sequence learning by honeybees. *J. Comp. Physiol. [A]* 172:693–706.
Couvillon, P.A., L. Arakaki, and M.E. Bitterman (1997) Intramodal blocking in honeybees. *Anim. Learn. Behav.* 25:277–282.
Davis, H., and J. Memmott (1982) Counting behaviour in animals: a critical evalutation. *Psychol. Bull.* 92:547–571.
Davis, H., and R. Perusse (1988) Numerical competence in aminals: definition issues, current evidence, and a new research agenda. *Behav. Brain Sci.* 114:561–615.
Davis, R.L. (1993) Mushroom bodies and *Drosophila* learning. *Neuron* 11:1–14.
de Belle, J.S., and M. Heisenberg (1994) Associative odor learning in *Drosophila* abolished by chemical ablation of mushroom bodies. *Science* 263:692–695.
Durst, C., S. Eichmüller, and R. Menzel (1994) Development and experience lead to increased volume of subcompartments of the honeybee mushroom body. *Behav. Neural. Biol.* 62:259–263.

References 363

Dyer, F.C. (1991) Honey bees acquire route–based memories but not cognitive maps in a familiar landscape. *Anim. Behav.* 41:239–246.

Dyer, F.C. (1996) Spatial memory and navigation by honeybees on the scale of the foraging range. *J. Exp. Biol.* 199:147–154.

Dyer, F.C., and J.L. Gould (1981) Honey bee orientation: a backup system for cloudy days. *Science* 214:1041–1042.

Erber, J. (1978) Response characteristics and after effects of multimodal neurons in the mushroom body area of the honey bee. *Physiol. Entomol.* 3:77–89.

Erber, J., U. Homberg, and W. Gronenberg (1987) Functional roles of the mushroom bodies in insects. In A.P. Gupta (ed.): Arthropod Brain: Its Evolution, Development, Structure, and Functions. New York: John Wiley and Sons, pp. 485–511.

Erber, J., R. Menzel, H. -J. Pflüger, and D. Todt (eds.) (1989) *Neural mechanisms of behavior.* Proceedings of the 2nd International Congress of Neuroethology.Georg Thieme Verlag, Stuttgart.

Esch, H.E., and J.E. Burns (1995) Honeybees use optic flow to measure the distance of a food source. Naturwissenschaffen. 82:38–40.

Esch, H.E., and J.E. Burns (1996) Distance estimation by foraging honeybees. *J. exp. Biol.* 199:155–162.

Estes, W.K. (1994) *Classification and Cognition.* Oxford University Press, Oxford.

Ewing, M.F., M.B. Larew, and A.R. Wagner (1985) Distribution–of–trials effects in pavlovian conditioning: an apparent involvement of backward inhibitory conditioning with short intertrial intervals. *J. Exp. Psychol. Anim. Behav. Proc.* 11:537–547.

Fahrbach, S.E., T. Giray, and G.E. Robinson (1995) Volume changes in the mushroom bodies of adult honey bee queens. *Neurobiol. Learn. Mem.* 63:181–191.

Frisch, K.V. (1914) Der Farbensinn und Formensinn der Biene. *Zool. Jb. Physiol.* 37:1–238.

Frisch, K.V. (1967) *The Dance Language and Orientation of Bees.* Harvard University, Press, Cambridge.

Frisch, K.V., and M. Lindauer (1954) Himmel und Erde in Konkurrenz bei der Orientierung der Bienen. *Naturwissenschatten,* 41:245–253.

Geiger, K., D. Kratzsch, and R. Menzel (1995) Target–directed orientation in displaced honeybees. *Ethology* 101:335–345.

Gelman, R, and C.R. Gallistel (1978) *The Child's Understanding of Number.* Harvard University Press, Cambridge.

Gerber, B., and J. Ullrich (1998) No evidence for olfactory blocking in honeybee classical conditioning. *J. Exp. Biol.* (press).

Giger, A.D., and M.V. Srinivasan (1995) Pattern recognition in honeybees: eidetic imagery and orientation discrimination. *J. Comp. Physiol. [A]* 176:791–795.

Giurfa, M. (1991) Colour generalization and choice behaviour of the honeybee *Apis mellifera ligustica. J. Insect Physiol.* 37:41–44.

Giurfa, M., W. Backhaus, and R. Menzel (1995) Colour and angular orientation in the discrimination of bilateral symmetric patterns in the honeybee. *Naturwissenschaften.* 82:198–201.

Giurfa, M., B. Eichmann, and R. Menzel (1996) Symmetry perception in an insect. *Nature* 382:458–461.

Giurfa, M., N. Müller–Deisig, D. Osoroi, R. Menzel (1998) A concept of symmetry in an insect. Abstract No. 252 from the *Fifth International Congress of Neuroethology*, University of California, San Diego, 1998.

Giurfa, M., J.A. Nunez, and W. Backhaus (1994) Odour and colour information in the foraging choice behaviour of the honeybee. *J. Comp. Physiol. [A]* 175:773–779.

Gould, J.L. (1985) How bees remember flower shapes. *Science* 227:1492–1494.

Gould, J.L. (1986) The locale map of honey bees: do insects have cognitive maps? *Science* 232:861–863.

Gould, J.L., and C.G. Gould (1982) The insect mind: physics or metaphysics? In D.R. Griffin (ed.): *Animal mind–Human Mind.* New York: Springer.

Greggers, U., and J. Mauelshagen (1997) Matching behavior of honeybees in a multiple–choice situation: the differential effect of environmental stimuli on the choice process. *Anim. Learn. Behav.* 25:458–472.

Greggers, U., and R. Menzel (1993) Memory dynamics and foraging strategies of honeybees. *Behav. Ecol. Sociobiol.* 32:17–29.

Gronenberg, W. (1986) Physiological and anatomical properties of optical input–fibres to the mushroom body in the bee brain. *J. Insect Physiol.* 32:695–704.

Hammer, M. (1993) An identified neuron mediates the unconditioned stimulus in associative olfactory learning in honeybees. *Nature* 366:59–63.

Hammer, M. (1997) The neural basis of associative reward learning in honeybees. *TINS* 20:245–252.

Hammer, M., and R. Menzel (1995) Learning and memory in the honeybee. *J. Neurosci.* 15:1617–1630.
Hateren, J.H.V., M.V. Srinivasan, and P.B. Wait (1990) Pattern recognition in bees; orientation discrimination. *J. Comp. Physiol. [A]* 167:649–654.
Heinrich, B. (1976) The foraging specializations of individual bumblebees. *Ecol. Monogr.* 46:105–128.
Heinrich, B. (1979) "Majoring" and "minoring" by foraging bumblebees, *Bombus vagans*: an experimental analysis. *Ecology* 60:245–255.
Heinrich, B. (1984) Learning in invertebrates. In P. Marler and H.S. Terrace (eds.): *The biology of learning (Dahlem Konferenzen)*. Springer Verlag, Berling, pp. 135–147.
Hellstern, F., R. Malaka, and M. Hammer (1997) Conditioned inhibition in honeybees depends on the us/cs–interal. In N. Elser and H. Wässle (eds.): *Proceedings of the 25th Göttingen Neurobiology Conference*. Thieme Verlag, Stuttgart, p. 645.
Hellstern, F., D. Wüstenberg, and M. Hammer (1995) Contextual learning in honeybees under laboratory conditions. In N. Elsner and R. Menzel (eds.): *Learning and Memory*. Proceedings of the 23rd Göttingen Neurobiology Conference. Georg Thieme Verlag, Stuttgart p. 30.
Hintzman, D.L. (1974) Theoretical implications of the spacing effect. In R.L. Solso (ed.): *Theories in Cognitive Psychology*. Hillsdale, New York, pp. 77–99.
Holland, P.C. (1990) Event representation in pavlovian conditioning: image and action. *Cogni* 37:105–131.
Holland, P.C. (1993) Cognitive aspects of classical conditioning. *Curr. Op in Neurobiol.* 3:230–236.
Homberg, U. (1984) Processing of antennal information in extrinsic mushroom body neurons of the bee brain. *J. Comp. Physiol. [A]* 154:825–836.
Howse, P.E. (1974) Design and function in the insect brain. In L. Barton-Brown (ed.): *Experimental Analysis of Insect Behaviour*. Springer, Berlin, pp. 180–194.
Howse, P.E. (1975) Brain structure and behavior in insects. *Annu. Rev. Entomol.* 20:359–379.
Jerison, H.J. (1969) Brain evolution and dinosaur brains. *Am. Nat.* 103:575–588.
Kamin, L.J. (1957) The retention of an incompletely learned avoidance response. *J. Comp. Physiol. Psychol.* 50:457–460.
Kamin, L.J. (1968) Attention–like processes in classical conditioning. In M.R. Jones (ed.): *Miami Symp. Predictability, Behavior and Aversive Stimulation*. University of Miami Press, Miami, pp. 9–32.
Kandel, E., and L. Squire (1992) Cognitive neuroscience. Curr. Opin. Neurobiol.2(2).
Kevan, P.G. and M.A. Lane (1985) Flower petal microtexture is a tactile cue for bees. *Proc. Natl. Acad. Sci. U.S.A.* 82:4750–4752.
Klopf, A.H. (1989) Classical conditioning: phenomena predicted by a drive-reinforcement model of neural function. In J.H. Byrne and W.O. Berry (eds.): *Neural Models of Plasticity: Experimental and Theoretical Approaches*. Academic Press, New York, pp. 94–103.
Kratzsch, D., M Giurfa, R. Menzel (1998) Sequence learning by honeybees. Abstract No. 296 from the *Fifth International Congress of Neuroethology*, University of California, San Diego, 1998.
Lachnit, H., and H.D. Kimmel (1993) Positiv and negative patterning in human classical skin conductance response conditioning. *Anim. Learn. Behav.* 21:314–326.
Lea, S.E.G. (1984) In what sense do pigeon learn concepts? In H.L. Roitblat, T.G. Bever, and H.S. Terrace (eds.): *Animal Cognition*. Lawrence Erlbaum Associates, Hillsdale, NJ.
LeDoux, J.E. (1992) Brain mechanisms of emotion and emotional learning. *Curr. Op. in Neurobiol.* 2:191–197.
Lindauer, M., and H. Martin (1972) Magnetic effect on dancing bees. In S.R. Galler et al. (eds.): *Symposium NASA SP-262, Animal Orientation and Navigation*. U.S Government Printing Office, Washington, D.C., pp. 559–567.
Mackintosh, N.J. (1975) A theory of attention: variations in the associability of stimuli with reinforcement. *Psychol. Rev.* 82:276–298.
Markl, H. (1985) Manipulation, modulation, information, cognition: some of the riddles of communication. *Exp. Behav. Ecol.* 31:163–194.
Maronde, U. (1991) Common projection areas of antennal and visual pathways in the honeybee brain, *Apis mellifera*. *J. Comp. Neurol.* 309:328–340.
Menzel, R. (1985) Learning in honey bees in an ecological and behavioral context. In B. Hölldobler and M. Lindauer (eds.): *Experimental Behavioral Ecology*. Gustav Fischer Verlag, Stuttgart, pp. 55–74.
Menzel, R. (1989) Bee–havior and the neural systems and behavior course. In T.J. Carew and D. Kelley (eds.): *Perspectives in Neural Systems and Behavior*. Alan R. Liss, New York, pp. 249–266.
Menzel, R. (1990) Learning, memory, and "cognition" in honey bees. In R.P. Kesner and D.S. Olten (eds.): *Neurobiology of Comparative Cognition*. Erlbaum Inc., Hillsdale, N.J., pp. 237–292.

Menzel, R., and W. Backhaus (1991) Colour vision in insects. In P. Gouras (ed.): *Vision and Visual Dysfunction. The Perception of Colour*. MacMillan Press, London, pp. 262–288.
Menzel, R., L. Chittka, S. Eichmüller, K. Geiger, D. Peitsch, and P. Knoll (1990) Dominance of celestial cues over landmarks disproves map–like orientation in honey bees. *Z. Naturforsch.* 45c:723–726.
Menzel, R., K. Geiger, L. Chittka, J. Joerges, J. Kunze, and U. Müller (1996) The knowledge base of bee navigation. *J. Exp.Biol.* 199:141–146.
Menzel, R., K. Geiger, U. Müller, J. Joerges, and L. Chittka (1998) Bees travel novel homeward routes by integrating separately acquired vector memories. *Anim. Behav.* 55:139–152.
Menzel, R., U. Greggers, and M. Hammer (1993) Functional organization of appetitive learning and memory in a generalist pollinator, the honey bee. In D. Papaj and A.C. Lewis (eds.): *Insect Learning: Ecological and Evolutionary Perspectives*. Chapman & Hall, New York, pp. 79–125.
Menzel, R., and U. Müller (1996) Learning and memory in honeybees: from behavior to neural substrates. *Ann. Rev. Neurosci.* 19:379–404.
Mobbs, P.G. (1982) The brain of the honeybee *Apis mellifera* I.The connections and spatial organization of the mushroom bodies. *Philos. Trans. R. Soc. Lond. Biol.* 298:309–354.
Mobbs, P.G. (1984) Neural networks in the mushroom bodies of the honeybee. *J. Insect Physiol.* 30:43–58.
Mobbs, P.G. (1985) Brain structure. In G.A. Kerkut and L.I. Gilbert (eds.): *Comprehensive Insect Physiology Biochemistry and Pharmacology*. Pergamon Press, Oxford, pp. 299–370.
Moller, A.P. (1990) Fluctuating asymmerty in male sexual ornaments may reliably reveal male quality. *Anim. Behav.* 40:1185–1187.
Moller, A.P. (1992) Female preferece for symmetrical male sexual ornaments. *Nature* 257: 238–240.
Moller, A.P. (1993) Patterns of fluctuating asymmetry in sexual ornaments predict female choice. *J. Evol. Biol.* 6: 481–491.
Morgan, C.L. (1894) *An Introduction to Comparative Psychology*, Scott, London, 1894.
Moscovitch, A., and V.M. Lolordo (1968) Role of safety in the pavlovian backward fear conditioning procedure. *J. Comp. Physiol. Psychol.* 66:673–678.
O'Keefe, J., and J. Nadel (1978) *The Hippocampus as a Cognitive Map*. Oxford University Press, New York.
Pearce, J.M. (1994) Discrimination and categorization. In N.J. Mackintosh (ed.): *Animal Learning and Cognition. Handbook of Perception and Cognition*. Academic Press, San Diego, pp. 109–134.
Rescorla, R.A. (1980) *Pavlovian Second-Order Conditioning* Lawrence Erlbaum Association, Hillsdale, N.J.,
Rescorla, R.A. (1988) Behavioral studies of pavlovian conditioning. *Annu. Rev. Neurosci.* 11:329–352.
Rescorla, R.A., and A.R. Wagner (1972) A theory of classical conditioning: variations in the effectiveness of reinforcement and non–reinforcement. In A.H. Black and W.F. Prokasy (eds.): *Classical Conditioning II: Current Research and Theory*. Appleton-Century-Crofts, New York, pp. 64–99.
Rieke, F., D. Warland, R. de Ruyter van Steveninck, and W. Bialek (1997) *Spikes: Exploring the Neural Code*. MIT Press, Cambridge, MA.
Rudy, J.W. (1996) Postconditioning isolation disrupts contextual conditioning: an experimental analysis. *Behav. Neurosci.* 110:238–246.
Rudy, J.W., and R.J. Sutherland (1992) Configural and elemental associations and the memory coherence problem. *J. Cogn. Neurosci.* 43:208–216.
Russel, I.S. (1979) Brain size and intelligence: a comparative perspective. In D.A. Oakley and H.C. Plotkin (eds.): *Brain Behaviour and Evolution*. Methuen, London, pp. 126–153.
Rybak, J., and R. Menzel (1993) Anatomy of the mushroom bodies in the honey bee brain: the neuronal connections of the alpha-lobe. *J. Comp. Neurol.* 334:444–465.
Ryback, J., and R. Menzel (1998) Integrative properties of the Pe1–neuron, a unique mushroom body output neuron. *Learn and Memory* 5:133–145.
Saavedra, M.A. (1975) Pavlovian conditioning in the rabbit. *Learn. Motivat.* 6:314–326.
Schultz, W., P. Dayan, and P.R. Montague (1997) A neural substrate of prediction and reward. *Science* 275:1593–1599.
Seeley, T.D. (1995) *The Wisdom of the Hive—The Social Physiology of Honey Bee Colonies*. Harvard University Press, London.
Singer, W., and C.M. Gray (1995) Visual feature integration and the temporal correlation hypothesis. *Annu. Rev. Neurosci.* 18:555–586.
Smith, B.H. (1991) The olfactory memory of the honeybee *Apis mellifera*. I. Odorant modulation of short- and intermediate-term memory after single–trial conditioning. *J. Exp. Biol.* 161:367–382.

Smith, B.H. (1996.) The role of attention in learning about odorants. *Biol. Bull.* 191:76–83.
Smith, B.H. (1997) An analysis of blocking in binary odorant mixtures: an increase but not a decrease in intensity of reinforcement produces unblocking. *Behav. Neurosci.* 111:57–69.
Smith, B.H., and S. Cobey (1994) The olfactory memory of the honey bee, *Apis mellifera*. II: blocking between odorants in binary mixtures. *J. Exp. Biol.* 195:91–108.
Spence, K.W. (1937) The differential response in animal to stimuli varying within a single dimension. *Psychol. Rev.* 44:430–444.
Squire, L.R. (1987) *Memory and Brain*. Oxford University Press, Oxford.
Srinivasan, M.V. (1994) Pattern recognition in the honeybee: recent progress. *J. Insect Physiol.* 40(3):183–194.
Srinivasan, M.V., S.W. Zhang, M. Lehrer, and T.S. Collett (1996) Honeybee navigation *en route* to the goal: visual flight control and odometry. *J. Exp. Biol.* 199:237–244.
Srinivasan, M.V., S.W. Zhang, and K. Witney (1994) Visual discrimination of pattern orientation by honeybees: performance and implications for "cortical" processing. *Philos. Trans. R. Soc. Lond. [Biol.]* 343:199–210.
Sutton, R.S., and A.G. Barto (1981) Toward a modern theory of adaptive networks: expectation and prediction. *Psychol. Rev.* 88:135–170.
Takeda, K. (1961) Classical conditioned response in the honey bee. *J. Insect Physiol.* 6:168–179.
Thinus-Blanc, C. (1987) The cognitive map concept and its consequences. In P. Ellen and C. Thinus-Blanc (eds.): *Cognitive Processes and Spatial Orientation in Animal and Man*. Martinus Nijhoff, Dordrecht, pp. 1–18.
Thomson, J.D. (1996) Trapline foraging by bumblebees: I. Persistence of flight–path geometry. *Behav. Ecol.* 7:158–164.
Thorpe, W.H. (1963) *Learning and Instinct in Animals*. Methuen, London.
Tolman, E.C. (1932) *Purposive Behavior in Animals and Men*. Century, New York.
Tolman, E.C. (1948) Cognitive maps in rats and men. *Psychol. Rev.* 55:189–208.
Vareschi, E. (1971) Duftunterscheidung bei der Honigbiene—Einzelzell-Ableitungen und Verhaltensreaktionen. *Z. vergl. Physiol.* 75:143–173.
Waddington, K.D. (1985) Cost–intake information used in foraging. *J. Insect Physiol.* 31:891–889.
Wagner, A.R. (1981) SOP: A model of Automatic memory processing in animal behavior. In N.E. Spear, R.R. Miller, A. Erlbaum, and N.J. Hillsdale (eds.): *Information Processing in Animals: Memory Mechanism*. Erlbaum, Hillsdale, NJ, pp. 5–47.
Wagner, A.R., and M.B. Larew (1985) Opponent process and pavlovian inhibition. In R.R. Miller and N.E. Spear (eds.): *Information Processing in Animals: Conditioned Inhibition*. Erlbaum, Hillsdale, NJ, pp. 233–265.
Wehner, R. (1981) Spatial vision in arthropods. In H.J. Autrum (ed.): *Handbook of Sensory Physiology* VIc. Springer, Berlin, pp. 287–616.
Wehner, R. (1992) Arthropods. In F. Papi (ed.): *Animal homing*. Chapman & Hall, London. pp. 45–144.
Wehner, R., S. Bleuler, C. Nievergelt, and D. Shah (1990) Bees navigate by using vectors and routes rather than maps. *Naturwissenschaften* 77:479–482.
Wehner, R., and R. Menzel (1990) Do insects have cognitive maps? *Annu. Rev. Neurosci.* 13:403–414.
Wehner, R., B. Michel, and P. Antonsen (1996) Visual navigation in insects: coupling of egocentric and geocentric information. *J. Exp. Biol.* 199:129–140.
Wehner, R., and S. Rossel (1985) The bee's celestial compass—case study in behavioural neurobiology. In B. Hölldobler and M. Lindauer (eds.): *Experimental Behavioral Ecology*. Gustav Fischer Verlag, Stuttgart, pp. 11–53.
Whitlow, J.W., and A.R. Wagner (1972) Negative patterning in classical conditioning: summation of response tendencies to isolable and configural components. *Psychon. Sci.* 27:299–301.
Withers, G.S., S.E. Fahrbach, and G.E. Robinson (1993) Selective neuroanatomical plasticity and division of labour in the honey bee (*Apis mellifera*). *Nature* 364:238–240.
Witthöft, W. (1967) Absolute Anzahl und Verteilung der Zellen im Hirn der Honigbiene. *Z. Morphol. Tiere* 61:160–184.
Woodbury, C.B. (1943) The learning of stimulus patterns by dogs. *J. Comp. Psychol.* 35:29–40.
Yang, E. C., and T. Maddess, (1997) Orientation–sensitive neurons in the brain of the honey bee (*Apis mellifera*). *J. Insect Physiol.* 43: 329–336.
Yuste, R., and D.W. Tank (1996) Dendritic integration in mammalian neurons, a century after. *Neuron* 16:701–716.

Chapter 12

INSECT BRAIN

Nicholas J. Strausfeld, Arizona Research Laboratories, Division of Neurobiology, University of Arizona

INTRODUCTION

By any measure, the insects are a success story. The evolution of highly maneuverable flight (Wootton et al., 1998), holometaboly (Truman and Riddiford, 1999), and eusociality (Trivers and Hare, 1976) have permitted them to exploit almost every type of environmental niche other than the sea, from which their progenitors emerged and which is the domain of their closest relatives, the crustaceans. In addition to their more obvious evolutionary acquisitions, the success of insects must also be attributed to the organization of their brains, which have evolved into compact and highly elaborate structures that support a behavioral diversity comparable to that of many land vertebrates, including mammals.

Insects and other arthropods belong to one of the two great protostome clades, the ecdysozoans—the other being the lophotrochozoans, which include the annelids. Like those of annelids, the brains of arthropods are situated dorsally above the gut as indeed are the brains of chordates. Paleontology, molecular phylogenetics, and the study of *Hox* gene complexes contribute to a modern consensus that the lophotrochozoans and ecdysozoans, along with the chordates, derive from a common bilateral ancestor (Knoll and Carroll, 1999; Rosa et al., 1999) and that this common origin is reflected in the early construction of chordate and arthropod nervous systems (Reichert and Simeone, 1999). Both comprise segmental entities (neuromeres) whose positional determination is under the control of orthologous regulatory genes. These genes were present more than 600 million years ago in the common ancestor to deuterostomes and protostomes; and, although no extant taxon is likely to represent the ancestral morph, developmental (Arendt and Nübler-Jung, 1994, 1996, 1997) and neural (Strausfeld, 1998) comparisons suggest enteropneusts or turbellarians as models. In this regard, it is of great interest that genes orthologous to those underlying axial patterning in the protocerebrum and forebrain of *Drosophila* and mouse have been identified in flatworms (Umesono et al., 1999).

Whereas the brains of polychaete annelids and the protocerebral ganglia of mollusks probably consist of a single neuromere, the brains of arthropods derive from two to three segments. In insects, the supraoesophageal ganglion is composed of the proto-, deuto-, and tritocerebra, also called preoral neuromeres because they are rostral to segments providing the mouthparts. Three postoral neuromeres (from the maxillary, mandibular, and labial segments) are also in the head but lie beneath the gut. These make up the postoral suboesophageal "ganglion," which, among other functions, receives sensory inputs from the mouthparts and provides motor neurons that control them.

In arthropods and annelids, no sensory or motor neurons have been thus far ascribed to the protocerebrum, and in this it seems to be genuinely different from other neuromeres and from the protocerebrum of annelids, which receives sensory afferents from the palps. Apart from that in onychophorans and diplopods (Strausfeld et al., 1995), it can be argued that the arthropod protocerebrum receives no direct sensory afferents except from the retina of the compound eye, which supplies the protocerebrum via, primitively, two lateral neuropils called the lamina and medulla. Although the segmental origin of these neuropils is still unresolved, in crown taxa a third visual neuropil (called the lobula) originates embryonically from an outgrowth of the protocerebrum (Elofsson and Dahl, 1970).

Neuropils in the protocerebrum are referred to as higher centers because of their synaptic distance from circuits that directly control motor neurons and because the integrity of the protocerebrum is necessary for complex behaviors. Arthropod and annelid protocerebra are unique in that one of their pairs of synaptic neuropils appears to be without a counterpart in other segments. These are the mushroom bodies (or their equivalent—the hemiellipsoid bodies of malacostracan crustaceans), which can also be identified in turbellarian flatworms (Hadenfeldt, 1929; Strausfeld, 1998). Historically, the paired mushroom bodies have been implicated in intelligence, in learning and memory functions, and in context-dependent sensory integration and choice (see Heisenberg, 1998). In contrast, the system of midline neuropils known as the central complex appears to be involved in supervising coordinated leg movements (Strauss et al., 1992) and may play an important role in goal-directed locomotion.

This chapter focuses on the mushroom bodies and the central complex (Figs. 12.1and 12.2) and discusses the relationship between these and other parts of the central nervous system.

GENERAL FEATURES OF SEGMENTAL GANGLIA

Before the unique attributes of the protocerebrum are discussed, it is useful to briefly summarize some of the salient features of metameric ganglia with which the protocerebrum should be compared.

The body of an insect has three thoracic ganglia followed by (primitively) 11 abdominal ganglia. In taxa representing evolutionarily basal insects (e.g., zygentomans, like firebrats; palaeopterans, like dragonflies and mayflies), most ganglia are discrete, being connected to their neighbors by paired nerve cords. An exception is the last two to three abdominal ganglia, which even in primitive insects can be fused, serving as a specialized integration center for sensory information provided by long caudal appendages, called cerci, which are used to detect air displacement (Edwards and Reddy, 1986).

General Features of Segmental Ganglia 369

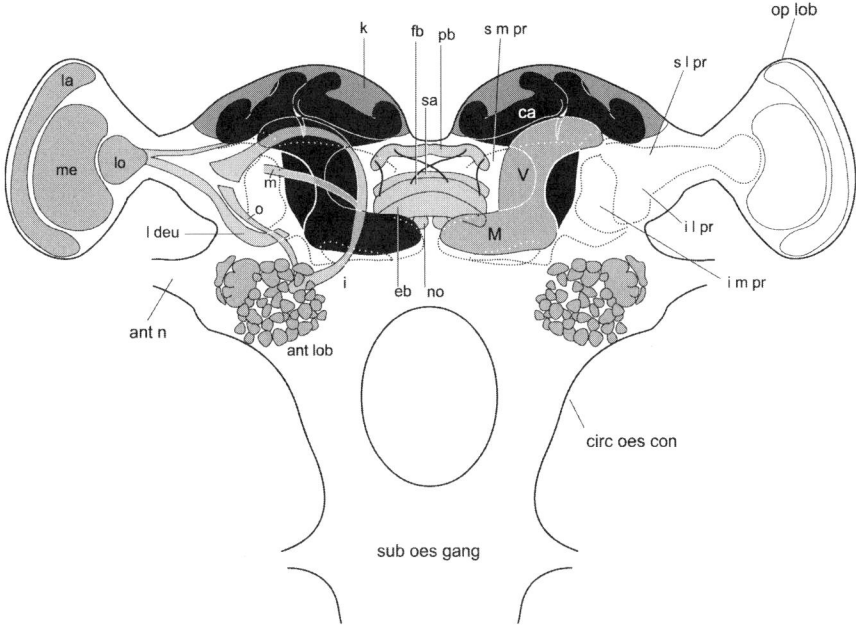

Figure 12.1. Front view of the supraoesophageal ganglia of the cockroach *Periplaneta americana*. The mushroom bodies and central complex dominate the brain. The paired mushroom bodies (black) consist of a vertical (V) and medial lobe (M) supplied from a pair of calyces (ca) above which lie many thousands of Kenyon cell bodies (k). The central complex consists of five main neuropils: the protocerebral bridge (pb), fan-shaped body (fb), superior arch (sa), ellipsoid body (eb), and the paired noduli (no). The brain is flanked lateroposteriorly by the optic lobes (op lob) and frontally by the antennal lobes (ant lob), which receive sensory axons from olfactory receptors via the antennal nerve (ant n). Axons from the antennal lobe glomeruli ascend to the calyces and superior (s l pr) and inferior lateral deutocerebra (i l pr) via the inner (i), medial (m), and outer (o) branches of the antennocerebral tract. The optic lobes consist of three neuropils: the lamina (la), which receives inputs from the compound retina (not shown); the medulla (me); and the lobula (lo). The latter provides most of its outputs to the lateral deutocerebrum (l deu). The supraoesophageal ganglia are connected to the postoral suboesophageal ganglion (sub oes gang) by the circumoesophageal connectives (circ oes con).

Separated ganglia are thought to be an evolutionarily primitive feature, whereas the converse, fused ganglia, is an advanced trait. Some hexapod groups, such as the Collembola, suggest an advanced feature because their thoracic ganglia can be completely fused. This trait also typifies "recent" neopteran insects such as cyclorrhaphan flies like *Drosophila*. In the fruit fly, three thoracic ganglia (the pro-, meso-, and metathoracic ganglia) and the compressed abdominal ganglia are coalesced into one mass, although it is still possible to discern segmentation. Social Hymenoptera, many Lepidoptera, Coleoptera, and cyclorrhaphan Diptera, all holometabolous insects, have fused supraoesophageal and suboesophageal ganglia pierced by a foramen that allows the passage of the gut through the brain. The advanced trait of ganglion fusion also typifies some malacostracan crustacean taxa, such as crabs.

Fused ganglia typify the chelicerates where the supraoesophageal and suboesophageal ganglia fuse with the thoracic ganglia into a single mass. The one exception

370 12 Insect Brain

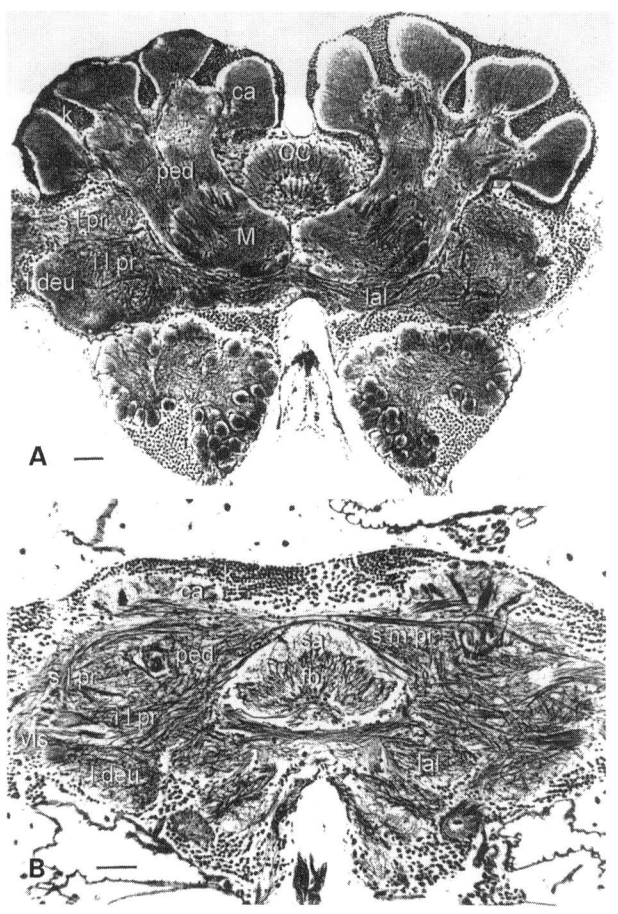

Figure 12.2. Hymenopterans and blattids have the largest mushroom bodies relative to the whole brain volume. (A) Frontal view of the brain of a female velvet ant *Dasymuttilus* showing the calyces (ca), pedunculus (ped), and medial lobes (M) of the paired mushroom bodies and the fan-shaped body of the central complex (CC). The superior lateral (s l pr) and inferior lateral protocerebra (i l pr) are relatively small and compact. The antennal lobes consist of two to three discrete populations of glomeruli. Note the size of the Kenyon cell bodies (k) above the calyces. Bar = 50 µm. (B) Frontal section through the brain of a fly (*Musca domestica*) at a level posterior to the antennal lobes and medial lobes. There are relatively few Kenyon cell bodies. The two calyces of each mushroom body are fused and are small, as is the pedunculus (ped). At this level the prominent central complex is represented by its fan-shaped body (fb) and superior arch(sa). Other protocerebral neuropils are the superior medial protocerebrum (s m pr), lateral accessory lobe (lal), superior lateral (s l pr), and inferior lateral protocerebra (i l pr). The lateral deutocerebrum (l deu) and i l pr are supplied by bundles of axons (vis) from the lobula (not

is in the Pycnogonida (sea spiders), where a pair of short connectives connects the suboesophageal ganglion to a chain of separate ganglia, one for each segment of the body, which is foreshortened. Scorpions and xiphosurans have discrete abdominal ganglia, but among the spiders only the "living fossil" *Heptathela kimura* has vestigial abdominal segmentation. This is entirely absent in three other chelicerate groups, the solpugids (sun spiders), uropygids (vinegaroons), and amblypygids (whip spiders). Because fossil evidence suggests that ganglion fusion was already accomplished in Ordovician eurypterids, either the chelicerates are older than the crustaceans and have had more time to evolve this trait or ganglion fusion evolved more rapidly in the chelicerates than in other groups.

As a rule, single, pairs, or groups of uniquely identifiable neurons are reiterated segmentally in each neuromere, irrespective of whether ganglia are fused. Erroneously referred to as segmentally homologous, ensembles of reiteratively equivalent neurons are often modified in certain segments by segment-specific cell death or hormonally controlled segment-specific elaboration of their dendrites and axons (Levine and Weeks, 1990). The affinities of segmentally equivalent neurons to antibodies raised against neuropeptides or transmitter substances are particularly useful for demonstrating such modifications as well as for demonstrating true homology between genera (Witten and Truman, 1998).

Often, modifications reflect peripheral effector and receptor structures that have been accentuated (or diminished) at that segment. For example, in diving Hemiptera, such as the backswimmer *Notonecta glauca*, the pair of metathoracic oarlike legs used for propulsion are served by metathoracic motor neurons and interneurons that have much larger diameters and more extensive dendritic trees than their equivalents in mesothoracic and prothoracic segments. In contrast, another hemipteran, the water strider *Gerris*, employs all three leg pairs for rowing. In this species, all three pairs of thoracic neuromeres appear to be equivalent with respect to leg motor neuropils. Another well-known example of local elaboration of segmentally equivalent neurons is in locusts, where circuits associated with the control of posture and walking have become highly modified for controlling the third leg pair, which is used for jumping as well as for walking (Pearson and Robertson, 1981; for reviews, see Pearson, 1983; Burrows, 1996). These circuits have also recruited neurons in the first two abdominal ganglia, which have become fused to the metathoracic ganglion. Together three fused ganglia provide specialized pathways that cock, prime, and release the jump response (Pearson, 1983; Gynther and Pearson, 1989).

What seem to be novel flight motor circuits in the mesothoracic and metathoracic ganglia are derived from neuronal lineages that already existed in primitive aptery gotes, before the evolution of wings (Truman and Ball, 1998). Additional neurons that provide unique segment-specific elements in pterothoracic flight circuits have arisen by expanding the number of neurons made by stem cells of those ancient lineages.

The same organizational rules pertain to each ganglion. Sensory axons enter the ganglion ventrally, and motor neuron axons leave the ganglion dorsally—a polarity and organization that is the inverse of that in the vertebrate spinal cord (Zawarzin, 1925) but retaining fundamental similarities between vertebrate and invertebrates regarding the control of walking and posture (Pearson, 1993). In ganglia, sensory endings from different sensory fields or different types of sensilla invade discrete islets of sensory neuropils where their terminals somatotopically map the peripheral arrangement of their sensory dendrites (Newland, 1991a,b; Merritt and Murphey, 1992). Topical representation of the sensory periphery supplied from tactile, taste, and odor receptors is also typical of circumscribed sensory neuropils in the tritocerebral and deutocerebral ganglia, supporting the idea that these are phylogenetically derived from postoral neuromeres (see below).

Studies on locusts have shown that in the thorax only a minority of sensory endings establishes monosynaptic inputs onto motor neurons. Most sensory afferents distribute onto the dendrites of local nonspiking and spiking interneurons whose processes have characteristic relationships with fields of sensory afferents (Siegler and Burrows, 1983, 1986; Burrows and Siegler, 1985; for review, see Burrows, 1996). These two types of local interneurons integrate sensory information and control the activity of motor neurons. Among these circuits are those that, with sensory feedback from the periphery, generate rhythmic action of muscles, as in respiration, walking, and flying. Such circuits are called central pattern generators (Getting, 1988). In insect ganglia, central pattern generators involve elements that are symmetrically connected to each side of the ganglion by commissural interneurons and are linked to those in adjacent segments by plurisegmental interneurons to provide segmental coordination (Laurent and Burrows, 1989). Dynamic modification of central pattern generators is afforded by sensory feedback from receptors in the same and adjacent segments.

Although these features were entirely unknown to scientists in the last century, it was a point of interest to two French ethologists (Faivre, 1857; Binet, 1894) that some insects, when decapitated, could organize short episodes of rhythmic activity, such as forward locomotion and other limited motor repertoires. These early researchers also noted that the supraoesophageal ganglion is necessary for adaptive and goal-directed motor actions that occur in response to novel sensory stimuli. Thus, it was recognized very early that the organization of behavior and the origin of novel motor repertoires must originate in the brain.

THE PROTOCEREBRUM AND THE PREORAL BRAIN

Evolutionary Considerations

The protocerebrum appears to be unique in that it contains neuropils that have no equivalents in the deutocerebrum and tritocerebrum, which have more similarity to postoral (suboesophageal and thoracic) ganglia than to the protocerebrum. Both the deutocerebrum and tritocerebrum receive peripheral sensory inputs and provide motor neurons as well as intersegmental interneurons to the ventral nerve cord.

The organization of brain segmentation is of some importance regarding the evolutionary affinities between onychophorans, chelicerates, and crustaceans because the number of preoral neuromeres in the brain distinguishes these groups (Fig. 12.3). The arrangement in onychophorans suggests that the segmented ancestor to the arthropods may have possessed only a single preoral neuropil and that additional neuromeres were added later. Onychophorans possess what appears to be a single supraesophageal neuromere that contains mushroom bodies and chelicerate-like central bodies. In addition to a protocerebrum, the chelicerate brain has one and the crustacean and insect brain has two postoral-like neuromeres in a preoral position. Possibly, these have been recruited by a caudal displacement of the mouth and gut

The Protocerebrum and the Preoral Brain 373

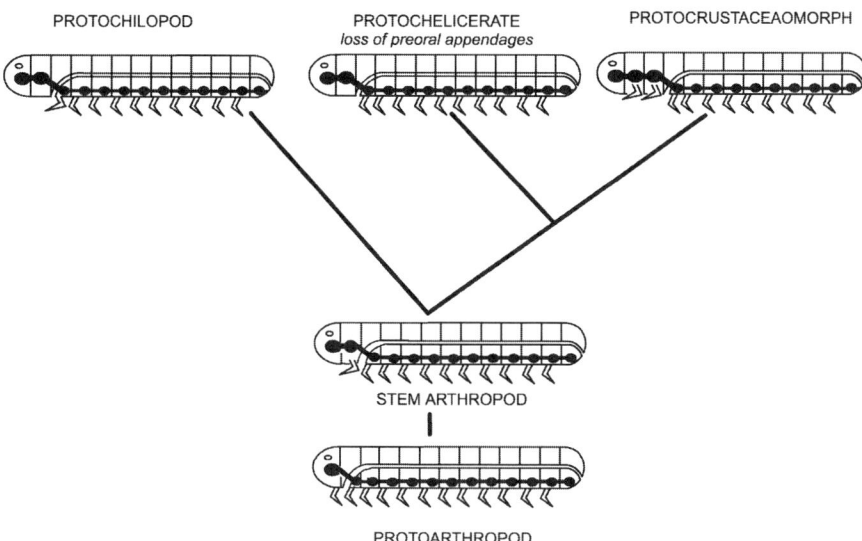

Figure 12.3. Originating from a stem condition in which there is a single preoral neuromere, the evolution of preoral ganglia may be associated with a successively more caudal segmental location of the mouth. This would allow the derived conditions of two (protochelicerates, protochilopods) or three (protocrustaceomorphs) preoral ganglia. Preoral appendages are not present in extant chelicerates.

(Fig. 12.3). An alternative explanation for these differences is that elaboration of the brain has arisen by the intercalation of novel neuromeres such that one additional neuromere has evolved in chelicerates and two in crustaceans and insects.

General Organization of the Protocerebrum

Protocerebral neuropils receive their inputs from interneurons. These carry information from the optic lobes and from neuropils of the deutocerebrum and tritocerebrum and from the suboesophageal, thoracic, and abdominal ganglia.

Interneurons to the protocerebrum report sensory events, as well as motor actions, after several layers of filtering and integration. Thus, visual inputs to the protocerebrum carry information not about simple visual stimuli (although these are often used to test for multimodality in protocerebral neurons) but about higher order stimuli, such as directional motion, texture, pattern orientation, and spectral organization of the retinal image. Likewise, recordings from efferent copy neurons in the protocerebrum encounter units that are activated by very specific motor events rather than general movement (Mizunami et al., 1998a). Recordings from the protocerebrum rarely encounter neurons that respond to only a single modality, although sensory interneurons do map discrete single modalities onto their own domains of protocerebral neuropils, as occurs in the calyces of the mushroom bodies (Mobbs, 1982). Neuroanatomy generally suggests, however, that multimodal convergence

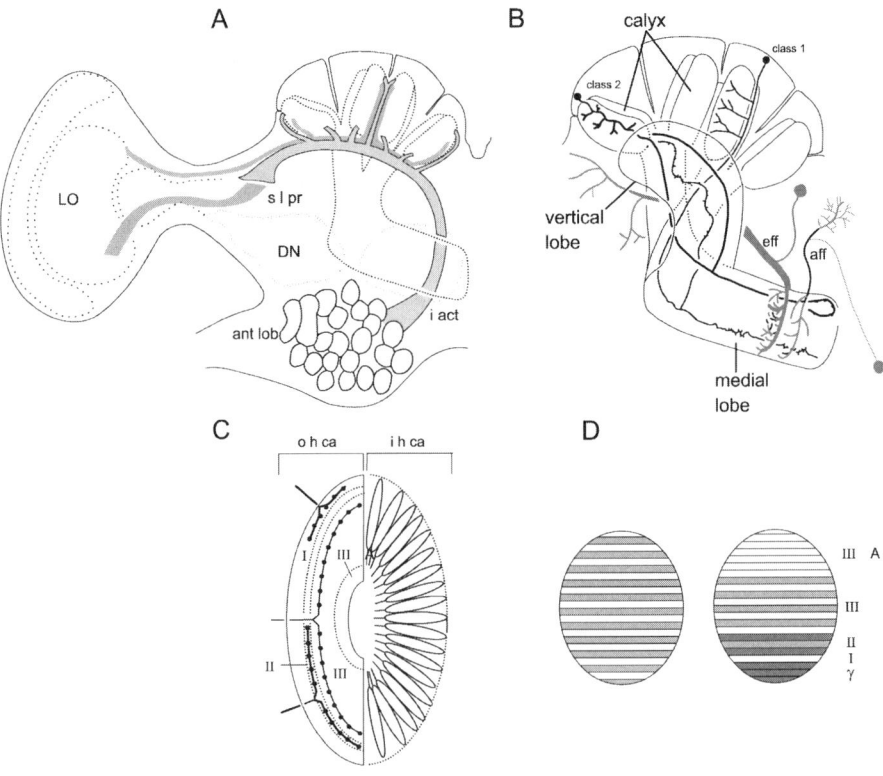

Figure 12.4. Organization in mushroom bodies. (A) Afferent supply to the calyces is from the visual system's lobula (LO) and olfactory neuropils (ant lob), the latter via the antennal cerebral tract (i act). Inputs to the calyces are the collaterals of antennal lobe projection neurons that terminate in the superior lateral protocerebrum (s l pr). This region also receives afferents from the lobula. (B) The bulk of the mushroom bodies is provided by two major classes of Kenyon cells, both having dendrites in the calyces and "axons" that bifurcate into the lobes. Axons are intersected by dendrites of efferent neurons (eff, extending to the protocerebrum; see Li and Strausfeld, 1997, 1999) and the terminals of afferents (aff, from protocerebral neuropils; Li and Strausfeld, 1997). (C) Efferents to the calyces map into discrete zones (I–IIIA in outer hemicalyx; o h ca), where they extend through folia of Kenyon cell dendrites (shown in inner hemicalyx; i h ca) (see Strausfeld and Li, 1999). (D) Cross sections of the lobes show two types of arrangements among Kenyon cell axons: dark and pale laminae (left) and layered groups of laminae that are immunopositive (or immunonegative) to antibodies against neuromodulators (here shown for antiFMRFamide). These layers represent the arrangement of zones in the calyces.

provides the basis for multimodal integration. This is seen in the superior lateral protocerebrum, which receives the terminals of projection neurons from two sources: from olfactory glomeruli in the antennal lobes and from relay neurons that originate in the lobula, a deep neuropil of the visual system (Fig. 12.4A). Furthermore, as is typical for protocerebral neuropils, the superior lateral protocerebrum does not merely integrate olfactory and visual information, but it also is reciprocally connected with other brain regions, suggesting its role in assessing odorant stimuli in other sensory contexts (Li and Strausfeld, 1997, 1999).

Unfortunately, however, apart from the two neuropil complexes described below, most protocerebral areas remain unexplored. This is because in the past their organization has been dismissed as "unstructured" and, understandably, because most observers have focused on regions that are easily distinguished (Flögel, 1876), like the mushroom bodies and central complex.

THE MUSHROOM BODIES

Structure

Mushroom bodies are paired neuropils, one on each side of the brain. As their name suggests, they have the appearance of fungi (Fig. 12.1). In neopteran insects, each mushroom body consists of two caps or cups (the calyces) at the back of the protocerebrum that are joined to a stalk (the pedunculus) extending to the front, there providing swollen roots or lobes. One or more lobes are directed toward the midline (medial lobes), while one or more extend upward to the roof of the brain (vertical lobes). In palaeopteran and zygentoman insects, mushroom bodies lack calyces.

The matrix of the mushroom body consists of thousands of extremely small neurons called globuli cells (Flögel, 1876). A mushroom body may possess more than a quarter of a million of these, as in the tarantula hawk wasp *Pepsis thisbe* and the cockroach *Periplaneta americana*, or only a few thousand, as in *Drosophila melanogaster*. Despite differences in cell number, the basic organization of the mushroom bodies is similar across the Insecta. Globuli cells are clustered above the pedunculus (Fig. 12.2), each cell providing a neurite that elongates into a slender axonlike process into the pedunculus and lobes (Fig. 12.4B). These processes are arranged approximately parallel to one another. In neopteran insects, globuli cells have dendrites in the calyces. In this manifestation, the cells are termed Kenyon cells, after the neurologist who first described them (Kenyon, 1896).

In many species, the mushroom body's lobes are subdivided longitudinally, as in *Drosophila*, where the medial lobes consist of three parallel subdivisions each corresponding to the axon projection of a specific morphological type of Kenyon cell. Genetic markers also reveal these subdivisions, two in the vertical lobe (called α and α') and three in the medial lobe (called β, β', and γ; Crittenden et al., 1998; Lee et al., 1999). One type of Kenyon cell branches into the α' and β' subdivisions of the vertical and medial lobes. Another sends its axons into the α and β subdivisions of the two lobes, while a third type provides unbranched axons to the γ subdivision of the medial lobe. Evidence that these subdivisions may be functionally independent is suggested by each having its own afferent terminals and efferent neuron dendrites (Ito et al., 1998).

Afferents supply the mushroom bodies at two levels: in the calyces and in the lobes (Figs. 12.4 and 12.5). The major input to the calyces is provided ipsilaterally by collaterals of olfactory projection neurons whose dendrites invade antennal lobe glomeruli and whose final terminal processes arborize through the superior lateral protocerebrum (Fig. 12.4A). In Hymenoptera (wasps, bees, ants), the calyces also

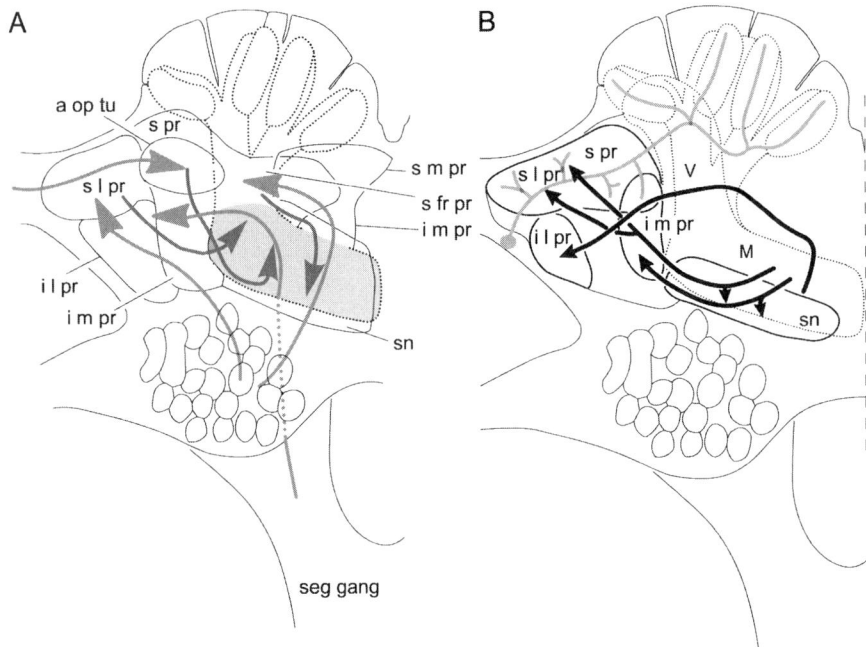

Figure 12.5. The mushroom body lobes receive and provide axons from and to the protocerebrum. (A) Discrete regions of the protocerebrum receive afferents (light gray arrows) from the antennal lobes and visual system, as well as ascending neurons from segmental postoral ganglia (seg gang). These regions provide inputs (gray arrows) to the mushroom body lobes (medial lobe shown shaded). s pr, superior protocerebrum; s m pr, i m pr, superior medial and inferior medial protocerebra; s fr pr, superior frontal protocerebrum; sn, satellite neuropil of the medial lobe. (B) The calyces are invaded by terminals of GABAergic neurons (light gray lines), the dendrites of which extend through protocerebral neuropils. Outputs (efferent neurons) from the medial lobes (black arrows) mainly terminate in lateral protocerebral regions and in satellite neuropil. Outputs from the vertical lobes (not shown) mainly end in medial protocerebrum.

receive bundles of axons from both optic lobes (Gronenberg, 1987, 1999), but in other insect groups visual inputs to the calyces are modest or absent.

In the calyces, visual and olfactory terminals segregate so as to subdivide the calyces into discrete zones distoproximally (Fig. 12.4C), each representing a different combination or class of afferent endings (Mobbs, 1982; Gronenberg, 1999). A second class of afferents to the calyces comprises inhibitory multimodal neurons whose dendrites arborize through protocerebral neuropils (Fig. 12.5B). In cockroaches, six types of these GABAergic afferents have been identified, each supplying a specific combination of calyx zones (Strausfeld and Li, 1999a). A third class of calyx afferents is made up of peptidergic neurons that are revealed by antibodies against octopamine or FMRFamide (Hammer, 1993; Strausfeld and Li, 1999a). Electron microscopy of the calyces demonstrates that Kenyon cells are postsynaptic to projection neurons from the antennal lobes as well as to other profiles, many of which contain dense-cored vesicles (Schürmann, 1987). These presumably belong to GABAergic and peptidergic elements.

In cockroaches and honey bees different zones of the calyces, defined by the identities of their afferent terminals (see below), are represented in the lobes by broad layers (also called bands; Mobbs, 1982) of Kenyon cell axons (Fig. 12.4D). In the cockroach each of these layers is composed of a number of smaller subunits called laminae that are arranged isomorphically across the lobes (Strausfeld and Li, 1999b). Each lamina is itself made up of thin sheets of Kenyon cell axons comprising the axons of a single type of Kenyon cell. The intrinsic organization of a single lamina thus compares with Kenyon cell-specific subdivisions of the entire *Drosophila* mushroom body, which could be viewed as representing a single lamina in the much larger cockroach. In honey bees and in cockroaches, layers are further divided into strata that are distinguished by their affinity to antibodies against FMRFamide, gastrin-cholecystokinin, or taurine (Schäfer et al., 1988; Bicker, 1991, Schürmann and Erber, 1990; Strausfeld and Li, 1999b; Strausfeld et al., 2000).

Evolution of Mushroom Bodies in Insects

Received opinion is that the calyces are the primary "input" neuropils of the mushroom bodies (for reviews, see Davis, 1993; Heisenberg, 1998). This view, however, needs revision because studies of phylogenetically basal hexapods suggest that the mushroom body lobes evolved long before the origin of the calyces and antennal lobes (Strausfeld, 1998). The most primitive representatives of the insects, the Archaeognatha, entirely lack mushroom bodies. Taxa that are thought to have evolved later, like the apterygote thysanurans or the palaeopteran dragonflies and mayflies, all lack olfactory (antennal) lobes even though chemosensory sensilla have been identified on their antennae (Bassemir and Hansen, 1980). They possess mushroom bodies, however, that lack calyces. Clusters of many thousands of globuli cells provide bundles of neurites, all devoid of dendrites, that extend from the back of the brain to the front, where each neurite bifurcates and then enlarges to provide an intrinsic element in the medial and vertical lobes (Strausfeld et al., 1998). The same organization is seen in aquatic insects that have vestigial antennae and have secondarily lost their antennal lobes, as in certain bugs (Hemiptera) and beetles. These taxa lack calyces, but their mushroom bodies possess vertical and medial lobes.

Thus, a crucial difference between palaeopteran and neopteran insects relates to the morphology of Kenyon cells, which in the Neoptera supply dendrites to outgrowths called the calyces, situated at the head of pedunculus. Nevertheless, both in palaeopterans and in neopterans, Kenyon cell "axons" in the lobes are equipped with presynaptic swellings and with postsynatic spines. Electron microscopic studies show that Kenyon cell "axons" are both pre- and postsynaptic in the lobes where they provide local circuits between afferent processes ending in the lobes and dendrites of efferent neurons leaving them (Strausfeld and Li, 1999b). The acquisition of a calyx by the Neoptera suggests a major evolutionary advance: the tuning of local circuits in the lobes by olfactory or visual neurons supplying the calyces with information about ambient olfactory and visual stimuli (Fig. 12.6).

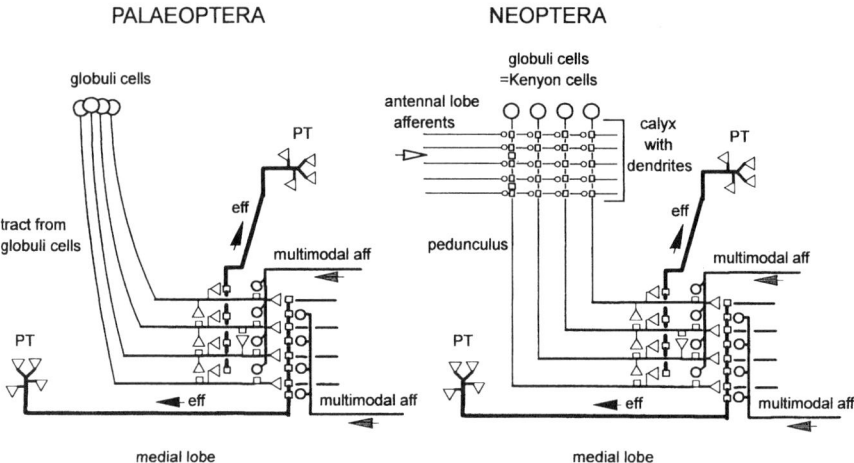

Figure 12.6. In both palaeopteran and neopteran insects, intrinsic processes in the lobes are equipped with presynaptic (triangles) and postsynaptic (boxes) sites. They receive multimodal afferent (aff) neurons from protocerebral neuropils and send efferent neurons (eff) to target areas in the protocerebrum (PT). In palaeopterans, globuli cells provide a tract linking them to the lobes (medial lobe shown only). In neopterans, globuli cells provide dendrites to an outer swelling of this tract, the calyx. The tract becomes the pedunculus. Thereby, the calyx is supplied with various afferents that synapse onto Kenyon cells to impose peripheral inputs on phylogenetically ancient circuits in the lobes.

In conclusion, comparisons between taxa representing the early insects with insects that arose during the Carboniferous era suggest that the lobes are the oldest part of the mushroom bodies and that they provide a unique system of local circuits for interactions between afferents and efferents. If the mushroom bodies indeed provide a substrate for learning and memory, then neural circuits underlying these attributes are likely to reside in phylogenetically "early" circuits rather than in the calyces. In certain groups of neopterans longitudinal subdivisions of the lobes, reflecting calycal zones (Strausfeld et al., 2000), suggests an additional evolutionary advance by longitudinal multiplexing of discrete integrative networks (Fig. 12.4D).

Relationships to Primary Sensory Neuropils

As has been outlined above, mushroom bodies are supplied by inputs to their calyces as well as to their lobes. These two levels of inputs are distinct and have different evolutionary origins. Whereas afferents supplying the lobes originate in protocerebral neuropils, afferents supplying the calyx (other than GABAergic neurons; see below) derive from primary sensory neuropils. These neuropils are composed of systems of neurons that receive inputs directly from sensory axons or systems of neurons that receive a map of the sensory periphery via only few intermediaries.

The antennal lobes. Except in hymenopterans (e.g., bees, ants and wasps), the major input to the calyces is from the antennal lobes. These are neuropils in the brain's second preoral segment (the deutocerebrum) that receive the axonal terminals of olfactory receptor neurons in the antenna's flagellum. Except in certain Orthoptera, such as the locust, antennal lobes are composed of glomeruli that have uniquely identifiable shapes and positions according to species and sex (Laissue et al., 1999; Rospars and Hildebrand, 1992). The cellular organization of a glomerulus involves three types of neurons whose synaptic connections with receptor terminals may vary little between species (Boeckh and Tolbert, 1993). In insects, projection neurons extend from the glomeruli to various parts of the protocerebrum via three major tracts called the antennocerebral pathways (Kanzaki et al., 1989). Projection neurons from two of these tracts (the inner and outer antennoglomerular tracts; Homberg et al., 1989) provide axon collaterals that invade the calyces. All the main axons of projection neurons go on, however, to end in lateral neuropils of the protocerebrum. It is these regions, among others, that both receive endings from neurons arising deeper in the mushroom bodies and provide interneurons that end in the mushroom body lobes. These regions are also connected by interneurons to dendrites of descending neurons leading to thoracic ganglia.

Most projection neurons have dendrites within a single glomerulus, where they receive synaptic inputs from olfactory receptor axons as well as from local interneurons, which also receive receptor inputs. Local interneurons are anaxonal neurons that provide connections among projection neurons (Christensen et al., 1993; Boeckh and Tolbert, 1993). There exist local neurons that have dendrites in one glomerulus and axons that terminate in several others, like the periglomerular neurons of vertebrates (Flanagan and Mercer, 1989). Information coding by projection neurons involves excitatory responses by uniglomerular output neurons preceded and followed by membrane hyperpolarization (Christensen et al., 1996). As cellular arrangements in insect glomeruli are similar to those in mammalian glomeruli in the olfactory bulb, these physiological events are remarkably similar to those observed in mammals and other vertebrates (Hildebrand and Shepherd, 1997).

Projection neurons respond to many features of the olfactory world. They may be tuned to specific odors or components of odor blends (Vickers et al., 1998). They may be tuned to specific frequencies of odor pulses, as would be encountered under natural conditions where an odor plume breaks up into discrete packets (Christensen et al., 1996). It is also of interest, however, that sustained odor presentation—which is a most "unnatural" stimulus—can evoke synchronous activity among projection neurons (Laurent and Davidowitz, 1994) and among Kenyon cells in the calyces that receive information from projection neurons (Laurent and Naraghi, 1994),

It has been shown in the cockroach that two different groups of glomeruli supply two different zones of the calyces (Strausfeld and Li, 1999a). Possibly, olfactory afferents parse the calyces into even smaller zones, which would suggest that there is some type of odortopic representation in the calyces as there is in the antennal lobes. Optical imaging of the antennal lobes has shown that glomeruli tuned to certain odors reside at invariant positions in the antennal lobes. Discrete groups of glomeruli seem to share similar properties with regard to their shared responses to a class of odors, and there is evidence that specific odorants belonging to that class activate individual glomeruli within the group (Galizia et al., 1998; Sachse et al., 1999). Again, there are great similarities between the insect and vertebrate olfactory systems. Recordings from zebrafish olfactory bulbs demonstrate odor-induced activity in identifiable ensembles of glomeruli responding to a class of odorants, with single glomeruli in the ensemble responding best to certain elements of that odor class (Friedrich and Korsching, 1998).

The optic lobes. Hymenopterans possessing compound eyes probably have about as much visual as olfactory input to their calyces. Tracer injections show that each mushroom body receives inputs from both optic lobes. This contrasts with the modality of olfaction: antennal lobe projection neurons to a mushroom body arise exclusively from the same side of the brain (Gronenberg, 1999).

Calyces derive their visual afferents from the optic lobe's medulla and lobula (Gronenberg, 1986). The medulla is comparable to a combination of a vertebrate retinal inner plexiform layer—albeit a highly stratified and complex one that is more like a bird's than a mammal's—and a simple geniculate body. The lobula region is a thick lenticular neuropil that consists of many levels of small retinotopic neurons that receive inputs from the medulla (Strausfeld, 1976).

The visual system of insects is divided into two major parallel pathways; one is achromatic and processes motion, and the other is thought to process information about color and texture (Strausfeld and Lee, 1991). The motion-sensitive pathway is highly conserved among taxa (Buschbeck and Strausfeld, 1996). It consists of groups of small retinotopic neurons that are distributed isomorphically beneath the retina, in the outer plexiform layer (called the lamina), and in the medulla. Neurons that receive their input from adjacent pairs of visual sampling points are sensitive to directional motion (Riehle and Franceschini 1982; Douglass and Strausfeld, 1995, 1997). Groups of these neurons terminate on wide-field interneurons that are presynaptic onto large tangentially organized dendrites that collate information about the direction and velocity of motion (Franceschini et al., 1989). In certain groups of insects (Coleoptera, Lepidoptera, and Diptera: beetles, butterflies/moths, flies) tangential collators are arranged in a tectum of neuropil called the lobula plate, which supplies axons that end on the dendrites of descending neurons in the deutocerebrum (Gronenberg and Strausfeld, 1992). With mechanosensory afferents from organs of balance, descending neuron axons synapse onto flight motor neuron circuits in the thoracic ganglia and thus contribute to the visual control of flight. In honey bees, analogous collator neurons lie in a special layer of neuropil deep in the lobula where they are visited by the same kinds of small-field inputs as in flies (Strausfeld, 1976).

The medulla receives primary receptor axons from the retina as well as interneurons from the lamina. Together, afferents to the medulla provide information about the spectral and contrast properties of the visual image. This information is integrated through layers in the medulla and then relayed via interneurons onto the dendrites of pyramidal cell-like neurons and small tangential neurons in the lobula. There are many morphological types of these small retinotopically organized cells, each type manifested by a discrete ensemble of several thousand identical neurons arranged at a characteristic depth in the neuropil (Strausfeld and Hausen, 1977). Each of these ensembles is thought to encode a specific property of the visual world. Each ensemble provides a bundle of axons that projects to a specific region of the deutocerebrum or protocerebrum. Some bundles converge with outputs from the lobula plate onto descending neurons that are involved in the control of flight. Others end on descending neurons involved in controlling leg movements. Still others send bundles of axons that ascend into the protocerebrum: these include projections to the calyces.

Injections of tracers into the lobula show that bundles of axons from the lobula provide afferents to the collar and basal ring regions of all four calyces (Gronenberg, 1999). Injections into the medulla reveal tangentially oriented elements that also provide axons to the calyces. It is not yet known if different types of lobula neurons terminate in different parts of the collar and basal ring, but there is some evidence to suggest this.

As has been described, the calyces are neopteran "inventions" in which sensory relays might modify the properties of Kenyon cell axons deeper in the lobes where they provide local circuits between inputs and outputs. While in palaeopterans, such as dragonflies, there are no connections analogous to those just described for the Hymenoptera, it is most likely that the optic lobes of palaeopteran insects provide indirect inputs to the mushroom body lobes via relays in the protocerebrum. This is what is found in neopterans where neurons arising in the protocerebrum carry information to the mushroom body's lobes about visual events as well as about olfactory and mechanosensory ones.

Mushroom Body Physiology

Recordings from the calyces have shown that already at this level antennal lobe projection neurons discriminate odors and that this information triggers activity in ensembles of Kenyon cells (Laurent and Naraghi, 1994). Each calyx also receives the terminals of GABAergic neurons that respond to a variety of multisensory stimuli (Strausfeld and Li, 1999a,b) and are likely to be presynaptic onto Kenyon cell dendrites. Because these GABAergic terminals invade specific zones of the calyces, the responses there by subsets of Kenyon cells to specific suites of odors should be conditional on other sensory contexts during olfactory stimulation.

Intracellular recordings demonstrate that afferent (input) and efferent (output) neurons in the lobes also respond to multimodal sensory stimuli, including odorants (Schildberger, 1981; Homberg, 1984; Rybak and Menzel, 1998; Li and Strausfeld, 1997, 1999). The activation of an efferent neuron is usually contingent on the sensory context or on the sequence of sensory stimuli in which the activating stimulus is embedded (Homberg and Erber, 1979; Schildberger, 1984; Li and Strausfeld, 1999). For example, a neuron responding to acoustic stimulation may do so only if the acoustic stimulus follows a tactile stimulus, but not if it occurs immediately after an olfactory stimulus. Other neurons may respond to visual stimuli only if presented during a mechanosensory stimulus.

Irrespective of whether the mushroom bodies possess calyces, the lobes can generally be considered to integrate multimodal sensory information depending on the context in which the stimuli are presented. By definition, context must include sensory events that antecede as well as succeed the stimulus. Context should also include current motor actions and, possibly, predicted motor output. The latter is suggested from extracellular recordings that demonstrate mushroom body units that anticipate specific motor actions (Mizunami et al., 1998b). In short, even as context-dependent sensory filters, memory is implicated in this function.

Outputs from the mushroom bodies distribute to many regions of the protocerebrum (Fig. 12.5), including those that provide inputs back to its calyces and lobes (Gronenberg, 1987; Grünewald, 1999a,b). Protocerebral regions that are supplied by mushroom body efferents also provide relays that extend to the central complex. It is this neuropil that appears to be crucial in supervising the control of leg motor neurons and in playing a cardinal role in directing locomotory behavior (Strauss and Heisenberg, 1991; Strauss et al., 1992; Leng and Strauss, 1997).

Roles of Mushroom Bodies

Evidence has been used to argue that the mushroom bodies play important roles in olfactory learning and memory as well as in sensory discrimination and association. Indeed, of any part of the brain it is the mushroom bodies to which the attribute "cognitive facilities" has been accorded (Heisenberg, 1998).

Dujardin (1850) first proposed this idea on the basis of comparative measurements of mushroom bodies. Dujardin suggested that they are largest and most elaborate in social species. Certainly the size of the mushroom bodies, relative to the rest of the brain, is probably greatest in some solitary wasps, but mushroom bodies appear to be most elaborate in species of social wasps and ants (Ehmer and Hoy, 2000; Gronenberg, 1999). Dujardin (1850) likened the folds of the mushroom bodies to sulci of the human cerebral cortex, echoing the bizarre claim of the Viennese phrenologist Franz Gall, who early in the nineteenth century proposed that the sulci of the cerebral cortex reflect mental faculties of humans. Three characters that distinguish the social Hymenoptera from other insects are the ability to relate things with places, the ability to learn, and the ability to be industrious (Dujardin, 1853).

Mushroom bodies have sustained interest since their rediscovery by Flögel in 1876, and their appeal has intensified during the last 15 years largely because of the finding that learning and memory mutants of *Drosophila* are attended by structural defects in the mushroom bodies (Heisenberg et al., 1985). Behavioral genetics has shown that components of biochemical pathways crucial to learning and memory, such as cAMP phosphodiesterase, protein kinase A, and guanyl cyclase, appear to be more concentrated in the mushroom bodies than elsewhere in the brain (Nighorn et al., 1991; Han et al., 1992; Skoulakis et al., 1993). Mutant flies lacking these substances have learning and memory defects (for review, see Heisenberg, 1998). One of these (the mutant *rutabaga*, which is deficient in adenyl cyclase), however, can be rescued by targeted gene expression of wild-type *rut* cDNA in one of the mushroom body's subdivisions (Zars et al., 2000). Nevertheless, if significance is to be attached to the absence of these components from the mushroom bodies of learning mutants, it needs to be shown that these substances are not present in other protocerebral regions that may also support learning and memory.

Even though chemical ablations of embryonic neuroblasts result in *Drosophila* imagoes that entirely lack mushroom bodies (de Belle and Heisenberg, 1994) and are incapable of forming olfactory memory, these experiments do not, however, support the hypothesis that the paired mushroom bodies themselves are the seat of learning and memory. They do show that mushroom bodies are essential to a neural system that allows memory formation.

Despite these reservations, it is generally agreed that certain learning and memory functions cannot occur without mushroom bodies. The vertical lobes appear to play a crucial role in olfactory associations (Erber et al., 1980), whereas the medial lobes and pedunculi appear necessary for place memory (Mizunami et al., 1998b). Results on heat avoidance in flies deprived of mushroom bodies show that these centers are also necessary for context-dependent memory (Liu et al., 1999).

The best evidence thus far that short-term memory might be established by the mushroom bodies comes from recordings of a uniquely identifiable efferent neuron in the honey bee that sends dendrites into the base of the vertical lobe and the pedunculus. This neuron, known as Pe-1 (Mauelshagen, 1993), progressively changes its responses to olfactory cues during conditioning. These changes in response thresholds and firing patterns persist for hours, suggesting that the cell is involved in the "learned" association.

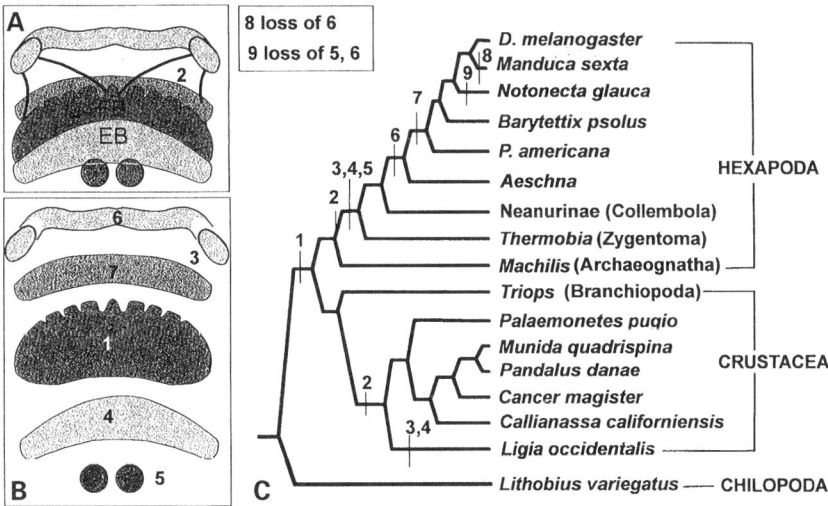

Figure 12.7. The central complex neuropils increase in number and complexity from stem to crown hexapods. The occurrence of these neuropils (A,B) is here mapped onto a phylogeny of the insects and crustaceans (C). Stem insects and crustaceans (archaeognathans and Branchiopoda) have a simple fan-shaped body (FB; 1). In the crustaceans this structure is retained with few additional components appearing, apart from in certain isopods (e.g., *Ligia occidentalis*) where there are buttresses and a chiasma linking them to the fan-shaped (2, 3) body and the ellipsoid body (EB; 4). Collembolans and zygentomans possess chiasmal fibers to the fan-shaped body (2), buttresses (3), ellipsoid bodies (4), and noduli (5). Palaeopteran and neopteran insects possess the complete protocerebral bridge (6), while neopterans have a superior arch (7). It is likely that the evolution of characters 2 to 4 is homoplastic to the crustaceans and insects.

THE CENTRAL COMPLEX

Evolutionary Considerations

The central complex (Fig. 12.7) consists of five interconnected neuropils in palaeopteran and neopteran insects. These are the protocerebral bridge and its buttresses; the fan-shaped body and superior arch; the ellipsoid body; and the paired noduli. In primitive apterygotes the protocerebral bridge is incomplete (*Thermobia*) or is absent, as are the noduli. In the archaeognathan *Machilis*, there is only a single midline neuropil (as there is in the basal branchiopod crustacean *Triops*) that may be homologous to the fan-shaped body (Strausfeld, 1998, and unpublished material) (Fig. 12.7). Comparative studies across the insects thus suggest that the fan-shaped body is the most primitive midline neuropil and that the superior arch may be the most recent one (Fig. 12.7). It is useful to consider this phylogenetic elaboration of a center in the insect's protocerebrum in the context of brain elaboration in craniates. Although genes that regulate segmental patterning of invertebrates and chordate brains are highly conserved (Reichert and Simeone, 1999), segmental genes in early chordates have apparently undergone duplication, clustering, and modification to provide major differences between the forebrains of primitive chordates and craniates (Williams and Holland, 1998; Puelles and Rubenstein, 1993). These differences among brains of animals with a notocord may parallel differences observed between the brains of archaeognathan and holometabolous insects. An unavoidable question is whether brain elaboration in neopteran insects may be due to analogous gene duplication events.

Organization of the Central Complex

Central complex neuropils originate embryonically from among neuroblasts of the protocerebrum (Boyan and Williams, 1997). In *Drosophila*, the origin and fate of individual neurons to their final participation in adult neuropil can be traced using enhancer-trap lines (Renn et al., 1999; Martin et al., 1999). The protocerebral bridge, fan-shaped body, and ellipsoid body, all unpaired midline neuropils (Figs. 12.2, 12.7, and 12.8), reach their greatest cellular elaboration in the Neoptera, particularly in dexterous taxa like the comb-building Vespidae (Fig. 12.8). The fan-shaped body is usually the largest neuropil, situated immediately behind, and confluent with, a smaller midline neuropil called the ellipsoid body. The latter is so named because in flies, where Flögel (1876) discovered the structure, its lateral margins fuse ventrally to form a torus. In most other insects the ellipsoid body is shaped like a shallow hillock. Both the fan-shaped body and ellipsoid body receive afferent terminals from many of the higher order neuropils of the protocerebrum (Fig. 12.8A). These end as bushy, comb-like, or fan-like arborizations that invade discrete modules that subdivide these neuropils each side of the midline.

Each module receives connections from the protocerebral bridge, which in neopterans links the left and right protocerebral hemispheres (Figs. 12.8 and 12.9A-C).

This arrangement has been secondarily modified in derived taxa (see below). In dexterous insects, such as locusts, wasps, and flies, small compact dendritic trees are arranged isomorphically across the protocerebral bridge, dividing the complex into 8 to 16 segments (Fig. 12.9E,F). This is also seen in the Odonata (Fig. 12.9A,B), whose aquatic larvae (although not the adults) are highly maneuverable.

Dendritic trees intersect parallel fibers that extend across the bridge from each protocerebral hemisphere. The parallel fibers originate from interneurons located in the back of the protocerebrum in areas that receive the terminals of plurisegmental interneurons that ascend to the brain from thoracic ganglia (Fig. 12.8B).

Dendritic trees in the bridge are connected to the fan-shaped body through an intricate warp of partially crossing axons (Figs. 12.8C and 12.9E). Groups of dendrites at two different locations across the bridge provide each module of the fan-shaped body with converging axons (Fig. 12.8C). This arrangement is highly ordered (Williams, 1975; Hanesch et al., 1989; Muller et al., 1997). In flies, for example, the most lateral dendritic tree on the left side of the protocerebral bridge has its terminal in the most lateral module of the left side of the fan-shaped body. This module also receives the ending from the most medial dendritic tree of the right side of the protocerebral bridge. In other words, the right-to-left arrangement of dendritic trees in the right half of the protocerebral bridge and the left-to-right arrangement in the left half overlap across the whole of the fan-shaped body (Fig. 12.8C). The paired interneurons then extend their axons further anteriorly into modules of the ellipsoid body. Modules also provide axons to the pair of ball-like noduli lying beneath or behind the fan-shaped body (Fig. 12.9E). Each nodulus consists of a mantel and core of terminals, the core being supplied mainly from the half of the fan-shaped body on the same side of the brain, the mantel supplied mainly by the other half. The significance of this elaborate organization is not yet understood, although the most likely interpretation relates to a dual role for the central complex: one in assessing motor imbalance on each side of the thorax, the other in supervising goal-directed locomotion.

Central Complex Function

Evidence from studies of *Drosophila* mutants suggests that the central complex plays an important role in the coordination of locomotion (Strauss et al., 1992; Strauss and Heisenberg, 1993; Strauss and Trinath, 1996). In normal *Drosophila*, the stride length of a leg depends on its frequency of stepping (Strauss and Heisenberg, 1990). In mutants that have discontinuities across their protocerebral bridge, however, stride lengths are almost independent of the step frequency. At low frequencies, short stride lengths are approximately the same as in normal flies and are maintained at high frequencies. Defects of the protocerebral bridge do not perturb the timing or the basic rhythm of stepping. This suggests that the bridge's role is likely to be for optimizing step lengths and walking speed. This is supported by other mutant strains, all having various bridge defects that generally interrupt the passage of axons across the bridge. During turning wild-type *Drosophila* execute smooth curves by reducing step lengths on the inside of the curve. Although this also occurs in protocerebral bridge mutants

386 12 Insect Brain

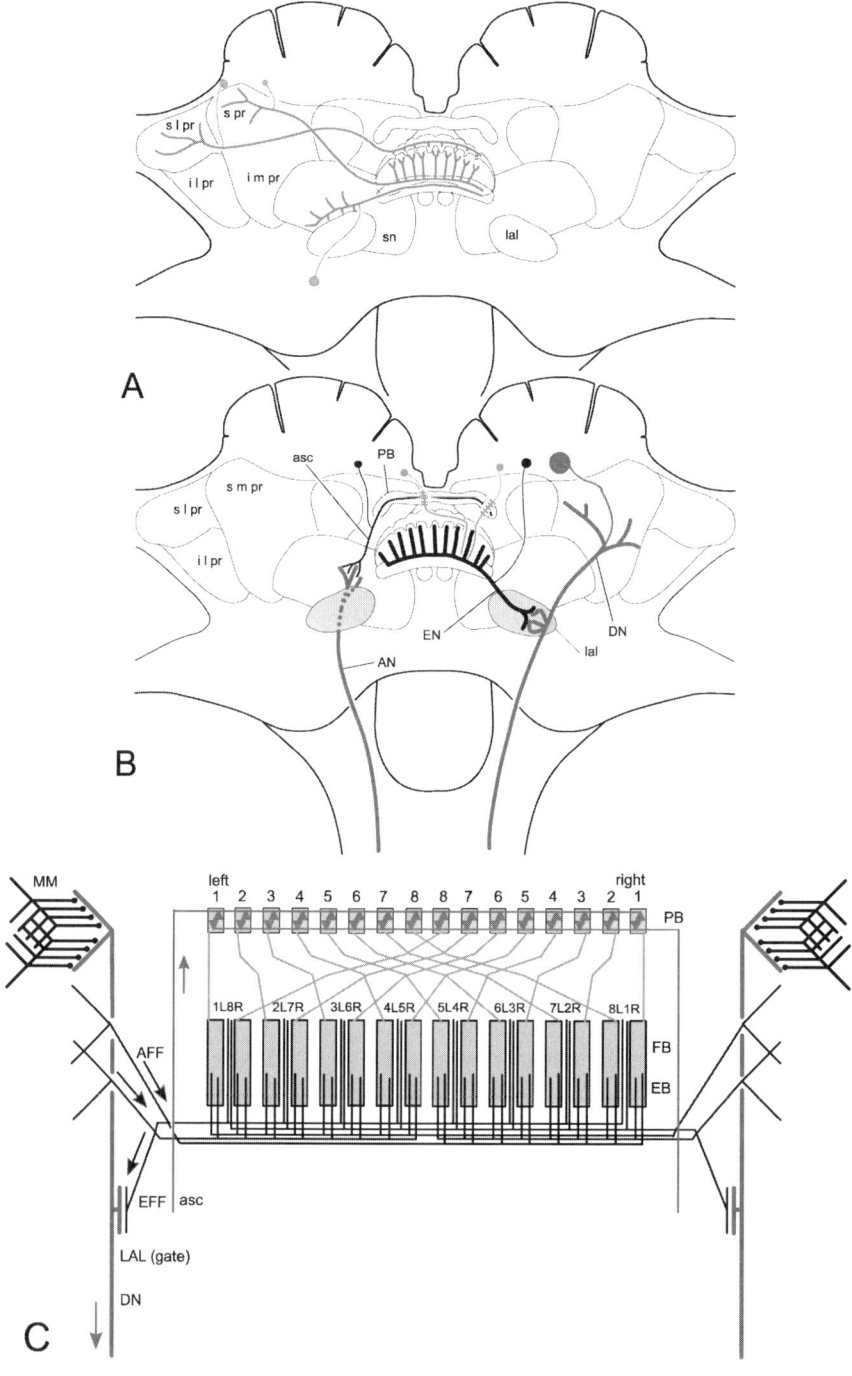

Figure 12.8. (legend on opposite page)

Figure 12.8. Relationship of the protocerebrum and central complex. (A) The fan-shaped and ellipsoid bodies receive afferents from a variety of protocerebral neuropils, themselves invaded by outputs from the mushroom bodies (Fig. 12.5B) and sensory neuropils. (B) Ascending plurisegmental neurons (AN) from the thoracic ganglia end in the inferior medial protocerebrum where they visit interneurons (asc) that ascend into the protocerebral bridge, these providing long terminals that cross from one side to the other. The bridge provides many small interneurons (two shown, gray), the axons of which invade the fan-shaped body (their further extensions to the ellipsoid body and noduli have been omitted for clarity). Outputs (EN) from the fan-shaped body and ellipsoid body extend to lateral protocerebral neuropils, including the lateral accessory lobe (lal), which is visited by axon collaterals of descending neurons (DN) that extend to thoracic and abdominal ganglia. (C) Summary diagram of central complex architecture. Clusters of dendrites (left 1 to 8, right 1 to 8) send crossing axons to modules in the fan-shaped body (other components omitted for clarity). The dendrites intersect the parallel endings of neurons (gray, arrowed) that relay information to the protocerebral bridge (PB) from ascending neurons that arrive in the brain from thoracic and abdominal ganglia. Branches of multimodal afferent neurons (AFF) that originate in other protocerebral neuropils also invade modules in the fan-shaped (FB) and ellipsoid bodies (EB). Efferent neuron dendrites (EFF) receive inputs in the modules. Certain efferents terminate in the lateral accessory lobe (LAL) where their endings branch among dendritic collaterals of descending neurons (DN). Central complex efferents are thought to gate descending neurons at this level. Descending neurons have other elaborately branched dendrites that receive inputs (MM) from the optic lobes, the deutocerebrum, and from protocerebral neuropils.

such as *no-bridge*, their steps are generally smaller than in wild type, and the swing speed is reduced by the legs on the inside of the turn. Episodes appear during which mutant flies are unable to position their legs appropriately during a goal-directed turn. As a consequence, the mutant fly trips over its own feet (Wannek and Strauss, 1998).

In wild-type flies, as in other species that are highly maneuverable in walking, the dendritic trees in the protocerebral bridge are arranged across the width of the bridge, including its buttresses that arise from the protocerebral hemispheres. In species that use their legs for clinging or clasping, however, but not for walking, the dendritic trees of neurons connecting the bridge and fan-shaped body are constrained laterally to each side of the bridge or are restricted to the buttresses only.

The organization of the central complex may relate less to maneuverability in flight than to maneuverability in walking. In the hummingbird hawkmoth *Macroglossum*, which maintains its hovering position in front of a moving target, motor adjustments are mediated by neurons in the optic lobes. These respond to the expanding or contracting image of the target and the movement of its image across its retina (Wicklein and Varju, 1999). This species of moth, which shows such precision in flight control, is hardly able to walk and uses its legs mainly for clinging. Although axons extend across the width of the moth's protocerebral bridge (Fig. 12.9C), dendrites in the bridge are restricted to each side. In *Macroglossum*, both the ellipsoid body and noduli are reduced in size compared with those in similar-sized brains of wasps, flies, and locusts. Also, modules in the fan-shaped body are barely delineated in the moth (Fig. 12.9D).

In species that are constrained to mainly symmetrical leg movements, as in the water strider *Gerris*, the two halves of the bridge are entirely separated. *Gerris* employs bilaterally symmetrical rowing movements, and turning employs synchronized leg movements to provide power strokes on one side of the body. There appears to be little modification of the swing phase of individual legs. Similarly in a related hemipteran, the backswimmer *Notonecta*, the protocerebral bridge is also reduced at the midline (Strausfeld, 1999).

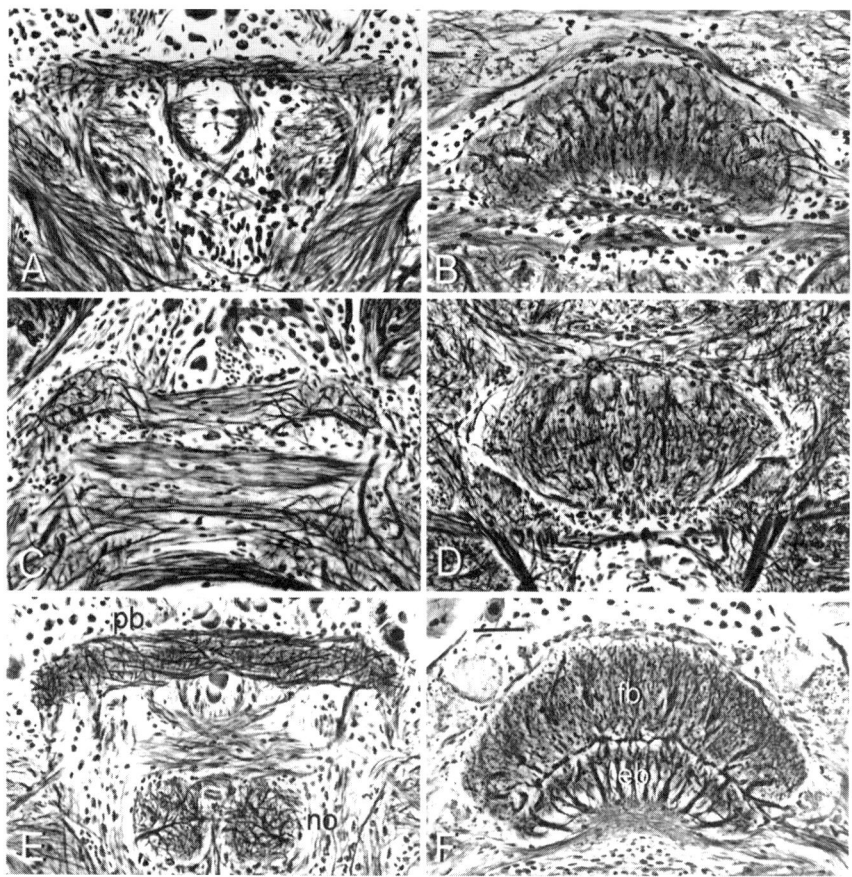

Figure 12.9. Comparisons of protocerebral bridges (Pb) and fan-shaped bodies (fb)/ellipsoid bodies (eb). (A,B). Palaeopteran dragonfly *Aeschna*. (C,D). Hummingbird hawkmoth *Macroglossum*. (E,F). Paper wasp *Polistes*. no noduli. Bar for all parts = 50 μm.

The evidence thus far suggests that the central complex is involved in both maintaining the direction of locomotion and supervising changes in direction. Insects turn toward attractive stimuli and away from noxious ones. This is accomplished by the brain appropriately biasing activity in motor neurons. Although it is not known which circuits determine how stimuli are chosen, current evidence suggests that the mushroom bodies play a crucial role in this (Li and Strausfeld, 1999; Strausfeld and Li, 1999b). The mushroom bodies provide inputs to protocerebral regions (Fig. 12.5B) that in turn send multimodal efferents to the central complex (Milde, 1988). These terminate across groups of modules in the fan-shaped and ellipsoid bodies (Fig. 12.8A). It is proposed that circuits intrinsic to the modules assess the weights of sensory stimuli provided to them by these protocerebral afferents. As a consequence, outputs from the fan-shaped and ellipsoid bodies (Fig. 12.8B) will asymmetrically (and appropriately) gate descending neurons supplying leg motor circuits (Strausfeld, 1999). These relationships are schematized in Fig. 12.8C.

COMPARISONS OF BRAIN REGIONS AMONGST ARTHROPODS

Mushroom Bodies

Mushroom bodies are found not only in arthropods but also in annelids and in planarians, suggesting that they may have arisen before the evolutionary divide to the lophotrochozoans and ecdysozoans. The organization of the crustacean brain, however, rather complicates this view.

Although molecular cladistics (Friedrich and Tautz, 1995) and phylogenetic analysis of brain structures (Strausfeld, 1998) support the view that crustaceans and insects are sister groups, studies on eumalacostracan crustaceans have thus far failed to recognize any lobed structure similar to the neopteran mushroom bodies. Instead, eumalacostracans possess hemiellipsoid bodies: dense and often stratified neuropils that are situated laterally in the protocerebrum near the origin of the optic peduncle. Each hemiellipsoid body derives from thousands or even hundreds of thousands of minute basophilic cell bodies. These provide intrinsic neurons that have dense spiny dendrites and extremely short axons (Mellon et al., 1992), rather like those described for the mushroom bodies of the chelicerate *Limulus* (Fahrenbach, 1979). Unlike Kenyon cells, intrinsic neurons of the hemiellipsoid body do not provide a pedunculus and lobes. Nevertheless, like the insect calyx, the hemiellipsoid body is supplied by projection neurons from primary olfactory neuropils.

In crustaceans, olfactory projection neurons originate in the antennular lobes, which are supplied by olfactory receptor axons from the first of two pairs of antennaform appendages, the antennules. Antennular lobe projection neurons characteristically differ from those of insect antennal lobes in having dendrites that invade many glomeruli and axons that bifurcate to both hemiellipsoid bodies (Schmidt and Ache, 1996). Projection neurons in insects supply calyces ipsilaterally (Homberg et al., 1989). Another difference is that axons from the antennular lobes have their final terminations in the hemiellipsoid bodies, whereas axons from antennal glomeruli send collaterals to the calyces but finally end more laterally in the superior lateral protocerebrum.

Hemiellipsoid bodies do not provide systems of parallel fibers as do insect mushroom bodies. Rather, they give rise to a small number of efferent neurons, the axons of which project into the protocerebrum (Mellon et al., 1992). This organization again differs from that of insect mushroom bodies where numerous efferents originate in the lobes. Another important difference is in decapod crustaceans where a large neuropil consisting of numerous small glomeruli lies in a region adjacent to each antennular lobe. This region, called the accessory lobe, is connected by tracts to the antennular lobe, as well as to the protocerebrum, and to the hemiellipsoid body. Insects do not possess a similar neuropil, although the gustatory lobe, which is a primary sensory neuropil receiving afferents from taste receptors, consists of many small glomeruli.

Mushroom bodies as defined by Flögel and Kenyon are found in planarians, annelids, onychophorans, diplopods, chelicerates, and chilopods (Strausfeld, 1998). In each of these taxa, clusters of globuli cells provide thousands of parallel axons that form lobes but no obvious calyces. Except in planarians, where afferent relationships to mushroom bodies are not yet known, the lobes of these taxa receive afferents from olfactory glomeruli and other sensory centers and provide efferents to other brain areas. Primary olfactory neuropils receiving terminals from olfactory glomeruli are either contiguous with the mushroom bodies (as in Onychophora) or are connected to them ipsilaterally by olfactory projection neurons. In annelids, onychophorans, and diplopods, olfactory glomeruli are situated in the protocerebrum. In chilopods they are in the first suboesophageal neuromere, equivalent to the preoral tritocerebrum of insects and crustaceans. In chelicerates, olfactory glomeruli occur in whichever postoral segment provides the olfactory appendage. Significantly, in all these groups the mushroom bodies reside in the most rostral neuromere, the protocerebrum.

The Central Complex

Agile fast-running isopods, such as the littoral species *Ligia occidentalis*, are crustaceans equipped with a central body comprising a bilayered midline neuropil, the appearance of which is most reminiscent of the fan-shaped body in apterygotes, such as *Thermobia*. In *Ligia*, this neuropil is supplied by a chiasmal arrangement of axons from a protocerebral bridge. The bridge comprises dendrites within the buttresses, which are connected by parallel fibers extending between them. In other crustaceans thus far investigated, the central complex consists of an elongated and columnar central body without obvious layers. A recent study on the crayfish *Cherax destructor* using dextran tracer injections (Utting et al., 2000), however, demonstrates a protocerebral bridge with uncrossed connections connected to a substantial midline neuropil in which antibodies against proctolin and dip-allatostatin reveal layered arrangements of endings from the protocerebrum. Dendritic trees in the central body send axons out to discrete regions in the posterior and lateral protocerebrum. Many of these projections are reminiscent of those identified in neopteran insects, such as in *Drosophila* (see Renn et al., 1999). These similarities imply that there has been convergent evolution between the central complexes of decapods and pterygotes if the primitive condition is represented by only a single midline neuropil, as in *Machilis* and *Triops*.

It is difficult to ascertain a clearly distinguished central complex in the brains of chilopods and diplopods because their brains show little lateralization. Other than the optic lobes and antennal lobes, many neuropils are contiguous across the midline. This organization contrasts with that of insects, crustaceans, and chelicerates, in which tracts of axons link discrete bilaterally symmetrical neuropils so that a midline region is readily visible. Although the onychophoran brain also consists of bilateral neuropils, neurons in one of these provide a system of layers and columns that is reminiscent of cellular arrangements in the single midline neuropil of the arachnid brain, (termed the central body by Hanström, 1928). The arachnid central body, however, looks very different from the central complex of neopteran insects and malacostracans, being a terraced neuropil distinguished by numerous strata and dense arrangements of columns (Strausfeld et al., 1993).

Although there is thus far no solid evidence that the chelicerate central body is homologous to the central complex of an insect, the role of the chelicerate central body in motor control nevertheless merits serious consideration. Comparative studies of arachnid brains have suggested that the central body is most elaborate in agile wandering spiders and least elaborate in web builders (Welzien and Barth, 1991). In other chelicerate groups, the central body is least elaborate in the amblypygids ("whip spiders") and is most elaborated in the solpugids ("sun spiders"). The latter are territorial, highly mobile, and extremely rapid predators that rely on their speed and agility for prey capture. Amblypygids are in contrast cautious predators, relying

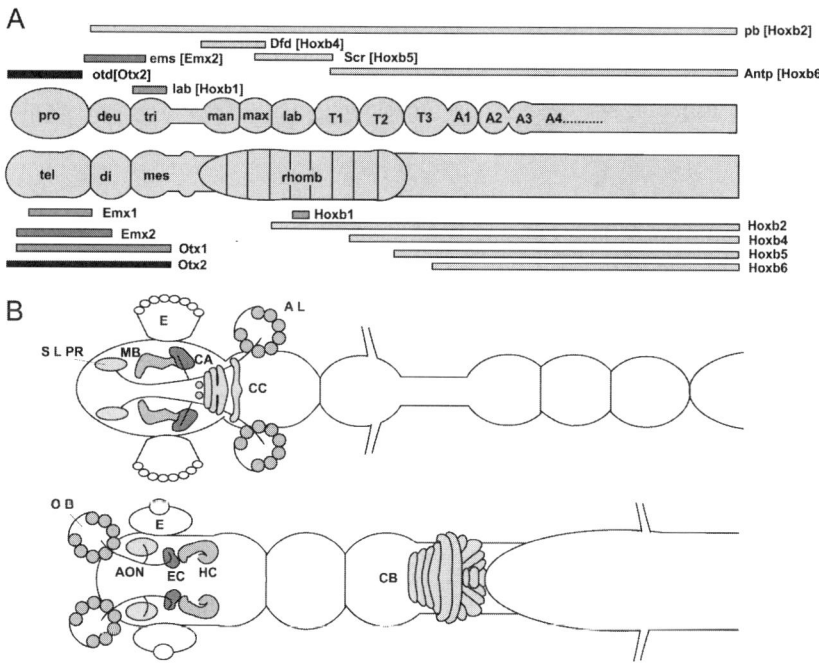

Figure 12.10. Orthologous gene expression compared with analogous neuropils in vertebrates and invertebrates. (A) Colinear expression of orthologous genes defines comparable segments of the insect (upper) and murine brain and central nervous system. (Adapted from Sharman and Brand, 1998; Williams and Holland, 1998). (B) Comparison of olfactory pathways and placement of central complex (CC)/cerebellum (CB) in a neopteran insect (upper) and mammal. In insects, efferents from the antennal lobe (AL) connect to the superior lateral protocerebrum (S L PR), sending collaterals to the calyces (CA). The calyces then send axons to the mushroom body lobes (MB), which share properties with mammalian hippocampus (Mizunami et al., 1998b). This pathway finds a counterpart in mammals where efferents from the olfactory bulb (OB) invade the anterior optic nucleus (AON) and entorhinal cortex (EC), which is connected to the hippocampus (HC). The central complex (CC) and cerebellum (CB) are both midline architectures involved in the control of movements.

on careful exploratory examination of potential victims using their elongated forelimbs. These provide chemoreceptors and tactile receptors whose axons supply hundreds of glomeruli associated with enormous mushroom bodies. The amblypygid mushroom bodies occupy most of the supraoesophageal ganglion at the expense of the central body and other neuropils, which are greatly reduced and even displaced postorally.

INSECT AND VERTEBRATE BRAINS COMPARED

Insect brains show a fascinating degree of structural and functional convergence with the brains of craniates. The question arises whether such convergence is homoplastic, a consequence of similar responses by the vertebrate and arthropod genome to similar evolutionary pressures to provide independent evolution of similar structures. Alternatively, do orthologous genes regulate suites of structural genes that have been recruited independently in vertebrates and invertebrates to encode comparable neuroanatomical and physiological motifs? Such appears to have occurred in the evolution of different eye types whose development is under the master regulatory gene *Pax6* (Callaerts et al., 1997).

Equivalence of Insect and Vertebrate Embryonic Forebrain

Because of its segmental position, the protocerebrum has been analogized with the vertebrate forebrain. Historically this comparison is based on circumstantial evidence (for review, see Strausfeld et al., 1995). Real genetic homology, however, is supported by recent studies of orthologous regulatory genes whose expression patterns (Fig. 12.10A) in the developing central nervous systems of insects and craniates are spatially and temporally colinear (for review, see Reichert and Simeone, 1999). Insect cephalic gap genes and homeotic genes (homeotic complex genes) are orthologous to craniate *Otx* and *Hox* genes, themselves an apparent elaboration of a simpler arrangement of regulatory genes present in cephalochordates and urochordates (Williams and Holland, 1998; Holland and Holland, 1999). That these genes are highly conserved across phyla finds support from comparable loss of function. Inactivation of the vertebrate *Hoxa1* and *Hoxb1* genes results in similar defects of segmental identity in vertebrates as does loss of the *Drosophila labial* gene (Studer et al., 1998; Hirth et al., 1998). Genes that pattern rostrocaudal identity of segments in the hindbrain and spinal cord can be matched to orthologous genes, which in *Drosophila* pattern identity caudally from the level of the protocerebrum and labial neuromeres (Hartmann and Reichert, 1998; Hirth et al., 1998; Sharman and Brand, 1998). Homology is further supported by recent studies showing that at least two orthologous genes are interchangeable across vertebrates and arthropods—phyla that diverged from a common ancestor 600 million years ago or longer (Wray et al., 1996).

Genes essential for the embryonic development of the protocerebrum are homologous and interchangeable with genes necessary for the development of the mammalian forebrain (Leuzinger et al., 1998). In *Drosophila*, the protocerebrum's development requires the expression of the homeobox gene *orthodenticle* (*otd*), which shares sequence homology with the murine homeobox gene *Otx 1* (Nagao et al., 1998). In mice, *Otx 1* is involved in the earliest stages of cortex development (Acampora et al., 1999). Protocerebral development fails in mutant *Drosophila* that do not express *otd*, but protocerebral development is rescued if murine *Otx* cDNA is expressed in the *otd*-deficient fly embryo (Leuzinger et al., 1998). Likewise, mice that are deficient in the *Otx 1* gene have cortex developmental defects. Corticogenesis in *Otx 1*-deficient mice can, however, be rescued by expression of *Drosophila otd* cDNA (Acampora et al., 1999).

The idea that vertebrates and arthropods share a common body plan is not new, having been first proposed by Geoffroy Saint-Hilaire in 1822 and debated many times since. A compelling number of arguments have now been mustered from already existing literature in favor of this hypothesis, including the observation that blastula fate maps are conserved among vertebrates, arthropods, and annelids (Nübler-Jung and Arendt, 1994, 1996; Arendt and Nübler-Jung, 1994, 1996, 1997). To achieve the chordate body plan from an ancestral invertebrate organization requires an inversion of the dorsoventral axis with a concomitant evolution of a new mouth, which according to Arendt and Nübler-Jung (1997) requires few steps. An inversion of the body, such that up in vertebrates is equivalent to down in arthropods while maintaining the neuraxis, is suggested by the expression of homologous genes that define dorsality in vertebrate embryos and ventrality in arthropods (Arendt and Nübler-Jung, 1996; Ferguson, 1996). Two genes cited are the *Drosophila* gene *decapentaplegic* and its vertebrate counterpart *BMP-4*. The former is expressed dorsally in the embryo and supports dorsalization, whereas the latter is expressed ventrally and supports ventralization. Likewise, a gene whose amphibian homologue encodes dorsalization (Holley and Ferguson, 1997) encodes ventralization in *Drosophila*. Arendt and Nübler-Jung (1997) point out that dorsal midline cells of vertebrates and ventral midline cells of insects, both crucial in the subsequent formation of the nerve cord, also share common gene expression.

The Adult Brain

There are profound similarities between the adult nervous systems of vertebrates and arthropods. Examples are the neuronal organization of the craniate spinal cord and arthropod segmental ganglia whose similarities have been explicitly proposed by Zawarzin (1925), Strausfeld (1976), and most recently by Pearson (1993). Cajal and Sanchez (1915) emphasized common organization of neurons in the vertebrate retina and insect optic lobes. Retzius (1890, 1891) also stressed the similarities of neuronal and neuropil organization in the segmental ganglia of annelids (lophotrochozoans) and crayfish (ecdysozoans).

There is compelling evidence that olfactory glomeruli in insects have evolved convergently with those of mammals to such a degree that synaptic organization and cell shapes are almost identical in both (Strausfeld and Hildebrand, 1999). Many organizational principles are shared between the visual systems of insects and mammals despite different strategies for forming an image on the photoreceptor layer, although one group of insects has been shown to have a compound eye composed of many image-forming vertebrate-like eyelets (Buschbeck et al., 1999). Neuronal arrangements and synaptic organization of the insect lamina and outer medulla are comparable to those of mammalian plexiform layers (Cajal and Sánchez, 1915). The lobula plate in the insect optic lobe is comparable to the optic tectum of lower vertebrates or the superior colliculus of mammals. Neuronal shapes and arrangements in the insect lobula are similar to those of pyramidal and stellate cells in primate primary visual cortex. In the protocerebrum, the central complex is implicated in orchestrating motor actions and can thus be thought analogous to the mammalian cerebellum. There are also tantalizing similarities between pathways linking the mammalian olfactory bulb to the anterior olfactory nucleus, piriform cortex, and hippocampus and pathways linking the antennal lobes to the superior lateral protocerebrum and the mushroom body calyces to the lobes (Fig. 12.10B). Certain nuclei of the protocerebrum, the roles of which are not yet known but which provide links between the mushroom bodies and central complex, may eventually be functionally and structurally compared with specific cortical or subcortical areas of the mammalian brain.

Two speculations might be drawn from these morphological similarities. One supports the idea that not only early gene expression similarly defines the neuraxis and neuromeric identity across craniates, lophotrochozoans, and ecdysozoans but that late genes common to these taxa may similarly orchestrate genetic programs for the formation of comparable circuits. Conversely, it could be argued that because orthologous segmental genes regulate transcription of other genes, they do not themselves play a role in determining neural structures but nevertheless orchestrate suites of heterologous structural genes that have been separately acquired during the divergent evolution of these groups. Thus, as in the case of eye development (Callaerts et al., 1997), neuropils sharing great similarity of architecture and computational properties could well have arisen independently from different groups of genes driven by homologous organizers.

Future anatomical and genetic studies will provide crucial data to show whether brain areas performing similar functions in mammals and insects require both similar wiring and similar genetic programs. Is it merely coincidental, for example, that the *Drosophila D-MEF2* gene, which is expressed in developing Kenyon cells of the mushroom bodies, has a murine homologue *mef2* that is expressed in neurons of the developing cortex, hippocampus, and hindbrain (Schulz et al., 1996)? This type of comparison represents the sightings of a new and fascinating continent of molecular and genetic studies. Furthermore, while exact replicas of the cerebral cortex, hippocampus, or cerebellum should not be sought in the brains of arthropods, evidence discussed in this chapter suggests that certain insect neuropils may provide fascinating albeit simpler counterparts to them.

ACKNOWLEDGMENTS

Support for the author's own work outlined in this chapter was provided by grants from the National Science Foundation, the National Institutes of Health National Center for Research Resources, and Fellowships from the John Simon Guggenheim Memorial Foundation and the John D. and Catherine T. MacArthur Foundation.

REFERENCES

Acampora, D., M. Gulisano, and A. Simeone (1999) Otx genes and the genetic control of brain morphogenesis. *Mol. Cell Neurosci.* 13:1–7.

Arendt, D., and K. Nübler-Jung (1994) Inversion of dorsoventral axis? *Nature* 371:26.

Arendt, D., and K. Nübler-Jung (1996) Common ground plans in early brain development in mice and flies. *BioEssays* 18:255–259.

Arendt, D., and K. Nübler-Jung (1997) Dorsal or ventral: similarities in fate maps and gastrulation patterns in annelids, arthropods and chordates. *Mech. Dev.* 61:7–21.

Bassemir, U., and K. Hansen (1980) Single-pore sensilla of damselfly-larvae: representatives of phylogenetically old contact chemoreceptors? *Cell Tissue Res.* 207:307–320.

Bicker, G. (1991) Taurine-like immunoreactivity in photoreceptor cells and mushroom bodies: a comparison of the chemical architecture of insect nervous systems. *Brain Res.* 568:201–206.

Binet, A. (1894) Contribution à l'étude du système nerveux sousintestinal des insectes. *J. Anat. Physiol.* 30:449–580.

Boeckh, J., and L.P. Tolbert (1993) Synaptic organization and development of the antennal lobe in insects. *Microsc. Res. Tech.* 24:260–280.

Boyan, G.S., and J.L.D. Williams (1997) Embryonic development of the pars intercerebralis/central complex of the grasshopper. *Dev. Genes Evol.* 207:317–329.

Burrows, M. (1996) *Function of an Insect Brain*. Oxford University Press, New York.

Burrows, M., and M.V.S. Siegler (1985) The organization of receptive fields of spiking local interneurones in the locust with inputs from hair afferents. *J. Neurophysiol.* 53:1147–1157.

Buschbeck, E.K., and N.J. Strausfeld (1996) Visual motion-detection circuits in flies: small field retinotopic elements responding to motion are evolutionarily conserved across taxa. *J. Neurosci.* 16:4563–4578.

Buschbeck, E., B. Ehmer, and R.R. Hoy (1999) Chunk versus point sampling: visual imaging in a small insect. *Science* 286:1178–1180.

Cajal, S.R., and D.S. Sanchez (1915) Contribucion al conocimiento de los centros nerviosos de los insectos. Parte I. Retina y centros opticos. *Trab. Lab. Invest. Biol. Uni. Madr.* 13:1–168.

Callaerts, P., G. Halder, and W.J. Gehring (1997) Pax-6 in development and evolution. *Annu. Rev. Neurosci.* 20:483–532.

Christensen, T.A., B.R. Waldrop, I.D. Harrow, and J.G. Hildebrand (1993) Local interneurons and information processing in the olfactory glomeruli of the moth *Manduca sexta*. *J. Comp. Physiol. [A]* 173:385–399.

Christensen, T.A., T. Heinbockel, and J.G. Hildebrand (1996) Olfactory information processing in the brain: encoding the chemical and temporal features of odors. *J. Neurobiol.* 30:82–91.

Crittenden, J.R., E.M.C. Skoulakis, K.-A. Han, D. Kalderon, and R.L. Davis (1998) Tripartite mushroom body architecture revealed by antigenic markers. *Learn. Memory* 5:38–51.

Davis, R. (1993) Mushroom bodies and *Drosophila* learning. *Neuron* 111:1–14.

deBelle, J.S., and M. Heisenberg (1994) Associative odor learning in *Drosophila* abolished by chemical ablation of mushroom bodies. *Science* 263:692–695.

Douglass, J.K., and N.J. Strausfeld (1995) Visual motion detection circuits in flies: peripheral motion computation by identified small field retinotopic neurons. *J. Neurosci.* 15:5596–5611.

Douglass, J.K., and N.J. Strausfeld (1997) Visual motion detection circuits in flies: parallel direction- and non-direction-sensitive pathways between the medulla and lobula plate. *J. Neurosci.* 16:4551–5562.

Dujardin, F. (1850) Mémoire sur le système nerveux des insectes. *Ann. Sci. Nat. Zool.* 14:195–206.
Dujardin, F. (1853) Quelques observations sur les abeilles et particulièrement sur les actes qui, chez ces insectes peuvent être rapportés à l'intelligence. *Ann. Sci. Nat. Zool.* 18:231–240.
Edwards, J.S., and G.R. Reddy (1986) Mechanosensory appendages and giant interneurons in the firebrat (*Thermobia domestica*, Thysanura): a prototype system for terrestrial predator evasion. *J. Comp. Neurol.* 243:535–546.
Ehmer, B., and R.R. Hoy (2000) Mushroom bodies of vespid wasps. *J. Comp Neurol.* 415:416:93–100.
Elofsson, R., and E. Dahl (1970) The optic neuropils and chiasmata of Crustacea. *Z. Zellforsch. Mikrosk. Anat.* 107:343–360.
Erber, J., T. Masuhr, and R. Menzel (1980) Localization of short-term memory in the brain of the bee, *Apis mellifera. Physiol. Entomol.* 5:343–358.
Fahrenbach, W.H. (1979) The brain of the horseshoe crab (*Limulus polyphemus*). III. Cellular and synaptic organization of the corpora pedunculata. *Tissue Cell* 11:162–200.
Faivre, E. (1857) Du cerveau des dytisques considéré dans ses rapports avec la locomotion. *Ann. Sci. Nat. (Zool).* 8:245–274.
Ferguson, E.L. (1996) Conservation of dorso-ventral patterning in arthropods and chordates. *Curr. Opin. Gen. Dev.* 6:424–431.
Flanagan, D., and A.R. Mercer (1989) Morphology and response characteristics of neurones in the deutocerebrum of the brain in the honeybee *Apis mellifera. J. Comp. Physiol. A.* 164:483–494.
Flögel, J.H.L. (1876) Über den feineren Bau des Arthropodengehirns. Tagbl. *Versamml. Dtschr. Naturforsch. Arzte. (Beilage)* 49:115–120.
Franceschini, N., A. Riehle, and A. Le Nestour (1989) Directionally selective motion detection by insect neurons. In D.G. Stavenga and R.C. Hardie (eds.): *Facets of Vision.* Springer, Berlin, pp. 360–390.
Friedrich, R.W., and S.I. Korsching (1998) Chemotopic, combinatorial, and noncombinatorial odorant representations in the olfactory bulb revealed using a voltage-sensitive axon tracer. *J. Neurosci.* 18:9977–9988.
Friedrich, M., and D. Tautz (1995) Ribosomal DNA phylogeny of the major extant arthropod classes and the evolution of myriapods. *Nature* 376:165–167.
Galizia, C.G., K. Nagler, B. Hölldobler, and R. Menzel (1998) Odour coding is bilaterally symmetrical in the antennal lobes of honeybees (*Apis mellifera*). *Eur. J. Neurosci.* 10:2964–2974.
Geoffroy, St-H.É (1822) Considérations générales sur la vertébre. *Mèm. Musée Hist. Nat.* 9:88–119.
Getting, P.A. (1988) Comparative analysis of invertebrate central pattern generators. In A.H. Cohen, S. Rossignol, and S. Grillner (eds.): *Neural Control of Rhythmic Movements in Vertebrates.* John Wiley & Sons, New York, pp. 101–127.
Gronenberg, W. (1986) Physiological and anatomical properties of optical input-fibers to the mushroom body of the bee brain. *J. Insect Physiol.* 32:695–704.
Gronenberg, W. (1987) Anatomical and physiological properties of feedback neurons of the mushroom bodies in the bee brain. *Exp. Biol.* 46:115–125.
Gronenberg, W. (1999) Modality-specific segregation of input to ant mushroom bodies. *Brain Behav. Evol.* 54:85–95.
Gronenberg, W., and N.J. Strausfeld (1992) Premotor descending neurons responding selectively to local visual stimuli in flies. *J. Comp. Neurol.* 316:87–103.
Grünewald, B. (1999a) Morphology of feedback neurons in the mushroom body of the honey bee, *Apis mellifera. J. Comp. Neurol.* 404:114–126.
Grünewald, B. (1999b) Physiological properties and response modulations of mushroom body feedback neurons during olfactory learning in the honeybee *Apis mellifera. J. Comp. Physiol. A.* 185:565–576.
Gynther, I.C., and K.G. Pearson (1989) An evaluation of the role of identified interneurons in triggering kicks and jumps in the locust. *J. Neurophysiol.* 61:45–57.
Hadenfeldt, D. (1929) Das Nervensystem von *Stylochoplana maculata* und *Notoplana atomota. Z. Wiss. Zool.* 133:586–638.
Hammer, M. (1993) An identified neuron mediates the unconditioned stimulus in associative olfactory learning in honeybees. *Nature* 366:59–63.
Han, P.-L., L.R. Levin, R.R. Reed, and R.L. Davis (1992) Preferential expression of the *Drosophila* rutabaga gene in mushroom bodies, neural centers for learning in insects. *Neuron* 9:619–627.
Hanesch, U., K.F. Fischbach, and M. Heisenberg (1989) Neuronal architecture of the central complex in *Drosophila melanogaster. Cell Tissue Res.* 257:343–366.

Hanström, B. (1928) *Vergleichende Anatomie des Nervensystems der Wirbellosen Tiere.* Springer, Berlin.
Hartmann, B., and H. Reichert (1998) The genetics of embryonic brain development in *Drosophila. Mol. Cell. Neurosci.* 12:194–205.
Heisenberg, M. (1980) Mutations of brain structure and function: what is the significance of the mushroom bodies for behavior. In O. Siddiqi, P. Babu, L.M. Hall, and J.C. Hall (eds.): *Development and Neurobiology of Drosophila.* Plenum, New York, pp. 373–390.
Heisenberg, M. (1998) What do the mushroom bodies do for the insect brain? *Learn. Memory* 5:1–10.
Heisenberg, M., A. Borst, S. Wagner, and D. Byers (1985) *Drosophila* mushroom body mutants are deficient in olfactory learning. *J. Neurogenet.* 2:1–30.
Hildebrand, J.G., and G.M. Shepherd (1997) Molecular mechanisms of olfactory discrimination: converging evidence for common principles across phyla. *Annu. Rev. Neurosci.* 20:595–631.
Hirth, F., B. Hartmann, and H. Reichert (1998) Homeotic gene action in embryonic brain development of *Drosophila. Development* 125:1579–1589.
Holland, L.Z., and N.D. Holland (1999) Chordate origins of the vertebrate central nervous system. *Curr. Opin. Neurobiol.* 9:596–602.
Holley, S.A., and E.L. Ferguson (1997) Fish are like flies are like frogs: conservation of dorsal-ventral patterning mechanisms. *BioEssays* 19:281–284.
Homberg, U. (1984) Processing of antennal information in extrinsic mushroom body neurons of the bee brain. *J. Comp. Physiol. [A]* 154:825–836.
Homberg, U., and J. Erber (1979) Response characteristics and identification of extrinsic mushroom body neurons of the bee. *Z. Naturforsch.* 34C:612–615.
Homberg, U., R.A. Montague, and J.G. Hildebrand (1989) Anatomy of antenno-cerebral pathways in the brain of the sphinx moth *Manduca sexta. Cell Tissue Res.* 254:255–281.
Ito, K., K. Suzuki, P. Estes, M. Ramaswami, D. Yamamoto, and N.J. Strausfeld (1998) The organization of extrinsic neurons and their implications in the functional roles of the mushroom bodies in *Drosophila melanogaster* Meigen. *Learn. Memory* 5:37–48.
Kanzaki, R., E.A. Arbas, N.J. Strausfeld and J.G. Hildebrand (1989) Physiology and morphology of projection neurons in the antennal lobe of the male moth *Manduca sexta. J. Comp. Physiol. [A]* 165:427–453.
Kenyon, F.C. (1896) The brain of the bee. A preliminary contribution to the morphology of the nervous system of the Arthropoda. *J. Comp. Neurol.* 6:133–210.
Knoll, A.H., and S.B. Carroll (1999) Early animal evolution: emerging views from comparative biology and geology. *Science* 284:2129–2137.
Laissue, P.P., C. Reiter, P.R. Hiesinger, S. Halter, K.F. Fischbach, and R.F. Stocker (1999) Three-dimensional reconstruction of the antennal lobe in *Drosophila melanogaster. J. Comp. Neurol.* 405:543–552.
Laurent, G., and M. Burrows (1989) Distribution of intersegmental inputs to nonspiking local interneurones and motor neurones in the locust. *J. Neurosci.* 9:3019–3029.
Laurent, G., and H. Davidowitz (1994) Encoding of olfactory information with oscillating neural assemblies. *Science* 265:1872–1874.
Laurent, G., and M. Naraghi (1994) Odorant-induced oscillations in the mushroom bodies of the locust. *J. Neurosci.* 14:2993–3004.
Lee, T., A. Lee, and L. Luo (1999) Development of the *Drosophila* mushroom bodies: sequential generation of three distinct types of neurons from a neuroblast. *Development* 126:4065–4076.
Leng, S., and R. Strauss (1997) Impaired step lengths common to three unrelated *Drosophila* mutant lines with common brain defects confirm the involvement of the protocerebral bridge in optimizing walking speed. In N. Elsner and H. Wässle (eds.): *Proceedings of the 25th Göttingen Neurobiology Conference, vol. II.* Thieme, Stuttgart, p. 294.
Leuzinger, S., F. Hirth, D. Acampora, A. Simeone, W.J. Gehring, R. Finkelstein, K. Furukubo-Tokunaga, and H. Reichert (1998) Equivalence of the fly orthodenticle gene and the human OTX genes in embryonic brain development of *Drosophila. Development* 125:1703–1710.
Levine, R.B., and J.C. Weeks (1990) Hormonally mediated changes in simple reflex circuits during metamorphosis in *Manduca. J. Neurobiol.* 21:1022–1036.
Li, Y.S., and N.J. Strausfeld (1997) Morphology and sensory modality of mushroom body extrinsic neurons in the brain of the cockroach *Periplaneta americana. J. Comp. Neurol.* 386:1–20.
Li, Y.S., and N.J. Strausfeld (1999) Multimodal efferent and recurrent neurons in the medial lobes of cockroach mushroom bodies. *J. Comp. Neurol.* 409:647–663.

Liu, L., R. Wolf, R. Ernst, and M. Heisenberg (1999) Context generalization in *Drosophila* visual learning requires the mushroom bodies. *Nature* 400:753–756.

Martin, J.-R., T. Raabe, and M. Heisenberg (1999) Central complex substructures are required for the maintenance of locomotory activity in *Drosophila melanogaster. J. Comp. Physiol. [A]* 185:277–288.

Mauelshagen, J. (1993) Neural correlates of olfactory learning paradigms in an identified neuron in the honeybee brain. *J. Neurophysiol.* 69:609–625.

Mellon, D., V. Alones, and M.D. Lawrence (1992) Anatomy and fine structure of neurons in the deutocerebral projection pathway of the crayfish olfactory system. *J. Comp. Neurol.* 321:93–111.

Merritt, D.J., and R.K. Murphey (1992) Projections of leg proprioceptors within the CNS of the fly *Phormia* in relation to the generalized insect ganglion. *J. Comp. Neurol.* 322:16–34.

Milde, J.J. (1988) Visual responses of interneurones in the posterior median protocerebrum and the central complex of the honey bee *Apis mellifera. J. Insect Physiol.* 34:427–436.

Mizunami, M., R. Okada, Y.-S. Li, and N.J. Strausfeld (1998a) Mushroom bodies of the cockroach: activity and identities of neurons recorded in freely moving animals. *J. Comp. Neurol.* 402:501–519.

Mizunami, M., J.M. Weibrecht, and N.J. Strausfeld (1998b) Mushroom bodies of the cockroach: their participation in place memory. *J. Comp. Neurol.* 402:520–537.

Mobbs, P.G. (1982) The brain of the honeybee *Apis mellifera*. 1. The connections and spatial organizations of the mushroom bodies. *Philos. Trans. R. Soc. Lond. [B]* 298:309–354.

Muller, M., U. Homberg, and A. Kuhn (1997) Neuroarchitecture of the lower division of the central body of the locust *(Schistocerca gregaria). Cell Tissue Res.* 288:159–176.

Nagao. T.,S. Leuzinger, D. Acampora, A. Simeone, R. Finkelstein, H. Reichert and K. Furukubo-Tokunaga (1998) Developmental rescue of *Drosophila* cephalic defects by the human Otx genes. *Proc. Natl. Acad. Sci. USA.* 95:3737–3742.

Newland, P.L. (1991a) Morphology and somatotopic organisation of the central projections of afferents from tactile hairs on the hind leg of the locust. *J. Comp. Neurol.* 312:493–508.

Newland, P.L. (1991b) Physiological properties of afferents from tactile hairs on the hindlegs of the locust. *J. Exp. Biol.* 155:487–503.

Nighorn, A., M.J. Healy, and R.L. Davis (1991) The cyclic AMP phosphodiesterase encoded by the *Drosophila* dunce gene is concentrated in the mushroom body neuropil. *Neuron* 6:455–467.

Nübler-Jung, K., and D. Arendt (1994) Is ventral in insects dorsal in vertebrates? *Rouxs Arch. Dev. Biol.* 203:357–366.

Nübler-Jung, K., and D. Arendt (1996) Enteropneusts and chordate evolution. *Curr. Biol.* 6:352–353.

Pearson, K.G. (1983) Neural circuits for jumping in the locust. *J. Physiol. (Paris)* 78:765–771.

Pearson, K.G. (1993) Common principles of motor control in vertebrates and invertebrates. *Annu. Rev. Neurosci.* 16:265–297.

Pearson, K.G., and R.M. Robertson (1981) Interneurons coactivating hindleg flexor and extensor motoneurons in the locust. *J. Comp. Physiol. [A]* 144:391–400.

Puelles, L., and J.L.R. Rubenstein (1993) Expression patterns of homeobox and other putative regulatory genes in the embryonic mouse forebrain suggest a neuromeric organization. *TINS* 16:472–479.

Reichert, H., and A. Simeone (1999) Conserved usage of gap and homeotic genes in patterning the CNS. *Curr. Opin. Neurobiol.* 9:589–595.

Renn, S.C., J.D. Armstrong, M. Yang, Z. Wang, X. An, K. Kaiser, and P.H. Taghert (1999) Genetic analysis of the *Drosophila* ellipsoid body neuropil: organization and development of the central complex. *J. Neurobiol.* 41:189–207.

Retzius, G. (1890) Zur Kenntnis des centralen Nervensystems der Crustaceen. *Biol. Untersuch. Neue Folge.* (Samson and Whalin, Stockholm) 1:1–50.

Retzius, G. (1891) Zur Kenntnis des centralen Nervensystems der Würmer. *Biol. Untersuch. Neue Folge.* (Samson and Whalin, Stockholm) 2:1–18.

Riehle, A., and N. Franceschini (1982) Response of a directionally selective movement detecting neurone under precise stimulation of two identified photoreceptor cells. *Neurosci. Lett. Suppl.* 10:5411–5412.

Rosa, R.D., J.K. Grenier, T. Andreeva, C.E. Cook, A. Adoutte, M. Akam, S.B. Carroll, and G. Balavoine (1999) Hox genes in brachiopods and priapulids and protostome evolution. *Nature* 399:772–776.

Rospars, J.P., and J.G. Hildebrand (1992) Anatomical identification of glomeruli in the antennal lobes of the male sphinx moth *Manduca sexta. Cell Tiss. Res.* 270:205–227.

Rybak, J., and R. Menzel (1998) Integrative properties of the Pe1 neuron, a unique mushroom body output neuron. *Learn. Memory* 5:133–145.

Sachse, S., C.G. Galizia, A. Rappert, and R. Menzel (1999) The conserved representation of different chemical structures in the honeybee antennal lobe: steps towards the spatial olfactory code. N. Elsner, U. Eysel (eds.): *Proc. German Neurosci. Soc II.* Thieme, Stuttgart, 1999:368.

Schäfer, S., G. Bicker, O.P. Otterson, and J. Storm-Mathison (1988) Taurine-like immunoreactivity in the brain of the honeybee. *J. Comp. Neurol.* 265:60–70.

Schildberger, K. (1981) Some physiological properties of mushroom body linked fibers in the house cricket brain. *Naturwissenschaften* 67:623.

Schildberger, K. (1984) Multimodal interneurons in the cricket brain: properties of identified extrinsic mushroom body cells. *J. Comp. Physiol. [A]* 154:71–79.

Schmidt, M., and B. Ache (1996) Processing of antennular input in the brain of the spiny lobster, *Panulirus argus*. II. The olfactory pathway. *J. Comp. Physiol. A.* 178:605–628.

Schürmann, F.W. (1987) The architecture of the mushroom bodies and related neuropils in the insect brain. In A.P. Gupta (ed.): *The Arthropod Brain*. Wiley Interscience, New York, pp. 2231–264.

Schürmann, F.W., and J. Erber (1990) FMRFamide-like immunoreactivity in the brain of the honeybee, *Apis mellifera*: a light- and electron microscopical study. *Neuroscience* 3:797–807.

Schulz, R.A., C. Chromey, M.-F. Lu, and E.N. Olson (1996) Expression of the D-MEF2 transcription factor in the *Drosophila* brain suggests a role in neuronal cell differentiation. *Oncogene* 12:1827–1831.

Sharman, A.C., and M. Brand (1998) Evolution and homology of the nervous system: cross-phylum rescues of *otd/Otx* genes. *TIG* 14:211–214.

Siegler, M.V.S., and M. Burrows (1983) Spiking local interneurons as primary integrators of mechanosensory information in the locust. *J. Neurophysiol.* 50:1281–1295.

Siegler, M.V.S., and M. Burrows (1986) Receptive fields of motor neurones underlying local tactile reflexes in the locust. *J. Neurosci.* 6:507–513.

Skoulakis, E.M.C., D. Kalderon, and R.L. Davis (1993) Preferential expression in mushroom bodies of the catalytic subunit of protein kinase A and its role in learning and memory. *Neuron* 11:197–208.

Strausfeld, N.J. (1976) *Atlas of an Insect Brain*. Springer, New York.

Strausfeld, N.J. (1998) Crustacean—insect relationships: the use of brain characters to derive phylogeny amongst segmented invertebrates. *Brain Behav. Evol.* 52:186–206.

Strausfeld, N.J. (1999) A brain region in insects that supervises walking. *Prog. Brain Res.* 123:273–284.

Strausfeld, N.J., and K. Hausen (1977) The resolution of neuronal assemblies after cobalt injection into neuropil. *Proc. R. Soc. Lond. [Biol.]* 199:463–476.

Strausfeld, N.J., and J.G. Hildebrand (1999) Olfactory systems: common design, uncommon origins? *Curr. Opin. Neurobiol.* 9:634–639.

Strausfeld, N.J. and J.K. Lee (1991) Neuronal basis for parallel visual processing in the fly. *Vis. Neurosci.* 7:13–33.

Strausfeld, N.J. and Y.S. Li (1999a) Organization of olfactory and multimodal afferent neurons supplying the calyx and pedunculus of the cockroach mushroom bodies. *J. Comp. Neurol.* 409:603–625.

Strausfeld, N.J., and Y.S. Li (1999b) Representation of the calyces in the medial and vertical lobes of cockroach mushroom bodies. *J. Comp. Neurol.* 409:626–646.

Strausfeld, N.J., P. Weltzien, and F.G. Barth (1993) Two visual systems in one brain: neuropils serving the principal eyes of the spider *Cupiennius salei. J. Comp. Neurol.* 328:63–75.

Strausfeld, N.J., E.K. Buschbeck, and R.S. Gomez (1995) The arthropod mushroom body: its roles, evolutionary enigmas and mistaken identities. In O. Breidbach, and W. Kutsch, (eds.): *The Nervous Systems of Invertebrates: An Evolutionary and Comparative Approach*. Birkhauser, Basel, pp. 349–381,

Strausfeld, N.J., U. Homberg, and P. Kloppenburg (2000) Parallel organization in honey bee mushroom bodies by peptidergic Kenyon cells. *J. Comp. Neurol.* 424:179–195.

Strausfeld, N.J., Y.S. Li, R. Gomez, and K. Ito (1998) Evolution, discovery, and interpretations of Arthropod mushroom bodies. *Learn. Memory* 5:11–37.

Strauss, R., and M. Heisenberg (1990) Coordination of legs during straight walking and turning in *Drosophila melanogaster. J. Comp. Physiol. [A]* 167:403–412.

Strauss, R., and M. Heisenberg (1991) Altered patterns of walking in *Drosophila* central complex central-body-defect mutants. *J. Neurogenet.* 7:147.

Strauss, R., and M. Heisenberg (1993) Higher control center of locomotor behavior in the *Drosophila* brain *J. Neurosci.* 13:1852–1861.

Strauss, R., and T. Trinath (1996) Is walking in a straight line controlled by the central complex? Evidence from a new *Drosophila* mutant. In N. Elsner and H.U. Schnitzler (eds.): *Proc. 24th Göttingen Neurobiol. Conf., vol. II*. Thieme, Stuttgart, p.135.

Strauss, R., U. Hanesch, M. Kinklein, R. Wolf, and M. Heisenberg (1992) *no-bridge* of *Drosophila melanogaster*—portrait of a structural brain mutant of the central complex. *J. Neurogenet.* 8:125–155.

Studer, M., A. Gavalas, L. Marshall, F. Ariza-McNaughton, M. Rijli, P. Chambon, and R. Krumlauf (1998) Genetic interactions between Hoxa1 and Hoxb1 reveal new roles in regulation of early hindbrain patterning. *Development* 125:1025–1036.

Trivers, R.L., and H. Hare (1976) Haploidploidy and the evolution of the social insect. *Science* 191:249–263.

Truman, J.W., and E.E. Ball (1998) Patterns of embryonic neurogenesis in a primitive wingless insect, the silverfish, *Ctenolepisma longicaudata*: comparison with those seen in flying insects. *Dev. Genes Evol.* 208:357–368.

Truman, J.W., and L.M. Riddiford (1999) The origins of insect metamorphosis. *Nature* 401:447–452.

Umesono, Y., K. Watanabe, and K. Agata (1999) Distinct structural domains in the planarian brain defined by the expression of evolutionarily conserved homeobox genes. *Dev. Genes Evol.* 209:31–39.

Utting, M., H.-J. Agricola, R. Sandeman, and D. Sandeman (2000) Central complex in the brain of crayfish and its possible homology with that of insects. *J. Comp. Neurol.* 416:245–261.

Vickers, N.J., T.A. Christensen, and J.G. Hildebrand (1998) Combinatorial odor discrimination in the brain: attractive and antagonist odor blends are represented in distinct combinations of uniquely identifiable glomeruli. *J. Comp. Neurol.* 400:35–56.

Wannek, U., and R. Strauss (1998) How flies perform turns—high resolution statistical analyses in normal and brain-defective *Drosophila melanogaster*. In N. Elsner and R. Wehner (eds.). *Proc. 26th Göttingen Neurobiol. Conf., vol. II.* Thieme, Stuttgart, p.258.

Welzien, P., and F.G. Barth (1991) Volumetric measurements do not demonstrate that the spider brain "central body" has a special role in web building. *J. Morphol.* 207:1–8.

Wicklein, M., and D. Varju (1999) Visual system of the European hummingbird hawkmoth *Macroglossum stellatarum* (Sphingidae, Lepidoptera): motion-sensitive interneurons of the lobula plate. *J. Comp. Neurol.* 408:272–282.

Williams, J.L.D. (1975) Anatomical studies of the insect nervous system: a ground plan of the midbrain and an introduction to the central complex in the locust, *Schistocerca gregaria* (Orthoptera). *J. Zool.* 176:67–86.

Williams, N.A., and P.W.H. Holland (1998) Molecular evolution of the brain of chordates. *Brain Behav. Evol.* 52:177–185.

Witten, J.L., and J.W. Truman (1998) Distribution of GABA-like immunoreactive neurons in insects suggests lineage homology. *J. Comp. Neurol.* 398:515–528.

Wootton, R.J., J. Kukalova-Peck, D.J.S. Newman, and J. Muzon (1998) Smart engineering in the Mid-Carboniferous: how well could Paleozoic dragonflies fly? *Science* 282:749–751.

Wray, G.A., J.S. Levinton, and L.H. Shapiro (1996) Molecular evidence for deep Precambrian divergences among metazoan phyla. *Science* 274:568–573.

Zars, T., M. Fischer, R. Schulz, and M. Heisenberg (2000). Localization of a short-term memory in *Drosophila*. *Science* 288:672–675.

Zawarzin, A.A. (1925) Der Parallismus der Strukturen als ein Grundprinzip der Morphologie. *Z. Wiss. Zool.* 124:118–212.

Chapter 13

CONSERVATION IN THE NEUROLOGY AND PSYCHOLOGY OF COGNITION IN VERTEBRATES

Euan M. Macphail, Department of Psychology, University of York

Comparative psychologists have found it difficult to demonstrate differences in cognition among vertebrate species. This seems odd in light of the clear differences in gross anatomical organization of vertebrate brains. Recent decades have, however, seen striking advances, led by neuroanatomists, in our understanding of the functional organization of vertebrate brains, and unexpected parallels in organization across different vertebrate classes have emerged. For example, birds have no six-layered neocortex, but the organization of sensory projections to the telencephalon suggests that regions within the avian neostriatal and hyperstriatal complexes may correspond functionally to regions within mammalian neocortex. Anatomical parallels have been supported by behavioral studies of avian telencephalic function: there are now data from lesion studies that suggest roles in learning comparable to those of their mammalian homologues for all the major divisions of the avian telencephalon (the archistriatal, paleostriatal, neostriatal, hyperstriatal, and hippocampal complexes). These data suggest that there has been conservation of the basic functional organization of the vertebrate forebrain through evolution and support the idea that there has been conservation also of basic cognitive processes.

INTRODUCTION: COMPLEXITY IN BRAINS AND BEHAVIOR

It is a commonplace that the evolution of vertebrates has seen advances in the complexity of both brain and behavior, and it is equally a commonplace that complexity in behavior accounts for complexity in brain. One of the most striking advances in behavioral complexity is seen in the chasm that exists between human general intelligence and the intelligence of nonhuman vertebrates. Reasonably enough, it is generally supposed that human intelligence is the product of a process of gradual evolution and that the ancestral species that appeared and disappeared in the history of human evolution would have shown gradual increases in intelligence as that evolution progressed. Correlated with these changes in intelligence there would have been changes in the brain, with a general tendency to show increases in both size and complexity of the later-evolving species.

Although no living species is ancestral to the human species, it is, again, reasonable to expect that we might see in living vertebrates a tendency toward increased complexity of brain and behavior in those species that are most closely related to humans. This expectation is readily realized by data on both the size and the organization of the brain. The brains of teleosts, for example, are approximately 10 times smaller than the brains of mammals of the same body weight; and the human brain is substantially larger than that of any other mammal of comparable body weight (Jerison, 1973). Most of the difference in size between the brains of bony fishes and of mammals is due to differences in size of the telencephalon—the region that seems most likely to be involved in intelligence. Congruent with this idea, the gross structural complexity of the mammalian telencephalon is strikingly greater than that of the teleost telencephalon: There are simply many more architectonically distinct regions in the mammalian brain.

SPECIES DIFFERENCES IN INTELLIGENCE

Differences between species in the size and the complexity of the telencephalon should lead us to expect corresponding differences, of both degree and kind, in the behavior served by the telencephalon—and, in particular, in intelligence. At first sight, this expectation is supported by informal observation. It seems obvious that the behavior of our closest relatives, nonhuman primates, is more flexible and intelligent than that of other mammals, rats, for example, and that mammals in general are more intelligent than such nonmammals as frogs and goldfish. There is, however, a problem with informal rankings of intelligence: Although it is obviously true that primates are more versatile than rats, it is not necessarily true that this versatility reflects a difference in intellect rather than differences in such noncognitive factors as sensory and motor capacities. A chimpanzee's vision is superior to that of rats, and its possession of hands with opposable thumbs considerably increases its dexterity.

It has proved remarkably difficult to show that genuine differences in intelligence exist among vertebrate species, and this is particularly true for claims that there are differences in kind—qualitative differences—as opposed to differences in degree—quantitative differences. So much so that, although the great majority of ethologists and psychologists believe that such differences exist, currently there is in fact no specific proposal for a qualitative difference in intellect among nonhuman vertebrates that enjoys overwhelming support. The difficulty in demonstrating intellectual differences has its origin not simply in the fact that it is difficult to design intelligence tests that are relatively free of contamination by sensory and motor factors but also in the repeated finding that supposedly less intelligent species succeed in mastering tasks originally supposed to be beyond their capacities.

It may, of course, be that psychologists have shown insufficient ingenuity in designing the tests used to explore species differences in intelligence. Another possibility is that such differences are in fact much less widespread than is generally supposed—that, in other words, there may be few, if any, differences in intelligence among vertebrate species. One problem with this conservative conclusion is that it seems to clash with the striking differences between the brains (and between telencephala in particular) of the various vertebrate groups. The object of this chapter is to argue that a reconciliation can be achieved between the contrasts seen in the neurological data and the parallels seen in the behavioral data. I argue that evidence obtained over recent decades has shown that major anatomical differences between telencephalic structures have evolved without there being any corresponding changes in the basic behavioral functions of those structures.

BIRDS AND MAMMALS COMPARED

I shall concentrate on data from birds, for a number reasons. Birds are very distant relatives of mammals and evolved from a quite different group of reptiles (the archosaurs) than that which gave rise to mammals (the pelycosaurs); for a common ancestor we need to go back to the earliest reptiles, some 300 million years ago. Comparisons between birds and mammals are, then, well-suited to test general questions about the evolution of brain and intelligence. As might be expected, there are indeed striking anatomical differences between the telencephala of birds and of mammals—there is, for example, no six-layered isocortex in birds. Birds have been widely regarded as being generally less intelligent than mammals. Darwin, for example, argued, with many others, that avian behavior is generally inflexible and dominated by instinct. Birds as a group have enjoyed more attention from neuroscientists and experimental psychologists than any other nonmammalian group so that there is by now a substantial body of both neurological and behavioral data.

A final reason for looking in some detail at birds is that behavioral data give good support to the contention that provides the rationale for this chapter, namely, that supposedly unintelligent animals frequently can be shown to be considerably more intelligent than expected. For, despite the widespread low reputation of the avian intellect (the phrase 'bird-brained' makes the point), comparative psychologists have found that birds perform with remarkable efficiency in a wide range of learning tasks. I have reviewed these data elsewhere (Macphail, 1982, 1987, 1996), and it will serve my purpose here simply to summarize some relevant findings. We now know that birds can show efficient performance in the following paradigms: learning-set formation (Kamil and Hunter, 1970); language acquisition (Pepperberg, 1994); the radial maze (Roberts and Van Veldhuizen, 1985); a "transitive inference" task (Von Fersen et al., 1991); and an avian analogue of "insight" (Epstein et al., 1984). By "efficient" here, I mean that avian performance is generally comparable with mammalian performance; the list is not, of course, exhaustive, but it does include tasks (such as learning-set formation) that have enjoyed support as potential tests of general intelligence and tasks (such as transitive inference) that might well have been supposed to tap capacities available only to animals with well-developed "higher" cognitive capacities.

Given that there are extensive parallels also between avian and mammalian performance on supposedly simpler tasks such as habituation and conditioning (Macphail, 1982), there is good support for a substantial commonality between the avian and the mammalian intellect and relatively little evidence of differences in cognitive capacities. The issue here is to reconcile this conclusion with the apparent divergence in avian and mammalian telencephalic neurology.

Early neuroanatomists (Ariëns-Kappers et al., 1936) supposed that most of the major structures of the avian telencephalon were comparable with the mammalian basal ganglia and labeled them accordingly as the *paleostriatum* and *neostriatum* (Fig. 13.1 shows the major anatomical divisions of the avian telencephalon). The paleostriatum was taken to correspond with the globus pallidus and the neostriatum, to the caudate nucleus and putamen. The supposed domination of the avian telencephalon by the basal ganglia agreed well with the general idea that birds' behavior was dominated by instincts—innately specified fixed patterns of motor activity. A further "striatal" region, the archistriatum, was believed (with, as we shall see, *some* justification) to be the avian correlate of the amygdala. Two other major telencephalic regions (the hyperstriatum and the ectostriatum) were labeled in a way that implied no mammalian equivalent. This agreed with the idea that there was in birds no equivalent of the mammalian isocortex: There was clearly no major laminated telencephalic structure, and it was also believed that the senses did not show orderly projections from the dorsal thalamus to any part of the telencephalon. Although there was a region labeled as *hippocampus*, this region did not show the

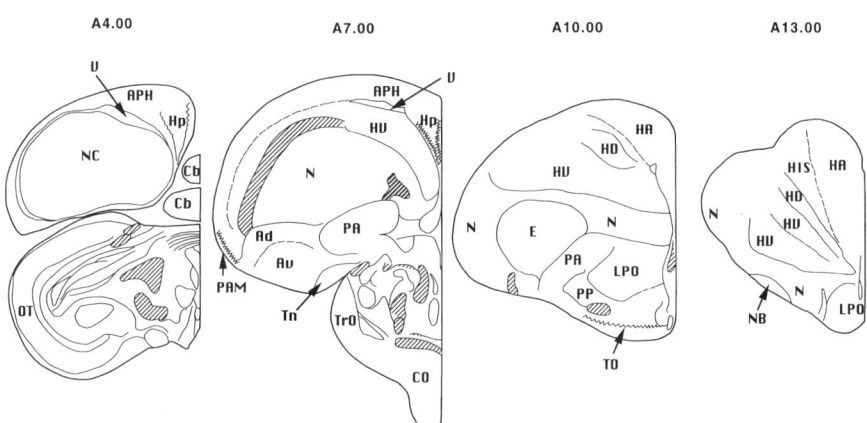

Figure 13.1. Transverse sections showing the major structures of the pigeon telencephalon. The numbers above of each drawing indicate the location of the section (in millimeters anterior to the interaural zero, using the vertical plane of the Karten and Hodos atlas). Ad, archistriatum dorsale; APH, parahippocampal area; Av, archistriatum ventrale; Cb, cerebellum; CO, chiasma opticum; E, ectostriatum; HA, hyperstriatum accessorium; HD, hyperstriatum dorsale; HIS, hyperstriatum intercalatus superior; Hp, hippocampus; HV, hyperstriatum ventrale; LPO, lobus parolfactorius; N, neostriatum; NB, nucleus basalis; NC, neostriatum caudale; OT, tectum opticum; PA, paleostriatum augmentatum; PAM, periamygdaloid cortex; PP, paleostriatum primitivum; Tn, nucleus taeniae; TO, tuberculum olfactorium; TrO, tractus opticus; V, lateral ventricle. (after Karten and Hodos, 1967.)

clear lamination of the mammalian hippocampus—which was, in any case, not supposed at that time to play a major role in cognition.

It has been primarily work by neuroanatomists that has, over recent decades, overthrown the traditional picture of the avian telencephalon. The key to the modern view is that the true avian representatives of the mammalian basal ganglia are to be found in the paleostriatal complex; the ectostriatum, the neostriatum, and the hyperstriatum are the avian representatives of the isocortical zone of mammals. I shall briefly review some of the relevant anatomical data here, as they provide the essential basis for the modern interpretation of correspondences between avian and mammalian telencephalic regions. I shall go on to discuss evidence that gives direct support to the idea that the parallels in anatomy are reflected in parallels in functions of corresponding regions. I shall concentrate on the roles played in learning, as this is clearly most relevant to the evolution of intelligence, and in selecting which experiments to describe I shall, of course, be guided by their overall interest and relevance. It will emerge that many of these experiments were carried out some years ago, and this reflects the regrettable fact that neuroanatomical advances have not always resulted in behavioral neuroscience research. I hope, then, that this chapter may also play a role in encouraging further exploration of the *behavioral* functions of avian telencephalic regions.

THE BASAL GANGLIA

The list of structures that should be included in the mammalian basal ganglia has varied over recent decades. Traditionally, its major components were the amygdala (known also as the *archistriatum*), the globus pallidus (the *paleostriatum*), and the caudate nucleus/putamen (the *neostriatum*). Now, however, the terms archistriatum and paleostriatum have fallen into disuse (in mammalian terminology), and the basal ganglia as a whole (excluding the amygdala) are commonly referred to as the *striatum*.

There have also been recent additions to the structures properly included in the basal ganglia, which are now divided into two major divisions, the dorsal and ventral divisions (Heimer et al., 1982); each of these divisions can in turn be divided into a striatum, with densely packed cells, and a pallidum, sparse in cells. The striatum of the dorsal division consists of the caudate nucleus and putamen; the dorsal pallidum consists of the globus pallidus and the entopeduncular nucleus. The ventral striatum consists of the nucleus accumbens and part of the olfactory tubercle; the ventral pallidum consists of the rostral part of the substantia innominata and a ventral extension of the globus pallidus.

The avian basal ganglia consist of the paleostriatum primitivum, the paleostriatum augmentatum, the lobus parolfactorius (LPO), and the olfactory tubercle (see Fig. 13.1). The parallels between the avian and the mammalian basal ganglia are the subject of an excellent review by Medina and Reiner (1995), and I can do no better than to summarize the central points of that review here. First, there are histochemical and embryological data that support a general homology between the avian and

13 Conservation in the Neurology and Psychology of Cognition in Vertebrates

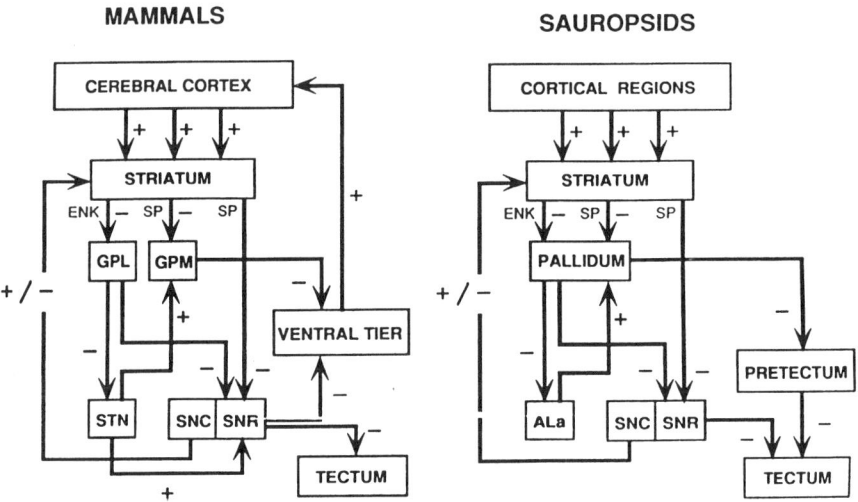

Figure 13.2. Simplified circuitry diagrams comparing the functional organization of the basal ganglia in mammals (left) and sauropsids (birds and reptiles) (right). The pluses and minuses indicate whether the specific projections of the basal ganglia circuitry use an excitatory (+) or an inhibitory (−) neurotransmitter. The +/− noted for the SNC-striatal projection indicates that the dopaminergic SNC input to the SP (substance P-containing) striatal neurons appears to be excitatory, while the dopaminergic SNC input to ENK (enkephalin-containing) striatal neurons appears to be inhibitory. In mammals and sauropsids, there are striatopallidal, striatonigral, nigrostriatal, nigrotectal, pallidosubthalamic, and pallidonigral pathways that use the same neurotransmitters, suggesting that these basal ganglia circuits play similar roles in the control of movement in all amniotes. ALa, anterior nucleus of the ansa lenticularis; GPL, lateral globus pallidus; GPM, medial globus pallidus; SNC, substantia nigra pars compacta; SNR, substantia nigra pars reticulata; STN, subthalamic nucleus. (From Medina and Reiner, 1995, by permission of Karger, Basel.)

mammalian basal ganglia. In both groups, for example, the basal ganglia are clearly distinguishable from the overlying cortical region by the relatively high concentration of acetylcholinesterase and dopamine; and there is evidence that comparable genes are expressed in mammals and birds in the neural primordia of the basal ganglia in embryonic animals. Second, there are parallels in the connections, both with cortical and with subcortical regions: Figure 13.2 shows in diagrammatic form the connections of the basal ganglia of, on the one hand, mammals and, on the other, sauropsids (birds and reptiles, whose gross brain anatomy more closely resembles that of birds than that of mammals).

I shall restrict detailed attention here to the structures of the dorsal division because there are no useful data for birds on the potential role of ventral structures in learning, the function of central interest to this chapter.

The dorsal striatum of birds consists of the paleostriatum augmentatum and the LPO. There are a number of close correspondences between the avian and mammalian regions. In both birds and mammals, for example, about 90 to 95% of dorsal striatal neurons contain γ-aminobutyric acid (GABA, an inhibitory neurotransmitter) and project outside the striatum. Projections to and from dorsal striatal regions are comparable in birds and mammals. There are projections to the mammalian striatum from sensory isocortical areas that process visual, auditory, and somatosensory input; the corresponding projections in birds arise from regions that are, as we shall see, comparable to the isocortex and that, similarly, process sensory input. There is also, in birds and mammals, a massive dopaminergic projection from the ventral tegmentum, as well as input from thalamic cell groups that are, again, comparable. There are major projections from the dorsal striatum to the dorsal pallidum and to the dopaminergic cell groups of the tegmentum; these projections are, again, strikingly similar in birds and mammals.

The dorsal pallidum is represented in birds by the paleostriatum primitivum. The great majority of these pallidal cells, in birds as in mammals, contain GABA and project outside the pallidum. The major input to the dorsal pallidum (in both birds and mammals) arises from the dorsal striatum; and both birds and mammals send a major projection from the pallidum to the dopaminergic cell groups of the tegmentum.

It is, then, apparent that there are compelling and detailed parallels between the mammalian basal ganglia and the paleostriatal complex (including the LPO) of birds. There is, moreover, evidence that damage to the avian paleostriatum may, like damage to the mammalian basal ganglia, cause disturbances in motor control (Rieke, 1980, 1981). What, then, of the role of the avian basal ganglia in learning?

PALEOSTRIATAL LESIONS AND CLASSICAL CONDITIONING IN THE PIGEON

Mitchell explored the effects of paleostriatal lesions on a number of learning tasks in pigeons (see Mitchell, 1983a,b; Mitchell and Hall, 1984). One intriguing feature of her results was that she found a number of paradigms in which the performance of the lesioned birds was actually *superior* to that of the controls. One of these paradigms was autoshaping, in which the illumination of a keylight is followed by food delivery. As is well-known, although the pigeon's behavior is irrelevant to the delivery or nondelivery of the food, hungry pigeons come to peck at the lit key. Pigeons with lesions targeted at the paleostriatum augmentatum responded more rapidly than controls in a conventional autoshaping procedure (Mitchell, 1983a). An increased response rate could, of course, reflect a motor problem, such as tremor, rather than improved learning. A motor explanation was ruled out, however, by experiments (Mitchell, 1983b; Mitchell and Hall, 1984) in which an alternation procedure was used, such that food followed key illumination (independent, again, of the bird's responses) on alternate trials only. As expected, the lesioned birds showed more rapid responding than controls on trials on which food was delivered. They also, however, learned to discriminate those trials from nonreward trials more rapidly than controls (which did not, in fact, master the discrimination); unlike controls, the paleostriatum-lesioned birds responded less rapidly on nonreward than on reward trials. The only way to respond appropriately in this task is to discriminate the aftereffects of nonreward trials from those of reward trials—to detect the difference, that is, between the two possible types of "trace" persisting from the most recent trial. The paleostriatum-lesioned birds were not, then, simply responding more rapidly than the controls; they were acquiring the appropriate associations—which involved *reducing* response rates on nonreward trials—more rapidly.

Why should a lesion to the basal ganglia *improve* the formation of associations? Mitchell proposed an account that appealed to the nature of the associations involved. Paleostriatum-lesioned pigeons, she suggested, show improved classical conditioning as a consequence of an impairment in processing information about responses—an impairment that should be reflected in disruption of performance on instrumental conditioning tasks. Classical conditioning involves the formation of an association between stimuli—in the case of autoshaping, of an association between the keylight and the food; instrumental conditioning involves an association between a response and a stimulus, between, for example, a lever-press and food, formed typically when the delivery of food is contingent upon the animal's response. In any given procedure, an event of significance, food delivery, in this instance, will necessarily occur in the presence of both some response of the animal and some environmental stimulation. The animal's task is to detect which event, which response or which environmental stimulus, is reliably correlated with food delivery. Mitchell's suggestion, congruent with the idea that the basal ganglia are involved in movement, was that paleostriatum-lesioned birds are relatively poor at using information about their own responses (perhaps because of reduced feedback from their responses) and that this lack of attention to responses enhanced the salience of environmental stimuli, thus facilitating classical conditioning.

A further experiment (Mitchell and Hall, 1984) was designed specifically to test the idea that the effectiveness of response cues was reduced in paleostriatum-lesioned pigeons. The procedure involved the use of an (instrumental) variable-interval schedule in which food was delivered for keypecks that occurred after the expiration of an interval that averaged 60 seconds; this type of schedule obtains a relatively steady rate of response from pigeons, as there is no cue that enables them to predict which responses will be effective. There was in this experiment a delay of 0.5 second between each effective peck and the delivery of the food reward, and in one condition, this delay was filled with a "flash" of the houselight, which otherwise was not lit. Control birds, as anticipated from an earlier report (Hall, 1982), showed a marked reduction in overall rate of response when the delay was filled by the houselight flash, but pigeons with paleostriatal lesions showed no change in rate. The rate reduction seen in intact pigeons has been interpreted (Hall, 1982) as reflecting a reduction in the strength of the response-reinforcer association that plays a role in instrumental responding. The reduction is supposed to reflect competition for associative strength between the (instrumental) response-reinforcer contingency and the (classical) stimulus (houselight flash)-reinforcer contingency—an instance of the overshadowing of one event (the response) by another event (the "flash") that is better correlated with reward.

If paleostriatum-lesioned pigeons show impaired instrumental conditioning, then their responding on interval schedules may reflect the formation of associations based on the classical (e.g., keylight-reinforcer) contingencies that inevitably exist in rewarded contexts. In that case, overshadowing of the response-reinforcer contingency should have little effect on response output, as was found.

The evidence that processing of information about responses is impaired in paleostriatum-lesioned pigeons gives general support to the idea that there are functional parallels between the avian paleostriatal complex and the mammalian striatum. One attraction of Mitchell's report, however, is that it gave rise to novel work on the mammalian striatum. Mitchell et al., (1985) reported an experiment that found that rats with caudate/putamen damage showed, compared with controls, a much reduced alteration in response rate on the introduction of a brief stimulus preceding each reward delivery.

THE ARCHISTRIATUM

The amygdala of mammals and the archistriatum of birds are both complexes containing many subdivisions. Amaral et al. (1992) describe 13 subdivisions of the primate amygdala, several of which may be further subdivided, and Zeier and Karten (1971) divided the pigeon archistriatum into 4 major regions, each of which showed from 4 to 8 subdivisions.

There is not enough information currently available on the detailed connections of subdivisions of the avian archistriatum—and, in particular, on intra-archistriatal connections—to allow homologies to be drawn between subdivisions of avian archistriatum and those of mammalian amygdala. The nuclei of the mammalian amygdala are commonly divided into two major groups, the basolateral and the corticomedial divisions (the latter division being taken here to include also the central nucleus). In general, information flows from the basolateral to the corticomedial division, which projects extensively to the hypothalamus, thus in effect equipping all of the amygdala with direct or indirect projections to the hypothalamus (Amaral et al., 1992). These connections in turn encourage the idea that the amygdala may be involved in motivation, and one of the best-known consequences of amygdalar damage is a reduction in fear; recent work on the rat amygdala has shown that both the basolateral and corticomedial amygdala play important but different roles in fear-motivated behavior (Killcross et al., 1997).

Posteromedial Archistriatum: Fear and Avoidance

Zeier and Karten (1971) established that only the posterior and medial divisions of the archistriatum projected to the hypothalamus and went on to propose that only this posteromedial division (Fig. 13.3) was homologous with the mammalian amygdala. Congruent with this idea, Reiner and Karten (1985) have shown that there are direct projections from the olfactory bulb to the posteromedial archistriatum but not to the anterior or intermediate archistriatum: similarly, in mammals, there are secondary olfactory projections to the amygdala.

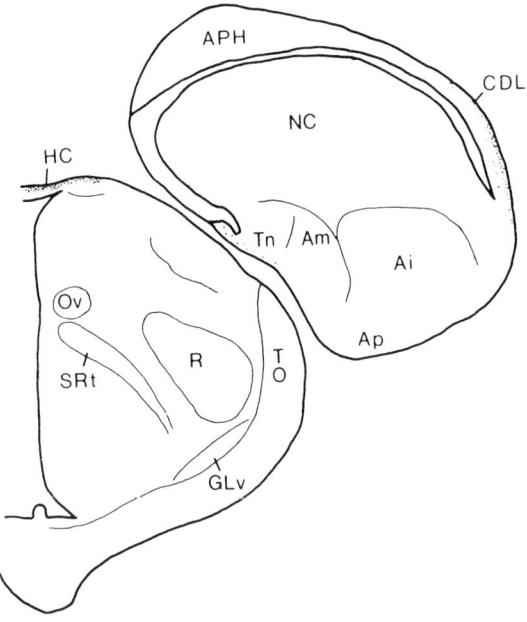

Figure 13.3. Line drawing of a transverse section through the caudal telencephalon of a pigeon, showing the general location of the major subdivisions of the archistriatum. Ai, Archistriatum intermedium; Am, Archistriatum mediale; Ap, Archistriatum posterior; APH, area parahippocampalis; CDL, Area corticoidea dorsolateralis; GLv, Nucleus lateralis geniculatus lateralis, pars ventralis; HC, habenular commissure; NC, Neostriatum caudale; Ov, Nucleus ovoidalis; R, Nucleus rotundus; SRt, Nucleus subrotundus; Tn, Nucleus taeniae; TO, Tractus opticus. (from Reiner and Karten, 1985, by permission of Karger, Basel.)

Support for a functional parallel between posteromedial archistriatum and the amygdala is found in the fact that lesions of the avian posteromedial archistriatum do (like amygdalar lesions) markedly reduce both fear and aggression (Phillips, 1964; Ramirez and Delius, 1979); Phillips (1944), for example, reported that mallard ducks (*Anas platyrhynchos*) were tamed by archistriatal lesions (so that they could readily be picked up); Dafters (1976) found that pigeons with posteromedial archistriatal lesions (unlike controls) showed very little suppression of food-motivated responding to a signal (a tone) that preceded an inescapable aversive shock; and Ramirez and Delius (1979) found reduced aggression by pigeons to a stick or a human hand inserted into the home cage.

Perhaps unsurprisingly, there is good evidence that, as in mammals with amygdalar lesions, avoidance learning is disrupted by archistriatal damage. Dafters (1975) found that archistriatal-damaged pigeons were severely impaired in both acquisition and retention of a task in which they had to learn to press a treadle to avoid a shock; and Lowndes and Davies (1994) found that chicks with archistriatal damage were impaired in a one-trial learning task in which controls learned not to peck an attractive colored bead that had been coated with an aversive-tasting substance.

These data support the idea that there may be substantial functional parallels between the roles in learning of the avian posteromedial archistriatum and the mammalian amygdala. The extent of those parallels is, however, not yet clear, because, whereas in mammals there have been many reports of the disruption by amygdalar damage of learning in tasks that have not involved aversive stimuli, there have been very few reports of the effects of posteromedial archistriatal lesions on tasks that have involved positive incentives. The dearth of useful data means that it is not currently possible to assess the comparability of the posteromedial archistriatum and the amygdala in learning tasks other than avoidance.

Anterior and Intermediate Archistriatum: Parallels with Isocortex

The intermediate and anterior regions of the archistriatum give rise to long descending projections to the brain stem and spinal cord, and these projections led Zeier and Karten (1971) to suggest that these parts of the archistriatum might be comparable with mammalian motor isocortex. A further anatomical parallel between the anterior archistriatum and mammalian isocortex is to be found in the fact that only the anterior region of the archistriatum contributes to the anterior commissure: in mammals, the anterior commissure consists of fibers joining the temporal isocortical regions, and the amygdala (like the posteromedial archistriatum) makes no contribution.

The functional role of the anterior and intermediate regions of the archistriatum is discussed in a later section, in which avian structures that now are taken to be comparable to parts of mammalian isocortex are discussed.

CORTEX

Traditionally, mammalian cortex has been assigned three divisions: paleocortex, represented by the (three-layered) olfactory cortex; archicortex, represented by the (three-layered) hippocampus; and the six-layered isocortex.

Olfactory Cortex

Nomenclature for mammalian olfactory cortex—those cortical regions that receive direct input from the olfactory bulbs—varies among neuroanatomists. Regions generally recognized include some that directly adjoin the bulb itself, such as the retrobulbar cortex and the prepiriform cortex, and, clearly separate from the bulb, the piriform cortex. Homologues of these areas have been proposed for birds. Ebinger et al., (1992) identified areas in the brains of anseriform species that corresponded to mammalian olfactory cortical regions in three ways: first, in general location; second, in architectonics—these regions are three layered; and third, in receiving direct projections from the olfactory bulb. They proposed that the areas adjoining the bulb should be regarded as the avian equivalents of the retrobulbar and prepiriform cortices and that an extensive area on the ventrolateral hemispheric surface, served by the lateral olfactory tract, should be regarded as periamygdaloid cortex (Fig. 13.4; this area has been referred to as *piriform cortex* by other authors—e.g., Bingman et al., 1994; and Reiner and Karten, 1985, whose anatomical study showed marked similarities between the afferent and efferent connections of avian and mammalian piriform cortex). Little is known of the role of the periamygdaloid (or piriform) cortex in birds: Lesions do not cause gross impairment of olfaction, but do disrupt navigation in pigeons in which olfaction is now known to play a major role (Gagliardo et al., 1997; Papi and Casini, 1990). Similarly, in mammals piriform cortex lesions do not cause gross impairment of olfaction, but do obtain subtle effects on learning (Staubli et al., 1987).

The extents of these olfactory cortical areas, like the size of the bulb itself, show (as in mammals) considerable variation, and the three layered structure seen in anseriform birds may be less prominent in other avian orders. As far as olfactory cortex is concerned, there seem to be no major systematic anatomical differences between avian and mammalian brains. This is, perhaps, not surprising, and it is of more interest to consider regions that are now thought comparable with the hippocampus and isocortex, regions that are, perhaps, more relevant to the neuroscience of intelligence.

Hippocampal Complex

The avian hippocampal complex, which lies in the dorsomedial region of the telencephalon, consists of the hippocampus and the parahippocampal area. There are good grounds for accepting the conventional proposal that these regions are homologous with the mammalian hippocampal complex: Both developed from the dorsomedial

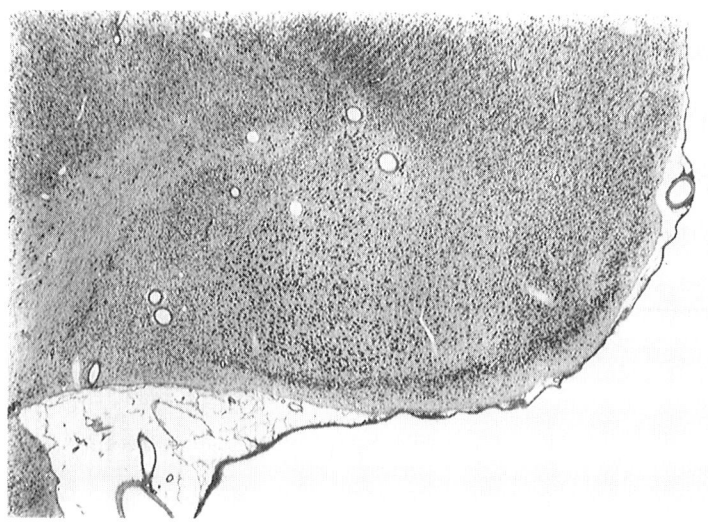

Figure 13.4. A cresyl violet–stained section of a ventrolateral region of the telencephalon of *Anas platyrhynchos*. The periamygdaloid cortex occupies the ventral surface, immediately subjacent to the archistriatum. (From Ebinger et al., 1992, by permission of Springer, Berlin.)

reptilian cortical area, and there are both neurochemical and hodological parallels between the avian and the mammalian hippocampal complexes (for review, see Macphail, 1993). The parallels should not be exaggerated: Although, for example, the avian hippocampus does project strongly to the septal region, there is no direct projection to the hypothalamus (and thus, no avian equivalent of the postcommissural fornix) and no direct input from the medial septal nucleus (which, in mammals, drives the theta rhythm). Moreover, despite the general homology between the regions, the gross anatomical appearance of the avian hippocampus is very different from the mammalian pattern. The avian hippocampus (Fig. 13.5) consists of a V-shaped band of cells that contains between the arms of the V a somewhat amorphous region and is regarded by some neuroanatomists (e.g., Ebinger et al., 1992) as exhibiting a three-layered structure. Erichsen et al., (1991), using parallels in neurochemistry and cell type, have suggested that the V-shaped band may correspond to the hippocampus proper of mammals and the amorphous region, to the dentate gyrus. We do not yet know, however, whether, as in the comparable structures of mammals, there is a major input from the amorphous region to the V-shaped band (corresponding to the mammalian mossy-fiber projection), nor is anything known of the inputs and outputs of the parahippocampal region (which may correspond to the mammalian subiculum).

The question of interest here is whether there are functional parallels between the avian and mammalian hippocampal complexes, in particular in their role in learning. There is in fact good evidence for significant functional similarities, much of it based on experiments concerned with the processing of spatial information.

One of the most striking consequences of hippocampal damage in mammals is the disruption of a variety of spatial tasks such as, for example, learning complex mazes. The precise cause of this disruption is still a matter of controversy; one fruitful hypothesis has been that the hippocampus contains a spatial map (O'Keefe and Nadel, 1978); but this proposal has been weakened by findings that indicate, first, that not all spatial tasks are disrupted and, second, that a number of nonspatial tasks are also susceptible to hippocampal damage (for review, see Macphail, 1993). Interpretation of the nature of the deficit need not concern us here, however, our interest is confined to asking whether the deficits induced by avian hippocampal damage resemble those induced by mammalian hippocampal damage.

Disruption of performance by hippocampal lesions in birds has been reported for several tasks with a strong spatial component (tasks such as pigeon homing, spatial delayed matching-to-sample, recovery of food caches; for review, see Macphail, 1993). Some of the most striking support for a role of the avian hippocampus in spatial processing, however, comes from quite another source. Reports by Krebs et al., (1989) and Sherry et al., (1989) established that the size of the hippocampus was larger in food-storing birds (of the parid, sittid, and corvid families) than in non–food-storing birds of the same family. Overall telencephalic size did not differ between storing and nonstoring species, and a plausible interpretation of this finding is that the demand made on spatial memory by the need to recover caches has encouraged the selective enlargement of the hippocampus in storing species; this interpretation is, of course, further supported by the finding that cache recovery is disrupted by hippocampal damage (Sherry and Vaccarino, 1989).

414 13 Conservation in the Neurology and Psychology of Cognition in Vertebrates

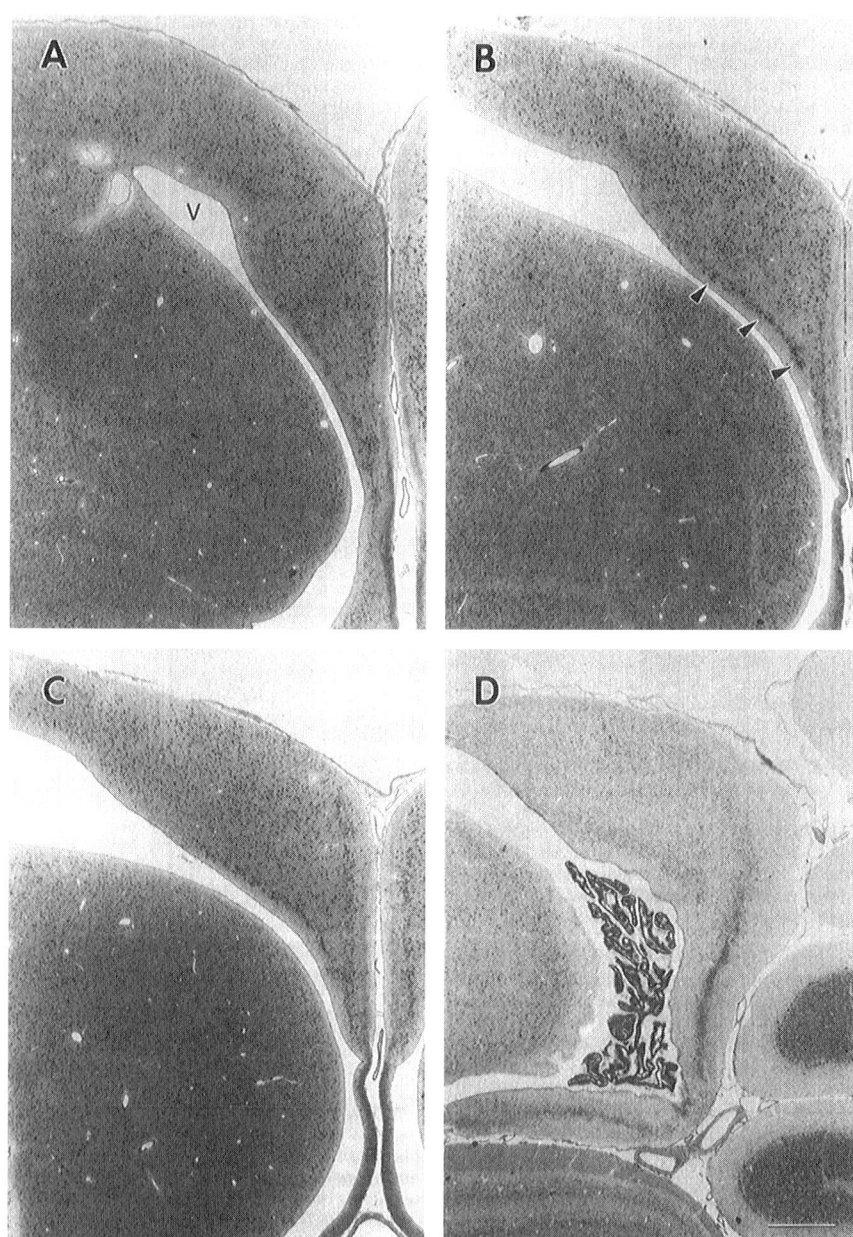

Figure 13.5. Four transverse Nissl- and Klüver-Barrera-stained section (A-D) through the hippocampal region of the pigeon at four successive rostro-caudal levels (9.00, 7.50, 6.00 and 3.75 mm) anterior to the zero of the Karten and Hodos (1967) atlas. V, ventricle; arrowheads, V-shaped bands of the hippocampus. (From Krebs et al., 1991.)

Selective hippocampal enlargement has also been found in birds associated with spatial demands independent of food storing. The hippocampus of homing pigeons is larger than that of pigeons that have not been bred for homing (Rehkämper et al., 1988), and the hippocampus of female cowbirds (*Molothrus ater*) is larger than that of male cowbirds (Sherry et al., 1993). The spatial significance of this sex difference is that cowbirds are a brood-parasitic species in which the females—but not the males—search for and identify suitable host nests in which to deposit their eggs, refinding those sites some time in the next few days.

A final piece of evidence linking avian spatial performance to the hippocampus concerns the phenomenon of long-term potentiation (LTP), first observed in the mammalian hippocampus. LTP has also been observed in cells of the avian hippocampus (Wieraszko and Ball, 1991). There is some variation in the mechanisms of LTP in mammals: in some cases (at synapses between the perforant path and the granule cells of the dentate gyrus, for example), LTP is mediated by NMDA receptors; at other sites (synapses between the mossy fibers and the pyramidal cells, for example), LTP is not NMDA-receptor dependent. Both NMDA-dependent LTP and NMDA-independent LTP have been established in pigeon hippocampal slices. There is evidence that in mammals hippocampal NMDA receptors may be involved in spatial learning (Morris et al., 1986), and hippocampal LTP in homing breeds of pigeon is mediated by NMDA receptors, whereas LTP established in nonhoming pigeons is not (Shapiro and Wieraszko, 1996). Oddly, however, intraperitoneal injections of the NMDA receptor blocker MK-801 disrupt radial maze performance in nonhoming but not in homing pigeons (Meehan, 1996).

These disparate sources of evidence do, then, converge on the conclusion that the avian hippocampus, like the mammalian hippocampus, is involved in processing of spatial information. As I noted above, however, there are tasks with no obvious spatial component that are, nevertheless, disrupted in mammals by hippocampal damage. Support for the parallel between avian and mammalian hippocampal function is considerably strengthened by work that has shown that some of those nonspatial disruptions are seen in birds too; I shall cite two examples here. The first concerns the effects of rewarded preexposure: When intact pigeons are rewarded for pecking two stimuli that are subsequently to be discriminated, discrimination is retarded compared with that seen in pigeons not having preexposure; hippocampal damage attenuated the disruptive effects of rewarded preexposure (Good and Macphail, 1994). The effects of rewarded preexposure parallel those seen in latent inhibition procedures (in which subsequent learning is retarded by nonrewarded preexposures); and latent inhibition is attenuated in mammals by hippocampal damage. The second example concerns the phenomenon of autoshaping—the classical conditioning procedure that was, it will be recalled, potentiated by paleostriatal damage. Reilly and Good (1989) found that autoshaping was significantly retarded in pigeons with hippocampal damage, and subsequent work (Good and Honey, 1991) has established that autoshaping in rats may, similarly, be disrupted by hippocampal damage. The Good and Macphail (1994) report provided further evidence of parallel function in nonspatial tasks: Neither overshadowing nor blocking was disrupted in hippocampus-lesioned pigeons, and these tasks are also immune in mammals to hippocampal damage.

Before leaving this discussion of avian hippocampal function, I shall make one further point with a view to encouraging behavioral neuroscience using birds: The avian work has led to novel hypotheses and findings in mammalian work. The discovery that hippocampal size varied with ecological demands on spatial memory has led to investigations of hippocampal size in mammals, and these investigations have revealed that in mammals also, hippocampal size varies with ecological niche (Sherry et al., 1992). Furthermore, the discovery that hippocampal damage disrupted autoshaping in pigeons led directly to the question whether a similar effect would be seen in rats. This initially seemed unlikely because, in general, hippocampal damage does not disrupt classical conditioning in mammals: but, as we have seen, the unexpected outcome was that, indeed, autoshaping in rats *was* disrupted by hippocampal damage (Good and Honey, 1991).

Isocortical Analogues/Homologues

Given that we now know that the avian neostriatum is *not* homologous to any part of the mammalian basal ganglia, we may now ask whether the neostriatum, along with the anterior archistriatum and the hyperstriatal complex, should not in fact properly be compared with the mammalian isocortex. Mammalian isocortical regions may be divided into three main categories: areas that are primarily devoted to analysis of sensory input and are predominantly unimodal; motor areas; and areas that receive highly processed input from all the senses, of which the most prominent is frontal cortex. We shall see that although there are no six-layered cortical regions in birds there are, nevertheless, neostriatal, archistriatal, and hyperstriatal regions that show general functional comparability to all three categories of mammalian isocortex.

Sensory areas We can achieve some idea of the revolution in thinking about nonmammalian vertebrate brains by considering the conclusions of two papers, both published in 1961, that were primarily interested in thalamic projections to the pigeon telencephalon. The first of these (Powell and Cowan, 1961) described the pattern of retrograde degeneration seen in the thalamus after destruction of the hemisphere: Three thalamic nuclei showed massive degeneration—the nucleus ovoidalis, the nucleus rotundus, and the nucleus dorsolateralis anterior. Subtotal hemispheric lesions pointed to the conclusion that the former two nuclei projected on the paleostriatum augmentatum and the latter (via the septomesencephalic tract) on the hyperstriatum accessorium. The second paper (Cowan et al., 1961) again used degenerative staining techniques, in this case to investigate the projection pattern of the pigeon retina on the thalamus. This report concluded that none of the thalamic regions that projected directly on the telencephalon received direct retinal projections. The authors concluded that "it appears that there is no direct relay of visual impulses from the thalamus to the telencephalon" (Cowan et al., 1961 , p. 557) and that the organization of the visual system in birds "is therefore completely different from that found in the higher mammals." Given that Erulkar (1955), using electrophysiological techniques, had concluded, similarly, that there were no thalamic relays for touch or hearing, the idea that there was a radical difference between the avian and the mammalian telencephalon received powerful support.

Advances in neuroanatomical techniques, however, rapidly overthrew the traditional picture in the late 1960s and during the 1970s. Research published then showed that in fact both the nucleus rotundus and the nucleus dorsolateralis anterior project visual information and that the nucleus ovoidalis projects auditory information; furthermore, all three nuclei project not to the paleostriatum but to regions within the neostriatal and hyperstriatal complexes. Because there is also now good evidence that somatosensory information is projected to neostriatal and hyperstriatal regions, it is evident that those regions, clearly not homologous with mammalian striatum, do, like mammalian isocortex, receive substantial sensory input from the thalamus.

The nucleus dorsolateralis anterior is one of a number of nuclei in the dorsal thalamus that receive direct retinal projections and that are now known collectively as the *principal optic nucleus* (OPT) of the thalamus. The OPT in turn projects to sites in the hyperstriatum accessorium and the hyperstriatum dorsale: These latter structures form the so-called Wulst, and those regions within the posterior Wulst that receive visual thalamic projections are the visual Wulst. The projection from the OPT to the visual Wulst clearly resembles the projection from the lateral geniculate nucleus to the striate cortex, and this system is known, in both birds and mammals, as the thalamofugal visual system. The visual input to the nucleus rotundus arises from the optic tectum/superior colliculus, and the projection from the nucleus rotundus to the ectostriatum resembles the projection from the lateral posterior nucleus (pulvinar, in primates) to extrastriate cortex (as the pulvinar also receives projections from the optic tectum/superior colliculus); this projection system is known as the *tectofugal visual system*. Figure 13.6 shows the organization of the thalamofugal and tectofugal visual systems in birds.

The projection from the nucleus ovoidalis (which receives projections from the nucleus mesencephalicus pars dorsalis, the avian homologue of the inferior colliculus) to a region (Field L) of the caudal neostriatum resembles the projection from the medial geniculate nucleus to auditory cortex; Figure 13.7 summarizes the organization of the avian auditory projection system. Similarly, somatosensory information in birds is carried by the dorsal column–medial lemniscal system to the dorsal thalamus, where two somatosensory regions have been identified, one, the caudal part of the nucleus dorsolateralis posterior (cDLP), the other, the nucleus dorsalis intermedius ventralis anterior (DIVA). Each of these regions projects to telencephalic areas that appear comparable to isocortex: DIVA projects to the anterior Wulst, and cDLP, to a medial region of neostriatum, including parts of both caudal and intermediate neostriatum (Delius and Bennetto, 1972; Wild, 1987). Figure 13.8 summarizes the somatosensory system in birds. The representation of somatosensory information in two separate telencephalic locations is reminiscent of the existence in mammals of two somatosensory isocortical areas, the primary area (S1) and the secondary area (S2); Wild (1987) provides a good discussion of the similarities and differences between avian and mammalian telencephalic organization of somatosensory input.

The functional parallels suggested by the similarities in anatomical thalamotelencephalic sensory projections have been supported by work using electrophysiological techniques: this is well illustrated by work on vision. Cells in the visual Wulst have a number of properties in common with cells in striate cortex: they show, for example,

418   13 Conservation in the Neurology and Psychology of Cognition in Vertebrates

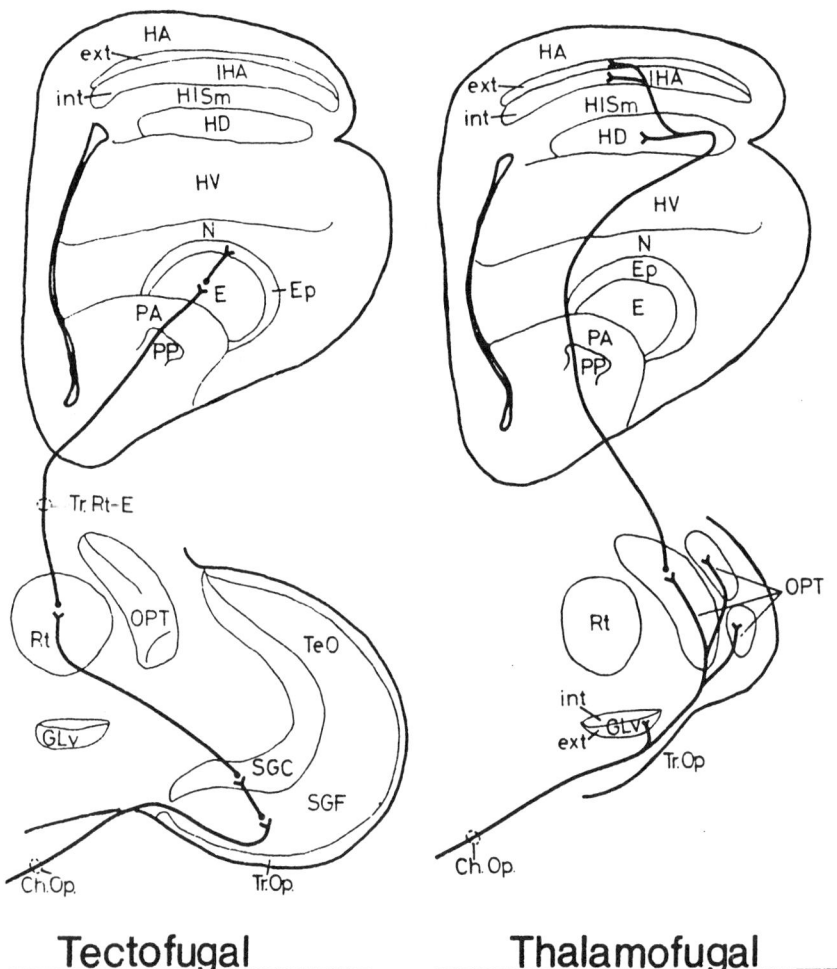

Figure 13.6. Schematic summary of the ascending tectofugal and thalamofugal visual pathways to the telencephalon. Ch.Op., chiasma opticum; E, ectostriatum (core region); Ep, zona periectostriatalis; GLv, nucleus lateralis geniculatus lateralis, pars ventralis: int, lamina internus; ext, lamina externus; HA, hyperstriatum accessorium; HD, hyperstriatum dorsale; HISm, hyperstriatum intercalatus suprema; HV, hyperstriatum ventrale; IHA, Nucleus intercalatus hyperstriatum accessorium, int, lamina internus; ext, lamina externus; N, neostriatum; OPT, nuclei optici principalis thalami dorsalis; PA, paleostriatum augmentatum; PP, paleostriatum primitivum; Rt, nucleus rotundus; TeO, tectum opticum; Tr.Op, Tractus opticus; Tr.Rt-E, tractus rotundo ectostriatalis; SGC, stratum griseum centrale; SGF, stratum griseum et fibrosum superficiale. (From Karten et al., 1973.)

columnar organization, have relatively small receptive fields, and are responsive to such features as narrow bars having a specific orientation and (in some species) binocular disparity. Cells in the ectostriatum, like cells in mammalian extrastriate visual cortex, have much larger receptive fields and are (like some extrastriate cells) peculiarly sensitive to movement.

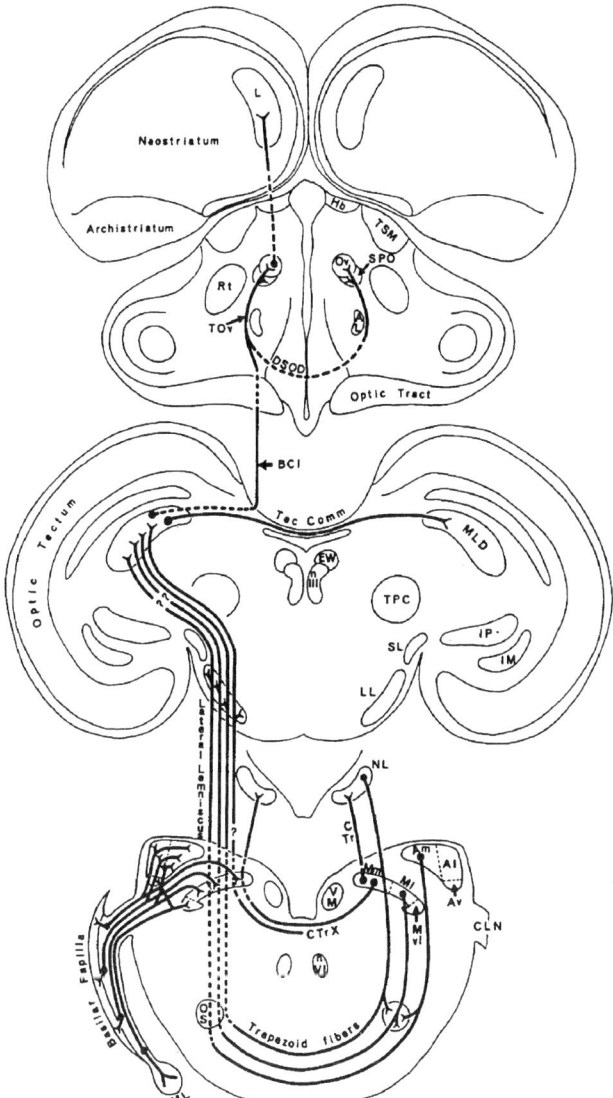

Figure 13.7. Diagram of the ascending auditory pathway from the peripheral receptor to the neostriatum of the pigeon. Al, Am, Av, nucleus angularis (lateral, medial, and ventral parts); BCI, brachium of inferior colliculus; CLN, cochlear and lagenar nerves; C Tr, uncrossed cochlear tract; CTrX, crossed cochlear tract; DSOD, dorsal supraoptic decussation; EW, Edinger-Westphal nucleus; Hb, habenula; IM, nucleus isthmi pars magnocellularis; IP, nucleus isthmi pars parvocellularis; L, Field L; LL, nucleus of lateral lemniscus; Mm, Ml, Mvl, nucleus magnocellularis (medial, lateral, and ventrolateral parts); ML, macula lagenae; MLD, nucleus mesencephali lateralis dorsalis; NL, nucleus laminaris; Ov, nucleus ovoidalis; OS, superior olive; Rt, nucleus rotundus; SL, nucleus semilunaris; SPO, nucleus semilunaris parovoidalis; Tec Comm, tectal commissure; TOv, tractus ovoidalis; TPC, nucleus tegmenti pedunculo-pontinus pars compacta; TSM, tractus septomesencephalicus; nIII, oculomotor nucleus; nVI, abducens nucleus; VM, medial vestibular nucleus. (From Campbell and Boord, 1974, by permission of Springer, Berlin.)

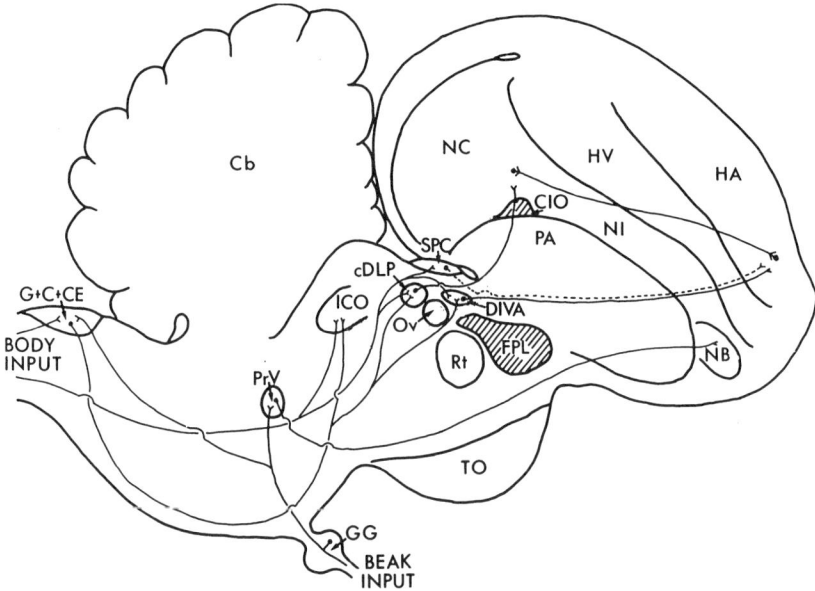

Figure 13.8. Connections of the somatosensory system of the pigeon. (The dashed line shows an additional potential somatosensory pathway to the hyperstriatum accessorium from the nucleus superficialis parvocellularis, which may receive somatosensory information). C, nucleus cuneatus; Cb, cerebellum; cDLP, nucleus dorsolateralis posterior, pars caudalis; CE, nucleus cuneatus externus; CIO, capsula internus occipitalis; DIVA nucleus dorsalis intermedius ventralis anterior; FPL, fasciculus prosencephali lateralis; G, nucleus gracilis; GG, gasserian ganglion; HA, hyperstriatum accessorium; HV, hyperstriatum ventrale; ICO, nucleus intercollicularis; NB, nucleus basalis; NC, neostriatum caudale; NI, neostriatum intermedium; Ov, nucleus ovoidalis; PA, paleostriatum augmentatum; PrV, nucleus sensorius pars principalis nervi trigemini; Rt, nucleus rotundus; SPC, nucleus superficialis parvocellularis; TO, tractus opticus. (Wild, 1987, by permission of Elsevier, Amsterdam.)

Damage to telencephalic visual areas does, as would be expected, lead, as in mammals, to impairments in visual discrimination. One notable contrast from the mammalian pattern is, however, that damage to the visual Wulst (comparable to striate cortex) has surprisingly little effect on performance: Riley et al., (1988), for example, reported little or no effect of visual Wulst lesions on retention of simultaneous discriminations based on color, brightness, or pattern; and psychophysical tests have found mild, transient elevations in intensity difference thresholds, and very little change in visual acuity (Hodos et al., 1984; Pasternak and Hodos, 1977). Damage to telencephalic targets of the tectofugal system generally produces more marked visual deficits than those seen after damage to thalamofugal system. Moderate ectostriatal damage disrupts retention of simultaneous discriminations based on color, brightness differences, or pattern (Hodos and Karten, 1970; Bessette and Hodos, 1989; Riley et al., 1988) and obtains elevations in psychophysical thresholds for brightness differences, acuity, and size (Hodos et al., 1984, 1986, 1988). There are, moreover, reports that suggest that certain types of concept formation may be disrupted by ectostriatal, but not by Wulst, damage (Watanabe, 1996, 1997). Ectostriatal lesions nevertheless appear to cause only a moderate disruption of visual processing: Preoperative levels of performance in simultaneous discriminations are usually reattained by ectostriatal birds after extensive retraining (e.g., Hodos and Karten, 1970), and smaller lesions confined to either the core or the belt region of the ectostriatum (see Fig. 13.6 for locations of these regions) do not disrupt visual discrimination performance (Bessette and Hodos, 1989).

There are, then, regions within the neostriatal and hyperstriatal complexes of the avian telencephalon that show detailed functional similarities to regions of sensory isocortex in mammals.

Motor areas. The mammalian isocortex contributes to movement via two major systems, known in primates as the *pyramidal* and the *extrapyramidal* systems.

Pyramidal system. Mammalian motor cortex projects via the pyramidal system extensively to brain stem motor regions, and, via the corticospinal tract, to the spinal cord: In some mammalian species, the corticospinal projections terminate on spinal motoneurons. There have been reports of long descending fibers (forming part of the septomesencephalic tract) from the anterior Wulst to the red nucleus and the reticular formation of the hindbrain and it has been suggested (Karten et al., 1973) that this projection is comparable with a component of the mammalian pyramidal tract. Whether there are in birds fibers from the anterior Wulst that progress as far as the spinal cord remains uncertain (Karten et al., 1973; Webster and Steeves, 1988; Webster, et al., 1990), and little is known of the nature of the involvement of the anterior Wulst in motor control.

There is, however, solid evidence for the involvement in motor activity of another telencephalic area, the archistriatum (excluding the posteromedial "limbic" archistriatum), which also has claims to be functionally analogous to mammalian motor cortex. The anterior and intermediate archistriatum is involved in at least three specific motor activities—bird song, feeding, and eye movements.

Neural control of bird song. Lesion studies in songbirds have established a system of telencephalic regions that play important roles in song. The two major efferent regions of this system are the nucleus robustus of the archistriatum, and the high vocal center (HVC). It was originally believed that the HVC was in a caudal part of the hyperstriatum ventrale (and it was labeled HVc as a result), but it seems that HVC should properly be regarded as part of the caudal neostriatum (Paton et al.,1981). The HVC receives input from Field L of the neostriatum, which, as we have seen, receives thalamic auditory projections. The HVC projects to the nucleus robustus, which in turn projects, via the occipitomesencephalic tract, directly onto motoneurons (in the hypoglossus nucleus) that innervate both the trachea and the syrinx (the avian vocal organ) (Fig. 13.9). There is an additional circuit, known as the *recursive loop*, that, although not necessary for the production of song, is necessary for song learning (Scharff and Nottebohm, 1991). That circuit also terminates in the robust nucleus of the archistriatum; it begins, however, with a projection from the HVC to a region (area X) of the parolfactory lobe, which in turn projects to the medial nucleus of the dorsolateral thalamus; this nucleus projects to the lateral magnocellular nucleus of the anterior neostriatum, from which the projection to the robust nucleus is derived.

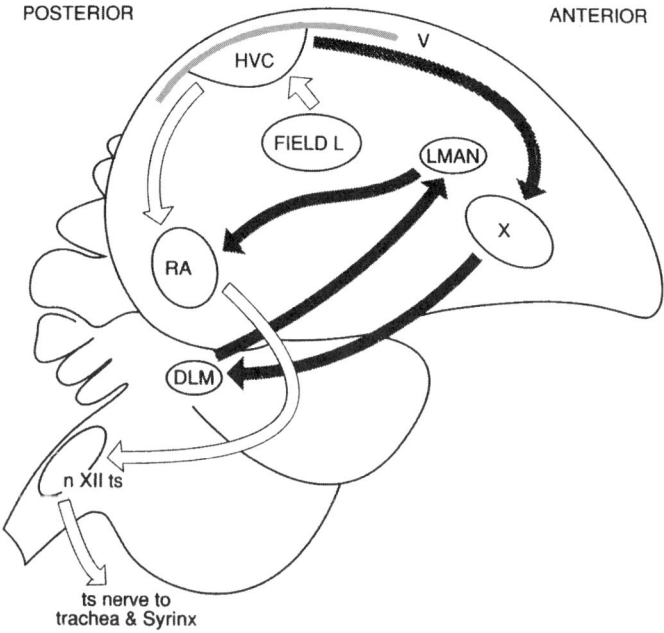

Figure 13.9. Schematic sketch of sagittal section through adult songbird brain showing the major pathways involved in the production and acquisition of learned song. Nuclei of the descending efferent pathway are connected with white arrows and those of the recursive loop, with gray arrows. DLM, medial nucleus of the dorsolateral thalamus; HVC, high vocal center; LMAN, lateral magnocellular nucleus of the anterior neostriatum; n XII ts, nucleus of the tracheosyringeal branch of cranial nerve XII ; RA, robust nucleus of the archistriatum; V, lateral ventricle; x, area X. (From Scharff and Nottebohm, 1991, by permission of Society for Neuroscience, Washington..)

There are data that suggest that there may be, in at least some nonsongbird species, pathways involving motor projections from the archistriatum that may be in some measure comparable with those seen in songbirds. In budgerigars, for example, there is an archistriatal nucleus, the central nucleus of the anterior archistriatum, that projects directly onto motoneurons in the hypoglossus nucleus concerned with vocalization and thus may be homologous with the nucleus robustus of songbirds; but in budgerigars this archistriatal nucleus receives auditory input not from HVC but from another telencephalic region, the nucleus basalis, that receives an auditory input which bypasses both the mesencephalon and the diencephalon (Striedter, 1994).

A feeding circuit. The archistriatum has also been found to form part of a "circuit" involved in the beak movements of feeding in pigeons (Wild et al., 1985); (Fig. 13.10). Sensory afferents from the oral region project to the main sensory trigeminal nucleus, which in turn projects to the nucleus basalis of the telencephalon. Efferents from the nucleus basalis run to the intermediate archistriatum, both directly and through a relay in the caudal neostriatum; this region of the archistriatum in turn projects to a region of the lateral reticular formation that contains premotor neurons that project directly upon beak muscle motoneurons in the trigeminal and facial cranial motor nerves.

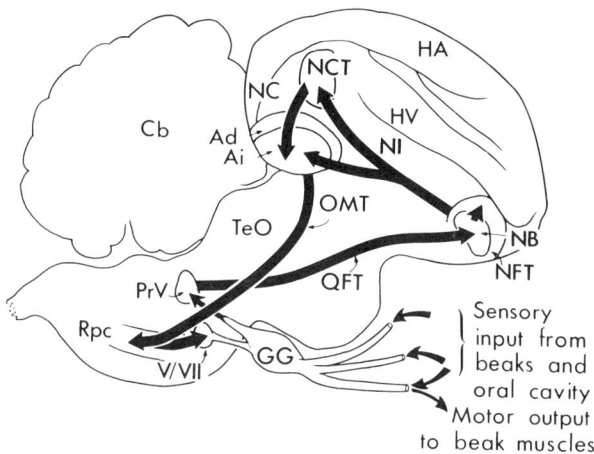

Figure 13.10. Afferent, efferent, and intratelencephalic connections of the trigeminal sensorimotor circuit in the pigeon. Ad, archistriatum, pars dorsalis; Ai, archistriatum intermedium; Cb, cerebellum; GG, gasserian ganglion; HA, hyperstriatum accessorium; HV, hyperstriatum ventrale; NB, nucleus basalis; NC, neostriatum caudale; NCT, neostriatum, pars caudalis (trigeminalis); NFT, neostriatum, pars rostralis (trigeminalis); NI, neostriatum intermedium; OMT, tractus occipitomesencephalicus; PrV, nucleus sensorius pars principalis nervi trigemini; QFT, tractus quintofrontalis; Rpc, nucleus reticularis parvocellularis; TeO, tectum opticum; V/VII, nucleus motorius nervi trigemini/nucleus nervi facialis. (From Wild et al., 1985.)

Gaze control. There is in the mammalian frontal cortex a region, separated from the motor cortex by premotor cortex, known as the *frontal eye field*. Stimulation of this region, as has been known since the last century, leads to conjugated saccadic eye movements toward the contralateral side. These movements are mediated by efferents from the frontal eye fields and carried in the pyramidal tract to interneurons in the pontine reticular formation that project directly onto motoneurons that control eye movements. A similar region has been discovered in the anterior archistriatum of the barn owl: stimulation of this region elicits eye (and head) saccades toward the side contralateral to the stimulation and efferents from this region run directly to brain stem regions concerned with the initiation of changes in direction of gaze. Moreover, this archistriatal region, like the mammalian frontal eye field, also projects to the optic tectum/superior colliculus (Knudsen et al., 1995).

Two candidates for avian "motor cortex". The parallels seen here between archistriatal efferents to motor centers have naturally encouraged the idea that they are comparable with components of the mammalian pyramidal tract. There are, then, in birds fibers arising from two regions, the anterior Wulst and the anterior and intermediate archistriatum, that show strong parallels in connectivity with components of the mammalian pyramidal motor system: In birds as in mammals, there is good evidence for a role in motor control of structures now widely regarded as analogous to cortex.

Extrapyramidal system. The extrapyramidal motor system of mammals centers on the basal ganglia, and all major regions of the isocortex project directly to the basal ganglia. We have seen that there is a strong correspondence between the avian and mammalian basal ganglia and that in birds, too, telencephalic regions that appear to correspond to sensory isocortex also project to the basal ganglia. And in birds as in mammals, there are also projections to the basal ganglia from telencephalic regions (the anterior Wulst and the somatomotor archistriatum) that send projections to motor regions within the brain stem and spinal cord. Since, as we have seen, paleostriatal damage in birds causes disturbances of motor control, there are good grounds for concluding that an extrapyramidal system including extensive cortical input, exists in birds as in mammals.

'Frontal' areas. A final, and perhaps the most startling, parallel between avian telencephalic structures and mammalian isocortex is to be found when we consider a possible avian analogue of the mammalian prefrontal association cortex. In 1982, Mogensen and Divac reported that an area in the posterodorsolateral neostriatum (PDLNS) of the pigeon was, like mammalian prefrontal cortex, richly innervated by dopaminergic fibers. Subsequent work, using increasingly refined techniques for demonstration of the presence of dopamine, has confirmed their claim and has shown also that the source of these fibers is to be found in cell groups in the midbrain that are clearly comparable with the cell groups (A9 and A10) of the mammalian nigral complex that give rise to the dopaminergic innervation of the frontal cortex.

Further support for the proposed analogy has been provided by evidence that the PDLNS plays a functional role similar to that of frontal cortex. The classical deficit following frontal damage in mammals is disruption of spatial tasks that involve a delay: In three separate reports, Divac and his colleagues have shown that lesions of PDLNS disrupt delayed spatial alternation in pigeons while having no effect on visual discriminations based on color, brightness, or pattern (Gagliardo et al., 1996; Mogensen and Divac, 1982, 1993).

Work on the primate frontal cortex suggests that it may contain several short-term memory stores for a variety of different types of information (Goldman-Rakic, 1987) and that the site for retention of spatial information is in fact restricted to a small part around the sulcus principalis (Butters and Pandya, 1969). One interesting finding has been that memory for the location of a light source to which a subsequent gaze is to be directed is disrupted by (unilateral) sulcus principalis lesions, lesions that do not affect the animal's ability to shift its gaze appropriately to a currently visible light (Funahashi et al., 1993); a similar outcome is obtained following unilateral frontal eye field lesions (Deng et al., 1986). This latter finding is relevant to avian brain function, because it is also the case that unilateral lesions of the archistriatal gaze field disrupt the ability of an owl to shift its gaze to a remembered sound source while not disrupting its ability to shift gaze toward a present sound (Knudsen and Knudsen, 1996). It seems, then, that birds, like mammals, have discrete brain regions concerned with the short-term storage of different types of information.

Homologues or analogues? The last three decades have seen a remarkable change in our understanding of the avian telencephalon, as a result of a series of demonstrations of anatomical and functional parallels between avian and mammalian telencephalic structures. These parallels have naturally led to speculation about possible homologies between avian and mammalian brain structures and about avian homologues for mammalian isocortex in particular. My object here has been to focus on functional parallels between avian and mammalian neurology, because it is comparability in function that is relevant to comparability in intelligence. This is not, therefore, the place for detailed discussion of proposed homologies (for specific proposals and critiques of alternative proposals see Butler, 1994; Karten, 1991), but there is one feature of some of the proposals that does have functional implications and should be introduced.

The parallels reviewed in this section are impressive but should not obscure the fact that all mammals possess a six-layered isocortex and that no similar layering is to be seen in any of the avian structures—archistriatal, neostriatal or hyperstriatal—that are so clearly comparable in other respects with mammalian isocortical regions (Reiner, 1986). Does this clear difference in anatomical organization not inevitably point to an important functional difference? Karten and Shimizu (1989) have suggested that this issue may be resolved if we regard avian "cortical" regions as comparable not to a isocortical region but to a specific layer of cells within an isocortical region: If we find different regions within the avian telencephalon that correspond to different layers of a given isocortical region, then we might well conclude that the functional equivalent of layered isocortex is indeed to be found in avian telencephalon.

Karten and Shimizu's suggestion (1989) is best made clear by considering vision. We may start by recognizing that, although birds do not have six-layered striate and extrastriate cortex, they do show extremely efficient vision—whether measured by psychophysics or by their capacities for learning about complex visual scenes; there is, in other words, no obvious functional deficit (or even difference) in avian as opposed to mammalian visual processing, which gives grounds for expecting parallels in neuronal organization. Karten and Shimizu (1989) (Fig. 13.11) find parallels of interest in the organization of the tectofugal visual system, which projects from the optic tectum/superior colliculus to the thalamus and from the thalamus to the telencephalon. The thalamic relay in birds is the nucleus rotundus and in mammals, the lateral posterior (pulvinar) nucleus; the telencephalic destination is, in birds, the ectostriatum and, in mammals, extrastriate cortex; more specifically, the telencephalic targets are the core of the ectostriatum (Ec) and layer 4 of the extrastriate cortex.

Cells in layer 4 of extrastriate cortex project in mammals to cells in layers 2 and 3 (within the extrastriate cortex); cells in Ec project to cells in the adjoining ectostriatal belt (Ep) and from there to adjoining neostriatum intermedium laterale (NIL). Cells in extrastriate layers 2 and 3 project to cells in layers 5 and 6, which in turn project, out of the extrastriate cortex, to the optic tectum/superior colliculus. Cells in NIL project to the intermediate archistriatum (Ai), which in turn projects to the optic tectum/superior colliculus. In both birds and mammals there is, then, a circuit that begins and ends in the optic tectum/superior colliculus: In terms of the role they play in this circuit, Ec cells correspond to cells in layer 4 of extrastriate cortex, Ep and NIL cells to cells in layers 2 and 3, and Ai cells to cells in layers 5 and 6.

It is possible, then, that the functional organization of mammalian isocortex, achieved by interconnections between the various layers of cortex, is achieved also in birds, but in the avian case, by connections between nuclear groups rather than between superimposed layers. The clear differences in neuroanatomy do not require us to suppose that there are significant differences in function.

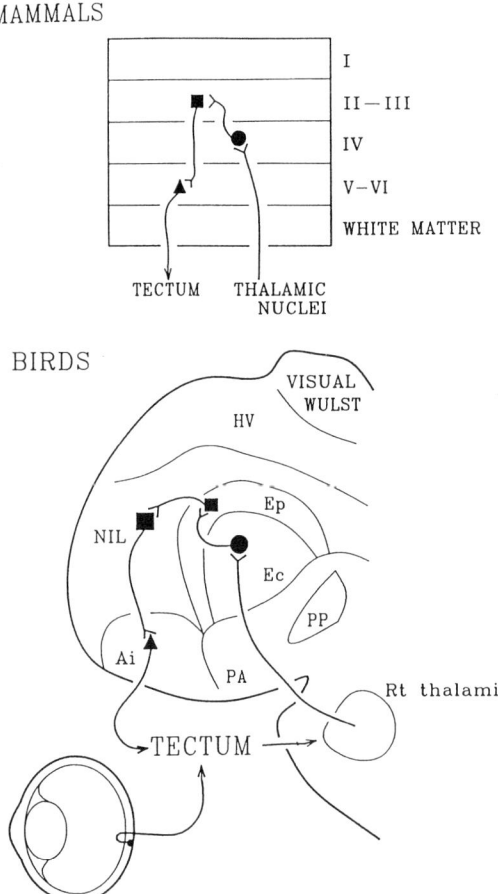

Figure 13.11. A comparison of visual-information circuits between the mammalian and avian brains. Circles indicate thalamic recipient neurons; squares indicate intrinsic neurons; triangles indicate neurons sending efferents to the optic tectum. Roman numerals indicate cortical layers. Ai, archistriatum intermedium; Ec, core region of ectostriatum; Ep, periectostriatal belt; HV, hyperstriatum ventrale; NIL, neostriatum intermedium laterale; PA, paleostriatum augmentatum; PP, paleostriatum primitivum; Rt thalami, nucleus rotundus thalami. (From Karten and Shimizu, 1989, by permission of MIT Press, Cambridge.)

CONCLUSIONS

The object of this chapter has been to challenge the assumption that cognitive complexity in vertebrates has evolved alongside neurological complexity. I have considered the case of birds, beginning with evidence that suggests that birds are not necessarily cognitively inferior to mammals (excluding humans). The evidence reviewed here shows that, contrary to the traditional view, the avian telencephalon shows extensive functional parallels to the mammalian telencephalon. To these parallels should be added one final fact, perhaps less well known than it should be: A bird's brain is, in general, roughly the same size as the brain of a mammal of the same body weight (Jerison, 1973). Birds have, then, brains that are the same size, and are organized in much the same way, as mammals. It may be that there are indeed significant differences (that remain to be demonstrated) between the avian and the mammalian intellect, but comparisons between their brains do not currently require us to suppose that there *must* be differences to be found. The widespread assumption that vertebrates have shown a progression in intellectual complexity that reaches its peak in mammals remains an assumption that awaits demonstrative proof.

REFERENCES

Amaral, D.G., J.L. Price, A. Pitkänen, and S.T. Carmichael (1992). Anatomical organization of the primate amygdaloid complex. In J.P. Aggleton (ed.): *The Amygdala: Neurobiological Aspects of Emotion, Memory, and Mental Dysfunction.* Wiley-Liss New York, pp. 1–64.

Ariëns-Kappers, C.U., G.C. Huber, and E.C. Crosby (1936) *The Comparative Anatomy of the Nervous System of Vertebrates, Including Man.* Hafner, New York.

Bessette, B.B., and W. Hodos (1989) Intensity, color, and pattern discrimination deficits after lesions of the core and belt regions of the ectostriatum. *Vis. Neurosci.* 2:27–34.

Bingman, V.P., G. Casini, C. Nocjar, and T.J. Jones (1994) Connections of the piriform cortex in homing pigeons (*Columba livia*) studied with fast blue and WGA-HRP. *Brain Behav. Evolu.* 43:206–218.

Butler, A.B. (1994) The evolution of the dorsal pallium in the telencephalon of amniotes—cladistic-analysis and a new hypothesis. *Brain Res. Rev.* 19:66–101.

Butters, N., and D. Pandya (1969) Retention of delayed-alternation: effect of selective lesions of sulcus principalis. *Science* 165:1271–1273.

Campbell, C.B.G., and R.L. Boord (1974) Central auditory pathways of non-mammalian vertebrates. In W.D. Keidel and W.D. Neff (eds.): *Handbook of Sensory Physiology, vol. 5, part 1: Auditory System.* Springer, Berlin, pp. 337–362.

Cowan, W.M., L. Adamson, and T.P.S. Powell (1961) An experimental study of the avian visual system. *J. Anat.* 945:545–563.

Dafters, R. (1975) Active avoidance behavior following archistriatal lesions in pigeons. *J. Comp. Physiol. Psychol.* 89:1169–1179.

Dafters, R. (1976) Effect of medial archistriatal lesions on the conditioned emotional response and on auditory discrimination performance of the pigeon. *Physiol and Behav.* 17:659–665.

Delius, J.D., and K. Bennetto (1972) Cutaneous sensory projections to the avian forebrain. *Brain Res.* 37: 205–221.

Deng, S.Y., M.E. Goldberg, M.A. Segraves, L.G. Ungerleider, and M. Mishkin (1986) The effect of unilateral ablation of the frontal eye fields on saccadic performance in the monkey. In E.L. Keller and D. S. Zee (eds.): *Advances in the Biosciences, vol. 57: Adaptive Processes in Visual and Oculomotor Systems* Pergamon, Oxford, pp. 201–208.

Ebinger, P., G. Rehkämper, and H. Schroder (1992). Forebrain specialization and the olfactory system in anseriform birds—an architectonic and tracing study. *Cell Tissue Res.* 268:81–90.

Epstein, R., C.E. Kirschnit, R.P. Lanza, and L.C. Rubin (1984). "Insight" in a pigeon: antecedents and determinants of an intelligent performance. *Nature* 308:61–62.

Erichsen, J.T., V.P. Bingman, and J.R. Krebs (1991) The distribution of neuropeptides in the dorsomedial telencephalon of the pigeon (*Columba livia*)—a basis for regional subdivisions. *J. Comp. Neurol.* 314:478–492.

Erulkar, S.D. (1955) Tactile and auditory areas in the brain of the pigeon. *J. Comp. Neurol.* 103:421–457.

Funahashi, S., C.J. Bruce, and P. S. Goldman Rakic (1993) Dorsolateral prefrontal lesions and oculomotor delayed-response performance: evidence for mnemonic "scotomas." *J. Neurosci.* 13:1479–1497.

Gagliardo, A., F. Bonadonna, and I. Divac (1996) Behavioral effects of ablations of the presumed prefrontal cortex or the corticoid in pigeons. *Behav. Brain Res.* 78:155–162.

Gagliardo, A., M. Mazzotto, and V.P. Bingman (1997) Piriform cortex ablations block navigational map learning in homing pigeons. *Behav. Brain Res.* 86:143–148.

Goldman-Rakic, P.S. (1987) Circuitry of primate prefrontal cortex and regulation of behavior by representational memory. In F. Plum (ed.): *Handbook of Physiology, Section 1, vol. 5: Higher Functions of the Brain, Part 1.* American Physiological Society, Bethesda, MD, pp. 373–417.

Good, M., and R.C. Honey (1991) Conditioning and contextual retrieval in hippocampal rats. *Behav. Neurosci.* 105:499–509.

Good, M., and E.M. Macphail (1994) Hippocampal lesions in pigeons (*Columba livia*) disrupt reinforced pre-exposure but not overshadowing or blocking. *Q. J. Exp. Psychol.* 47B:263–291.

Hall, G. (1982) Effects of a brief stimulus accompanying reinforcement on instrumental responding in pigeons. *Learn. Motivat.* 13:26–43.

Heimer, L., R.D. Switzer, and G.W. Van Hoesen (1982) Ventral striatum and ventral pallidum: components of the motor system? *Trends Neurosci.* 5:83–87.

Hodos, W., and H.J. Karten (1970) Visual intensity and pattern discrimination deficits after lesions of ectostriatum in pigeons. *J. Comp. Neurol.* 140:53–68.

Hodos, W., K.A. Macko, and B.B. Bessette (1984) Near-field acuity changes after visual system lesions in pigeons. II. Telencephalon. *Behav. Brain Res.* 13:15–30.

Hodos, W., S.R. Weiss, and B.B. Bessette (1986) Size-threshold changes after lesions of the visual telencephalon in pigeons. *Behav. Brain Res.* 21:203–14.

Hodos, W., S.R. Weiss, and B.B. Bessette (1988) Intensity difference thresholds after lesions of ectostriatum in pigeons. *Behav. Brain Res.* 30:43–53.

Jerison, H.J. (1973) *Evolution of the Brain and Intelligence.* Academic Press, New York.

Kamil, A.C., and M.W. Hunter (1970) Performance on object-discrimination learning set by the greater hill myna *(Gracula religiosa). J. Comp. Physiol. Psychol.* 73:68–73.

Karten, H.J. (1991) Homology and evolutionary origins of the "neocortex". *Brain Behav. Evolu.* 38:264–272.

Karten, H.J., and W. Hodos (1967) *A Stereotaxic Atlas of the Brain of the Pigeon (Columba livia).* Johns Hopkins University Press, Baltimore, MD.

Karten, H.J., W. Hodos, W.J.H. Nauta, and A.M. Revzin (1973) Neural connections of the "visual Wulst" of the avian telencephalon. Experimental studies in the pigeon (*Columba livia*) and owl (*Speotyto cunicularia*). *J. Comp. Neurol.* 150:253–278.

Karten, H.J., and T. Shimizu (1989) The origins of neocortex: connections and lamination as distinct events in evolution. *J. Cogn. Neurosci.* 1:291–301.

Killcross, S., T.W. Robbins, and B.J. Everitt (1997) Different types of fear-conditioned behavior mediated by separate nuclei within amygdala. *Nature* 388:377–380.

Knudsen, E.I., Y.E. Cohen, and T. Masino (1995) Characterization of a forebrain gaze field in the archistriatum of the barn owl—microstimulation and anatomical connections. *J. Neurosci.* 15:5139–5151.

Knudsen, E.I., and P.F. Knudsen (1996) Disruption of auditory spatial working-memory by inactivation of the forebrain archistriatum in barn owls. *Nature* 383:428–431.

Krebs, J.R., J.T. Erichsen, and V.P. Bingman (1991) The distribution of neurotransmitters and neurotransmitter-related enzymes in the dorsomedial telencephalon of the pigeon (*Columba livia*). *J. Comp. Neurol.* 314:467–477.

Krebs, J.R., D.F. Sherry, S.D. Healy, V.H. Perry, and A.L. Vaccarino (1989) Hippocampal specialization of food-storing birds. *Proc. Natl. Sci. U.S.A.* 86:1388–1392.

Lowndes, M., and D.C. Davies (1994) The effects of archistriatal lesions on one-trial passive-avoidance learning in the chick. *Eur. J. Neurosci.* 6:525–530.

Macphail, E.M. (1982) *Brain and Intelligence in Vertebrates.* Clarendon Press, Oxford.

Macphail, E.M. (1987) The comparative psychology of intelligence. *Behav. Brain Sci.* 10:645–696.

Macphail, E.M. (1993) *The Neuroscience of Animal Intelligence: From the Seahare to the Seahorse.* Columbia University Press, New York.

Macphail, E.M. (1996) Cognitive function in mammals: the evolutionary perspective. *Cogn. Brain Res.* 3:279–290.

Medina, L., and A. Reiner (1995) Neurotransmitter organization and connectivity of the basal ganglia in vertebrates—implications for the evolution of basal ganglia. *Brain Behav. Evol.* 46:235–258.

Meehan, E.F. (1996) Effects of MK-801 on spatial memory in homing and nonhoming pigeon breeds. *Behav. Neurosci.* 110:1487–1491.

Mitchell, J.A. (1983a) Autoshaping and paleostriatal lesions in the pigeon. *Physiol. Behav.* 31:45–55.
Mitchell, J.A. (1983b) Paleostriatal lesions in the pigeon (*Columba livia*) potentiate classical conditioning—evidence from fixed-interval responding, free-operant go no-go discrimination, and alternation. *Behav. Neurosci.* 97:171–194.
Mitchell, J.A., S. Channell, and G. Hall (1985) Response reinforcer associations after caudate-putamen lesions in the rat—spatial discrimination and overshadowing potentiation effects in instrumental learning. *Behav. Neurosci.* 99:1074–1088.
Mitchell, J.A., and G. Hall (1984) Paleostriatal lesions and instrumental learning in the pigeon. *Q. J. Exp. Psychol.* B36:93–117.
Mogensen, J., and I. Divac (1982) The prefrontal "cortex" in the pigeon. Behavioral evidence. *Brain Behav. Evol.* 21:60–66.
Mogensen, J., and I. Divac (1993) Behavioral effects of ablation of the pigeon equivalent of the mammalian prefrontal cortex. *Behav. Brain Res.* 55:101–107.
Morris, R.G.M., E. Anderson, G.S. Lynch, and M. Baudry (1986) Selective impairment of learning and blockade of long-term potentiation by an *N*-methyl-*D*-aspartate receptor antagonist, AP5. *Nature* 319:774–776.
O'Keefe, J., and L. Nadel (1978) *The Hippocampus as a Cognitive Map*. Clarendon Press, Oxford.
Papi, F., and G. Casini (1990) Pigeons with ablated pyriform cortex home from familiar but not from unfamiliar sites. *Proc. Natl. Acad. Sci. U.S.A.* 87:3783–3787.
Pasternak, T., and W. Hodos (1977) Intensity difference thresholds after lesions of the visual Wulst in pigeons. *J. Comp. Physiol. Psychol.* 91:485–497.
Paton, J.A., K.R. Manogue, and F. Nottebohm (1981) Bilateral organization of the vocal control pathway in the budgerigar, *Melopsittacus undulatus*. *J. Neurosci.* 1:1279–1288.
Pepperberg, I.M. (1994) Vocal learning in gray parrots (*Psittacus erithacus*)—effects of social interaction, reference, and context. *Auk* 111:300–313.
Phillips, R.E. (1964) "Wildness" in the mallard duck: effect of brain lesions and stimulation on "escape behavior" and reproduction. *J. Comp. Neurol.* 122:139–155.
Powell, T.P.S., and W.M. Cowan (1961) The thalamic projection upon the telencephalon in the pigeon (*Columba livia*). *J. Anat.* 95:78–109.
Ramirez, J.M., and J.D. Delius (1979) Aggressive behavior of pigeons: suppression by archistriatal lesions. *Aggress. Behav.* 5:3–17.
Rehkämper, G., E. Haase, and H.D. Frahm (1988) Allometric comparison of brain weight and brain structure volumes in different breeds of the domestic pigeon, *Columba livia f.d.* (Fantails, Homing pigeons, Strassers). *Brain Behav. Evol.* 31:141–149.
Reilly, S., and M. Good (1989) Hippocampal lesions and associative learning in the pigeon. *Behav. Neurosci.* 103:731–742.
Reiner, A. (1986). Is prefrontal cortex found only in mammals? *Trends Neurosci.* 9:298–300.
Reiner, A., and H.J. Karten (1985) Comparison of olfactory bulb projections in pigeons and turtles. *Brain Behav. Evol.* 27:11–27.
Rieke, G.K. (1980) Kainic acid lesions of pigeon paleostriatum: a model for study of movement disorders. *Physiol Behav.* 24:683–687.
Rieke, G.K. (1981) Movement disorders and lesions of pigeon brain stem analogs of basal ganglia. *Physiol. Behav.* 24:379–384.
Riley, N.M., W. Hodos, and T. Pasternak (1988) Effects of serial lesions of telencephalic components of the visual system in pigeons. *Vis. Neurosci.* 1:387–394.
Roberts, W.A., and N. Van Veldhuizen (1985) Spatial memory in pigeons on the radial arm maze. *J. Exp. Psychol. Anim. Behav. Processes* 11:241–259.
Shapiro, E., and A. Wieraszko (1996) Comparative, in-vitro, studies of hippocampal tissue from homing and non-homing pigeon. *Brain Res.* 725:199–206.
Scharff, C., and F. Nottebohm (1991) A comparative study of the behavioral deficits following lesions of various parts of the zebra finch song system: implications for vocal learning. *J. Neurosci.* 11:2896–2913.
Sherry, D.F., M.R.L. Forbes, M. Khurgel, and G.O. Ivy (1993) Females have a larger hippocampus than males in the brood-parasitic brown-headed cowbird. *Proc. Natl. Acad. Sci. U.S.A.* 90:7839–7843.
Sherry, D.F., L.F. Jacobs, and S.J.C. Gaulin (1992) Spatial memory and adaptive specialization of the hippocampus. *Trends Neurosci.* 15:298–303.

Sherry, D.F., and A.L. Vaccarino (1989) Hippocampus and memory for food caches in black-capped chickadees. *Behav. Neurosci.* 103:308–313.

Sherry, D.F., A.L. Vaccarino, K. Buckenham, and R.S. Herz (1989) The hippocampal complex of food-storing birds. *Brain Behav. Evol.* 34:308–317.

Staubli, U., F. Schottler, and D. Nejat Bina (1987) Role of dorsomedial thalamic nucleus and piriform cortex in processing olfactory information. *Behav. Brain Res.* 25:117–129.

Striedter, G.F. (1994) The vocal control pathways in budgerigars differ from those in songbirds. *J. Comp. Neurol.* 343:35–56.

Von Fersen, L., C.D.L. Wynne, J.D. Delius, and J.E.R. Staddon (1991) Transitive inference in pigeons. *J. Exp. Psychol. Anim. Behav. Processes* 17:334–341.

Watanabe, S. (1996) Effects of ectostriatal lesions on discriminations of conspecific-species and familiar objects in pigeons. *Behav. Brain Res.* 81:183–188.

Watanabe, S. (1997) Visual discrimination of real objects and pictures in pigeons. *Ani. Learn. Behav.* 25:185–192.

Webster, D.M., and J.D. Steeves (1988) Origins of brainstem-spinal projections in the duck and goose. *J. Comp. Neurol.* 273:573–583.

Webster, D.M.S., L.J. Rogers, J.D. Pettigrew, and J. D. Steeves (1990) Origins of descending spinal pathways in prehensile birds—do parrots have a homolog to the corticospinal tract of mammals? *Brain Behav. Evolu.* 36:216–226.

Wieraszko, A., and G.F. Ball (1991) Long-term enhancement of synaptic responses in the songbird hippocampus. *Brain Res.* 538:102–106.

Wild, J.M. (1987). The avian somatosensory system: connections of regions of body representation in the forebrain of the pigeon. *Brain Res.* 412:205–223.

Wild, J.M., J.J.A. Arends, and H.P. Zeigler (1985). Telencephalic connections of the trigeminal system in the pigeon (*Columba livia*): a trigeminal sensorimotor circuit. *J. Comp. Neurol.* 234:441–464.

Zeier, H., and H.J. Karten (1971). The archistriatum of the pigeon: organization of afferent and efferent connections. *Brain Res.* 31:313–326.

Chapter 14

MULTIMODAL AREAS OF THE AVIAN FOREBRAIN—BLUEPRINTS FOR COGNITION?

Onur Güntürkün and Daniel Durstewitz, Biopsychologie, Fakultät für Psychologie, Ruhr-Universität Bochum

THE THEME

Is it possible to disentangle the neuronal circuits with which we are perceiving the world, with which we are thinking, with which you are reading these lines? And, if it were possible, would we discover the neural processes underlying these functions to be radically different from the mental mechanisms of other species? Or would we have to come to the conclusion that evolution crafted comparable biological solutions for similar cognitive demands? This chapter outlines some approaches to answer these questions.

Animals can be investigated on many different levels of organization, reaching from molecules to cognition. Neurobiologists today are able to describe an unprecedented amount of molecular events that interconnect intracellular processes from the synaptic input up to the finely tuned genetic response that alters the morphology and thus ultimately the function of single neurons. For example, they study how single membrane ion channels undergo structural changes resulting in altered electrophysiological behavior of the cell. Cognitive psychologists, on the other hand, study the mental mechanisms with which humans disambiguate sensory material, process information, create memory stores, and perform complex movement plans. Cognitive psychologists generally think of the human brain as a system of functional units, connected with each other in form of flow charts. Although psychologists are quite successful in describing the functional processes going on within such single units, they naturally fail when it comes to outlining the neuronal mechanisms that govern these functions. Molecular neurobiologists have the inverse problem. Despite great advantages in the last decade, the gap from single neurons studied by neurobiologists to the functional units characterized by cognitive psychologists still is too wide to be easily overcome.

A possible way to bridge this gap would be to concentrate on a single neural structure of a nonhuman species and to study the neural events leading to the emergence of a single cognitive operation on the cellular, neural network and behavioral level. This chapter describes experiments that were born out of this idea. The neural structure in focus is the prefrontal cortex (PFC) in humans, monkeys, and pigeons, and the relevant cognitive operation is working memory, a key function of the PFC.

WORKING MEMORY AND PREFRONTAL CORTEX

Working memory is the capability to store and to process for a short time information that is relevant to the behavioral goals of the organism. This information is usually forgotten after goal achievement. Looking into a telephone book and dialing a number involves working memory because the sequence of numbers is temporaly stored until the call is placed. If the telephone book is far away from the telephone, the number has to be rehearsed until it is dialed. Converging points of evidence from brain-damaged patients, animal experimentation, and neuroimaging studies show that the mammalian PFC is an essential structure for working memory.

Lesions of the PFC lead to incapabilities to maintain this short-term storehouse with devastating effects on everyday life. Most aspects of thinking need a temporal information buffer. If this buffer fails, behavior cannot be planned ahead. Shallice and Burgess (1991) constructed a list of everyday tasks for their prefrontal patients, like shopping for certain items and being at a certain place at a certain time. The patients had problems organizing these simple everyday demands; they entered shops without buying anything, forgot to ask for information they had to gather, did not show up at their rendezvous, and so forth.

Several laboratory tests are able to quantify these failures in ordinary life. A very telling one is the Tower of London, a game consisting of three vertical pegs and three colored disks of different sizes that have a central hole for the pegs (Shallice, 1982). At the beginning the three disks are positioned on one peg, the largest one at the bottom and the smallest at the top. The task is to pile up the three disks in the same order onto another peg. Only one disk can be moved per trial. The problem is that a larger disk cannot be placed on a smaller one. The task can be solved in seven moves if the subject makes use of the three pegs in the correct sequence. It is possible to plan the whole sequence of actions ahead and then move the disks, but this then involves a temporal information buffer in which the virtual moves made have to be stored. Prefrontal patients have lost this buffer to a good extent and fail remarkably in this simple task. They are at the same time generally not handicapped in cognitive operations that are not in need of working memory processes.

A comparable way to test working memory functions in monkeys is the delayed alternation task. Here, the monkey has to choose between two food wells that both are covered with identical lids. At the beginning of a session both wells are baited with a peanut, and the monkey is reinforced regardless of which well he decides to uncover. After removing a lid and eating the peanut a screen is lowered so that the animal can no longer look at the wells. After a delay time the screen is raised again, and the monkey is free to remove one of the lids, but now only the well not chosen before is baited. This schedule goes on for the whole session so that the animal always has to alternate between wells. Normal monkeys have no problem remembering the well avoided just before for long intervals. Monkeys with PFC lesions, however, perform nearly at chance level, even after short delays. If no delay is imposed, they act perfectly.

A further experiment that is reminiscent to the shopping study described above is the spatial search task in which monkeys are faced with 25 food wells, arranged in five rows of five. Each well is baited with a peanut and is covered by a small door that can be opened but that closes again therafter. The monkey has to collect the peanuts, a task that the animal likes. Removing a peanut from a well renders it empty, and therefore returns to this well make no sense. Prefrontal-damaged monkeys forget which well they had chosen before and make many errors in returning to empty locations (Passingham, 1985). It is important to note that errors in working memory are often accompanied by other "prefrontal symptoms," including perserverations (i.e., an incapability to suppress false responses) combined with reversal deficits, that is, an inflexibility to switch to another option when the option that was correct before turns out now to be incorrect.

One hallmark of the neuroanatomical definition of the mammalian PFC is the dense dopaminergic input into this area. Dopamine is a catecholaminergic neuromodulator that acts mainly via dopamine D1 receptors. The main neural targets of dopaminergic inputs seem to be excitatory pyramidal cells. The dopaminergic midbrain system of rats consists of only 45,000 cells, but a single one of these neurons makes up to 200,000 synapses on tens of thousands of cells in the cortex and the basal ganglia. If a single cell synapses on such a vast amount of diverse neurons, it is very unlikely that dopamine conveys specific sensory information. Rather, it probably changes working parameters of its efferent structures during those events that induce intense activities of dopaminergic neurons. Schultz and coworkers (1995) discovered that all kinds of cues and situations that are of potential biological significance and for which the animal has no ready-to-run program activate the dopaminergic system. If, for example, a light source consistently starts signaling the occurrence of food, dopaminergic cells that first were only activated by the sight of food start firing action potentials at the onset of the light signal and no longer care for the food stimulus itself. If, after a while, the animal has perfectly learned to associate this light signal with food occurrence, the dopaminergic neurons stop firing at all. Thus, they seem to be switched on during the learning process itself and are switched off after the memory trace has become established.

Besides, their role in the acquisition of learning tasks, dopaminergic neurons play a prime role in delay tasks. If, in the delayed alternation task described above, the animal has to memorize a certain well during a delay to obtain food after delay offset, the dopaminergic neurons fire at the onset of the delay, but not during the whole delay period. Remarkably, pyramidal cells within PFC seem to need this dopamine burst at delay onset to turn into working memory cells: They are now active during the whole delay period, probably keeping information relevant for the next response. Some of these cells continue to fire even if the delay is extended for as long as 60 seconds (Fuster, 1989). The learning-promoting effect and the ability to trigger high levels of activity during the delay period in cortical pyramidal cells is probably at the heart of the mechanism with which the dopaminergic system enables the animal to acquire and to perform working memory tasks. Consequently, lesions of the dopaminergic system cause dramatic deficits in delay tasks.

AVIAN BRAIN AND COGNITION

Birds show remarkable cognitive capacities, with some avian species being on par with nonhuman primates. Even the ordinary pigeon is capable of memorizing 725 different visual patterns, is able to learn concepts like "man-made," "different," or "cubistic style of painting" is able to symbolically communicate, to "lie," and to recognize transitive relations in a learned rank order of visual symbols (Güntürkün, 1996). Birds, of course, have working memory competence, and especially food-hoarding species seem to be real masters in that. But do birds have a PFC? Traditionally, nonmammalian vertebrates were not conceived at all to have an isocortex typical of mammals. Studies of the last three decades, however, make it likely that birds have very similar neural forebrain systems as mammals, although not arranged in six layers.

It seems as if the principle organization and connectivity of the forebrain emerged very early in vertebrate evolution but that this schema was molded into a six-layered arrangement in the branch leading to modern mammals. If this is true, we have a good chance to find an avian version of the PFC, although it might look very different. Following this line of reasoning, Divac and Mogensen (1985) looked for regions in the pigeon's forebrain that are especially densely innervated by axons containing tyrosine hydroxylase, an enzyme that catalyzes an early step in the transmitter synthesis of catecholaminergic neurons. Catecholaminergic cells use dopamine, noradrenaline, or adrenaline as a transmitter. Divac and Mogensen found, as expected, a dense meshwork of fibers in the basal ganglia, where the majority of dopaminergic axons project to. In addition, they observed a semilunar area in the caudalmost part of the forebrain, the neostriatum caudolaterale.

Indeed, with an antibody specifically directed against dopamine Waldmann and Güntürkün (1993) confirmed that axons with this transmitter densely innervate the neostriatum caudolaterate (Fig. 14.1). Some of these fibers form a very peculiar arrangement, namely, the "baskets". Baskets consist of dopaminergic fibers that coil repeatedly around single neuronal cell bodies and the initial dendrites so that somata are completely wrapped by dopaminergic axons. Functionally, baskets create a condition in which the postsynaptic neuron is under tight control of the dopaminergic system. Apart from baskets, a large number of dopaminergic fibers within the neostriatum caudolaterate were observed traversing the tissue with numerous small branches and boutons-en-passant, which probably contact dendrites. These en-passant fibers may have less dramatic effects on postsynaptic physiology than the baskets.

The dense dopaminergic innervation of the neostriatum caudolaterale suggests similarities to the mammalian PFC, although it is thus far only a single point of equivalence. More information is needed before conclusions on the nature of this forebrain

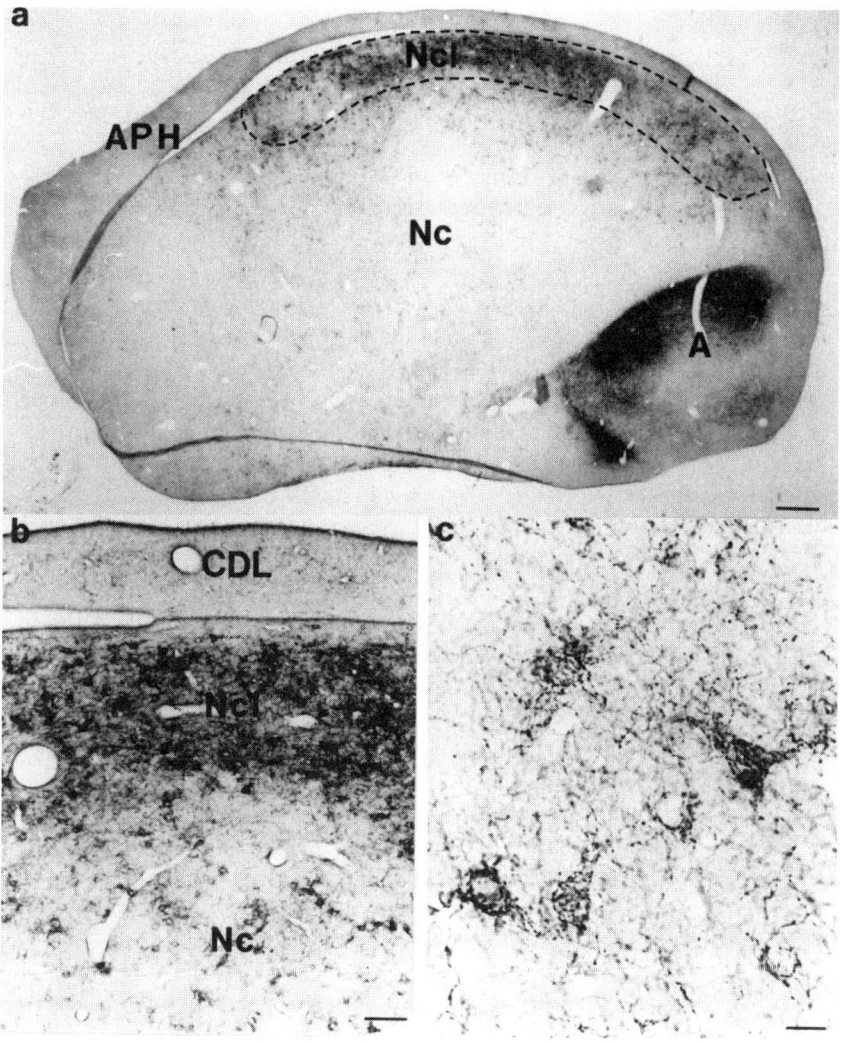

Figure 14.1. Photomicrographs of frontally oriented brain sections depicting the dopaminergic innervation of the pigeon caudal telencephalon. The other region with a large number of dopaminergic fibers is the lateroventrally situated archistriatum (A). Dorsal is upward and medial is to the left. (a) Section at level of the neostriatum caudolaterale (Ncl) with its dense dopaminergic fiber structure. Baskets are only visible as small dots. Bar = 500 μm (b) Magnification of a part of a Bar = 100 μm (c) Dopaminergic baskets at the border between Ncl and Nc Bar = 15 μm. APH, area parahippocampalis; CDL, area corticoidea dorsolateralis; Nc, neostriatum caudale. (From Waldmann and Güntürkün, 1993.)

region can be drawn. If the neostriatum caudolaterale is equivalent to the mammalian PFC, lesions of this area should cause deficits similar to those observed in prefrontal mammalian species, including humans. Meanwhile, numerous behavioral studies have indeed shown that lesions of the pigeon's neostriatum caudolaterale lead to deficits in delayed alternation, but left performance in various visual discrimination tasks intact (Mogensen and Divac, 1993; Güntürkün, 1997). Thus, such lesioned birds have severe difficulties with memorizing for a few seconds the side of the pecking key that they had just pecked, but are on par with control animals even in extremely demanding discriminations of visual objects. Additionally neostriatum caudolaterale–lesioned birds perseverate in go/no-go tasks (i. e., they cannot stop responding despite the fact that the no-go signal is shown (Güntürkün, 1997). These lesioned pigeons likewise have difficulties "unlearning"; thus, they easily learn that "A" is correct and "B" is incorrect, but face problems in reversal tasks, in which the previously learned values of A and B have to be inverted. These cognitive deficits are also typical of PFC-lesioned mammals.

In mammals, the PFC represents a multimodal sensorimotor interface because it receives afferents from the association cortices of all sensory modalities and projects to different premotor and motor areas. This anatomical arrangement probably enables the prefrontal cortex to play its prominent role in the selection and planning of actions on the basis of available sensory information and past experiences. If the pigeon's neostriatum caudolaterale indeed corresponds to the PFC, it should be characterized by afferents from all sensory association fields and project to motor areas of the birds telencephalon. Several investigators have meanwhile accumulated evidence to chart the blueprints of the input/output relations of the neostriatum caudolaterale, and the emerging picture is astoundingly similar to the mammalian pattern (Rehkämper and Zilles, 1991). According to these studies, visual thalamofugal, visual tectofugal, auditory, somatosensory, and trigeminal pathways are all organized according to the same pattern: The primary sensory telencephalic regions project to the respective secondary sensory association areas, which in turn project to the neostriatum caudolaterale. Thus, this structure is a multimodal area that represents the third step in each chain of sensory intratelencephalic projections. The efferents of the neostriatum caudolaterale can be followed to premotor and motor areas of the archistriatum and to the basal ganglia, and this is exactly the pattern observed in mammals.

One further important aspect of the definition of the mammalian PFC are its afferents from the mediodorsal nucleus of the thalamus. The mediodorsal nucleus is a polysensory structure with close anatomical and functional relationships to the PFC. This is demonstrated by behavioral studies showing deficits after mediodorsal nucleus lesions to be similar to those after ablations of the PFC (Fuster, 1989). These lesion studies are additionally supported by experiments demonstrating increased metabolic activity of neurons of the mediodorsal nucleus during delay tasks. In pigeons, the main thalamic afferent structure to the caudolateral neostriatum is the nucleus dorsolateralis posterior thalami (Waldmann and Güntürkün, 1993), a structure that integrates visual, auditory, and somatosensory information (Korzeniewska and Güntürkün, 1990). Although the multimodal character of the nucleus dorsolateralis posterior thalami is very promising for a potential equivalency to the mediodorsal nucleus, a detailed comparison of the connectivities of these two thalamic structures shows that they are very likely not homologous (Güntürkün, 1997). Is it conceivable, however, that the avian nucleus. dorsolateralis posterior thalami may be different from the mediodorsal nucleus due to its subcortical connectivities but nevertheless subserve similar functions? The answer seems to be partly "yes." Dorsolateralis posterior thalami lesions cause deficits in delayed alternation experiments, but have no effect on go/no-go performance (Güntürkün, 1997). Thus, at least for the working memory component of prefrontal functions, this thalamic nucleus with its projections to the neostriatum caudolaterale seems to subserve similar functions as the mammalian mediodorsal nucleus.

Summarizing these studies, we can conclude that mammals and birds have in common a very similar forebrain structure subserving the same kind of cognitive processes. These similarities are inspiring because they open the possibility that mammals and birds, while being separated from each other during evolution for more than 200 million years, not only share equivalent sensory and motor processing structures but also have remarkable similarities in at least one forebrain structure subserving cognitive integration.

DETAILS OF THE MACHINE

Until now we have followed a rather broad approach to the functional anatomy of the prefrontal cortex of mammals and birds. To really understand how function emerges from a cellular network, the neuronal circuitry has to be traced in much more detail. Cortical structures such as the PFC are made of repetitive cellular circuits, each of them crafted with the same basic design. Thus, a single circuit may be viewed as a simple uniform machinery, repeated over and over, like molecules in a crystal. Therefore, the starting point of any inquiry into neuronal function should be the single circuit. Millions of these circuits wired in parallel could generate modes of operation that are hard to follow by imagination. Therefore, computational neuroscientists simulate the activity of assemblies of neurons on computers. For these simulations to be biologically realistic, the virtual neurons and their connectivities should be implemented according to neuroanatomical and neurophysiological results. If this is done in an appropriate way, computer simulations can be a very powerful tool to understand how complex functions are generated by sets of cells. This is addressed in the upcoming parts of this chapter. First, the principal circuits of the neostriatum caudolaterale are characterized anatomically and compared with those in the mammalian PFC. Then, behavioral experiments are described that analyze the cognitive deficits after a short time blockade of some neurons within neostriatum caudolaterale. Finally, computer simulations of cellular interactions within this structure are discussed in order to understand the possible neuronal basis of working memory and the observed behavioral pertubations after pharmacological interventions.

A possible starting point for uncovering the principle circuits of the neostriatum caudolaterale are the baskets. As outlined before, they represent dopaminergic fibers that densely coil around single neuronal cell bodies so that the function of this cell is probably an important extent under the control of the dopaminergic system. If we could find out which cell type is located within baskets, an important insight into functional circuits of the neostriatum caudolaterale could be gained.

The D1 receptor is the prevailing dopamine receptor subtype in the mammalian cortex. Therefore, our first question was whether the avian dopaminergic baskets coil around cells that posses D1 receptors. Their activation through dopamine can alter for up to several seconds the working parameters of diverse ion channels, but is also able to trigger the activation of genetic responses of the neuron. Thus, activation of D1 receptors has profound effects on the short-term but partly also on the long-term functions of neurons. One well-characterized phosphoprotein specifically enriched in D1 receptor–positive neurons is DARPP-32 (*d*opamine- and cyclic *A*MP-*r*egulated *p*hospho*p*rotein). DARPP-32 acts as an intracellular third messenger after D1 receptor activation and anatomically shows virtually the same distribution as the D1 receptor.

Using an antibody against DARPP-32, we analyzed the distribution of this phosphoprotein and, thus, of D1 receptor–expressing neurons in the pigeon's forebrain. The neostriatum caudolaterale was not only rich in DARPP-32 labeled neurons, but many axonal baskets specifically coiled around them (Durstewitz et al., 1998). The caudal neostriatum and further associative structures displayed the largest percentage of DARPP-32–positive cells being targets of dopaminergic baskets, namely, 30%. Thus, the neostriatum caudolaterale is characterized by the presence of D1 receptor–possessing neurons, and about one third of them receive the basket-type dopaminergic input.

From a functional perspective it would be important to know whether the D1 cells within baskets are excitatory or inhibitory. The vast majority of inhibitory cells in the central nervous system utilize γ-aminobutyric acid (GABA) as a transmitter. To test the assumption that D1 cells in baskets are inhibitory, the possible colocalization of DARPP-32 and glutamate decarboxylase (GAD), the critical enzyme in the GABA synthesis pathway, was studied. None of the DARPP-32–labeled neurons examined was positive for GAD; and none of the GAD-positive neurons could be labeled with DARPP-32. Additionally, despite looking for a co-occurence in more than 1000 GAD-labeled neurons, in no case could we find a basket coiling around a GAD-labeled cell. Thus, dopaminergic baskets do not contact GABAergic neurons, at least not via baskets and D1 receptors. From this result it is likely that the dopaminergic baskets within the neostriatum caudolaterale primarily modulate the physiological properties of excitatory units. Additional experiments make it further likely that the neurons inside baskets do not project back to secondary sensory areas, from where sensory inputs are received. Also at least the majority of cells within baskets do not seem to project out of the neostriatum caudolaterale to motor structures like the archistriatum. Thus, these results corroborate the view that dopaminergic baskets primarily modulate the activity of excitatory, intrinsic neostriatum caudolaterale neurons via D1 receptors (Fig. 14.2).

In principle, this picture is similar to that in mammals, where dopaminergic terminals are found mainly on dendritic spines of glutamatergic pyramidal cells. Occasionally, however, dopaminergic contacts on nonspiny, nonpyramidal cells were also observed, possibly hinting at dopaminergic effects on GABAergic interneurons (Smiley and Goldman-Rakic, 1993). Additionally, it is likely that the pyramidal cells receiving a dopaminergic input in mammals project to structures outside the PFC, a condition seemingly different than in birds. The experiments in pigeons described thus far, however, concentrated on basket-innervated cells. Dopaminergic baskets seem to be an anatomical arrangement to tightly control a subset of avian forebrain

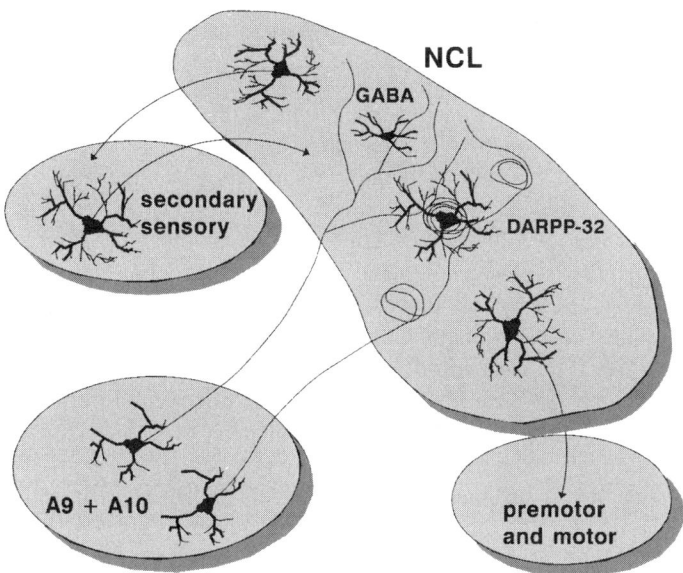

Figure 14.2. Schematic overview of the principal circuit of the neostriatum caudolaterale (NCL). A9 and A10 depict the dopaminergic tegmental cell groups. Note the two different types of dopaminergic innervation types (basket, en-passant fibers) of the neostriatum caudolaterale.

cells and do not seem to have a counterpart in the mammalian PFC. It is, therefore, possible that those dopaminergic fibers in pigeons that do not form baskets may, similar to mammals, innervate cells projecting out of the neostriatum caudolaterale.

THE DECLINE OF A MEMORY STORE

The tight coupling of dopaminergic baskets and D1 receptor–positive neurons makes it likely that an important part of the cognitive capacities mediated by the neostriatum caudolaterale depends on the appropriate activation of D1 receptors. In monkeys, microinjections of the D1 antagonist SCH23390 into PFC leads to deficits in working memory (Sawaguchi and Goldman-Rakic, 1991). As outlined above, some PFC neurons turn into "working memory cells" during the delay period of delay tasks. Williams and Goldman-Rakic (1995) recorded these neurons and demonstrated altered activity patterns of these cells after iontophoretic application of SCH39166, another D1 antagonist. Taken together, D1 receptor–mediated modulation seems to play a key role in the maintenance of working memory in monkeys. Is there a similar pattern in pigeons?

To answer this question, we devised in our laboratory a "shopping test" similar to that used in the study of Passingham (1985). A pigeon labyrinth with 16 chambers was constructed. At the front wall of each chamber a cup was positioned. There were two different kinds of cups, red and white ones. While the white cups always contained a few grains at the beginning of the experiment, the red ones were always empty. The pigeons were free to move around in the halls of the labyrinth to peer into any cup they wanted. After finishing the grains of one of the white cups it of course made no sense to return to this chamber. The animals were removed only after consuming all grains from all white cups. Within a few sessions the pigeons learned never to enter chambers with red cups. Learning never to return to white cup chambers took considerably longer, but finally all animals managed this task. The pigeons were always placed alternately in one of the opposite start positions in consecutive sessions. Probably this contributed to the pigeons mostly not adopting a certain individual route through the labyrinth but always following a different path.

The animals had to use two different memory stores to finish the task. One was reference memory, that is, a long-term storehouse of acquired information. For this task, the relevant information in the reference memory of the pigeons were "red cups are always empty" and "white cups are always baited at the beginning of one session." Thus, it was sufficient to enter chambers with white cups only. To prevent the animal from returning to white cup chambers, however, a second type of memory is needed. This kind of memory has to store information during an individual session, and it is only useful during this one session. The content of this second type of memory store could be "I'm finished with white cup chamber 3, now lets turn to 7, followed by 1"; then "I'm finished with 3 and 7, next to 1"; and so on. Thus, similar to a mental shopping list the pigeon may hold a mental list of next labyrinth goals. This is of course working memory as outlined in the beginning of this chapter.

If the computational principles of the neostriatum caudolaterale are equivalent to those of the PFC, blocking of D1 receptor–positive cells should lead to a decline of working memory without affecting reference memory. To test this hypothesis, at the beginning of training we placed two tiny injection cannulas into the neostriatum caudolaterale of each hemisphere and closed them tightly. After the pigeons had perfectly acquired the task, 0.5 µl of the D1 receptor blocker SCH23390 was slowly injected through each cannula into the neostriatum caudolaterale. This amount of substance affects less than 1 mm^3 neural tissue at the tip of the cannula; hence, only a portion of the D1 receptors of the neostriatum caudolaterale were blocked. The effects were nevertheless clear cut. The pigeons made four times more working memory errors in the D1-blocking sessions than under baseline conditions. Sometimes, the injected animals directly returned to a white cup chamber that they just had left. More often, they returned to white chambers that they had visited several moves before (Fig. 14.3). Some other pigeons made two correct visits first, then circled a little bit in front of different white chambers, and then stood silently for a while, just looking around. After about 30 minutes, the effect of the drug seemed to diminish because after this time only few errors were recorded. Despite all these problems with the white chambers, the SCH23390-injected animals had no difficulties avoiding the red cups. Thus, reference memory was not affected by the drug. To control for the effect of the injection as such, in different sessions saline instead of SCH23390 was injected into the cannulas. Under this condition, working memory errors also slightly increased, but were significantly below those in the D1

control session

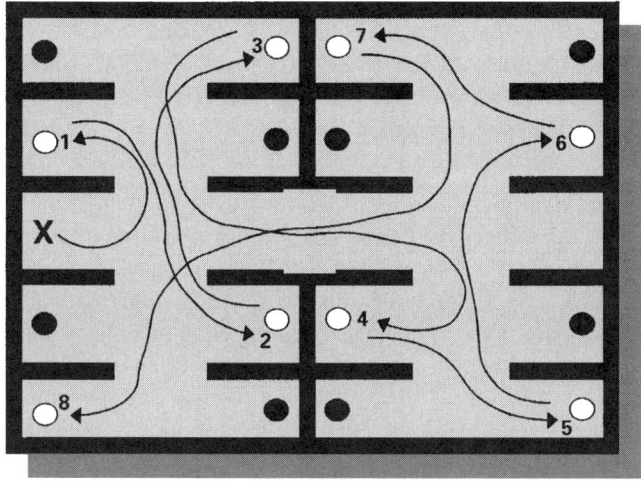

session with D1-blocker

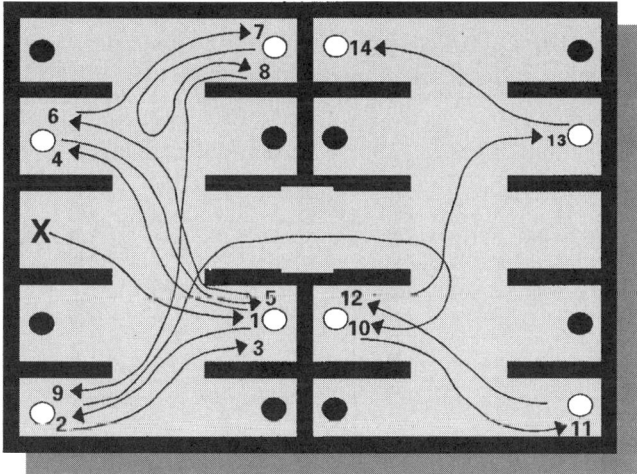

Figure 14.3. The labyrinth experiment with two different types of cups. The white ones were baited at the beginning of each session, while the red ones (shown in black) were always empty. Two representative sessions of the same pigeon are shown, one without microinjections (control session) and one with injections of SCH23390 (session with D1 blocker). The arrows depict the paths of the animal, with numbers giving the sequence of visits. "X" indicates the startpoint.

receptor–blockade sessions. Thus, the slight compression of neural tissue in neostriatum caudolaterale during injection seems to have a small effect, but only the prevention of D1 receptor–activation creates the full-blown working memory deficit.

SIMULATION OF THE MACHINE

What are the neural mechanims responsible for keeping and utilizing information in working memory? How does the perturbed dopaminergic system interfere with these mechanisms to produce the observed deficits? To investigate such questions in detail, adequate computer models serve as valuable scientific tools because all variables governing the behavior of the system can be accessed or manipulated at any time and in any way. Figure 14.4 depicts our network model, which captures some essential neuroanatomical properties of the prefrontal cortex and presumably also the neostriatum caudolaterale. We constructed a net of locally connected excitatory neurons, termed the *pyramidal cell layer*, as well as inputs from other telencephalic association areas, represented by an *input layer* (Durstewitz and Güntürkün, 1996). Thus, each pyramidal neuron receives two kinds of excitatory inputs: one from other pyramidal cells in the local neighborhood and the other one from neurons in the input layer. Furthermore, about 10 to 30 % of neurons in the avian forebrain and the mammalian cortex utilitize the inhibitory transmitter GABA. In our model these neurons are located in "GABA pools," which become activated by pyramidal neurons and distribute inhibitory feedback throughout the whole pyramidal cell net. The two

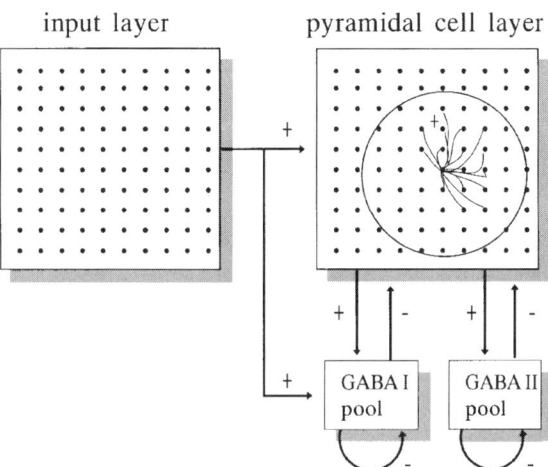

Figure 14.4. Structure of the network model that captures some essential anatomical properties of the Prefrontal cortex/neostriatum caudolaterale. The circle in the pyramidal cell layer indicates the range of excitatory connections of a single neuron. +, excitatory, and - inhibitory, synaptic effects. (From Durstewitz and Güntürkün, 1996.)

groups are distinguished by their GABA receptor mechanisms. The first utilizes $GABA_A$ receptors, which open chloride ion channels in the postsynaptic membrane and thereby provide a fast and efficient "shunting" inhibition. The second group uses $GABA_B$ receptors by which GABA indirectly opens potassium channels, resulting in a slower and less effective but longer lasting hyperpolarizing postsynaptic event. These two effector mechanisms are associated with different populations of cells in neocortex and are termed *GABA I pool* (fast shunting inhibition) and *GABA II pool* (slow, long-lasting inhibition) in the model. Finally, afferent connections from the input layer terminate on "GABA I" cells, providing a fast feed-forward inhibition.

The electrophysiological dynamics of virtual single neurons are simulated by membrane potential equations, which take into account different intrinsic and extrinsic sources of current. *Intrinsic* means voltage-gated and leakage membrane currents, whereas *extrinsic* means excitatory and inhibitory synaptic currents provided by other neurons in the network. With these currents, the virtual single neurons electrically behave like real cells.

Other basic aspects of network function are the mechanisms of learning. Processing of information in neural networks is highly dependent on the learning history of the net. Learning is associated with structural modifications of neural tissue. Thus, real networks are not static. There are two well-known phenomena, called *long-term potentiation* (LTP) and its counterpart *long-term depression* (LTD), that describe long-lasting changes in the efficiency of excitatory synapses. LTP means that the amplitude of excitatory postsynaptic potentials is increased for a long time period, whereas LTD means just the opposite. Various physiological conditions can evoke LTP or LTD. For example, activation of a presynaptic terminal, together with strong depolarization of the postsynaptic cell, leads to LTP of the respective synapse (Fig. 14.5). Therefore, LTP can strengthen the synaptic efficacy of weak fiber inputs, if these fibers are coactivated with axons giving rise to a strong excitatory input. Activation of weak fibers alone, however, does not sufficiently depolarize the postsynaptic cell and leads to LTD, that is, to a further reduction in synaptic efficacy. In general, strong coactivation of a presynaptic and a postsynaptic neuron is followed by LTP of the respective synapse, while strong activation of only one of the two neurons is followed by LTD. This "correlational" condition conforms broadly to Hebb's law, which was proposed in 1949 by the American psychologist Donald O. Hebb. The physiological details are, however, a little bit more complicated.

Artola and Singer (1993), for example, provided a more precise description of synaptic long-term modifications. From experimental results, they derived a learning rule that depends on presynaptic activity and local postsynaptic calcium concentration, which in turn depends on gating of voltage-dependent calcium channels and, thus, on postsynaptic membrane potential. Equipped with such a learning rule, a neural network (whether artificial or real) can learn several patterns of neural activity. To make sense of such activity patterns, however, we first have to talk about how different perceptual objects such as labyrinth chambers or different behavioral goals like finding food in cups might be represented by the nervous system.

One central idea is that neurons use a time code. As put forward by von der Malsburg (1981) and experimentally shown by Singer and co-workers (see Singer,

444   14 Multimodal Areas of the Avian Forebrain—Blueprints for Cognition?

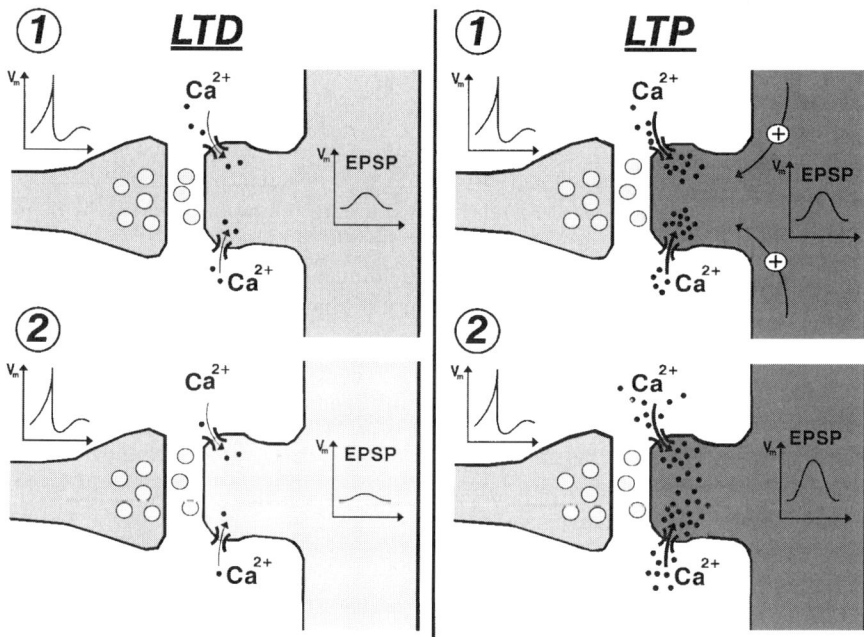

Figure 14.5. Physiological conditions under which synaptic long-term modifications are induced. The four pictures show a presynaptic terminal emitting transmitter into the synaptic cleft on the left hand side and a patch of postsynaptic membrane including a spine with membrane-bound Ca^{2+} channels on the right hand side. If an action potential arrives at the presynaptic terminal as indicated by the voltage trace inserted on the left, transmitter is released and depolarizes the postsynaptic membrane, thereby inducing an excitatory postsynaptic potential (EPSP) as indicated by the voltage trace on the right. Whether the postsynaptic response is enhanced (LTP) or reduced (LTD) depends on calcium influx through calcium channels. Because these channels open with depolarization, the total amount of calcium influx depends on postsynaptic depolarization. Strong postsynaptic depolarization may occur in response to presynaptic transmitter release if the postsynaptic cell is at the same time depolarized by intracellular current as indicated by the arrows in the LTP 1 part of the figure. After enhancement of the synapse (LTP 2), the EPSP alone depolarizes the postsynaptic membrane sufficiently to induce high Ca^{2+} influx.

1993), neurons that code for different aspects of the same object fire synchronously, whereas neurons belonging to different objects fire out of phase, that is, they emit their action potentials at different time points (Fig. 14.6). By these means, different perceptual or mental objects can be kept active simultaneously in working memory without intermingling. For example, in the labyrinth experiments, pigeons could keep active in their neostriatum caudolaterale representations of goals. These representations may encode labyrinth locations that the pigeon has to encounter next to find food. To explain these basic working memory functions, we first have to know under which circumstances neurons synchronize their activity, how synchronous activity is protected against noise, and when neurons desynchronize. These questions can be answered with the help of simulations of the network model introduced thus far. We come back later to the question of how blockade of dopaminergic receptors interferes with these processes.

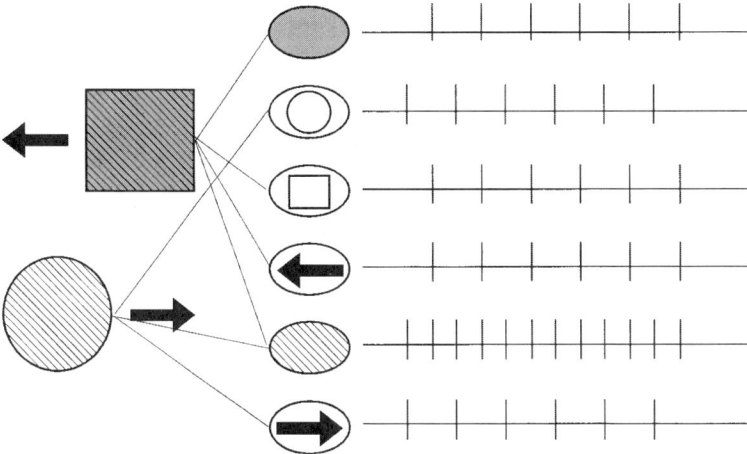

Figure 14.6. The idea of cortical neurons using a time code. If several objects are present in a visual scenery, for example, a gray striped square moving to the left and a white striped circle moving to the right, both objects could be represented by the neural system simultaneously by assemblies of neurons firing action potentials at different times. All neurons encoding features of one object emit action potentials at the same time, whereas neurons encoding features of the second object fire at different times. Also, neurons encoding features present in both objects may fire simultaneously in both representations.

Consider the case in which all excitatory synapses in the pyramidal cell layer have small weights (efficiencies) of similar strength. A certain amount of random variance in synaptic weights is permitted. Now we activate three groups of neurons at three successive time steps (2 to 4 msec apart in time) and document what happens. As illustrated in Figure 14.7, the three groups of neurons tend to synchronize over time. This effect occurs entirely automatically, although variance in weights could be expected to counteract synchronization. The basic explanation for this pheneomenon is that pyramidal neurons that are more advanced in their phase become inhibited more strongly by GABA II feedbacks because synaptic current depends on postsynaptic membrane potential, which is more depolarized in more advanced cells. This means that these neurons are reset more in their phase than neurons further away from spike threshold. GABA II feedbacks are more effective than GABA I feedbacks in synchronizing neurons because they extend over a much longer period of time. In contrast, fast GABA I feedbacks prevent different neural representations from collapsing in time. If two groups of neurons are activated with a time delay crossing a certain threshold, fast GABA I feedbacks provoked by the first group ensure that the second group does not merge with the first one. The two groups may even become more separated in time. This is due to the short but very efficient inhibitory phase provided by GABA I feedbacks. In summary, there is a critical time window within which neurons tend to synchronize, whereas neurons activated with time delays exceeding this window tend to desynchronize even further.

What do these results mean for the labyrinth example? As described above, the PFC of mammals is involved in behavioral planning. A behavioral plan may consist

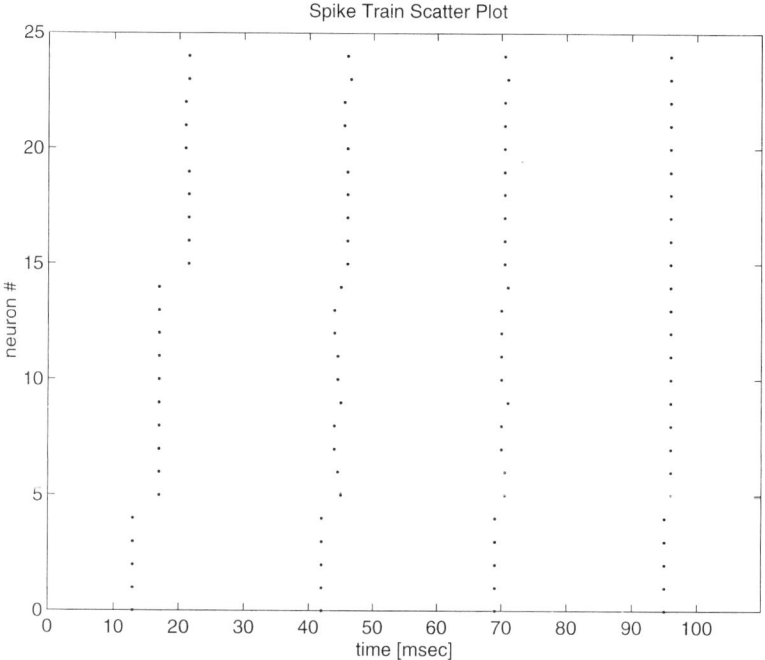

Figure 14.7. Synchronization of neurons by inherent dynamics of a model network. Each dot in a column represents the action potential time of a different neuron. With increasing time, initially desynchronized neurons synchronize with each other as can be seen by the dots lining up vertically.

of a sequence of successive goal states that is generated in working memory, triggered by the actual situation and the current needs of the animal. In the present context, a neural goal state representation comprises an assembly of neurons coding for different sensory and motor aspects of a certain labyrinth arm, together with the related sight of food and the anticipated consummatory behavior. If these neurons become active very close in time, as one would expect for neurons responding to different aspects of the same situation, the network maintains their synchronous activity and compensates for small perturbations. If, on the other hand, neurons representing another goal state become active at another time, the temporal separation of the latter representation from the former one is also ensured by inherent network mechanisms. This occurs without any prior learning or specificity in the synaptic weight matrix. Problems may arise, however, when not all neurons belonging to the same representation are activated at the same time. The converse case is also possible, that is, features belonging to different representations being activated simultaneously, for example, if there arises a conflict between different next goals. The question of how a neural net copes with these situations is addressed next. The solution rests on the fact that, in general, neural networks have some prior learning history and that synaptic weights are not evenly distributed but that some connections will be very strong and others will be weak.

Assume that the network—due to prior exposition—has learned two partly overlapping patterns (Loc1 and Loc2; see Fig. 14.8), which may encode two different labyrinth locations and their associations with food. Hence, as a result of synaptic learning as described above, there are two neural groups in the pyramidal cell network within which neurons are interconnected by strong excitatory weights, whereas only weak excitatory synapses exist toward neurons outside the group (Figure 14.8). Each group consists of neurons responding to general features of the labyrinth situation, of cells representing sensory features of one of the two locations, and of neurons encoding motor acts suitable for reaching food reward in one of the respective locations.

Now let us place the pigeon in the starting position of the labyrinth. The labyrinth context evokes "labyrinth feature"–neurons in the neostriatum caudolaterale. Because several labyrinth arms could be selected initially, probably neurons of different goal state representations will be activated together. One of these various goal states may, however, be associated most strongly with the starting position in the labyrinth, and therefore most of the activated neurons may belong to this representation. Thus, in the example of Figure 14.8, 60% of the Loc1 neurons become activated by the labyrinth starting position, whereas only a few Loc2 and some other neurons fire action potentials. As illustrated in Figure 14.8, after a short while the whole Loc1 assembly has been activated via excitation from initially stimulated Loc1 cells, whereas all neurons not engaged in Loc1 become dissociated in time. Hence, Loc1 stands out as a unique pattern in the network activity.

One could say that the pigeon has "decided" to encounter location 1 first and to initiate the appropiate motor acts. Why do non-Loc1 neurons, which had been coactivated with the initial stimulus, desynchronize their activity? The reason lies in the connectivity of the cells activated by the stimulus. Neurons that, due to their learning history, are interconnected with high synaptic weights with other neurons activated by location 1, receive a much higher excitatory input than do neurons that are weaker coupled. This strong imbalance in excitatory inputs for different neurons overrides synchronizing forces and drives neurons apart in time. If, by learning or by chance, more Loc2 neurons than Loc1 neurons would have been activated initially, the network would have singled out the Loc2 pattern first. It can be concluded that synchronization and desynchronization phenomena depend on the stimulus conditions and the structure of the synaptic weight matrix. The significance of labyrinth locations changes throughout a trial, because locations once visited are no longer associated with food. If the pigeon visits one labyrinth arm, the respective goal representation may be inhibited by negative feedback elicited by the consummatory act and by the perception that there is no more food in the cup. This may enable a successive goal-state to become dominant. In this way, a sequence of goal states may be carried out in the neostriatum caudolaterale, until all food cups have been cleared.

How can a finished goal state be prevented from being activated again and again by the sight of respective labyrinth features? To put it more generally, how can goal states in the neostriatum caudolaterale or the PFC be protected against interfering processes such as response tendencies elicited by other stimulus configurations in the environment? This is the point where we come back to dopamine.

448   14 Multimodal Areas of the Avian Forebrain—Blueprints for Cognition?

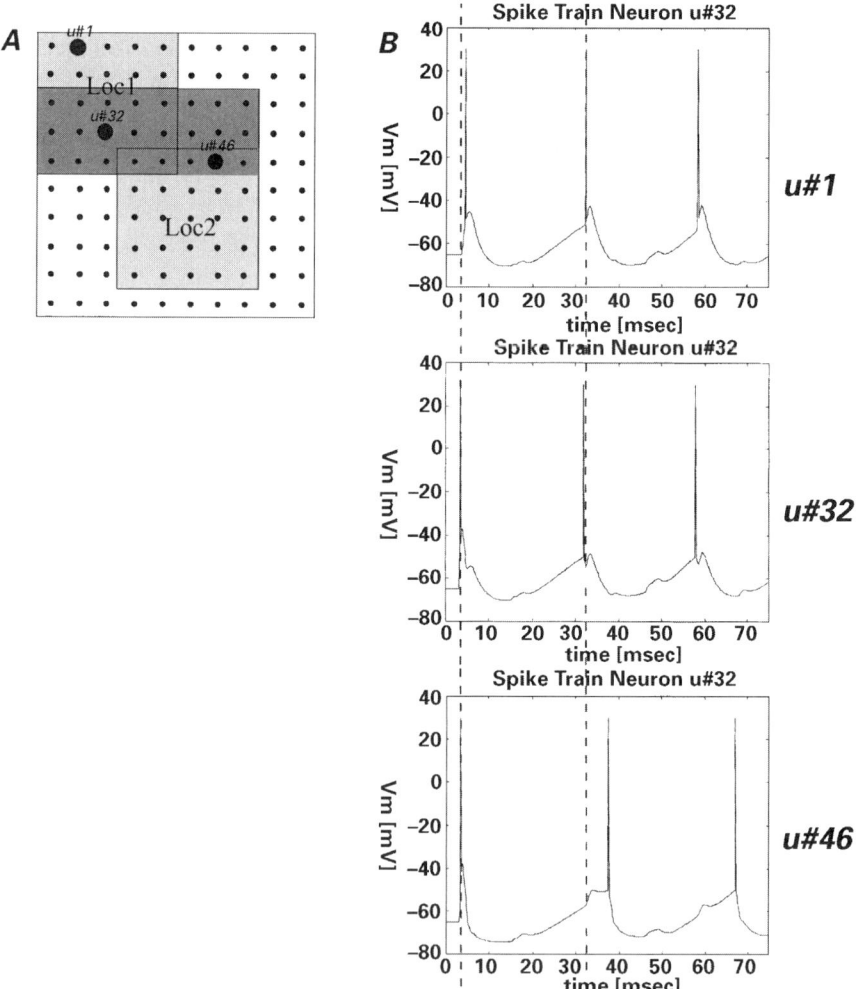

Figure 14.8. Synchronization and desynchronization in a network model with specific learning history. (A) The two light gray squares termed "Loc1" and "Loc2" represent two patterns imprinted in the synaptic weight matrix of the pyramidal cell layer. Each dot represents a neuron, with bigger dots representing those neurons whose activity is shown in B. The dark gray bar illustrates the group of neurons activated by the initial stimulus, that is, the starting labyrinth situation. (B) Membrane potential of three representative neurons. Neurons u#32 and u#46 are coactivated by the stimulus at about t = 3.5 msec. Neuron u#1 is activated shortly thereafter due to strong excitation spreading from the initially stimulated Loc1 neurons. Loc2 neurons do not receive sufficient excitation. Neuron u#46, which receives significantly less excitation than Loc1 neurons, becomes desynchronized in its spike activity from the other neurons.

As has been described earlier in this chapter, the dopaminergic innervation of the neostriatum caudolaterale or PFC plays an essential role in learning and working memory functions. Dopaminergic midbrain tegmental neurons are·active in new and biologically significant situations. In vivo, dopamine mainly seems to inhibit cortical pyramidal cells, that is, the firing frequency of pyramidal cells is reduced when dopaminergic fibers are stimulated or when dopamine is applied directly (Ferron et al., 1984). It has been found that dopamine does not "inhibit" cells in a classic sense, as GABA does, but it reduces excitatory synaptic transmission and changes the conductances and time characteristics of several voltage-gated membrane ion channels (Yang and Seamans, 1996). The latter modification of ion channels results in reducing the effect that synaptic inputs impinging on distal parts of the apical dendritic tree of pyramidal cells exert on soma potential. In contrast, the cell responses to inputs to the proximal dendritic parts are enhanced. To appreciate the functional significance of this modification, one has to know that axons from other cortical areas terminate on the distal dendrites in the PFC, and local feedbacks and thalamic inputs terminate on the proximal dendrites. Hence, local excitatory interactions are reinforced by dopamine, while inputs from other cortical areas are diminished due to reduced synaptic transmission and the weaker effects of distal postsynaptic potentials on soma potential. As a consequence, dopamine helps to keep current goal state activity in the PFC upright and protects this activity against interfering perceptual or memory influences. Under the control of dopamine, it becomes very difficult for perceptual features of the environment to evoke new goal states or to evoke finished goal states again and thus to override the presently active goal states in working memory. This becomes possible, however, if dopaminergic receptors are blocked. Then the probability increases that current goal states get lost from working memory and the pigeon is attracted by already visited labyrinth arms again.

LOOKING INSIDE

If a pigeon's walk through a few chambers of a labyrinth really involves processes of such complexity, will we ever be able to understand the machinery of human thought, or will the human brain fail in understanding itself? Presently we do not know the answer to this question, but sometimes the quest to comprehend our own mind indeed seems to be beyond realistic chances. The human brain is not unique, however, but just one variation of a typical vertebrate brain from which the pigeon brain is another. Both were crafted based on the very same *Bauplan*, having most of their blueprints in common. From this perspective, a scientific inquiry into the neuronal operations guiding a pigeon's walk through a labyrinth might provide us windows onto the cellular basis of our own cognitive processes.

ACKNOWLEDGMENTS

This work was supported by the Alfried Krupp zu Bohlen und Halbach-Stiftung and the Deutsche Forschungsgemeinschaft through its Graduiertenkolleg KOGNET and the Sonderforschungsbereich NEUROVISION.

REFERENCES

Artola, A., and W. Singer (1993) Long-term depression of excitatory synaptic transmission and its relationship to long-term potentiation. *Trends Neurosci.* 16:480–487.

Divac, I., and J. Mogensen (1985) The prefrontal "cortex" in the pigeon—catecholamine histofluorescence. *Neuroscience* 15:677–682.

Durstewitz, D., and O. Güntürkün (1996) The possible function of dopamine in associative learning: a computational model. In C. von der Malsburg, W. von Seelen, J. C. Vorbrüggen, and B. Sendhoff (eds.): *Lecture Notes in Computer Science: Artificial Neural Networks.* ICANN 1996. Springer, Berlin, pp. 667–672.

Durstewitz, D., S. Kröner, H.C. Hemmings, Jr., and O. Güntürkün (1998) The dopaminergic innervation of the pigeon telencephalon: distribution of DARPP-32 and coocurrence with glutamate decarboxylase and tyrosine hydroxylase. *Neuroscience* 83:763–779.

Ferron, A., A.-M. Thierry, C. Le Douarin, and J. Glowinski (1997) Inhibitory influence of the mesocortical dopaminergic system on spontaneous activity or excitatory response induced from the thalamic mediodorsal nucleus in the rat medial prefrontal cortex. *Brain Res.* 302:257–265.

Fuster, J.M. (1989) *The Prefrontal Cortex.* Raven Press, New York.

Güntürkün, O. (1996) Lernprozesse bei Tieren. In J. Hoffmann and W. Kintsch (eds.): *Enzyklopädie der Psychologie, Themenbereich C: Theorie und Forschung, Serie II: Kognition, Band 7: Lernen.* Hogrefe, Göttingen, pp. 85–129.

Güntürkün, O. (1997) Cognitive impairments after lesions of the neostriatum caudolaterale and its thalamic afferent: functional similarities to the mammalian prefrontal system? *J. Brain Res.* 38:133–143.

Korzeniewska, E., and O. Güntürkün (1990) Sensory properties and afferents of the n. dorsolateralis posterior thalami (DLP) of the pigeon. *J. Comp. Neurol.* 292:457–479.

Mogensen, J., and I. Divac Behavioural effects of ablation of the pigeon-equivalent of the mammalian prefrontal cortex. *Behav. Brain Res.* 55:101–107.

Passingham, R.E. (1985) Memory of monkeys (*Macaca mulatta*) with lesions in prefrontal cortex. *Behav. Neurosci.* 99:3–21.

Rehkämper, G., and K. Zilles (1991) Parallel evolution in mammalian and avian brains: comparative cytoarchitectonic and cytochemical analysis. *Cell Tissue Res.* 263:3–28.

Sawaguchi, T., and P.S. Goldman-Rakic (1991) D1 dopamine receptors in prefrontal cortex: involvement in working memory. *Science* 251:941–950.

Schultz, W., R. Romo, T. Ljungberg, J. Mirenowicz, J.R. Hollerman, and A Dickinson. (1995) Reward-related signals carried by dopamine neurons. In J.C. Houk, J.L. Davis, and D.G. Beiser (eds.): *Models of Information Processing in the Basal Ganglia.* MIT Press, Cambridge, pp. 233–248.

Shallice, T. (1982) Specific impairments of planning. *Philos. Trans. R. Soc. Lond. Biolo.* 298:199–209.

Shallice, T., and P. Burgess (1991) Specific impairments of planning. *Brain* 114:727–741.

Singer, W. (1993) Synchronization of cortical activity and its putative role in information processing and learning. *Annu. Rev. Physiol.* 55:349–374.

Smiley, J.F., and P.S. Goldman-Rakic (1993) Heterogeneous targets of dopamine synapses in monkey prefrontal cortex demonstrated by serial section electron microscopy: a laminar analysis usingsilver-enhanced diaminobenzidine sulfide (SEDS) immunolabeling technique. *Cerebral Cortex* 3:223–238.

von der Malsburg, C. (1981) *The Correlation Theory of Brain Function.* Internal Report. Max-Planck-Institute for Biophysical Chemistry, Göttingen, Germany.

Waldmann, C.M., and O. Güntürkün (1993) The dopaminergic innervation of the pigeon caudolateral forebrain: immunocytochemical evidence for a "prefrontal cortex" in birds? *Brain Res.* 600:225-234.

Williams, G.V., and P. Goldman-Rakic (1995) Blockade of dopamine D1 receptors enhances memory fields of prefrontal neurons in primate cerebral cortex. *Nature* 376:572–575.

Yang, C.R., and J. K. Seamans (1996) Dopamine D1 receptor actions in layers V–VI rat prefrontal cortex neurons in vitro: modulation of dendritic-somatic signal integration. *J. Neurosci.* 16:1922–1935.

Chapter 15

COGNITIONS OF BIRDS AS PRODUCTS OF EVOLVED BRAINS

Juan D. Delius, Martina Siemann, Jacky Emmerton and Li Xia
Allgemeine Psychologie, Universität Konstanz (J.D.D., M.S., L.X.)
and Department of Psychology, Purdue University (J.E.)

Evolution does not work logically with a long term perspective on the design of the neural structures, but rather selects the most successful behavior from generation to generation (Dumont and Robertson, 1986).

INTRODUCTION

What counts as a cognitive competency is by no means a well-defined matter. Many behavioral feats of animals and humans that older textbooks labeled as learning, for example, are found under the heading of cognition in newer books (e.g., Domjan, 1993; Pearce, 1997). Psychologists studying human learning and performance in the late 1950s and early 1960s rekindled the interest in cognition as a reaction to the then dominant behavioristic psychology. They drew attention to the Latin root "cognoscere," meaning "to know," and considered that the defining feature of cognitive processes was the involvement of information processing based on mental representations. The "mental" substrate alluded to was merely another word for the brain and "representations" another word for memory contents that encoded past experiences. The topics of recent cognitive psychology handbooks accordingly range widely, including almost every process that can intervene between the initial sensing of stimuli and the final emission of behaviors. Indeed, the recurrence of the term cognition is simply a modern way of emphasizing the importance of these mediating processes that were studiously ignored for so long by behaviorist psychologists.

For the purposes of this chapter, the word "cognitive" is used as an adjective that identifies relatively complex behavioral competencies that are assumed to require these mediating processes for their performance. The stimuli to which an animal is exposed, the behavioral actions that it produces, the outcomes of these activities, and even the motivational states that accompany them may be coded and stored as integrated sets of information. These representations of past experience may be operated on further off-line toward bringing them into more efficient formats. In species, or more precisely individuals, that are cognitively highly endowed, this conversion may operate to the extent that they end up possessing a more or less complete mental model of their environment and of their "self." Regardless of the perfection of the resulting representations, the causation of any cognitive behavior is deemed to involve a recourse to these representations of past experience as well as to the codes signaling the immediate situation.

Despite the difficulty of defining precisely what cognitive behavior is, there is consensus that the information-processing capacity, or intelligence, for short, needed by animal species to show such behavior is largely dependent on the evolutionary status that their brains have achieved. A reliance on cognition as an intermediary stage of processing principally characterises the behavior of the two anagenetically most progressive vertebrate classes, the avians and the mammals. Along with mammals (Mammalia), birds (Aves), although often said to be dominated by instincts, have been shown in the last 50 years or so to be capable of behaviors that now readily fall into the cognitive category. Often they perform complex behavioral tasks with more proficiency than mammals of comparable body and, more importantly, brain size. Indeed, in several instances they show abilities comparable with those of nonhuman primates of considerably larger brain size. Birds in any case undoubtedly do better on cognitive tasks than representatives of the anamniotes and reptiles, arguments to the contrary notwithstanding (Macphail, 1985). Bees (Apidae), as exceptionally gifted insects, possibly come cognitively closer to them than any of the fish (Pisces), anuran (Anura) or reptile (Reptilia) species (Siemann et al., 1998).

Birds have a brain morphology that differs markedly from that of mammals and that is arguably more similar to that of reptiles, with whom they indeed share the clade Sauropsida (Ariens-Kappers et al., 1936). The avian brain does not possess a structure that can squarely compare with the isocortex of mammals. Its dorsal pallium, although massive and probably equivalent to it, is not nearly as architecturally differentiated as the mammalian isocortex (Karten, 1991; Rehkämper, et al., and Zilles, 1991; Veenman, 1997; Medina and Reiner 2000). Instead, birds have a sophisticated tectum opticum that is arguably the most complex neural structure extant (Ramón y Cajal, 1911). As a result, the overall information-processing capabilities of birds may be generally on a par with those of equal-sized mammals.

Both mammals and avians ultimately descend phylogenetically from a common cold-blooded reptilian ancestor living some 310 million years ago (Kumar and Hedges, 1998). Why, then, do the two groups show such marked differences in their brains, besides, of course, all the other distinguishing characters? Perhaps this is in part because as proper mammals and birds they emerged from two already divergent reptilian-saurian stocks: Triassic therapsids about 250 million years ago, the ancestors of mammals (Ahlberg and Milner, 1994), and Jurassic theropodans about 150 million years ago, the ancestors of birds, probably had brains that already differed somewhat. Possibly a more incisive reason, however, is that the evolutionary scenarios during the Jurassic and Cretaceous eras threw the two lineages into radically different ecological niches (Feduccia, 1996). The ancestral mammalian brains were apparently selected for a nocturnal habitat while maintaining a terrestrial life. This combination placed diminished demands on their visual system and increased demands on their olfactory system, which promoted an early shift from a relative mesencephalization to a relative telencephalization in terms of altered volumes and histological differentiation of these structures. The ancestral avian brains, on the other hand, continued to be selected for an aerial habitat together with a persisting diurnal life that placed strongly enhanced demands on their visual system and their locomotor-navigational abilities. These demands presumably resulted in the maintenance of a relative mesencephalization and the emergence of the relative cerebellarization that still characterises them today (Dubbledam, 1998). Indeed, the newer view, that the cerebellum is concerned with much more than motor control and is very probably centrally involved in cognitive operations (Akshoomoff and Courchesne, 1992; Schmahmann, 1997), could partially help to explain why birds are as intelligent as we shall argue they are.

Similarities in the energetic necessities of both the nocturnal and the aerial niche promoted a convergent warm bloodedness in mammals and avians (Ruben, 1995). This homoeothermy in turn enhanced the potency of neural functioning and thus expanded the repertoire of behavioral options. For mammals and avians, flexible behavior became the key device underlying their advances in Darwinian fitness, and this again presumably fostered a relative telencephalization. The emphasis on behavioral adaptability also caused the relative (allometric) brain-to-body size of both avians and mammals to rise above that of the reptiles, which are still today handicapped by poikilothermy (Van Dongen, 1998; Wyles Kunkel and Wilson, 1983). Among the very first consequences would be complex behavior sequences dedicated to the optimization of pelage and plumage insulatory functions. Birds' preening would be more demanding than mammals' grooming because feathers were also essential for flight (Delius, 1988). The divergent and complicated reproductive strategies of brooding and lactating emerged not least because of the need to release into independence offspring with brains too large to mature intrauterinely or intraovally, but which nevertheless had to achieve a fully functioning state. These strategies in turn demanded differentiated parental care behaviors, for which these same brains had to evolve new capabilities. The accompanying birth or hatching at an early stage of embryological development caused the brains of the offspring to be exposed at an immature stage to an environment to which they eventually had to match their behavior. This undoubtedly enhanced the role of neural plasticity in the adjustment of the behavioral repertoire in both avians and mammals and advanced the development of brain structures specialized for learning and memory, resulting in a relative dorsopallialization in both classes. The heavier parental investment in offspring production generated demands for an intelligent selection of sexual mates. In turn the behavioral bond between parents and offspring furthered the evolution of sociality. This eventually converted the ecological niches in which birds and mammals operated into socioecological niches that encouraged the evolution of capabilities for highly flexible social behaviors. There is reason to believe that the need to manage the complexities of social relationships is the prime mover for the evolution of advanced intelligence (Whiten and Byrne, 1997; Wyles et al., 1983). With the massive extinction of many saurian and, incidentally, also avian lineages right at the end of the Cretaceous about 65 million years ago, some of the mammalian lineages began to move into the diurnal habitat. Their thalamotelencephalic visual system proceeded to expand in volume within the cortex cerebri, which was partially relieved from olfactory functions. In avians, meanwhile, the tecto-thalamic-telencephalic visual pathway expanded massively within the dorsal pallium, converting it into a highly developed sensory system (Güntürkün, 1991; Veenman et al., 1995).

Speculative and inadequate as this brief phylogenetic account may be, it serves to emphasize that the evolution of the brain is not a self-contained process that obeys laws unto itself, as it would sometimes appear from the writings of some comparative anatomists, but rather, like the evolution of all other organismic characters, it has to be understood as the product of a history of selection pressures operating on a stream of random mutation opportunities or rather on the behavioral competencies that this genetic material enabled (Dumont and Robertson, 1986). Of course, the ensemble of selection pressures that operated at any time would only partly originate from the current ecosocial niche as sketched above. The persistence of any mutation that might arise depends on whether it can first satisfy more basal demands. Whatever biochemical-developmental cascade the mutation might trigger, this causal cascade must not appreciably interfere with either the metabolic pathways or the embryological mechanisms maintained by the genome existing at that time (Berezeney et al., 1995; Bohley, 1995; Chan and Jan, 1999). In other words, the effects of a mutation must not impair to any significant degree the Darwinian fitness that an organism has already achieved if it is to spread through the population. This represents an intrinsic selection pressure that maintains a flowing state of genomic coadaptation. It guarantees a measure of evolutionary conservatism that in turn makes it reasonable for comparative anatomists and physiologists to search, among other things, for equivalencies between the brain structures of avians and mammals. Still, adaptation to the environment is what in the end must mainly drive the evolution of organisms' characteristics. Brains are certainly no exception, but they are perhaps somewhat special. What is decisive for their fitness is, vegetative regulation aside, the somatic behavior that they can produce, although even today we can say rather little about the correspondence between the gross appearance of brain structures and the characteristics of the behavioral responses that they can implement. When it comes to behaviors that are complex enough to be labeled cognitive, these correlations often become desperately tenuous. With such behaviors, it is the still poorly understood functional interconnectivities of neuronal assemblies, often belonging to many diverse brain structures, rather than the gross size and layout of any particular brain structures, that are the decisive features. It is these neural networks that define the complex information processing that is characteristic of cognitive behaviors (Gazzaniga, 1995).

Domestic pigeons (*Columba livia*, var. *domestica*), pigeons, for short, in the remainder of this chapter, are the preferred bird species for research both on avian cognition and on the avian brain, simply because of their convenience as laboratory animals (Abs, 1983). Birds evince about as much cladogenetic radiation in morphology as mammals, however, although the cognitive capacities of birds probably do not range as widely as those of the mammals. Bird species may not marshal any behavioral and neural differentiations as drastic as those between, say, hedgehogs (Erinacidae), whales (Cetacea), and humans (Hominidae). Still, with rock pigeons (*Columba livia*, var. *livia*), the wild species from which the domestic pigeon derives, being just one among some 9700 extant birds species, and indeed one among some 310 existing and varied pigeon species (Columbidae), it cannot claim to be representative of all of them. Similarly, that other popular research subject, the laboratory variety of Norwegian rat (*Rattus norvegicus*), cannot be claimed to be representative of the roughly 4300 existing mammalian species. The class Aves after all includes divergent groups such as ostriches (Rheidae), penguins (Spheniscidae), moundbirds (Megapodidae), oilbirds (Steatornithidae), keas (Nestorinae), birds of paradise (Paradisiaeinae), and hummingbirds (Trochillidae), to mention a few. Pigeons can certainly not be a universal stand-in for any of these or for the many other avian species. There is even reason to doubt that the pigeon is among the most cognitively endowed or intelligent birds. Species of the crow family (Corvidae) and the parrot family (Psittacidae) have, for example, already been shown to out-do pigeons in some cognitive tasks (see later). Even within the pigeon species there are good grounds for believing that the artificial domesticating selection that has affected pigeons for several thousand generations might have tended to blunt their intelligence (Rehkämper et al., 1988). Subvarieties that were selectively bred for the ability of fast, long-range homing (homing pigeons; Levi, 1977) or in which the domestication effect may have been partly reversed by a return to a predominantly feral existence (street pigeons; Simms, 1979) can be expected to do better in cognitive tasks than subvarieties that have been selected for special looks (e.g., pouter pigeons) or for peculiar behaviors (for example, tumbler pigeons). Whether pigeon subvarieties that were bred primarily for meat productivity (e.g., Silver King and White Carneaux pigeons; Levi, 1977), which are often used for experiments in North American laboratories because of their convenient commercial availability, are the most suitable to explore the limits of pigeon intelligence is somewhat doubtful.

Regardless of these concerns, it is the case that like most other birds, the pigeon is a highly visual animal. The sophistication of the pigeon's visual system is indexed anatomically by the relatively large eyes (Fig. 15.1), an effectively bifoveate retina, a partly binocular field of vision (Güntürkün et al., 1989; Remy and Güntürkün, 1991), about 2.5 million optic nerve fibers, a massive, 15 layered tectum opticum, a sizeable optic thalamus, and large telencephalic visual structures (Güntürkün, 1991). This sophistication is reflected behaviorally in the complexity of the color vision system, which is at least tetrachromatic and ranges in sensitivity from ultraviolet to red wavelengths (300 to 700 nm; Emmerton and Delius, 1980; Palacios and Varela, 1992), in a probable sensitivity to the polarization of light (Delius et al., 1976; Able and Able, 1997; but see Coemans et al., 1990), a high degree of motion sensitivity (Emmerton, 1986; Martinoya and Delius, 1990; Neiworth and Rilling, 1987), and in an excellent invariant pattern recognition (Delius and Hollard 1995; Jitsumori and Ohkubo, 1996). Gross estimates suggest that about one third of the pigeon's nervous system, with its about 2.5 ml volume and 10^9 neurons, is mainly engaged in visual functions. This provides pigeons with a visual neural network involving perhaps some 10^{11} synaptic connections that potentially equips them with information-processing capacities for the most sophisticated visuocognitive performances conceivable. That these capacities are primarily visual is an advantage for the conduct

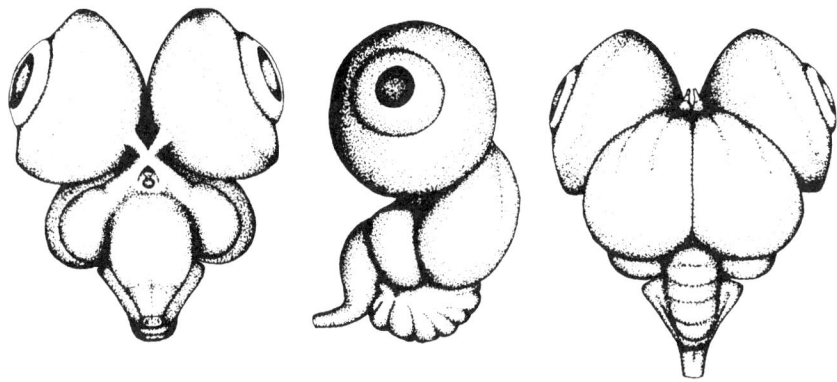

Figure 15.1. Ventral, lateral and dorsal aspect of the pigeon's brain and eyes to illustrate the relative importance of the visual system.

of cognitive experiments by human experimenters who are themselves visually disposed and who are aided by a technology that is biased toward vision. That the pigeon appears to cognitively outperform the popular mammalian experimental animal, the laboratory rat, may largely be due to the fact that the latter species, by being nocturnal and, even worse, being often albino, is conversely specialized for olfactory information processing, a modality that is not particularly accessible to humans or their technology. It may also be the reason why pigeons' cognitive performances are mostly compared with those of nonhuman primates that share with us the primacy of the visual sense but are of course a notch above most of the nonprimate mammals and indeed birds, regarding the brain-to-body size relation (Jerison, 1973).

Following these lofty theoretical considerations, we now turn to an overview of what an avian brain is capable of by discussing some examples of cognitive competencies of pigeons and comparing them with those of mammals.

CATEGORIZATION

It is generally recognized that in vertebrates the information influx through the sensory systems by far exceeds both the information throughput capacities of the nervous system and the range of motor-output options. Central representations of different stimuli that unify these inputs according to their physical similarity and/or functional significance to a smaller set of stimulus classes can certainly contribute to a reduction of the informational load. For example, pigeons may benefit in this way from classing food types, pigeon varieties, tree species, nesting sites, and predator species into such categories or concepts. It has been shown that they can indeed do so, and it can even be argued that the research on such classing of stimuli has advanced further in pigeons than it has in primates, including humans.

Already in 1964, Herrnstein and Loveland demonstrated that pigeons could be trained to discriminate pictures containing humans from pictures not containing humans and that pigeons would generalize this distinction to a new set of pictures that were characterized by the presence or absence of humans. These investigators did this by successively and repeatedly back-projecting onto a translucent pecking key a set of 80 randomly ordered color slides of a great variety of scenes, half of which contained a human figure and the other half of which did not. Both types of slides followed each other in random order. Several pecks by the hungry pigeons to the slides which contained humans led to a food reward. Pecks to a slide that did not contain a human never led to a reward. After about 700 slide presentations the pigeons pecked significantly more often at the positive slides than at the negative slides. They were then tested with a set of 80 human and no-human slides that had not been used for training. The pigeons showed an immediate pecking preference for the new slides containing humans, that is, they applied the distinction between two stimulus categories that they had learned with one collection of pictures to another, different set of pictures that also represented these categories. Using similar procedures, it was shown that pigeons could learn to distinguish in this generalizing way among other categories. The stimuli they have successfully categorized so far include pictures of trees from pictures of nontrees, pictures of fish from pictures of other animals, pictures of water from pictures without water, and even pictures of a particular person from pictures of other people or pictures of a particular scenic site from pictures of other scenic sites (Herrnstein, 1985; Honig and Stewart, 1988). Pigeons have also proved capable of learning to categorize such unnatural stimuli as workshop tools, letters of the alphabet, and painting styles with which they are certain to have had no preexperimental experience (Morgan et al., 1976; Lubow, 1974; Watanabe et al., 1995). Bhatt et al., (1988) showed that pigeons were even able to learn to categorize concurrently pictures of cats, flowers, cars, and chairs with similar facility.

Although much of the work on categorization has employed pictorial stimuli, this ability is not limited to the visual modality. Pigeons, not renowned for the musicality of their own vocalizations, have nevertheless been trained to discriminate variable, brief portions of Bach organ music from analogous portions of Stravinsky's 'Rite of Spring' (Porter and Neuringer, 1984). In subsequent tests involving novel excerpts from work played on different instruments or by other composers, the birds generalized their conditional discrimination and categorized in ways similar to humans who were analogously tested. The birds thus responded to excerpts from other baroque composers by preferentially pecking the "Bach" response key and to a different piece by Stravinsky and to excerpts from compositions by other modernistic composers by pecking the "Stravinsky" key.

Using a special conditioning apparatus, Delius (1992) trained pigeons to categorize small three-dimensional objects according to the somewhat abstract physical property of being spherical or nonspherical (Fig. 15.2). The apparatus allowed the successive presentation of different object triplets. If a bird grasped a spherical shape, it received a reward of several grains whereas its grasping of nonspherical objects yielded a period of darkness. The animals learned the discrimination task very quickly, probably because of the realism of the stimuli that, among other things, offered tactile as well

458 15 Cognitions of Birds as Products of Evolved Brains

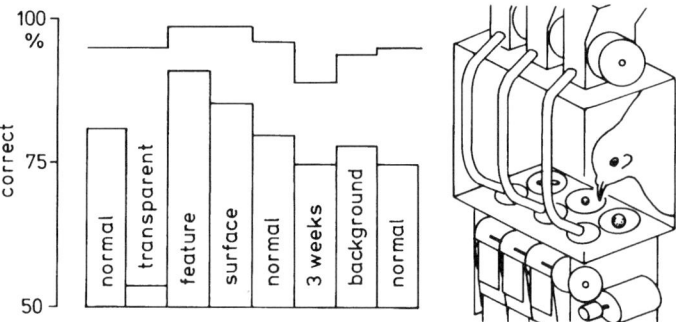

Figure 15.2. Categorization of spherical and nonspherical objects by pigeons. (Right) Apparatus with which objects were successively presented in triplets (one sphere vs. two nonspheres or vice versa). The pecking of spherical objects was rewarded with grain deliveries. (Left): Staircase: discrimination of standard training objects. Columns: preference for spheres in different sets of novel stimuli; normal: standard novel objects; transparent: glassy objects, all with nonspherical inclusions; feature: objects differing only by the sphericity criterion; surface: objects with novel surfaces; background: familiar objects on a novel background; 3 weeks: test after an experimental pause. (Modified from Siemann et al., 1998.)

as visual cues. Familiar training objects presented on novel backgrounds were readily discriminated by the pigeons. Tests with sets of new spherical and nonspherical objects showed that they could also generalize their categorization to these, except when the novel set consisted of transparent objects all containing nonspherical opaque inclusions. After some training with these latter objects, however, even they were discriminated correctly. Though not shown in Figure 15.2 the study revealed that the pigeons would, without any special training, also categorize objects on a relative basis, meaning that when exclusively presented with nonspherical objects they would choose preferentially those that human observers judged as the roundest, most spherical-like. Also, the pigeons immediately categorized pictures of spherical and nonspherical objects but, interestingly, they did significantly better with black and white than with color photographs. As already mentioned, the color vision system of pigeons is at least pentachromatic and thus is clearly different from the merely trichromatic system of humans (Emmerton and Delius, 1980; Palacios and Varela, 1992). This means that these birds are very likely to perceive color pictures that are adjusted to human color vision as false color images. It may therefore be unwise to confuse, for example, the earlier mentioned categorization of the color pictures of scenes with the categorization of the scenes themselves, a caveat that is only sometimes taken into account (Dawkins et al., 1996; Delius et al., 1999).

Delius and Nowak (1982) trained pigeons to discriminate a set of various black and white decorative-geometrical patterns that were successively projected on to a pecking key according to whether their shape was axially symmetrical or asymmetrical. They rewarded responses to one type of stimulus and penalized responses to the other type of stimulus. When the animals had learned to perform correctly to these stimuli they were confronted with sets of unreinforced novel test patterns, some of them stylistically very different from the patterns used for training. The pigeons displayed a consistently high level of categorization transfer to these novel sets (but see Huber et al., 1999). When pigeons were alternatively trained by intermittently but indiscriminately rewarding responses to both symmetrical or asymmetrical patterns they showed a weak but still significant spontaneous preference for asymmetrical patterns, which may indicate that they have a preexperimental, perhaps even innate capacity for categorizing such stimuli. This supposition has recently gained some interest in the sense that a faulty genetic constitution of an individual of a given species is liable to result in an asymmetrical growth of somatic features. Indeed, some experiments have shown that at least some bird species prefer sexual mates of a regular, symmetrical body build (Møller, 1993). The fact that pigeons showed evidence of having a weak preexperimental capacity of judging the symmetricity of visual patterns may be seen as supporting this view, but the preference for asymmetrical patterns associated with it does not fit in well. Rensch (1973) has, however, reported a more fitting spontaneous preferences for symmetry in corvids.

The mechanisms that underlie the capacity to form categories have not as yet been completely identified. Note that when learning to categorize a set of items into two or more classes, pigeons could be doing so by memorizing how to respond to each of the relevant items by rote (Herrnstein, 1990). Only a few years ago it was thought that the memory capacities of pigeons were too reduced to be capable of storing more than one or two dozen different individual pictures in this way. It is now known that pigeons can learn to recognize up to several hundreds, possibly even thousands of pictures in such a one-by-one manner (Vaughan and Greene, 1984). Fersen and Delius (1989), for instance, showed that pigeons could learn to reliably discriminate an arbitrary selection of 100 different decorative-geometric black and white patterns from another analogous selection of 625 patterns. It is also well known that animals that have been conditioned to respond to a specific stimulus (e.g., the green color of 530 nm light) in a particular way will respond, although with less strength, to physically similar stimuli (e.g., to the yellow-green of 550 nm or the blue-green of 510 nm). This phenomenon of stimulus generalization is partly attributable to the limited discriminatory capabilities of sensory systems but is also a result of the way in which perceptual recognition systems are designed to allow for a certain degree of stimulus variability (Blough, 1972). Thus at least some of the novel test items that did not differ by much in physical appearance from the training items would be spontaneously responded to in a category-adequate manner (Pearce, 1987).

Another mechanism can further broaden the inclusiveness of categorization. Complex stimuli, such as those used in the categorization studies described above, are composed of many separate components or features. This polymorphic nature of the stimuli raises the possibility that no one single set of features is both necessary and sufficient to determine the category and that variable combinations of features may determine choices toward training and test stimuli by the pigeons. Fersen and Lea (1990) trained pigeons with sets of slides showing buildings. Each slide was characterized by five features, each in one of two possible versions: building type (public house, university building), orientation (upright, oblique), lighting (sunny, cloudy), angle of view (seen from high above, or from ground level), and distance (close by or far away). One version of each feature was designated as positive, the other as negative. The pigeons were rewarded for pecking slides in which three of the five features were positive and were not rewarded for pecking when conversely three of the five stimuli were negative. Only four of the eight pigeons trained ended up by attending to all five discriminative features. A further three, however, did so only after additional corrective training. In any case, these pigeons exhibited proportionally higher peck rates to the slides containing more positive feature variants, that is, the birds responded proportionally to the sum of positive feature variants. Fersen and Lea ascribed this result to the employment of naturalistic stimuli because in an earlier experiment Lea et al., (1993), using artificially constructed stimuli (drawings of seedlike items also incorporating five dichotomous features), had found that pigeons ended up reacting to only one or two of five dichotomous feature dimensions and failed to sum all the relevant features. Huber and Lenz (1993), however, who used schematic faces, and Jitsumori (1993), who used geometric stimuli, found that pigeons attended to all features of their artificial stimuli in an additive fashion. The assessment of presence or absence of feature variants in test stimuli alluded to above could be seen as a kind of feature generalization that adds to the stimulus generalization alluded to before. A difficulty remains in deciding what is the actual set of elementary features that the pigeon's visual system selects to process. Attempts to identify the nature of features used by pigeons when categorizing nonconstructed stimuli have not been overly successful, and even with constructed stimuli it is not always certain that the pigeons' visual system analyzes the compound stimuli in the manner intended by the experimenters (Herrnstein, 1990).

Neurophysiological data on the processing of visual stimuli by optic tectum neurons, analogous to what is known about such processing by visual cortex neurons in mammals, could be useful, but such an analysis has not yet provided much insight as far as our understanding of pigeons' perceptions are concerned. Nevertheless, Delius and Nowak (1982) suggested that the categorization of visual patterns according to their axial symmetry or asymmetry could depend on the interaction of Gabor detector neurons (bar and edge detectors) of the type found in the mammalian visual cortex (De Valois and De Valois, 1988) and that perhaps exist in the optic tectum of pigeons in a modified form (Jassik-Gerschenfeld, 1979). In mammals these Gabor detectors are spatial frequency selective, exist in cosine or sine modulated varieties, and occur in sets coaligned for orientational sensitivity (Pollen and Ronner, 1981). Similarly the sphericity categorization of objects reported by Delius (1992) could rely on the activation of Bessel detectors (doughnut detectors) that are found in the avian and mammalian visual thalamus (Jassik-Gerschenfeld et al., 1979). It would be helpful for the further pursuit of this approach to know what brain structures are involved at all in categorization processes. Watanabe (1996) has presented evidence that lesions in the ectostriatum, the dorsopallial structure that is the telencephalic target of the tecto-thalamic visual system in birds, impair the categorization of visual stimuli. The few data that there are about the responsiveness of ectostriatal neurons could fit with the categorization function implied. The neurons there have been described as having wide receptive fields but containing smaller feature detecting regions (Engelage and Bischof, 1996). A neuron-by-neuron physiological account of how pigeons achieve categorization performances such as those described earlier is still in any case only a remote perspective. Lamentably, there are generally relatively few single unit studies being done on pigeons, although probably they would bring ample returns (see, e.g., Sun and Frost, 1998). That enterprise is at a far more advanced stage with respect, for example, to recognition of faces by rhesus monkeys (*Macaca mulatta*; Bayliss, et al., 1985; Perrett, et al., 1987).

More theoretically, however, it can be shown that such performances can be obtained with adaptive neural networks consisting of only two layers of artificial neurons if the input layer is already a suitable collection of feature detectors. Gluck (1991), for instance, has proposed a neuronal network with an input layer of units that each represent, elementary cues (a, b, c) or cue combinations (ab, ac, bc). All these input units are linked through modifiable connections with each of two output units, one yielding a category x response and the other yielding a category y response. The connection weights are modified by the occurrence of reinforcing feedback on correct category outputs. The cue-recognizing units can be in turn thought of as the output layer of a nonadaptive, preprocessing, multilayer network that can extract the relevant cues from the pixel-like luminosity raster input at the retinal receptor level. Nevertheless, the details of the actual performance of Fersen and Lea's pigeons, for example, appear to be better simulated by a postfeatural three-layer neural network containing a so-called hidden, intermediary layer (Watanabe, et al., 1993). Pearce (1994) has described such a network where the hidden units act as units recognizing feature configurations, that is, units whose output is maximal if a certain configuration of simultaneously occurring stimulus features is present. The network operates according to the so-called exemplar model of categorization in which each stimulus instantiation with which the organism has had experience is separately coded. In any case, the 15 neuronal layers of the avian tectum opticum alone, without the additional retinal, ectostriatal, and postectostriatal layers, allow scope for almost unlimited networking fantasies.

Coming back to reality and to the comparison between mammals and avians, Roberts and Mazmanian (1988) had pigeons, squirrel monkeys (*Saimiri sciureus*), and humans learn to categorize a set of slides that had to be discriminated at different levels of abstraction. They used pictures in which the various experimental subjects were required to distinguish kingfishers from other bird species, birds species from other animals, and then mixed bird and mammal species from inanimate objects. Although humans had no trouble with generalizing the categorizations to novel sets of pictures at all three levels of abstraction, pigeons and monkeys only coped with the first two levels of abstraction. After additional training, the monkeys, but not the pigeons, managed even the most abstract level of categorization involving animal and nonanimal pictures.

CONCEPTS

The ability to learn to discriminate exemplars belonging to classes of stimuli and to apply this discrimination to novel exemplars without additional training was for a long time considered as sufficient evidence of concept formation. Lea (1984), however, pointed out that the term concept is used in a more restrictive sense in the realm of human psychology and argued that the above animal evidence did not warrant its use. He argued that this term would only be valid if stimuli categorized together were additionally shown to belong to a functional equivalence class. Indeed, according to this definition it is not even necessary that the stimuli to be discriminated are perceptually distinct between classes and perceptually similar within classes, as they had to be for the categorization described in the preceding section. Instead, all that was essential for stimuli to be classed together as a concept was that they must control responding in a unitary fashion. Vaughan (1988) trained pigeons with slides that all depicted trees but that were arbitrarily divided into a set of 20 positive, rewarded and another set of 20 negative, nonrewarded slides. When the pigeons had learned to distinguish these arbitrary sets well, the allocation of reward and nonreward between the two sets of slides was exchanged. As soon as the animals had switched their discriminative responding to criterion level, the reinforcement allocations were exchanged again and so on until the birds became proficient at switching their responding upon each reinforcement reversal between the slide sets. At this point, Vaughan could show that experience with reinforcement reversal with only half of the slides of each set was sufficient to induce the pigeons to immediately respond correctly to the remaining half. That is, the birds had conceptualized the stimuli of each set as belonging together in the sense that, when they noticed that some of the slides of the sets had exchanged their functional significance, the birds spontaneously extended the adequate mode of responding to the remainder of the slides. Note that an element of induction is involved: the pigeons appeared to have inferred that, if some members of a conceptual class have acquired a new meaning, then other members were bound to have done so too. Although such an experiment was not actually done, Vaughan's pigeons would thus be expected to transfer their conceptual manner of responding if the same sets of stimuli had been employed as discriminanda in, say, a punishment-reinforced task.

Notice that a conceptualization in the functional equivalence sense is not necessarily restricted to an arbitrary grouping of stimuli. It can be expected to arise also, and perhaps more readily, with stimuli that can be categorized according to perceptual similarity. Indeed, Bhatt and Wasserman (1989) and Fersen and Lea (1990) attempted to demonstrate concept formation with the reinforcement reversal paradigm as extensions of their categorization experiments described above. In fact, their pigeons failed to show the required response reversal, but, differently from Vaughan, they exposed their animals to only a single training reversal. A complication that needs to be kept in mind, though, is that while the reversal in Vaughan's study (1988) and Bhatt and Wasserman's study concerned whole stimuli, those in Fersen and Lea's concerned only component features. More generally, the use of complex stimuli, whether naturalistic or artificial, tends to hamper the understanding of what is involved in the formation of functional concepts because responding to such stimuli usually allows the application of multiple classificatory options.

Delius et al. (1995), therefore, attempted to employ a minimum number of single-featured stimuli. Four different color stimuli were used in a paired manner: red-green and yellow-blue. The pigeons began by learning to discriminate both pairs concurrently using a simultaneous, two-key presentation paradigm r+g–, y+b– where the plus sign means that pecks at the stimulus were rewarded and the minus sign means that responses to the stimulus were penalized. As soon as the animals had learned this task, the reinforcement allocations of both pairs were reversed to r–g+, y–b+ and were again reversed as soon as they had learned this new task. This repeated reversal procedure continued until they became proficient in switching their responding to the stimuli. Then they were tested for the equivalencies r ≡ y and g ≡ b that the training was meant to have established. Test sessions invariably involved reinforcement reversals but were special in that only one of the stimulus pairs was presented during their initial 8 to 12 trials. During these trials the birds had time to adopt correct responding to this pair. During the remainder of the session the other reversed pair was also presented. In these latter trials the second pair occurred more frequently than the first pair. The pigeons' behavioral adaptation to the reversal was on average faster for the second pair than for the first pair, as would be expected by the equivalence hypothesis. In another kind of test session with intermixed pair presentations, a reinforcement reversal was arranged to affect only one stimulus pair and not the other pair instead of both as during the routine reversal sessions. The pigeons showed a worse readjustment learning performance during such half-reversal sessions than during the standard full-reversal sessions. This also suggests that the stimuli r and y and also g and b had been associated together according to their concordant reinforcement consequences during training. The linkage effects, however, were not particularly strong, despite the many preparatory reversals to which the pigeons were exposed before testing (cf. Fersen and Delius, 2000; dolphins, *Tursiops*).

In the above study stimulus generalization might have intervened through the fact that spectrally red is next to yellow and green next to blue on the wavelength spectrum, and the results of the leading-pair/trailing-pair test sessions could have been caused by a within-session warm-up effect. Siemann and Delius (1998a) carried out a study that avoided these defects. Instead of color discriminanda they used two pairs of stimuli selected to be all quite dissimilar physically. The pigeons were conditioned using intelligence panels that were attached to their home cages and that enabled sessions consisting of several hundred trials to be run (Xia et al., 1996). Reinforcement reversals came into effect during these long sessions whenever the pigeons had reached a criterion performance of 70% correct choices in a block of 40 preceding trials. Even though this procedure avoided the shortcomings of the previous study, it still revealed functional equivalence linkages between quite dissimilar stimuli. The effects were again, however, comparatively small.

Recently, Jitsumori et al., (2000) used the same basic procedure as Siemann and Delius but employed more stimuli involved in more pairings and a modified form of testing. Pigeons were taught to discriminate concurrently two sets of four pairs of shapes each a+e–, b+e–, a+f– and b+f– or c+g–, d+g–, c+h– and d+h–. For one group of pigeons the shapes within the a, b, c, d and within the e, f, g, h series were selected to be physically somewhat similar to each other so as to allow potentially a degree of within-series generalization, for another group they were chosen to be quite dissimilar so as to minimise such generalization. When they had achieved a learning criterion of 80% or more correct responses in a block of 80 trials, the reinforcement allocations to the various stimuli were reversed and the pigeons trained again up to criterion and so on until they had undergone more than 16 in-step reversals with both sets. Unreinforced tests for equivalence using novel pairs assembled from the above stimuli (e.g., pairs a*oho* or c*ofo*) revealed that stimulus similarity had facilitated the formation of equivalence concepts a ≡ b ≡ c ≡ d and $e \equiv f \equiv g \equiv h$, although the birds trained with dissimilar stimuli also showed weaker transfer effects. The better concept formation achieved by the former group presumably related to the fact that concepts acquired by organisms in nature are likely to concern mostly stimuli that, because they share equivalent functional properties, are also likely to have some physical similarities with each other (natural concepts; Rosch, 1978).

Neuronal networks may be helpful in explaining why the equivalence effects obtained in the various studies mentioned are rather variable. Generally a three-layer adaptive network is necessary to account for the formation of perceptual concepts of the functional type, where the hidden layer units are those mainly mediating the coding of concepts (Watanabe et al., 1993). Hidden units, however, are only effectively recruited in this way if the training stimulus set is complex enough (many stimuli, many features) and the reversals occur often enough for their concept-adequate activation to yield a processing advantage. Otherwise such neural networks have a tendency to settle on a by-rote categorization, two-layer manner of processing that does not really incorporate a true conceptualization. Of the abovementioned studies producing such variable results, Vaughan's study involved more stimuli and reversals than Bhatt and Wasserman's. Our own studies employed again only a small number of stimuli and features, but very many reversals.

Instead of using coherent reinforcement outcomes, another way of establishing stimulus equivalencies between stimuli is based on a so-called symbolic variant of the matching-to-sample discrimination procedure. With the more usual nonsymbolic form, a trial begins with the presentation of a sample stimulus a on the middle key of a three-key conditioning chamber. Pecks to this stimulus trigger the presentation of comparison stimuli on the side keys, one of them identical to the sample stimulus, a, the other different from it, b. The pigeon has to peck the identical comparison stimulus a to receive the reward. In the symbolic variant of the matching procedure none of the comparison stimuli are identical to the sample. If, for example, the shape a is presented as a sample stimulus on the middle response key, and both shape α and shape β are presented on side keys, the subject is arbitrarily required to choose the α comparison stimulus to obtain reward. On the other hand, if b is the sample stimulus in another trial, β rather than α is defined as the correct comparison stimulus. A symmetry of the equivalence would be demonstrated if the subject trained with this task would spontaneously choose a from among the comparison stimuli after being presented α as sample and b after being presented β as sample in test trials. Equivalence transitivity would be demonstrated if, after having learned the equivalence a ≡ α and also the equivalence α ≡ A according to the above plan, subjects would spontaneously recognise the equivalence between a and A in suitably arranged tests. The symmetry of transitivity would be demonstrated if the animals would similarly recognize the equivalence between stimuli A and a, that is, when the stimuli were presented with reversed sample and comparison roles (Sidman, 1992). Earlier attempts to demonstrate transitive equivalence in pigeons using this method failed (e.g., Lipkens et al., 1988) but recently Kuno, et al. (1994) had success with at least one pigeon. Note also that Yamamoto and Asano (1995) found that a chimpanzee (*Pan troglodytes*) had problems with the symmetry of the equivalence relations and only mastered it after special training. The chimpanzee then demonstrated equivalence transitivity during tests, but still had difficulties with the test on the symmetry of transitivity relations. Normal humans master all these relationships quite easily at the age of 5 years, quite probably because they can bring their linguistic abilities to bear on them (Sidman, 1992).

With logical concepts rather than the perceptual concepts treated thus far, there is no possible confusion with categorization because these concepts are based on quite abstract and general relationships between, in principle, any stimuli. A classic example is the concept of identity versus nonidentity. The straightforward version of the matching-to-sample procedure explained earlier, or indeed its converse, the oddity-from-sample procedure, is used to demonstrate this concept. In the identity task, the pigeon has to peck the physically identical comparison stimulus to receive reward, while in the nonidentity task it has to peck the physically different comparison stimulus to receive reward. A training phase, with stimulus triplets assembled from a given set of stimuli, continues until the pigeons respond mainly correctly. Then they are presented with triplets made from a set of novel stimuli. These serve to check whether they are able to transfer the recognition of the same or different relation between sample and comparisons to novel stimuli. The results of earlier studies seemed to indicate that pigeons could not master this principle but that monkeys could. Zentall and colleagues showed, however, that pigeons that had learned the identity task with one set of stimuli found it easier to relearn the identity task rather than learn the nonidentity task, with a novel set of stimuli. Conversely, pigeons that had learned the nonidentity task found it easier to relearn this task with a novel set of stimuli than to learn the other task (Zentall et al., 1984).

Clearer evidence for an identity/nonidentity concept in pigeons was obtained by Lombardi et al. (1984). They used either 5 or 20 stimuli to train two groups of pigeons on the oddity-from-sample task. The group that learned with more stimuli showed a better transfer performance during tests run under extinction conditions. Under extinction, there was no possibility of learning anything about sets of novel stimuli, including stimuli that were quite different in pictorial style from those used during training (Fig. 15.3). Based on this result Wright et al., (1988) trained one group of pigeons with 152 different stimuli. The pigeons now showed no performance decrement when they were confronted with a variety of novel stimuli. A group of pigeons trained with only two stimuli showed no transfer at all when tested with such stimuli. This result confirms that pigeons are more likely to apply conceptlike rules if the task they have to cope with is constructed so that it strains their considerable capacities for rote learning (Fersen and Delius, 1989; Vaughan and Greene, 1984). Pigeons may be somewhat backward even among birds, however, with gull (Laridae; Benjamini, 1983), crow (Wilson et al., 1985), and parrot (Pepperberg, 1987a) species being certainly more gifted than pigeons at conceptualizing the identity/nonidentity relation, supporting the general assumption that at least the latter two groups may be endowed with cognitive abilities superior to those of pigeons.

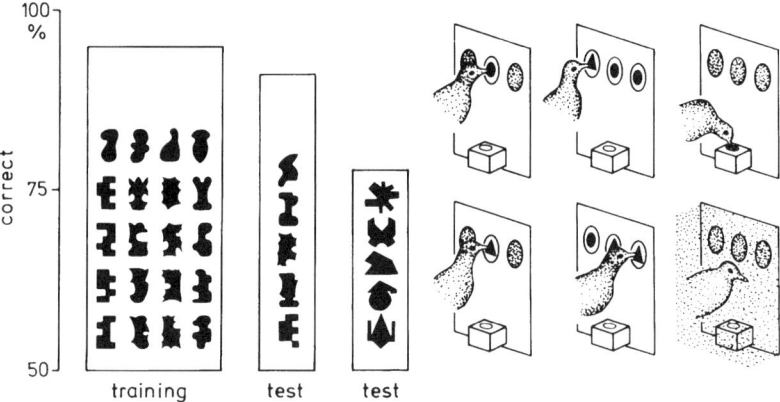

Figure 15.3. Oddity recognition by pigeons. Right: Oddity from sample procedure with a correct trial and an incorrect trial as examples. Left: Performance during test phase with a set of 25 training stimuli and two sets of 5 novel test stimuli each, one similar to the training stimuli and another different from them. (Modified from Lombardi et al., 1984.)

The identity–oddity decisions of pigeons, and perhaps of other species, may be based on judgements about the relative familiarity–novelty of stimuli. By being identical to the previously pecked sample, the identical comparison stimulus is relatively more familiar than the nonidentical stimulus (Delius, 1994). Macphail and Reilly (1989; see also Todd and Mackintosh, 1990) had pigeons learn to discriminate novel, scenic slides they had never seen before from familiar, already seen, scenic slides through rewarding them for pecking the former and not rewarding them for pecking the latter. The pigeons learned to do this in only about 100 trials. They obviously used a familiar/unfamiliar concept that is related to a same/different concept. The competence for distinguishing between familiar and unfamiliar stimuli appears to be widespread among animals, including invertebrates, in the sense that stimulus-specific habituation is a common form of learning. A model originally proposed by Sokolov (1975) to account for several habituation phenomena has been adapted to deal with this phenomenon. A neural network version of it has information about incoming stimuli bifurcating into a specific recognition system and an unspecific arousal system. The recognition system can be instantiated by an associative network capable of memorising many different stimuli (Kohonen, 1984). When this system recognizes a stimulus as one that it has already experienced, it broadcasts a signal that the stimulus is familiar. This signal inhibits the arousal system that otherwise would issue a signal that the stimulus is novel, which normally generates an orienting response. If furnished with a short- as well as a long-term stimulus storage, as well as a forgetting-by-disuse process, the network differentiates between relative familiarity and relative novelty and thus also functions as an identity–oddity detector system. It is conceivable that this mechanism is based on the interplay between the reticular activating system and the dorsopallial cortex-equivalent of birds, but as yet there is no proper evidence on this.

As to a comparison with mammals, it is certain that capuchin monkeys (*Cebus apella*) are quicker than birds at learning matching-to-sample tasks and are more proficient at showing transfer of performance to new stimuli (D'Amato et al., 1985). Neiworth and Wright (1994) furthermore demonstrated that rhesus monkeys could match stimuli belonging to the same categories like faces and flowers. Taking the matter further, Thompson and Oden (1996) have compared the performances of rhesus monkeys, chimpanzees, and humans on physical identity recognition tasks of the kind described above, as well as on another, even more abstract task involving the recognition of the identity of identity relations. Given that a pair of simultaneously presented sample stimuli involve two identical items *aa*, then they bear, at this higher level of abstraction, an identity relation with another pair of comparison items also composed of two identical stimuli *bb*, but bear an oddity relation with a comparison pair composed of two different stimuli *cd*. Rhesus monkeys could only learn to cope with physical identity tasks, but not with ones of the latter relational identity type. Normal chimpanzees were similarly able to recognize physical identity but were unable to recognize relational identity. Chimpanzees previously trained to master a minimal symbolic language, however, could also cope with relational identity tasks (Premack, 1988). Human infants, by contrast, can recognize the relational identity or nonidentity existing between pairs of objects long before they have acquired any use of language (Tyrrell et al., 1993).

TRANSITIVITY

In humans, transitive inference is considered to be a form of deductive thinking. Given, for example, that a rational individual compares for quality a series of items, a, b and c, and he finds out that a is better than b and b is better than c, we expect him to conclude that a is better than c without further comparisons. Pigeons have been shown to do so too. For them the premise information was arranged as a multiple stimulus discrimination task. Five different visual shapes were displayed in four overlapping pairs according to the scheme a+b−, b+c−, c+d−, d+e− using two keys of a conditioning chamber (Fig. 15.4). The right/left key allocation of the stimuli within the pairs and the presentation order of the four pairs were randomized. Pecks to the + stimuli were rewarded with food, and pecks to the − stimuli were penalized with a period of darkness. The training was meant to convey to the pigeons the premises a>b, b>c, c>d, d>e. Note that, whereas the end stimuli a and e were scheduled to be either always rewarded or always penalized, the middle stimuli b, c, and d were meant to be equally often rewarded and penalized.

Four of six pigeons reached a criterion of 80% correct trials within 5000 training trials. They were then occasionally presented the unreinforced conclusion pair bodo interspersed among the training trials. Responses during test trials were neither rewarded nor penalized. All four pigeons nevertheless preferred to peck stimulus b rather than stimulus d, on average on 87.5% of the test trials. The pigeons thus behaved as if they ranked the stimuli according to the inequality b>d, derivable from

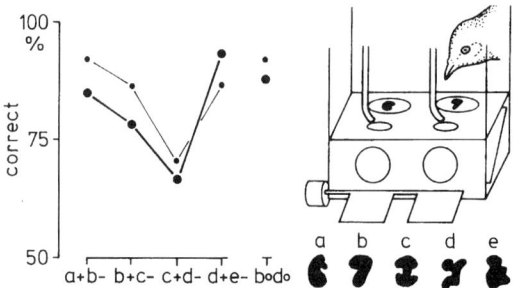

Figure 15.4. Right: Apparatus and stimuli employed to demonstrate transitive responding in pigeons. Left: Large circles: Discrimination performance on the premise pairs and the conclusion pair during the test phase. (Modified from Fersen et al., 1991.) Small circles: Simulation results obtained with Luce's algebraic model. The 50% baseline corresponds to chance choices. (Modified from Delius and Siemann, 1998.)

the inequalities implied by the premise pairs (Fersen et al., 1991; Fig. 15. 4). After the series of premise pairs was expanded by also training the pigeons with an x+a– and an e+f– pair until they reattained criterion, they were tested again with unreinforced conclusion pairs $a_o c_o$, $a_o d_o$, $a_o e_o$, $b_o d_o$, $b_o e_o$, and $c_o e_o$. All these test pairs once more yielded choice preferences that were consistent with transitive inference.

The pigeons in the previous experiment had learned the various premise pairs to unequal levels of proficiency (Fig. 15.4). This fact partially invalidates the design's intention to equate the reinforcements for the critical stimuli b and d. Siemann et al., (1996) replicated part of that study using a different and faster procedure. The pigeons were trained with the usual a+ to e– series, but the stimuli were five different types of grit. These stimuli were offered in a pair of plastic cups with the positive grit concealing grain and the negative grit not hiding anything. The presentation frequencies of the four training pairs were adjusted so that those that had yielded worse discrimination in Fersen's experiment were shown more often than those that had yielded better discrimination. The 4 times a+b–, 6 times b+c–, 7 times c+d–, and 1 time d+e– proportions that were used yielded a fairly even performance across the premise pairs after a total of some 2700 training trials. The pigeons still showed a strong preference for grit b (91% choices) over grit d when confronted with the grainless b–d– test pair. Note that now, however, by design, stimulus b was being relatively more often rewarded than d so that a conditioning account could still not be excluded.

Roberts and Phelps (1994; see also Davis, 1992) trained rats in an arena with pairs of odor-cued boxes, one of which gave access to food and another which did not, according to the a+ to e– scheme using five different odors. When the pairs were set up according to a linear spatial order, with the a>b>c>d>e hierarchy implied by the premise pairs, the rats learned the training pairs to a criterion of 80% correct choices in about 100 trials and exhibited transitivity with test pairs, even when the latter were presented in a spatial layout that differed from the linear order used in training. When the training did not involve a congruent spatial ordering, the rats still managed to learn the premise pairs but, interestingly, failed to pass the transitivity test.

Nonhuman primates have also proved capable of transitive responding. McGonigle and Chalmers (1992) trained squirrel monkeys with the usual scheme of premise pairs consisting of five differently colored tins. For half of the subjects the positive tin of each pair was heavier and hid a peanut, while the negative tin was lighter and hid nothing. For the other half of the animals this arrangement was reversed. Seven of eight monkeys progressively learned the various training pairs up to a level of 90% correct choices in an unspecified but obviously large number of trials. When tested with an equal-weight b+d+ conclusion pair, they showed a 90% preference for b rather than d. Treichler and van Tilburg (1996) trained six macaque monkeys with two initially independent but concurrent tasks (a+ to e–; f+ to j–) using 10 small junk objects. Both series yielded transitive responding with b+d– and g+i– test pairs. The two series were then linked by training with an additional e+f– pair. A large number of novel test pairs could be assembled from within the resulting a+ to j– series, and all of these yielded above-chance transitive responding results.

Boysen et al., (1993; see also Gillan, 1981) trained three chimpanzees on the transitivity task using again five differently colored containers with the usual a+ to e– premise pair scheme to an average 85% correct level in an unspecified number of trials. All three individuals showed a very strong (average 94%) preference for b in b+d+ and b–d– tests. When numerals 1 to 5 replaced the colors as cues, the performance deteriorated, and only one animal passed the conclusion tests, even though all the chimpanzees had been trained successfully before to equate the numerals with corresponding quantities. With further numerosity and transitivity task experience two animals eventually also passed the conclusion test using numerals. In short, a number of advanced animal vertebrate species seem capable of transitive responding when adequately trained with premise pairs and suitably tested with conclusion pairs.

The results of older studies on humans cannot easily be compared with those on animals because they used verbal tasks. Chalmers and McGonigle (1984), however, carried out much the same experiment with 6-year-old children as they had with squirrel monkeys. They found that the children yielded 70% transitive choices in the b+d+ tests and so did not do much better than the squirrel monkeys. Siemann and Delius (1993, 1996) reported a series of nonverbal transitive responding experiments done with university students. To ensure good motivation, the transitivity tasks were presented as computer games. In one experiment 24 student subjects had to navigate a small figure through a castlelike labyrinth. Pairs of swing-doors bore pairs of polygon shapes according to an a+b–, b+c–, c+d–, d+e–, e+f– design. If the positive door was chosen there was a symbolic reward consisting in a coin from a treasure chest. If a negative door was chosen there was a symbolic penalty consisting in having to give a coin to a beggar. All subjects learned the premise pairs within an average of 395 trials to a criterion of at least 70% correct choices. Only 15 subjects, however, responded transitively (at least 70% transitive choices) when faced with the conclusion tests $bodo$, $boeo$ and $codo$ by preferring polygons b and c at well above chance levels (92% average preference). The remaining 9 subjects failed to show transitivity despite having learned the premises. Pigeons, in contrast, only rarely fail to respond transitively if they have discriminated the premise pairs (e.g., Higa-King and Staddon, 1993). We return to this remarkable relative weakness of humans later.

An overall analysis suggests that none of these organisms, not even humans, respond with what might be called deliberative reasoning involving rules of logic. Rather, they seem to do so by processes that are well captured by simple mathematical learning models (Luce operator model: Wynne, et al., 1992; Siemann and Delius, 1998b). These models in turn can be cast into a neuronal network format. One such minimalistic network capable of learning to respond transitively consists of an input, an intermediate, and an output layer that all contain the same number of units. This number must not be less than the number of stimuli occurring in the premise pairs (Fig. 15.5). The input units j are conceived of as reacting specifically to each of these stimuli and the output units l as issuing responses that are directed to each of these stimuli. The o_j output of a j unit equals 1 if the corresponding stimulus is present and 0 if it is not. The input units are connected one-to-one to the intermediate units k. The net input component of a k unit, due to the input from its j unit, is $n_{j,k} = o_j * w_{j,k}$ where the strength or weight $w_{j,k}$ of the connection will be specified soon. This net input component persists for a period of time in the corresponding k unit but also yields an immediate output $o_k = n_{j,k}$.

Each hidden unit k is connected to all output units l so as to form a forward lateral inhibition network. The net input of the l units is thus $n_l = \Sigma o_k * w_{k,l}$ with $w_{k,l} = 1$ when k = l, but $w_{k,l} = -1$ when k ≠ l. The output of each l unit is either $o_l = 1$, a response to when stimulus i = l is present, or $n_{k,l} > 0$, or else $o_l = 0$, a no-response when $n_{k,l} < 0$. That is, there is an exclusive response to one of the stimuli, namely, the one that activates the path with the strongest connection $w_{k,l}$ of a given pair on a given trial. Depending on whether the response issued corresponds to a stimulus scheduled to

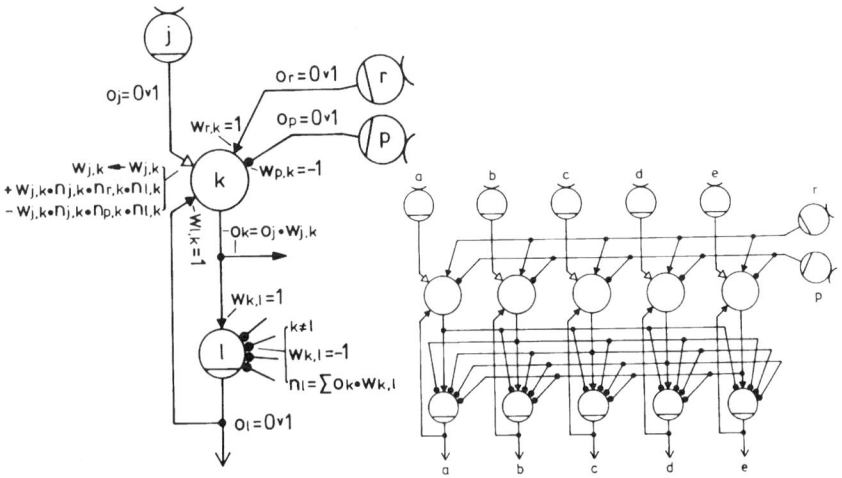

Figure 15.5. Adaptive neuronal net for transitive responding. Right: Overall network. Large circles are neuronal units; arcs designate input units (j); arrows designate output units (l); bars designate units with thresholds. Triangles indicate excitatory connections; circles, inhibitory connections. Open triangles are connections with variable weight. Left: The detailed network allocates the algebraic functions explained in the text to the various network components. The symbol ∨ stands for "or"; the remaining symbols are explained in the text. (Modified from Siemann and Delius, 1998b.)

yield a reward or corresponds to a stimulus scheduled to yield a penalty, either input unit r or input unit p is activated with a small time delay so that either $o_r = 1$ and $o_p = 0$, or else $o_p = 1$ and $o_r = 0$. These outputs are relayed to all hidden layer units. This corresponds to the widely distributed reinforcement-mediating systems found in vertebrate brains (Rolls, 1975; Delius and Pellander, 1982). The reward and penalty signals contribute to delayed latent net-input components in the hidden k units with the activations $n_{r,k} = w_{r,k} * o_r$ where $w_{r,k} = 1$, and $n_{p,k} = w_{p,k} * o_p$ where $w_{p,k} = -1$. These signals initiate a $w_{j,k}$ increment/decrement only in the stimulus-response link that was instrumental in bringing about either the reward or the penalty consequence. This link specificity is ensured by recurrent feedback connections from the output units l to the corresponding units k. The feedbacks activate with a brief time delay the k units according to $n_{l,k} = o_l$. This activation equals 1 in the k units for which $k = i$, corresponding to the stimulus i that was responded to, and equals 0 in all the $k \neq i$ units, corresponding to the stimuli i not responded to. The $n_{l,k}$ activation acts as a gating factor that permits or does not permit the reinforcement messages o_r or o_p to bring about a Hebbian-like $w_{j,k}$ change (Kandel et al., 1991). In conjunction with the delayed net-input components specified earlier, $n_{r,k}$, $n_{p,k}$ and $n_{j,k}$, the activation $n_{l,k}$ occasions an updating of the relevant j to k connections according to the update function $w_{j,k} \leftarrow w_{j,k} + (w_{j,k} * n_{j,k} * n_{r,k} * n_{l,k}) - (w_{j,k} * n_{j,k} * n_{p,k} * n_{l,k})$. This operation only modifies the weight of the connection and does not lead to any immediate k unit output. All net-input components reset $n_{z,k} = 0$ as soon as the weight adjustment has taken place.

Recurrent pathways of the kind used by the model are frequent in real brains (Durand et al., 1997; Vates et al., 1997; Veenman, 1997), but the idea that they may be subserving the allocation of reinforcement effects on stimulus-response links is probably new. They represent a neurally realistic replacement for the commonly used, but neurally unrealistic, error back-propagation scheme (Churchland and Sejnowski, 1993). In any case, when trained according to the usual experimental scheme, the network very soon produces a perfect transitive performance on all the training and test pairs. To mimic the less than perfect performance of real organisms, the finished model has to include a noise variable much as real neurons actually do (Kandel et al., 1991). The reader is referred to Siemann and Delius (1998b) for the demonstration that this "noisy" network comes close to simulating the behavior of most animal and many human subjects performing in nonverbal transitive responding tasks. Here we should mention the possibility that a learning process, embodied in the so-called value-transfer theory originally advocated by Fersen et al. (1991), may also intervene in bringing about transitive-like responding. This process differs from the instrumental discrimination learning of stimuli incorporated in the above network and seems to operate under certain special training arrangements (Steirn et al., 1995). The value-transfer process is akin to classical conditioning. The existence of such a conditioning process is undisputed, but the question is whether it intervenes to any appreciable degree in a standard transitive responding task (Siemann et al., 1996). In any case, the addition of this mechanism into the above network signifies only a minor modification (Siemann and Delius, 1998b).

We thus assume that a real neuronal network, structured much as that described above, underlies transitive competencies, but, beyond suspecting that the adaptive intermediate layer is likely to be located at the corticostriatal interface, we cannot say more about the correspondence of the model network to brain structures. We (Siemann and Delius, 1998b; see also Wynne, 1995) have, however considered why it is that often animals, and occasionally humans (see above), learn to discriminate the premise pairs but fail to respond transitively to the conclusion pairs. The assumption is that humans, but more particularly animals, can bring into play an additional layer of so-called configural units that respond to the stimulus combinations (a+b−), (b+c−), (c+d−), (d+e−) rather than to the individual stimuli a to e. When the premises are exclusively learned on the basis of these configural units, the network can indeed not respond transitively to the test pair bodo because it has previously learned nothing about this particular configuration. Superficially this might be seen as a regression in cognitive competency but it ignores the fact that transitivity is a generally valid property only of linear relational structures between stimuli. Whenever there are exceptions to such linearity in a structure these can only be captured through configural units. In experiments involving the pairwise learning of, for example, circular relational structures and comparing pigeons and humans, Siemann and Delius (1994) found that birds could not cope with the task while people could. Delius and Siemann (1998b) argued more generally that the transitive responding of pigeons, in the manner of the above neural network, represented little more than the application of a basic stimulus discrimination mechanism capable of dealing with the simple social hierarchies of birds. The responding of humans, and probably apes, accords with the more complex network that can cope with nonlinear structures. This, they suggest, is the evolutionary result of the more sophisticated structures and thus more demanding characteristics of primate social groups (De Waal, 1988).

NUMEROSITY

Koehler (1941) and his students were among the first to investigate experimentally and systematically the numerosity capabilities of several avian and mammalian species. They showed that birds (pigeons, corvid, and parrot species) could discriminate between numbers of items, such as seeds or ink-blobs, up to about six versus seven items, depending on the species. They tested the birds in the quasinaturalistic settings of aviaries rather than in the more tightly controlled, high-tech environment of modern training chambers. Nevertheless, Koehler went to considerable lengths to control for stimulus factors that could potentially be confounded with numerosity and to guard against observers unintentionally cueing the animals' performance. Modern research has confirmed several of Koehler's findings and has also extended the work on numerosity discrimination. For instance, Emmerton and Delius (1993) report an experiment in which pigeons learned to choose between two simultaneously projected visual displays containing different numbers of dots. When the animal pecked the key displaying more items it was rewarded, whereas if it pecked the key displaying the lesser number it was penalized by timeout. The difference between the number of items in the pairs of displays was progressively reduced to one, and then ranged between one versus two and seven versus eight. After this, test trials were introduced in which the new displays differed from the familiar ones in the size and arrangement of the items. The brightness of each display within the novel pairs was also equated. On these test trials, the pigeons were able to transfer their discrimination of choosing the greater number without difficulty but the accuracy of their discrimination depended on the number of items in each pair. They were about 80% correct in their choices for one versus two items, but their performance level dropped systematically to about 55% correct with the seven versus eight comparison. This latter score was no longer significantly different from the 50% chance level.

More evidence that it is the numerosity, rather than any other dimension of the stimuli, that is important was provided by Emmerton et al., (1997). They trained pigeons to discriminate successively presented displays containing one or two ("few") small items from displays containing six or seven ("many") small items. When a "few" item display was presented on a given trial, the pigeons had to peck one side-key to obtain reward. If a "many" item display was shown, they had to peck the other side-key for reward. If the animals chose the wrong key they were penalized with timeout. When the pigeons' performance reached at least 85% correct they were given interspersed test trials involving the presentation of displays containing new amounts of three, four or five items, as well as novel displays for the numerosities used for "few" and "many." There were more choices of the side-key corresponding to "few" when three items were seen and increasingly more than chance level choices of the "many" side-key for four and five items. For five, six, and seven items, the discrimination performance leveled off, indicating that the birds could not differentiate among these larger amounts as well as they did the smaller quantities. These results were maintained when the birds were shown additional displays that varied in brightness, contrast, item size, and arrangement so as to exclude cues other than numerosity. The numerosity of items thus seems to be represented in an orderly manner by pigeons.

The type of task and the data obtained in this experiment were reminiscent of those in an earlier study of rats' discrimination of stimuli that varied either in time or number. Meck and Church (1983) trained rats to press one lever following a series of two sound tones that lasted in all for 2 seconds and another lever following a series of eight tones lasting eight seconds. In test trials, the duration of all series of sounds was held constant at 4 seconds but their number varied. Like pigeons, rats distributed their responses to the two levers in a systematic fashion as the number of tones in a series varied between two and eight.

The discrimination of numerosity is not confined to these relatively small numbers of items, however. Honig (1993) has shown that pigeons can still perform numerosity discriminations even when the number of elements ranges up to 64. In one study, the birds had to discriminate differences in the total numbers of dots, for example, 16 versus 25, in successively presented displays. In another, they had to discriminate according to the proportion of different items (e.g., red vs. blue dots) within successively presented arrays, each containing a constant total number of items (Honig and Stewart, 1989). In the latter experiment, when there were relatively more red dots than blue, for instance, the birds had to peck the key through which they saw the display and were rewarded for doing so. When the proportions were reversed, however, they received no reward for pecking so that responding to these arrays ceased at some point.

What may be more important than the absolute differences in number between displays is the relative difference (but see Honig, 1993). In a recent experiment (Emmerton, 1998a), pigeons were again trained to choose between simultaneously presented groups of dots. Irrespective of the absolute numbers of dots in the paired displays, for some birds, choice of "more" was always rewarded and choice of "less" led to timeout, whereas for other birds these contingencies were reversed. There was apparently a preference for choosing "more" items so that the birds for which this relative quantity was correct yielded better discrimination results to begin with than those for which "less" was correct. With extended training, this bias was no longer apparent, although it reemerged when novel displays were introduced on nonreinforced trials. Once both groups of animals had reached similar levels of performance, their discrimination scores, when expressed on a logarithm-related scale, increased as the relative discrepancy in numerosity of the paired displays increased. This is one line of evidence that suggests that Weber's law may apply to the discrimination of numerosity in these birds. Basically, this law tells us that, as the base number of items increases, so too there is a proportional increase in the size of the difference between this reference amount and another number that can just be discriminated from it. Other results from pigeons also seem to fit this law, for instance, the earlier findings that small numbers in the range one to four are better discriminated than numbers in the range five to seven (Emmerton et al., 1997), as well as some of Honig's findings that pigeons can discriminate the proportion of elements, even when the absolute numbers vary (Honig and Stewart, 1989). Weber's law may generally characterize numerical differentiation in other animals too, because species varying from rats to chimpanzees seem to base their discrimination of numerosities more on relative than on absolute differences (rats: Meck and Church, 1983; chimpanzees: Boysen et al., 1996).

Although the above experiments on pigeons demonstrate a numerical-like apprehension of item quantities, they still lack the demonstration of a one-to-one linkage of these quantities to representations such as the numerical symbols that play such a prominent role in the counting performance of educated humans. Xia et al., (2000a) reports an experiment in which pigeons learned to peck at a number of visual items that were presented on a computer monitor and that varied on a trial-by-trial basis. Having pecked these items, the birds had to report the number of items they had seen by choosing one of several symbols presented at the end of each trial, where each symbol represented an exact number of items. Thus the birds had to learn a one-to-one correspondence between number of items and specific symbols. The pigeons were successively trained session by session to respond in this manner to one item and one symbol, one and two items and two symbols, and so on. In the final situation, five birds were able to respond to varying, trial-by-trial presentations of one, two, three, or four items and to choose one of four symbols corresponding to these numbers. Two of these birds were also able to learn this correspondence for five items. The pigeons chose correctly among these symbols at levels that were significantly above the chance level of 20%. The five birds that learned one to four items scored 63% correct on average. The two birds given additional training scored 70% correct on trials with five items. Xia showed furthermore that the pigeons continued to evince such counting behavior with novel forms of items (squares or butterflies rather than circles), even if the novelty transitorily depressed performance. One cannot however, overlook the fact that it took the pigeons up to some 18,000 trials to cope with the five item task. On the other hand, it is not certain that five is the maximum that pigeons could potentially count in this manner. Perhaps with further training they would have managed to count six or more items. Alex, an African gray parrot (*Psittacus erithacus*), has been taught to produce vocal numerical labels for groups of up to six objects (Pepperberg, 1987b; cf. Smirnova et al., 2000.). This performance has been slightly exceeded in chimpanzees that have been trained to use Arabic numerals to label arrays containing up to eight objects (Boysen, 1993).

Xia (1997) and Xia et al. (2000b) also gradually trained another group of pigeons in an experiment that involved making specific numbers of key-pecks following given symbols. First the birds had to peck a symbol when it was presented at the beginning of the trial. Then they had to peck one key a particular number of times before pecking a different one to receive reward. Six birds were able to learn this task up to a limit of five pecks, and for four of these birds this limit was extended to six pecks after further training. The symbol presented on a given trial was thus one of six and the number of subsequent pecks required varied between one and six, depending on the symbol presented at the beginning of any trial. If the pigeons pecked too few times on the response key before calling up the reward on the other key or pecked once too many on the response key, they were penalized with a timeout period (Fig. 15.6). Again the training progressed from using only the symbol corresponding to one within a session to finally using one of five or else six different symbols from trial to trial to signal the number of pecks to be made. For the four birds that completed the task for up to six pecks, the mean percentages of correct trials for the one to six pecks required were well above the corresponding chance levels. These decreased because of the mounting

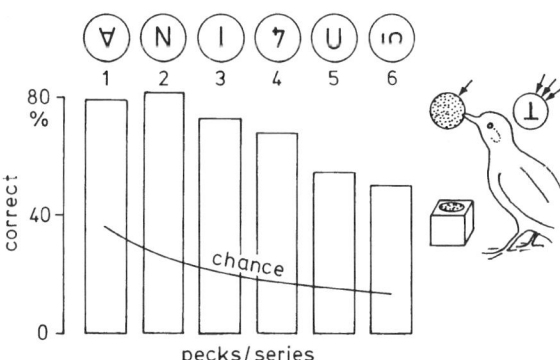

Figure 15.6. Production of responses numerosities depending on symbolic label instructions in pigeons. (Right) Example of a correct trial involving the symbolic instruction 3 on the business key, that number of pecks to it, and a peck on the end key followed by grain reward. (Left) Percent correct peck series on business key as a function of instruction stimulus. The chance level is determined by the number of possible alternative series. (Modified after Xia, et al., 2000b.)

number of erroneous choices possible with the increasing numerosities. When the birds made errors, they tended to do so by issuing a number of pecks close to the correct number. So here, performance accuracy decreased as the target number of pecks increased. The birds had more experience with the low numerosities than with the higher ones, however, and the chance of producing random correct choices was higher for smaller than for larger numerosities. It must be noted that to attain this final performance level, the pigeons needed an average of over 30,000 trials. Again it is well possible that the pigeons could have coped with higher numerosities if given even more training. For comparison, Lögler (1959) managed to train an African gray parrot with a task that involved somewhat less symbolic instruction than that used by Xia et al. (2000b) to selectively produce up to 8 responses, depending on the visual cues given.

What kind of neural mechanism could underlie these kinds of numerical abilities? One possibility is the neural network model proposed by Dehaene and Changeux (1993). It consists of a sensory layer that represents the items perceived as size-varying so-called blobs. A second layer normalizes these blobs so that their size is no longer a critical factor. In a third layer, activity from the second layer is summated and compared with threshold settings. Then a fourth layer consists of numerosity clusters. A specific numerosity is detected when one of these clusters responds to a limited range of activity that it receives as input from the previous threshold-setting layer. All stages involve network operations that are reasonably well understood. The model is particularly suitable for explaining how the numerosity of items in visual arrays may be abstracted by parallel processing, although Dehaene and Changeux (1993) also affirm that it would apply to serially presented auditory stimuli if an additional sensory memory stage is assumed.

A timing and sequential counting model based on different principles has been developed by Meck and Church (1983; see also Roberts and Mitchell, 1994). It incorporates a pacemaker that emits regular pulses, one or more gated accumulators that can be switched to operate in either a timing or counting mode, and one or more working memory units that store updated timing or counting information. The accumulator stage collects pulses from the pacemaker. When the system is operating in a counting mode, the start of each event is marked by a limited number of pulses reaching the accumulator. This accumulated information is passed to working memory and is subsequently compared with more permanent information from reference memory for a behavioral decision to be made about whether or not a predetermined "count" has been achieved yet. A specific number is thus represented by a function based on number of pulses accumulated.

Staddon and Higa (1998) have recently proposed an alternative multiple time-scale model that accounts for a variety of timing effects, some of which the above pacemaker-accumulator model has difficulties explaining. Because of its mode of processing time intervals, the model can also be applied to the counting of stimulus events, such as occurrences of food rewards or of light flashes. Any stimulus event is assumed to produce an internal marker or short-term memory trace that decreases in strength as a function of time. Multiple events will boost the strength of a fading trace. Thus this model does not assume the presence of a clock pacemaker, but represents a memory-based explanation for timing and counting operations. Organisms are assumed to learn to differentiate memories of different strengths in order to discriminate the times between events or the numbers of stimulus occurrences. They thus come to perform different behavioral responses (such as "peck this key rather than that one") on the basis of changing memory trace magnitudes.

All these models probably account for the Weber style degradation of discrimination accuracy with increasing numerosities, although the pacemaker-accumulator model requires some special assumptions in order to do so. As described previously, these effects refer to a decrease in discriminability with increasing numerosity of items in stimulus arrays or series. The neural network model (Dehaene and Changeux, 1993) can best deal with numerosity discrimination of simultaneous stimulus arrays whereas the other two models seem more suited for discrimination of sequentially presented stimuli. This difference may, however, be less critical than it appears. Some recent data from pigeons suggest they might successively "scan" simultaneous arrays of dots, processing these elements one by one (Emmerton, 1998b). These birds were trained on a simultaneous discrimination between paired arrays of dots and they always had to choose the array with the smaller number of items to obtain a food reward. Although discrimination accuracy mainly depended on the numerosity differences between arrays, performance level was also affected when the spacing between the dots within arrays was altered. In particular, if the dots were spaced further apart in the "incorrect," larger number array, more errors were made, as if the birds scanned each array for the number of dots present and erroneously pecked at such an array prematurely before it had noticed all the dots.

To what extent the models proposed thus far accurately reflect the way the brain processes number remains debatable. Dehaene and Changeux's model (1993) has the advantage of neural plausibility, but it is easier to see how it could function under conditions of parallel uptake of visual input. The pacemaker-accumulator model (Meck and Church, 1983; Roberts and Mitchell, 1994) unites timing and counting processes, but it is not clear how its component parts could be realized neuronally. The multiple time-scale model (Staddon and Higa, 1998) also applies to both timing and counting and, while not postulating specific neural mechanisms, it is based on realistic properties of memory trace decay. In fact, the only evidence thus far for neurons that "count" comes from a study by Thompson et al. (1970) of cells in the cat's (*Felis catus*) association cortex. They found a few cells that responded with increased firing rate to, for instance, the sixth stimulus in a series. Other cells seemed to encode the numbers 2, 5, and 7. The stimulus item's ordinal number was important for triggering a response in these neurons, but neither the stimulus intensity nor modality (auditory or visual), nor, within limits, the temporal gap between stimuli in a series, seemed to be critical.

EPILOGUE

In the preceding sections we have described the capabilities of pigeons in categorization, conceptualization, transitivity, and numerosity tasks. Where feasible we have compared their competencies with those of other birds and mammals, including humans. We may summarize the above sections by asserting that pigeons do quite well in a number of behavioral tasks that are widely considered to involve cognitive processing of information. Some corvid and parrot species are known (see above), or suspected, however, to do even better on the same kinds of tasks. The cognitive anagenesis of these species, much as in primate species, is likely to have been primarily driven by the intricacies of the selfish and altruist strategies that determine the inclusive Darwinian fitness game (Hamilton, 1974) and which are fostered by the complex interactions in social systems (Trivers, 1985). Whether the performance of pigeons is better or worse than that of mammals of similar brain size remains uncertain because we largely lack the empirical basis for a valid comparison. Rats resemble pigeons in brain and body size, but their olfactory rather than visual dispositions make them an inconvenient species for the comparison enterprise. Moreover, their competencies on the kind of cognitive tasks that we have reviewed are still poorly investigated. Among the diurnal primate species that compare for visuality with pigeons, those that have been studied in any detail are all much larger brained than pigeons. From capuchins through chimpanzees to humans, though, all primate species seem fairly clearly to out-do pigeons in the speed with which they learn the relevant cognitive tasks, in the degree of task abstractness with which they can cope, and/or in the range of transfer to other contexts that they exhibit; but then all the better studied primate species have markedly larger brains (absolutely) than the pigeon has.

Still, as stressed many times but as equally often ignored, the course of evolution is arguably more importantly determined by the process of cladogenesis (specialization) than it is by that of anagenesis (advancement). The peak cognitive competencies of birds may differ from those of mammals, and also the cognitive peaks of pigeons might not be the same as those of other bird species. The point is that, almost by definition, different species inhabit differing socioecological niches. Evolution functions to progressively adapt each species to each of these differing habitats, as long as this adaptation is not held back by a conserving selection exerted by the existing intragenomic environment. This means that to gauge the cognitive capacities of a given species we really should test it with tasks that correspond closely to those that they are more likely to encounter in their natural environment. Possibly because of having been guided from the outset by naturalistic field work (Frisch, 1965), experimentation with the honeybee (*Apis mellifica*) has revealed remarkable cognitive capacities for such a tiny-brained insect (Menzel, Giurfa, Gerber, and Hellstern, this volume, Chapter 11).

It may thus be worth considering particularly those competencies in which some bird species, because of the special environmental demands that they acutely face, must be expected to excel. Their flying ability is one such competency that we have already linked to the relative cerebellarization of the avian brain (Dubbledam, 1998), but we can at present only guess what, for example, the aerodynamically remarkable wave-riding, gliding-flight of albatrosses (Diomedidae) requires in terms of cognitive skills (Sachs, 1993). The increase in mobility that the capacity of flying entails, however, enhances the need for navigational abilities, and about these more is known. Migration, often over long distances, is yet another evolutionary adaptation to seasonal stresses that is found in many avian species (Berthold, 1996). Past experience is known to determine their goal-directed navigation to their winter quarters. Starlings (*Sturnus vulgaris*), for instance, can only maintain an innate fixed-compass orientation during their first autumn migration and thus cannot correct for wind or experimentally induced lateral drifts from their route. During their first spring migration, however, they can truly navigate to end up quite close to the birthplace to which they imprinted as youngsters. In their subsequent autumn migrations they also navigate their return to their habitual wintering area (Perdeck, 1958). For the plain-compass orientation, starlings and other daylight migrants rely on a sun-compass mechanism involving a solar azimuth compensated by circadian time computation. Birds are also sensitive to the polarization patterns of skylight that are sun-azimuth related, and daytime migrants use these as an additional source of navigational information. In night migrating species, a star compass provides directional cues (Kramer, 1961). In addition they use polarized light patterns at dusk (between sunset and the time the first stars appear) as primary navigational information through which their magnetic compass is then calibrated (Able and Able, 1997). This in-built magnetic compass relies on the inclination rather than polarity properties of the earth's magnetic field for the discrimination of north from south (Wiltschko and Wiltschko, 1971). The targeted homing navigation demonstrated by migrating birds, but also by nonmigrating species when displaced from their breeding site and released, naturally requires more than a compass. Pigeons of the homing variety that have long been selectively bred for this ability have been subjects of much research on this problem without it being clear what principle they use for its solution. Even though it is difficult to imagine how it might work in detail, evidence has accumulated that pigeons require experience with olfactory stimuli at their home loft and exposure to the same stimuli at the release site to head for and arrive at home (Wallraff, 1991). This may relate to the fact that their telencephalon is well provided with olfactory projection areas (Wenzel, 1981). The fact that lesions of the hippocampal formation markedly impair homing could also have to do with this but could also have to do with the fact that at short range pigeons clearly depend on previously acquired visual knowledge about navigational cues (Bingman and Jones, 1994).

Seasonal stress, mentioned earlier, is countered by some bird species with food hoarding during the autumn. When food is abundant these birds collect food items and hide them in a variety of sites that they visit later when food is scarce. This behavior has been well studied in titmice (Paridae) and in jays (Corvidae; Clayton and Dickinson, 1998). The important finding is that the hoards, of which tits may install hundreds and jays thousands, are undoubtedly found again under the guidance of memory and not simply by searching in likely places. This requires a remarkably extensive long-term spatial memory. An interesting fact is that among closely related species some species store food and others do not. This affords the opportunity to look for neural specialization among brains that are otherwise highly similar. In fact, storing species not only exhibit a basically larger hippocampus but this structure also swells as storing occurs (Healy, 1996; Krebs, 1990). This may again relate to the finding that this formation seems to be involved in the spatial abilities of pigeons too. It is of course interesting that the hippocampus has also been strongly implicated in the spatial learning competencies of rats and other mammals (McNaughton and

Morris, 1987). That jays out-do tits in remembering food stores may again reflect the fact that, as corvids, they may be more gifted. One should not forget, however, that their brains are about three times as large as those of titmice. Though they do not demonstrate it as impressively as these tits and jays during their normal life, pigeons nevertheless have a capacious memory for hundreds of visual stimuli (Vaughan and Greene, 1984; Fersen and Delius, 1989), which may underlie the fact that, as mentioned above, a familiarity with the relevant terrain aids their homing navigation (Braithwaite and Guilford, 1991). Interestingly, both pigeons and tits show evidence of memorizing with a left hemisphere bias (Fersen and Güntürkün, 1990; Clayton and Krebs, 1995). Such lateralization of cognitive functions was formerly seen as the hallmark of human cognition but it seems to be widespread in birds and to affect many behavioral competencies (Rogers, 1995; Güntürkün, 1997).

The extravagant breeding strategies to which some bird species resort can also be suspected to call for cognitive competencies. Even though, for example, South American ovenbirds (*Furnarius*) mostly manage to build their mud-walled, two-chambered nest under largely instinctive control when they do so for the first time as yearlings, the quality of the nest ovens and the speed with which they are built improves markedly as the birds gain in experience with age (Hermann, 1965). The attachment between parents and offspring based on imprinting, a very rapid learning during a limited age phase that occurs particularly in geese and chickens (Anatidae, Phasianidae), is known to be associated with the activation of circumscribed telencephalic areas (Honey et al., 1995). Of special interest is the fact that imprinting, although undoubtedly a learning process, is normally channelled by largely innate predispositions about what to imprint to. This may reflect the presence of adaptive networks that have been half assembled by evolutionary adaptation but are only completely specified by ontogenetic learning, presumably to ensure the express and faultless learning that is essential for the survival of the nidifugous offspring of the relevant species (Bolhuis, 1996). It is also interesting that this learning, which initially subserves filial attachments, later comes to control, often in a sex-differentiated way, the mate choices of the adult birds (Oetting and Bischof, 1996).

The key significance of mate selection for the fitness of offspring can easily trigger sexual selection processes. These in turn can involve cognitive operations. The song of most of the 4500 or so species of songbirds (Oscines) is acquired through imitative learning involving auditory imprinting. The song heard from the father, sometimes also from the neighbors, or played in experiments by a tape recorder, is memorized during a juvenile, sensitive age-phase lasting a few days or weeks. Later the grown-up males, when their vocal apparatus has fully developed, learn through trial and error to match stepwise and quite closely their vocal output to this memorized auditory template (Kroodsma and Miller, 1996). Some species, such as the nightingales (*Luscinia*), acquire in this way hundreds of song syllables that are then produced in a variety of constrained, nonrandom song sequences (Hultsch and Todt, 1989). In such specially gifted species, sensitive periods for the acquisition of new auditory templates tend to recur each year. Song reception and production are mediated by several interconnected telencephalic, diencephalic, and mesencephalic nuclei (Wild, 1997). Much is known about the neurophysiological functioning of this circuitry (Mello and Clayton, 1994; Wallhäusser-Franke et al., 1995; Vates et al., 1997). Because of the essentially imitative transmission of bird song, it has led de facto to a profusion of different song traditions. These song cultures presumably began about 40 million years ago when the common ancestor of present-day songbirds appeared (Delius, 1991). In common with human language, bird song leads to the formation of dialects (Catchpole, 1986) and is controlled principally by the left brain hemisphere (Saito and Maekawa, 1993). Not only do birds out-do mammals in the number of species capable of vocal learning (several thousand birds against a bare hundred mammals), but also they have turned out to be different from the mammals in that telencephalic neurons of adult birds are subject to massive yearly renewal. In songbirds there is good evidence that this may serve to replace saturated memory banks by blank ones, allowing thus the periodic refreshment of song repertoires (Alvarez-Buylla and Kirn, 1997).

Remarkably, though, despite all the complexities birdsong can attain, its communicative functions are very limited. This is probably not so for the vocalizations of parrots, which are among the few nonsongbird species that are capable of vocal learning. The African gray parrot Alex gradually learned, through imitation and reward, to answer questions about the names, attributes, and actions connected with about 100 different small objects. Terms that he had learned to apply to a series of training objects, he also regularly applied correctly to a collection of new objects. He can answer questions about the presence or absence, similarity or difference, and size relations of a selection of these novel objects (Pepperberg and McLaughlin, 1996; Pepperberg, 1996). Alex was asked, for instance, how many blue keys there were within a collection of six objects shown to him on a tray that also contained green keys and blue corks. He usually answered such questions with more than 80% accuracy (Pepperberg, 1994). Alex only performs when in close social contact with the experimenter, however, a fact that has raised the criticism that his achievements might be aided by unintended but artifactual signaling by the experimenter. Manabe et al. (1995) have begun to develop a method that excludes the intervention of such an effect. Budgerigars (*Melopsittacus undulatus*) spontaneously produce a variety of vocalizations that can be recognized by a suitably equipped computer. Through reward conditioning the birds can be brought to produce the individual calls only in the presence of particular visual stimuli. The repertoire of the probably less gifted budgerigars is still, however, quite limited (see, however Manabe et al., 1997). The reverse problem of letting them learn to select specified visual stimuli with corresponding vocalizations has not yet been tried. From a phylogenetic point of view, however, it is interesting, and in agreement with convergent evolution, that the vocalization-controlling neural substrates of parrots differ somewhat from those of songbirds (Striedter, 1994; Durand et al., 1997).

The design of laboratory experiments, however, is often dictated by research traditions and by technological conveniences rather than by ecological validity. It is thus risky to deny to a given species a particular kind of competency only because it failed to show it in a highly rational, but hare-brained rather than bird-brained experiment. As elsewhere in science, negative evidence is unfortunately a poor basis on which to base safe conclusions. As cognitive tasks are fashioned to fit the peculiarities of a given species however, they become less suitable as tools for across-species comparisons. To the extent that it may be desirable to assess the general intelligence of a species rather than its quaint specializations, it may be reasonable to test it with contrived, non-natural, laboratory problems. It is part of the definition of intelligence that it concerns a competency that largely determines the performance of many different cognitive tasks. In humans, intelligence is arguably best measured with tests that set problems having minimal ecological validity because their solution is not helped by expertise (Carpenter et al., 1990). Intelligence refers to the aspects of speed and quality of information-processing that are least influenced by experience, even though its functional value lies in the fact that it improves the utilization of information arising from experience.

These characteristics of intelligence are thought to be instantiated by a serially operating neural processor that controls the behavioral output of an individual over some brief period of time. It is considered to be closely associated with short-term memory, or working memory as it is more usually called nowadays (Baddeley, 1997). It is worth mentioning a study that compared pigeons, macaques, and humans for the capacity and dynamics of short-term memory (Wright, 1989). Over many trials, these species were presented, for brief instants and in quick succession, a series of four different pictorial stimuli that were drawn without repetitions from a very large collection of photographic slides. After a retention interval that varied in duration from trial to trial, they were presented with either one of the slides that had been part of the series or a novel stimulus. The subjects then had to press either a "same stimulus" or an "odd stimulus" key to receive a reward. If they pressed the incorrect one they were penalized with a period of darkness. The three species exhibited quite similar patterns of so-called primacy-recency effects. Depending on the length of the retention interval, pictures shown at the beginning (primacy) and/or at the end (recency) of the series were better remembered. This indicates that the task was tapping a similar mechanism in pigeons, macaques, and humans. The retention intervals at which the various serial position patterns emerged differed between the species, however, ranging up to 10 seconds in pigeons, up to 30 seconds in macaques, and up to 100 seconds in humans. With humans, incidentally, it was important to use meaningless kaleidoscope pictures because otherwise they could name the slides and achieve near perfect recall performance, regardless of sequence position. In short, a species' intelligence may be partly determined by the capacity and the persistence of its working memory. In primates the working memory function has been more or less convincingly ascribed to parts of the prefrontal cortex (Goldman-Rakic, 1992). This has lead to a search for an equivalent of the prefrontal cortex in pigeons. The neostriatum caudolaterale is at present considered a possible candidate on the basis of both anatomical and behavioral evidence (Güntürkün and Durstewitz, this volume, Chapter 14; Aldavert-Vera et al., 1998).

Cognitive performances shown by an individual, as with any other phenotypic characteristics that it may show, are the end product of its phylogeny, ontogeny, and physiogeny, in that order. Perhaps more than in any of the other characteristics, the detailed causal pathways involved in this process are obscured by the almost arbitrary nature of the selective forces that drove their phylogeny, the lifelong plasticity of the brain that enabled their ontogeny, and the endless intricacies of the layout and functioning of the nervous circuitry that underlies their physiogeny. This chapter has stressed that the evolution of brains is driven by natural selection operating on the behavioral products that they can produce and that the layout of neural microcircuits, rather than gross brain structures, are the relevant substrates of behavior in general and of cognition in particular (Nieuwenhuys et al., 1998). Finally, however, the crucial selection is not of behaviors but of the genes that control the ontogenetic development of the relevant neural circuitry. It is regrettable that we know even less about the neurogenetics of neural ensembles that underlie cognitive performance in birds than we do in mammals (Lasalle, 1996) and that we have no information about what artificial selection for cognitive functions does to the structuring of neural circuits (Hauserr-Zarmakuppi et al., 1996). Indeed, even with regard to the responding of single neurons in birds, our knowledge is still remarkably patchy. In any case, it may be illusory to hope that we may come to understand cognitive competencies as neurophysiological processes in view of the sheer complexity of the undertaking. Artificial neural nets, particularly those kinds that are arranged to evolve in a quasi-Darwinian manner, may represent the heuristically most efficient way to advance our understanding of how cognition is produced by the nervous system and how again it steers the evolution of brain structures (Churchland and Sejnowski, 1993). They may help us to understand among other things the refined balance that birds seem to have struck between the ready-made, phylogenetically adapted, ontogenetically largely fixed behaviors and the demand-tailored, phylogenetically enabled, ontogenetically highly adaptable behaviors that in the past made birds classical study subjects for both instinct and learning (Tinbergen, 1951; Ferster and Skinner, 1957).

ACKNOWLEDGMENTS

Much of our own research reported here was supported by the Deutsche Forschungsgemeinschaft, Bonn. While co-authoring this chapter, J.E. was on sabbatical leave from Purdue University and was a visiting professor in Konstanz University. We thank Rita Leydel for much help with the manuscript preparation.

REFERENCES

Able, K.P., and M.A. Able, (1997) Development of sunset orientation in a migratory bird: no calibration by the magnetic field. *Anim. Behav*. 53:363–368.
Abs, M. (ed.) (1983) *Physiology and Behaviour of the Pigeon*. Academic Press, London.
Ahlberg, P.E. and A.R. Milner, (1994) The origin and early diversification of tetrapods. *Nature* 368:507–514.
Akshoomoff, N.A., and E. Courchesne, (1992) A new role for the cerebellum in cognitive operations. *Behav. Neurosci*. 106:731–738.

Aldavert-Vera, L., D. Costa-Miserachs, I. Divac, and J.D. Delius (1999) Presumed "prefrontal cortex" lesions in pigeons: effects on visual discrimination performance. *Behav. Brain Res.* 102: 165—170.

Alvarez-Buylla, A., and J. Kirn, (1997) Birth, migration, incorporation and death of vocal control neurons in adult song birds. *J. Neurobiol.* 33:508–601.

Ariens-Kappers, C.U., C.C. Huber, and E.C. Crosby, (1936) *The Comparative Anatomy of the Nervous System of Vertebrates.* Macmillan, New York.

Baddeley, A.D. (1997) *Human Memory: Theory and Practice.* Erlbaum, London.

Baylis, G.C., E.T Rolls, and C.M. Leonard, (1985) Selectivity between faces in the responses of a population of neurons in the cortex in the superior temporal sulcus of the monkey. *Brain Res.* 342:91–102.

Benjamini, L. (1983) Studies in the learning abilities of brown-necked ravens and herring gulls. I. Oddity learning. *Behaviour* 84:173–194.

Berezeney, R., M.J. Mortillaro, H. Ma, and X. Wei, (1995) The nuclear matrix: a structural milieu for genomic function. *Int. Rev. Cytol.* 162A:1–65.

Berthold, P. (1996) *Control of Bird Migration.* Chapman and Hall, London.

Bhatt, R.S., and E.A. Wasserman, (1989) Secondary generalization and categorization in pigeons. *J. Exp. Anal. Behav.* 52:213–224.

Bhatt, R.S., E.A. Wasserman, W.F. Reynolds, and K.S. Knauss, (1988) Conceptual behavior in pigeons: categorization of both familiar and novel examples from four classes of natural and artificial stimuli. *J. Exp. Psychol: Anim. Behav. Proc.* 14:219–234.

Bingman, V.P., and T.J. Jones (1994) Sun compass-based spatial learning impaired in homing pigeons with hippocampal lesions. *J. Neurosci.* 14:6687–6694.

Blough, P.M. (1972) Wavelength generalization and discrimination in the pigeon. *Percept. Psychophys.* 12:342–348.

Bohley, P. (1995) The fates of proteins in cells. *Naturwissenschaften.* 82:544–550.

Bolhuis, J.J. (1996) Development of perceptual mechanisms in birds: predispositions and imprinting. In C.F. Moss and S.J. Shettleworth (eds.): *Neuroethological Studies of Cognitive and Perceptual Processes.* Westview, Boulder, pp. 84–112.

Boysen, S.T. (1993) Counting in chimpanzees: nonhuman principles and emergent properties of number. In S.T. Boysen and E.J. Capaldi (eds.): *The development of numerical competence: animal and human models.* Erlbaum, Hillsdale, pp. 39–60.

Boysen, S.T., G.G. Berntson, M.B. Hannan, and J.T. Cacioppo (1996) Quantity-based interference and symbolic representations in chimpanzees (*Pan troglodytes*). *J. Exp. Psychol. Anim. Behav. Proc.* 22:76–86.

Boysen, S.T., G.G. Berntson, T.A. Shreyer, and K.S. Quigley (1993) Processing of ordinality and transitivity by chimpanzees (*Pan troglodytes*). *J. Comp. Psychol.* 107:208–215.

Braithwaite, V.A., and T. Guilford (1991) Viewing familiar landscapes affects pigeon homing. *Proc. R. Soc. Lond. Biol.* 245:183–186.

Carpenter, P.A., M.A. Just, and P. Shell (1990) What one intelligence test measures: a theoretical account of the processing in the Raven progressive matrices test. *Psychol. Rev.* 97:404–439.

Catchpole, C.K. (1986) The biology and evolution of bird songs. *Perspect. Biol. Med.* 30:47–62.

Chalmers, M., and B. McGonigle (1984) Are children any more logical than monkeys on the five-term series problem? *J. Exp. Child Psychol.* 37:355–377.

Chan, Y. M. and Y. N. Jan, (1999) Conservation of neurogenic genes and mechanisms. *Curr. Opin. Neurobiol.*, 9:582—88.

Churchland, P.S., and T.J. Sejnowski (1993) *The Computational Brain.* MIT Press, Cambridge.

Clayton, N.S., and A. Dickinson (1998) Episodic-like memory during cache recovery by scrub jays. *Nature* 395:272–274.

Clayton, N.S., and J.R. Krebs (1995) Lateralization in memory and the avian hippocampus in food storing birds. In: E. Alleva (ed.): *Behavioural Brain Research in Naturalistic and Semi-naturalistic Settings.* Kluwer, Amsterdam, pp. 139–157.

Coemans, M.A.J.M., J.J. Vos, and J.F.W. Nuboer (1990) No evidence for polarization sensitivity in the pigeon. *Naturwissennschaften* 77:138–142.

D'Amato, M.R., D.P. Salmon, and M. Colombo (1985) Extent and limits of the matching concept in monkeys (*Cebus apella*). *J. Exp. Psychol. Anim. Behav. Proc.* 11:31–51.

Davis, H. (1992) Transitive inference in rats (*Rattus norvegicus*). *J. Comp. Psychol.* 106:342–349.

Dawkins, M.S., T. Guilford, V.A. Braithwaite, and J.R. Krebs (1996) Discrimination and recognition of photographs of places by homing pigeons. *Behav. Proc.* 36:27–38.

Dehaene, S., and J.P. Changeux (1993) Development of elementary numerical abilities: a neuronal model. *J. Cogn. Neurosci.* 5:390–407.
Delius, J.D. (1988) Preening and associated comfort behavior in birds. *Ann. N. Y. Acad. Sci.* 525:40–55.
Delius, J.D. (1991) The nature of culture. In M.S. Dawkins, T.R. Halliday, and R. Dawkins (eds.): *The Tinbergen Legacy.* London, Chapman and Hall, pp. 75–99.
Delius, J.D. (1992) Categorical discrimination of objects and pictures by pigeons. *Anim. Learn. Behav.* 20:301–311.
Delius, J.D. (1994) Comparative cognition of identity. In P. Bertelson, P. Eelen, and G. d'Ydewalle (eds.): *International Perspectives on Psychological Science: Leading Themes.* Erlbaum, Howe, pp. 25–40.
Delius, J.D., M. Ameling, S.E.G. Lea, and J.E.R. Staddon (1995) Reinforcement concordance induces and maintains stimulus associations in pigeons. *Psychol. Rec.* 45:283–297.
Delius, J.D., J. Emmerton, W. Hörster, R. Jaeger, and J. Ostheim, (1999) Picture-object recognition in pigeons. *Curr. Psychol. Cogn.*, 18: 621—656.
Delius, J.D., and V.D. Hollard (1995) Orientation invariance in pattern recognition by pigeons (*Columba livia*) and humans (*Homo sapiens*). *J. Comp. Psychol.* 109:278–290.
Delius, J.D., and B. Nowak (1982) Visual symmetry recognition by pigeons. *Psychol. Res.* 44:199–212.
Delius, J.D., and K. Pellander (1982) Hunger dependence of electrical brain self-stimulation in the pigeon. *Physiol. Behav.* 28:63–66.
Delius, J.D., R.J. Perchard and J. Emmerton (1976) Polarized light discrimination by pigeons and an electroretinographic correlate. *J. Comp. Physiol. Psychol.* 90:560–571.
Delius, J.D., and M. Siemann (1998) Transitive inferences in animals and humans: adaptation or exaptation? *Behav. Proc.* 42:107–137.
De Valois, R.L., and K.K. De Valois (1988) *Spatial Vision.* Oxford University Press, New York.
De Waal, F. (1988) Chimpanzee politics. In R. Byrne and A. Whiten (eds.): *Machiavellian Intelligence* Clarendon, Oxford, pp. 122–131.
Domjan, M. (1993) *The Principles of Learning and Behavior,* 3rd. ed. Brooks/Cole, Pacific Grove.
Dubbledam, J.L. (1998) Birds. In R. Nieuwenhuys, H.J. Ten Donkelaar, and C. Nicholson (eds.): *The Central Nervous System of Vertebrates.* Springer, Berlin, pp. 1526–1636.
Dumont, J.P., and R.M. Robertson (1986) Neuronal circuits, an evolutionary perspective. *Science* 233:849–853.
Durand, S.E., J.T. Heaton, S.K. Amateau, and S.E. Brauth (1997) Vocal control pathways through the anterior forebrain of a parrot (*Melopsittacus undulatus*). *J. Comp. Neurol.* 377:179–206.
Emmerton, J. (1986) The pigeon's discrimination of movement patterns (Lissajous figures) and contour-dependent rotational invariance. *Perception* 5:573–588.
Emmerton, J. (1998a) Biases in pigeons' responses to numerosity: discrimination of "more" versus "less." Submitted.
Emmerton, J. (1998b) Numerosity differences and effects of stimulus density on pigeons' discrimination performance. *Animal Learn. Behav.* 26:243–256.
Emmerton, J., and J.D. Delius (1980) Wavelength discrimination in the "visible" and ultraviolet spectrum by pigeons. *J. Comp. Physiol.* 141:47–52.
Emmerton, J., and J.D. Delius, (1993) Beyond sensation: visual cognition in pigeons. In H.P. Zeigler and H.-J. Bischof (eds.): *Vision, Brain, and Behavior in Birds.* MIT Press, Cambridge, pp. 377–390.
Emmerton, J., A. Lohmann, and J. Niemann (1997) Pigeons' serial ordering of numerosity with visual arrays. *Anim. Learn. Behav.* 25:234–244.
Engelage, J., and H.J. Bischof (1996) Single cell responses in the ectostriatum of the zebra finch. *J. Comp. Physiol. A.* 179:785–795.
Feduccia, A. (1996) *The Origin and Evolution of Birds.* Yale University Press, New Haven.
Fersen, L. von, and Delius, J.D. (1989) Long-term retention of many visual patterns by pigeons. *Ethology.* 82:141–155.
Fersen, L.v., and J.D. Delius, (2000) Acquired equivalences between auditory stimuli in dolphins (*Tursiops truncatus*). *Anim. Cogn.* (in press).
Fersen, L. von, and O. Güntürkün (1990) Visual memory lateralization in pigeons. *Neuropsychologia.* 28:1–7.
Fersen, L. von, and S.E.G. Lea (1990) Category discrimination by pigeons using five polymorphous features. *J. Exp. Anal. Behav.* 54:69–84.
Fersen, L. von, C.D.L. Wynne, J.D. Delius, and J.E.R. Staddon (1991) Transitive inference formation in pigeons. *J. Exp. Psychol. Anim. Behav. Proc.* 17:334–341.
Ferster, C.B., and B.F. Skinner (1957) *Schedules of Reinforcement.* Appleton Century Crofts, New York.

Frisch, K. von (1965) *Tanzsprache und Orientierung der Bienen* [Dance-Language and Orientation of Bees]. Springer, Berlin.

Gazzaniga, M.S. (1995) On neural circuits and cognition. *Neurol. Comp.* 7:1–12.

Gillan, D.J. (1981) Reasoning in the chimpanzee: II. Transitive inference. *J. Exp. Psychol. Anim. Behav. Proc.* 7:150–164.

Gluck, M.A. (1991) Stimulus generalization and representation in adaptive network models of category learning. *Psychol. Sci.* 2:50–55.

Goldman-Rakic, P.S. (1992) Working memory and the mind. *Sci. Am.* 92:72–79.

Güntürkün, O. (1991) The functional organization of the avian visual system. In R.J. Andrew (ed.): *Neural and Behavioral Plasticity.* Oxford University Press, Oxford, pp. 92–105.

Güntürkün, O. (1997) Visual lateralization in birds: from neurotrophins to cognition? *Eur. J. Morphol.* 35:290–302.

Güntürkün, O., J. Emmerton, and J.D. Delius, (1989) Neural asymmetries and visual behavior in birds. In H. Lüttgau and R. Necker (eds.): *Biological Signal Processing: Cellular and Integrative Aspects.* Verlag Chemie, Weinheim, pp. 122–145.

Hamilton, W.D. (1974) The evolution of social behavior. *J. Theor. Biol.* 7:1–52.

Hausherr-Zarmakuppi, Z., D.P. Wolfer, M.C. Leisinger-Trigona, and H.P. Lipp (1996) Selective breeding for extremes in open-field activity of mice entails a differentiation of hippocampal mossy fibers. *Behav. Genet.* 26:167–176.

Healey, S.D. (1996) Ecological specialization in the avian brain. In: C.F. Moss and S.J. Shettleworth (eds.): *Neuroethological Studies of Cognitive and Perceptual Processes* Westview, Boulder, pp 84–112.

Herrmann, H. (1965) Das Brutverhalten des Südamerikanischen Töpfervogels *Furnarius rufus* (The breeding behavior of the Southamerican ovenbird *Furnarius rufus*) *Abhand. Verhand. Naturwiss. Vereins Hamburg* 10:117–152.

Herrnstein, R.J. (1985) Riddles of natural categorization. In: L. Weiskrantz (ed.): *Animal Intelligence* Clarendon Press, Oxford, pp. 129–144.

Herrnstein, R.J. (1990) Levels of stimulus control: a functional approach. *Cognition* 37:133–166.

Herrnstein, R.J. and D.H. Loveland (1964) Complex visual concept in the pigeon. *Science* 146:549–551.

Higa-King, J.J., and J.E.R. Staddon (1993) "Transitive inference" in multiple conditional discrimination. *J. Exp. Anal. Behav.* 59:265–291.

Honey, R.C., G. Horn, P. Bateson, and M. Walpole (1995) Functionally distinct memories for imprinting stimuli: behavioral and neural dissociations. *Behav. Neurosci.* 109:689–698.

Honig, W.K. (1993) Numerosity as a dimension of stimulus control. In S.T. Boysen and E.J. Capaldi (eds.): *The Development of Numerical competence: Animal and Human Models* Erlbaum, Hillsdale, pp. 61–86.

Honig, W.K., and K.E. Stewart (1988) Pigeons can discriminate locations presented in pictures. *J. Exp. Anal. Behav.* 50:541–551.

Honig, W.K., and K.E. Stewart (1989) Discrimination of relative numerosity by pigeons. *Anim. Learn. Behav.* 17:134–146.

Huber, L., and R. Lenz (1993) A test of linear feature model of polymorphous concept discrimination with pigeons. *Q. J. Exp. Psychol.* 46B:1–18.

Huber, L., U. Aust, G. Michelbach, S. Ölzant, M. Loidolt, and R. Nowotny, (1999) Limits of symmetry conceptualization in pigeons. *Quart. J. Exper. Psychol*, 52B:351–379.

Hultsch, H., and D. Todt (1989) Memorization and reproduction of songs in nightingales (Luscinia megarynchos): evidence for package formation. *J. Comp. Physiol. A.* 165:197–203.

Jassik-Gerschenfeld, D. (1979) Single-neuron responses to moving sine-wave gratings in the pigeon optic tectum. *Vis. Res.* 19:993–999.

Jassik-Gerschenfeld, D., J. Teulon, and O. Hardy, (1979) Spatial interactions in the visual receptive fields of the nucleus dorsolateralis anterior of the pigeon thalamus. In A.M. Granda and J.H. Maxwell (eds.): *Neural Mechanisms of Behavior in the Pigeon.* Plenum, New York, pp. 145–164.

Jerison, H.J. (1973) *Evolution of the Brain and Intelligence.* Academic Press, New York.

Jitsumori, M. (1993) Category discrimination of artificial polymorphous stimuli based on feature learning. *J. Exp. Psychol. Anim. Behav. Proc.* 19:244–254.

Jitsumori, M., and O. Ohkubo (1996) Orientation discrimination and photographs of natural objects by pigeons. *Behav. Proc.* 38:205–226.

Jitsumori, M., M. Siemann, M. Lehr, and J.D. Delius (2000) The formation and expansion of equivalence classes in pigeons. Submitted.

Kandel, E.R., J.H. Schwartz, and T.M. Jessell, (1991) *Principles of Neural Science*, 3rd ed. Prentice-Hall. London.

Karten, H.J. (1991) Homology and evolutionary origins of the "neocortex." *Brain Behav. Evol.* 38:264–272.

Koehler, O. (1941) Vom Erlernen unbenannter Anzahlen bei Vögeln. [About the learning of unnamed numbers by birds]. Naturwissenschaften, 29:201–218.

Kohonen, T. (1984) *Self-Organization and Associative Memory*. Springer, Berlin.

Kramer, G. (1961) Long-distance orientation. In A.J. Marshall (ed.): *Biology and Comparative Physiology of Birds*. Academic Press, New York, pp. 341–371.

Krebs, J.R. (1990) Food-storing birds: adaptive specialization in brain and behavior? *Philos. Trans. R. Soc. Lond.* 329B:153–160.

Kroodsma, D.E., and E.H. Miller, (eds.) (1996) *Ecology and Evolution of Acoustic Communication in Birds*. Comstock, Ithaca.

Kruska, D. (1988) Mammalian domestication and its effect on brain structure and behavior. In H.J. Jerison and I. Jerison (eds.): *Intelligence and Evolutionary Biology*. Springer, Berlin. pp. 211–251.

Kumar, S., and B. Hedges (1998) A molecular timescale for vertebrate evolution. *Nature* 392:917–920.

Kuno, H., T. Kitadate, and T. Iwamoto, (1994) Formation of transitivity in conditional matching to sample by pigeons. *J. Exp. Anal. Behav.* 62:399–408.

Lasalle, J.M. (1996) Neurogenetic basis of cognition: facts and hypothesis. *Behav. Proc.* 35:5–18.

Lea, S.E.G. (1984) In what sense do pigeons learn concepts? In H.L. Roitblat, T. Bever and H.S. Terrace (eds.): *Animal Cognition*. Erlbaum, Hillsdale. pp. 263–277.

Lea, S.E.G., Lohmann, A., and C.M. Ryan, (1993) Discrimination of five-dimensional stimuli by pigeons: limitations of feature analysis. *Q. J. Exp. Psychol. Comp. Physiol. Psychol.* 46B:19–42.

Levi, W.M. (1977) *The Pigeon*. Levi, Sumter.

Lipkens, R., P.F.M. Kop, and W. Matthijs, (1988) A test of symmetry and transitivity in the conditional discrimination performances of pigeons. *J. Exp. Anal. Behav.* 49:395–409.

Lögler, P. (1959) Versuche zur Frage des "Zähl"—Vermögens an einem Graupapagei und Vergleichsversuche an Menschen [On the question of the "counting" ability of a grey parrot and comparative experiments on humans]. *Z. Tierpsychol.* 16:179–217.

Lombardi, C., C. Fachinelli, and J.D. Delius, (1984) Oddity of visual patterns conceptualized by pigeons. *Anim. Learn. Behav.* 12:2–6.

Lubow, R.E. (1974) Higher-order concept formation in the pigeon. *J. Exp. Anal. Behav.* 21:475–483.

Macphail, E.M. (1985) Vertebrate intelligence: the null hypothesis. In L. Weiskrantz (ed.): *Animal Intelligence* Oxford, Clarendon, pp. 37–51.

Macphail, E.M., and S. Reilly, (1989) Rapid acquisition of a novelty versus familiarity concept by pigeons (*Columba livia*). *J. Exp. Psychol. Anim. Behav. Proc.* 15:242–252.

Manabe, K., T. Kawashima, and J.E.R. Staddon (1995) Differential vocalization in budgerigars: towards an experimental analysis of naming. *J. Exp. Anal. Behav.* 63:111–126.

Manabe, K., Staddon, J.E.R., and J.M. Cleaveland, (1997) Control of vocal repertoire by reward in budgerigars (Melopsittacus undulatus)., *J. Comp. Psychol.*, 111: 50–62.

Martinoya, C., and J.D. Delius, (1990) Perception of rotating spiral patterns by pigeons. *Biol. Cybernet.* 63:127–134.

McGonigle, B., and M. Chalmers (1992) Monkeys are rational. *Q. J. Exp. Psychol.* 45B:189–228.

McNaughton, B.L., and R.G.M. Morris (1987) Hippocampal synaptic enhancement and information storage within a distributed memory system. *Trends Neurosci.* 10:408–415.

Meck, W.H., and R.M. Church (1983) A mode control model of counting and timing processes. *J. Exp. Psychol. Anim. Behav. Proc.* 9:320–334.

Medina, L., and A. Reiner, (2000) Do birds possess homologues of mammalian primary visual, somatosensory and motor cortices? *Trends Neurosci.*, 231:1–12.

Mello, C.V., and D.F. Clayton (1994) Song-induced zenk gene expression in auditory pathways of songbird brain and its relation to the song control system. *J. Neurosci.* 14:6652–6666.

Møller, A.P. (1993). Female preference for apparently symmetrical male sexual ornaments in the barn swallow *Hirundo rustica*. *Behav. Ecol. Sociobiol.* 32:371–376.

Morgan, M.J., M. Fitch, J. Holman, and S.E.G. Lea (1976) Pigeons learn the concept of an "A." *Perception* 5:57–66.

Neiworth, J.J., and M.E. Rilling (1987) A method for studying imagery in animals. *J. Exp. Psychol. Anim. Behav. Proc.* 13:203–214.

Neiworth, J.J., and A.A. Wright, (1994) Monkeys (*Macaca mulatta*) learn category matching in a nonidentical same-different-task. *J. Exp. Psychol. Anim. Behav. Proc.* 20:429–435.

Nieuwenhuys, R., H.J. Ten Donkelaar, and C. Nicholson (1998) The meaning of it all. In R. Nieuwenhuys, H.J. ten Donkelaar, and C. Nicholson (eds.): *The Central Nervous System of Vertebrates*. Berlin, Springer, pp 2135–2195.

Oetting, S., and H.-J. Bischof (1996) Sexual imprinting in female zebra finches: changes in preferences as an effect of adult experience. *Behaviour* 133:387–397.

Palacios, A.G., and F.J. Varela (1992) Color mixing in the pigeon (*Columba livia*). II. A psychophysical determination in the middle, short and near-UV wavelength range. *Vis. Res.* 32:1947–1953.

Pearce, J.M. (1987) A model for stimulus generalization in pavlovian conditioning. *Psychol. Rev.* 94:61–73.

Pearce, J.M. (1994) Similarity and discrimination: a selective review and a connectionist model. *Psychol. Rev.* 101:587–607.

Pearce, J. M. (1997) *Animal Learning and Cognition, an Introduction,* 2nd ed. Psychology, Hove.

Pepperberg, I.M. (1987a) Acquisition of the same/different concept by an African grey parrot (*Psittacus erithacus*): learning with respect to categories of color, shape, and material. *Anim. Learn. Behav.* 15:423–432.

Pepperberg, I.M. (1987b) Evidence for conceptual quantitative abilities in the African grey parrot: labelling of cardinal sets. *Ethology*, 75:37–61.

Pepperberg, I.M. (1994) Numerical competence in an African grey Parrot (*Psittacus erithacus*). *J. Comp. Psychol.* 108:36–44.

Pepperberg, I.M. (1996) Categorical class formation by an African grey parrot (*Psittacus erithacus*). In T.R. Zentall and P.M. Smeets (eds.): *Stimulus Formation in Humans and Animals*. Elsevier, Amsterdam, pp. 71–90.

Pepperberg, I.M., and M.A. McLaughlin (1996) Effects of avian-human joint attention on allospecific vocal learning by grey parrots (*Psittacus erithacus*). *J. Comp. Psychol.* 110:286–297.

Perdeck, A.C. (1958) Two types of orientation in migrating starlings, *Sturnus vulgaris*, and chaffinches, *Fringillla coelebs*, as revealed by displacement experiments. *Ardea* 46:1–37.

Perrett, D.I., A.J. Mistlin, and A.J. Chitty (1987) Visual neurones responsive to faces. *Trends Neurosci.* 10:358–364.

Pollen, D.A., and S.F. Ronner (1981) Phase relationships between adjacent simple cells in the visual cortex. *Science* 212:1409–1411.

Porter, D., and A. Neuringer (1984) Music discriminations by pigeons. *J. Exp. Psychol. Anim. Behav. Proc.* 10:138–148.

Premack, D. (1988) Minds with and without language. In L. Weiskrantz (ed.): *Thought Without Language* Oxford, Clarendon, pp. 46–65.

Ramón y Cajal, S. (1911) Histologie du système nerveux de l'homme et des vertébrés [Histology of the Nervous System of Humans and Vertebrates]. Maloine, Paris.

Rehkämper, G., H.D. Frahm, and K. Zilles (1991) Quantitative development of brain and brain structures in birds (Galliformes and Passeriformes) compared to that in mammals (Insectivores and Primates). *Brain Behav. Evol.* 37:125–143.

Rehkämper, G., E. Haase, and H.D. Frahm (1988) Allometric comparisons of brain weight and brain structure in different breeds of domestic pigeons, *Columba livia* (fantails, homing pigeons, strassers). *Brain. Behav. Evol.* 31:141–149.

Remy, M., and O. Güntürkün (1991) Retinal afferents of the tectum opticum and the nucleus opticus principalis thalami in the pigeon. *J. Comp. Neurol.* 305:57–70.

Rensch, B. (1973) *Gedächtnis, Begriffsbildung und Planhandlungen bei Tieren [Memory, Concept Formation and Planned Behaviour]*. Parey, Berlin.

Roberts, W.A., and D.S. Mazmanian (1988) Concept learning at different levels of abstraction by pigeons, monkeys, and people. *J. Exp. Psychol. Anim. Behav. Proc.* 14:247–260.

Roberts, W.A., and S. Mitchell (1994) Can a pigeon simultaneously process temporal and numerical information? *J. Exp. Psychol. Anim. Behav. Proc.* 20:66–78.

Roberts, W.A., and M.T. Phelps (1994) Transitive inference in rats: a test of the spatial coding hypothesis. *Psychol. Sci.* 5:368–374.

Rogers, L.J. (1995) *The Development of Brain and Behaviour in the Chicken*. CAB, Wallingford.

Rolls, E.T. (1975) *The Brain and Reward*. Pergamon, Oxford.

Rosch, E. (1978) Principles of categorization. In E. Rosch and B. Lloyd (eds.): *Cognition and Categorization*. Erlbaum, Hillsdale. pp. 27–48.
Ruben, J. (1995) The evolution of endothermy in mammals and birds: from physiology to fossils. *Annu. Rev. Physiol.* 57:69–95.
Sachs, G. (1993) Minimum wind strength for dynamic soaring of albatrosses. *J. Ornith.* 134:435–445.
Saito, N., and M. Maekawa (1993). Birdsong: the interface with human language. *Brain Dev.* 15:31–40.
Schmahmann, J.D. (ed.) (1997) *The Cerebellum and Cognition*. Academic Press, San Diego.
Sidman, M. (1992) *Equivalence Relations and Behavior: A Research Story*. Authors Cooperative, Boston.
Siemann, M., and J.D. Delius (1993) Implicit deductive responding in humans. *Naturwissenschaften*. 80:364–366.
Siemann, M., and J.D. Delius (1994) Processing of hierarchic stimulus structures has advantages in animals and humans. *Biol. Cybernet.* 71:531–536.
Siemann, M., and J.D. Delius (1996) Influences of task concreteness upon transitive responding in humans. *Psychol. Res.* 59:81–93.
Siemann, M., and J.D. Delius (1998a) Induction of stimulus associations by reinforcement concordances in pigeons. In N. Elsner and R. Wehner (eds.): *Göttingen Neurobiology Report 1998*. Thieme, Stuttgart, p. 525.
Siemann, M., and J.D. Delius (1998b) Algebraic learning and neural network models for transitive and nontransitive responding in humans and animals. *Eur. J. Cogn. Psychol.* 10:307–334.
Siemann, M., J.D. Delius, D. Dombrowski, and S. Daniel (1996) Value transfer in discriminative conditioning with pigeons. *Psychol. Rec.* 46:707–728.
Siemann, M., J.D. Delius, and A.A. Wright (1996) Transitive responding in pigeons: influences of stimulus frequency and reinforcement history. *Behav. Proc.* 37:185–195.
Siemann, M., L. Fersen, von and J.D. Delius (1998) Kognition bei Tieren. In E. Irle and H.J. Markowitsch (eds.): *Vergleichende Psychobiologie, Enzyklopädie der Psychologie*. Hogrefe, Göttingen, pp. 695–738.
Simms, E. (1979) *The Public Life of the Street Pigeon*. Hutchinson, London.
Smirnova, A.A., O.F. Lazareva, and Z.A. Zorina, (2000) Use of number by crows: investigation by matching and oddity learning. *J. Exp. Anal. Behav.*, 73:177–193.
Sokolov, E.N. (1975) The neuronal mechanisms of the orienting reflex. In: E.N. Sokolov and O.S. Vinogradova (eds.): *Neuronal Mechanisms of the Orienting Reflex*. Erlbaum, Hillsdale, pp. 217–235.
Staddon, J.E.R., and J.J. Higa (1999). Time and memory: towards a pacemaker-free theory of interval timing. *J. Exp. Anal. Behav.* 71:215–251.
Steirn, J.N., J.E. Weaver, and T.T. Zentall (1995) Transitive inference in pigeons: simplified procedures and a test of value transfer theory. *Anim. Learn. Behav.* 23:76–82.
Striedter, G.F. (1994) The vocal pathways in budgerigars differ from those in songbirds. *J. Comp. Neurol.* 343:35–56.
Sun, H., and B.J. Frost (1998) Computation of different optical variables of looming objects in pigeon nucleus rotundus neurons. *Nature Neurosci.* 1:296–303.
Thompson, R.K.R., and D. L. Oden (1996) A profound disparity revisited: perception and judgement of abstract identity relations by chimpanzees, human infants, and monkeys. *Behav. Proc.* 35:149–161.
Thompson, R.F., K.S. Mayers, R.T. Robertson, and C.J. Patterson (1970) Number coding in association cortex of the cat. *Science* 168:271–273.
Tinbergen, N. (1951) *The Study of Instinct*. Oxford: University Press, Oxford.
Todd, I.A., and N.J. Mackintosh (1990) Evidence for perceptual learning in pigeons' recognition memory for pictures. *Q. J. Exp. Psychol.* 42B:385–400.
Treichler, F.R., and D. van Tilburg (1996) Concurrent conditional discrimination tests of transitive inference by macaque monkeys: list linking. *J. Exp. Psychol. Anim. Behav. Proc.* 22:105–117.
Trivers, R. (1985) *Social Evolution*. Benjamin/Cummings, Menlo Park.
Tyrrell, D.J., M.C. Zingaro, and K.L. Minard (1993) Learning and transfer of identity-difference relationships by infants. *Infant. Behav. Dev.* 16:43–52.
Van Dongen, P.A.M. (1998) Brain size in vertebrates. In R. Nieuwenhuys, H.J. ten Donkelaar, and C. Nicholson (eds.): *The Central Nervous System of Vertebrates*. Springer, Berlin, pp. 2099–2134.
Vates, G.E., D.S. Vicario, and F. Nottebohm (1997) Reafferent thalamo-"cortical" loops in the song system of oscine songbirds. *J. Comp. Neurol.* 380:275–290.

Vaughan, W. (1988) Formation of equivalence sets in pigeons. *J. Exp. Psychol. Anim. Behav. Proc.* 14:36–42.
Vaughan, W., and S.L. Greene (1984) Pigeons' visual memory capacity. *J. Exp. Psychol. Anim. Behav. Proc.* 10:256–271.
Veenman, C.L. (1997) Pigeon basal ganglia: insights into the neuroanatomy underlying telencephalic sensorimotor processes in birds. *Eur. J. Morphol.* 35:220–233.
Veenman, C.L., J.M. Wild, and A. Reiner (1995) Organization of the avian "corticostriatal" projection system: a retrograde and anterograde pathway tracing study in pigeons. *J. Comp. Neurol.* 354:87–126.
Wallhäusser-Franke, E., B.E. Nixdorf-Bergweiler, and T.J. DeVoogd, (1995) Song isolation is associated with maintaining high spine frequencies on zebra finch LMAN neurons. *Neurobiol. Learn. Mem.* 64:25–35.
Wallraff, H.G. (1991) Conceptual approaches to avian navigation systems. In P. Berthold (ed.): *Orientation in Birds.* Birkhäuser, Basel, pp. 128–165.
Watanabe, S. (1996) Effects of ectostriatal lesions on discrimination of conspecific, species and familiar objects in pigeons. *Behav. Brain Res.* 81:183–188.
Watanabe, S., S.E.G. Lea, and W.H. Dittrich (1993) What can we learn from experiments on pigeon concept discrimination? In H.P. Zeigler and H.-J. Bishof (eds): *Vision, Brain and Behavior in Birds.* Cambridge, MA: MIT Press. pp. 351–376.
Watanabe, S., Sakamoto, J. and Wakita, M. (1995) Pigeons' discrimination of paintings by Monet and Picasso. *J. Exp. Anal. Behav.* 63:165–174.
Wenzel, B.M. (1981) Functional status and credibility of avian olfaction. In F. Papi and H. G. Wallraff (eds.): *Avian Navigation.* Springer, Berlin.
Whiten, A., and R.W. Byrne (eds.) (1997) *Machiavallian Intelligence: Evaluations and Extensions.* Cambridge University Press, Cambridge.
Wild, J.M. (1997) Functional anatomy of neural pathways contributing to the control of song production in birds. *Eur. J. Morphol.* 35:303–325.
Wilson, B., N.J. Mackintosh, and R.A. Boakes (1985) Matching and oddity learning in the pigeon: transfer effects and the absence of relational learning. *Q. J. Exp. Psychol.* 37B:295–311.
Wiltschko, R, and R. Wiltschko, (1971) Magnetic compass of European robins. *Science* 176:62–64.
Wright, A.A. (1989) Memory processing by pigeons, monkeys and people. *Psychol. Learn. Mem.* 2:25–70.
Wright, A.A., R. Cook, J. Rivera, S. Sands, and J.D. Delius (1988) Concept learning by pigeons: matching-to-sample with trial-unique video picture stimuli. *Anim. Learn. Behav.* 16:436–44.
Wyles, J.S., J.G. Kunkel, and A.C. Wilson (1983) Birds, behavior, and anatomical evolution. *Proc. Nat. Acad. Sci.* U.S.A. 80:4394–4397.
Wynne, C.D.L. (1995) Reinforcement accounts for transitive inference performance. *Anim. Learn. Behav.* 23:207–217.
Wynne, C.D.L., L. von Fersen, and J.E.R. Staddon (1992) Pigeons' transitive inferences are the outcome of elementary conditioning principles: a response. *J. Exp. Psychol. Anim. Behav. Proc.* 18:313–315.
Xia, L. (1997) *Numerische Fähigkeiten bei Tauben* [Numerical Competencies in Pigeons]. Dissertation, Universität Konstanz.
Xia, L., J.D. Delius, and M. Siemann (1996) A multistimulus intelligence platform for pigeon conditioning. *Behav. Res. Methods. Instrum. Comp.* 28:49–54.
Xia, L., M. Siemann, and J. D. Delius, (2000b) Matching of numerical symbols with number of responses by pigeons. *Anim. Cogn.*, 3:35–43.
Xia, L., J. Emmerton, M. Siemann, and J.D. Delius, (2000a) Pigeons learn to link numerosities with symbols. *J. Comp. Psychol* (in press).
Yamamoto, J., and T. Asano (1995) Stimulus equivalence in a chimpanzee. *Psychol. Rec.* 45:3–21.
Zentall, T.R., Hogan, D.E. and Edwards, C. A. (1984) Cognitive factors in conditional learning by pigeons. In: H.L. Roitblat, T. Bever and H.S. Terrace (Eds.), *Animal Cognition* (pp. 389–408). Hillsdale: Erlbaum.

Chapter 16

WHAT CAN THE CEREBRAL CORTEX DO BETTER THAN OTHER PARTS OF THE BRAIN?

Almut Schüz, Max-Planck-Institut für biologische Kybernetik, Tübingen

INTRODUCTION

One of the most striking results of mammalian evolution is the development of a large cerebral cortex. A cortex or pallium, a planar piece of nerve tissue at the surface of the forebrain, is there in most vertebrates, but its size (relative to the rest of the brain) usually does not reach that in mammals. In all mammals, the cortex is the most impressive subdivision of the brain. In mice, for example, the cortex amounts to about 40% of the brain weight (estimated from measurements on cortical volume; Schüz and Palm, 1989); in humans it reaches nearly 80% (gray and white matter taken together) of the brain weight (estimated from the 76% isocortical volume in Frahm et al., 1982). This raises the question as to the evolutionary advantage of this part of the brain. It can be assumed to be related to the fact that the cerebral cortex is responsible for higher cognitive functions as is evident from neurological deficits in humans.

A comparison among various mammalian species shows that it is mainly the dorsal part of the cortex, the isocortex, that increases along the mammalian evolutionary scale. The surrounding parts, considered to be homologues to most of the reptilian cortex (e.g., Desan, 1988) and often described by the term *allocortex*, remain relatively small. In humans, 96% of the cortical surface area belongs to the isocortex, while in hedgehogs it is only 32% (Filimonov, 1949, quoted in Blinkov and Glezer, 1968). A clue to the understanding of the enlargement of the dorsal part may be the fact that this part of the cortex receives input from all the sensory systems (preprocessed in other parts of the brain). In reptiles, too, there is a small dorsal region, which receives polysensory input (e.g., Hoogland and Vermeulen-Van der Zee, 1988). Thus, when seeking the evolutionary advantage of the enlargement of the cerebral cortex, one may assume that it is connected to the possibility of coordinating the various sensory systems. This is certainly a prerequisite for higher cognitive functions.

The very fact that the cortex is a place where the sensory systems meet, however, is probably not a sufficient explanation for its special development. There are other parts of the brain, where at least some of the sensory systems are represented close to each other, for example, the thalamus or the cerebellum. This leads to the suspicion that, in addition to polysensory input, there is something in the intrinsic connectivity of the cortex that is advantageous to higher cognitive functions.

Indeed, microscopic observations indicate that the various parts of the brain, besides being characterized by their input and output relationship and their relative size, also show characteristic differences in their intrinsic structure. Some parts of the brain, for example, the olfactory bulb or the cerebellum, have so typical a structure that they can be recognized at first sight in the microscope. In other cases more time and practice is required, but it is possible in principle. One may assume that the typical appearance of the various parts of the brain reflects different kinds of connectivity and, consequently, different kinds of information processing.

Thus, with respect to the success of cortical evolution, the question arises: What is the typical connectivity of the cerebral cortex, and what made it so particularly suited for higher cognitive functions? This has been a long-standing question in our group (Braitenberg, 1977, 1978a, 1986; Palm, 1982; Braitenberg and Schüz, 1991, 1998), and the main points are summarized in this chapter.

BASIC CONNECTIVITY OF THE ISOCORTEX

The cortex, like the rest of the brain, consists mainly of nerve cells, the processes of which (axons and dendrites) are interwoven at the highest possible packing density. In the case of the cerebral cortex, this compact mass forms a flat sheet and is separated into a superficial gray matter in which the neurons have their synaptic connections and a white matter that consists of long axonal processes, forming a kind of cable system underneath the gray matter. The thickness of the gray matter does not vary much between species: about 1 mm in mice and about 3 mm in humans. Under $1mm^2$, the number of neurons is of the order of 10^5 (Rockel, 1980), with some variability between areas or species. The surface area differs, however, by a factor of 1000 between these species. As a consequence, the cortex is folded in larger brains.

The entire isocortex can be viewed as a continuous network despite the fact that it can be subdivided morphologically into different areas. These areas constitute local variations of the common basic connectivity, which is described below. Fibers emanating from the sensory systems radiate into the cortex and project the various sensory surfaces onto separate areas.

The various parts of the brain can usually be characterized by the presence of particular cell types. These are classified mainly by the shape or size of their cell bodies, by the shape and size of their dendritic and axonal ramifications, or by the outlines of their dendrites, which can be smooth, beaded, or spiny.

Typical of the cerebral cortex is the so-called pyramidal cell (Fig. 16.1). Its cell body is often pyramidal in shape, and its dendritic tree is usually elongated, its long axis directed perpendicularly toward the surface of the cortex. The axon is directed in the opposite direction and enters the white matter. The dendrites are densely studded with spiny processes, each of which carries a synapse. About 85% of cortical neurons are pyramidal cells (Peters and Kara, 1985; Braak and Braak, 1986). The other

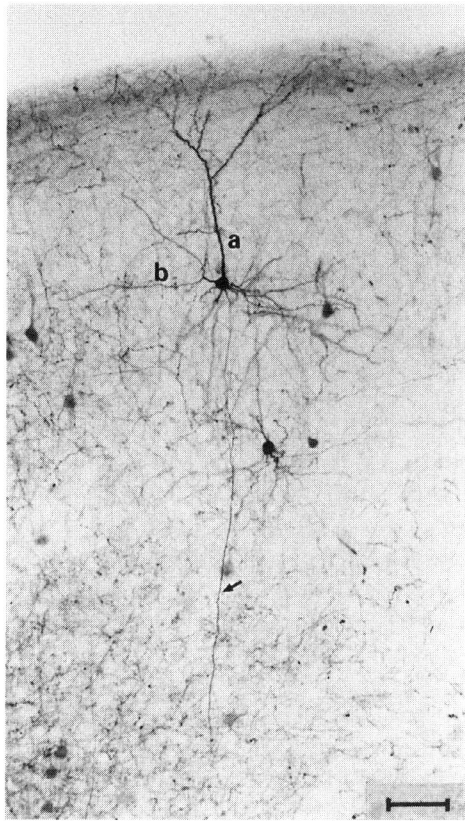

Figure 16.1. Pyramidal cell in the cortex of the mouse, stained by retrograde tracing with biotinylated dextran amine. a, Apical dendrite, reaching the surface of the cortex; b, basal dendrites, emananting from the cell body; arrow, main axon, running toward the white matter. Bar = 50 µm.

neurons in the cortex are loosely interspersed among the pyramidal cells. Their dendrites are smooth, and their axons do not leave the gray matter.

The connectivity of a given part of the brain normally cannot be derived directly from its light or electron microscopical appearance. This is particularly difficult in the cerebral cortex, where, under the microscope, one is confronted with thousands of fibers crossing each other with no obvious order or aim. Combinations of methods are, thus, necessary. Our approach relied on a quantitative assessment of the cell parts (cell bodies, spines, synapses, axons, dendrites) that can be visualized in the microscope with various histological methods (summarized in Braitenberg and Schüz, 1991, 1998). In the next few paragraphs, the most important results are summarized and compared with those from other parts of the brain (see also the review by Nieuwenhuys, 1994).

The neurons in the cortex are mainly connected to other cortical neurons. The axons of the pyramidal cells give off collaterals during their course toward the white matter and connect to neurons in their neighborhood. The axons then leave the gray matter, and most of them run through the white matter to a distant place, where they reenter the gray matter and connect to neurons there. Only a small proportion of the pyramidal cells are true output neurons (probably below 10% in humans) that send their axons to other parts of the central nervous system. Input fibers from the sensory systems and from other parts of the brain to the cortex are also much lower in number than the reentering axons of pyramidal cells.

In the cortex of the mouse, a pyramidal cell receives on average about 8000 synapses on its dendrite and makes about the same number of synapses with its axonal ramifications. About 85% of the synapses connect the neuron to other pyramidal cells, about 11% to nonpyramidal cells, and a few percent of the synapses on the dendrites come from input neurons. A pyramidal cell usually makes only one or a few synpases with each of its postsynaptic neighbors. *Thus, the individual pyramidal cell is connected to thousands of other pyramidal cells.*

The synapses made by the axons of pyramidal cells are of a special morphological type (type I), which is known to be *excitatory* (e.g., Peters and Jones, 1984). When the postsynaptic neighbor is another pyramidal cell, the synapse is usually *located on a dendritic spine* (for review see White, 1989). If it is a nonpyramidal cell, the synapse is located directly on the dendrite or on the cell body. The axons of non-pyramidal cells make inhibitory synapses (e.g., Houser et al., 1984). They are usually located directly on the dendrites (or the cell bodies) of the postsynaptic neurons. There is indirect evidence that the dendritic spines play a role in the regulation of the strength of the synapse located on them (summarized by Horner, 1993).

A glance at the other relatively large parts of the brain, the cerebellum, the striatum, and the thalamus, shows that some of the properties of the cortex also appear in these and perhaps other parts of the brain. The entire set of properties mentioned above, however, is unique to the cortex. This indicates that the role of the cortex must be quite different from that of the other brain parts (Fig. 16.2). For example, the striatum also consists mainly of one type of neuron and, as in the cortex, these neurons are connected among each other. They are, however, connected by inhibitory synapses (for review and functional interpretation, see Wickens, 1993; Plenz and Aertsen, 1996). In the thalamus, the majority of the neurons seem to be excitatory, as in the cortex. These, however, relay the sensory input to the cerebral cortex and do not seem to be directly connected to each other (Steriade et al., 1990; for functional interpretation, see Miller, 1996). Dendritic spines are also a typical feature of neurons in the cerebellum, the Purkinje cells. These spines do not, however, receive synapses from the same type of neurons, but from granular cells. In the cerebellar cortex, there is no intrinsic positive feedback either (Braitenberg et al., 1997). Inhibitory interneurons are present both in the cerebellar cortex and in the thalamus.

THE CEREBRAL CORTEX AND COGNITION

What could be the functional role of the kind of connectivity typical of the cerebral cortex? The answer is that it is particularly well suited for functions that are essential for cognitive processes (viz., for storing, retrieving, and handling correlations).

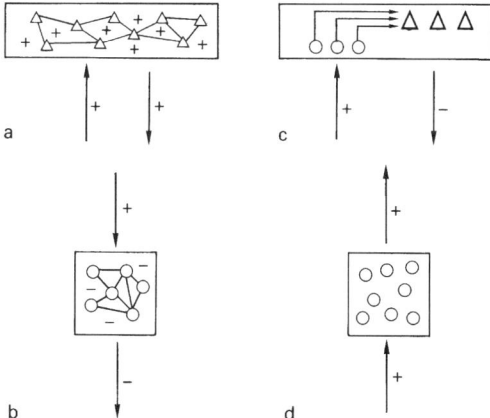

Figure 16.2. Sketches characterizing some aspects of the connectivity of four brain regions. (a) Cerebral cortex. The main input and the output are excitatory. The main cell type forms an excitatory network. (b) Striatum. The input from the cortex is excitatory, the output is inhibitory, and the main cell type forms an inhibitory network. (c) Cerebellar cortex. The input is excitatory, the output inhibitory. The input is relayed by granular cells (round) to the output neurons, the Purkinje cells (triangular), in a typical geometrical arrangement. (d) Thalamic relay nucleus. Input and output are excitatory. The projection neurons do not form a network among themselves.

A mechanism for the storage of correlations was proposed by Hebb (1949) in his theory of cell assemblies, a concept that was taken up again by Legendy (1971) and further elaborated by Braitenberg (1978b). According to this theory, learning is achieved by strengthening the connections between those neurons that are often active together. When a child is exposed to a new object, the various properties of the object, such as its particular color, shape, consistency, and so forth, will be projected onto the cortex by the sensory input systems and will excite a certain set of neurons there. This set will be more or less the same, whenever this or a similar object reappears. If there happen to be connections between members of this set, these connections might be strengthened whenever the neurons fire together. After a while, the connections will have become strong enough to ignite the whole set when only some of its members are activated from outside. By then, the new object will have a representation in the brain, and the concept of it can be evoked relatively independently from the input. Such "cell assemblies" might constitute the units of cognition (Fig. 16.3).

According to this theory, individual neurons of a cell assembly might be part of other cell assemblies representing concepts with similar properties. A train of thoughts could then result from the successive ignition of overlapping cell assemblies. It is difficult to prove this theory, but it turned out to be a very promising starting point whenever trying to pin down cognitive functions to the neuronal level (Braitenberg, 1985; Palm, 1990; Miller and Wickens, 1991; Braitenberg and Pulvermüller, 1992; Braitenberg and Schüz, 1992; Pulvermüller, 1992; Wickelgren, 1992).

16 What can the Cerebral Cortex do Better than other Parts of the Brain?

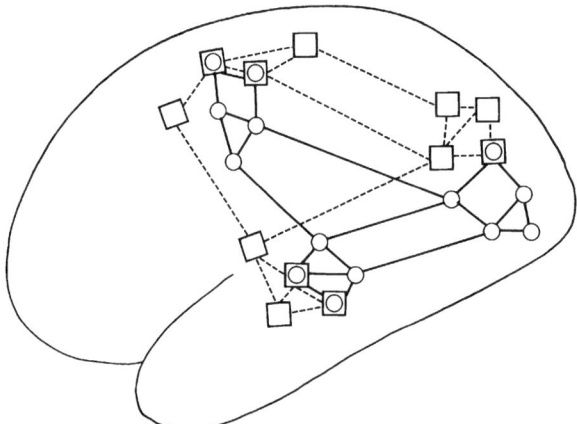

Figure 16.3. Scheme of two overlapping cell assemblies in a human brain. The neurons, indicated by circles or squares, respectively, are representative of neurons in higher (not primary) sensory areas (visual, acoustic, somatosensory).

When seeking the properties required by a piece of nervous tissue for the Hebbian kind of learning, one would end up with the connectivity typical of the cerebral cortex (Table 16.1). The tissue should receive input from the various sensory systems and should be composed of many neurons of the same kind. The neurons should be connected into a network. The synapses between the neurons should be modifiable in strength. This can be assumed to be the case for the synapses between pyramidal cells, most of which are located on dendritic spines. The connections should be excitatory in order to translate correlated activity in the input into correlated activity in the network. The network should be large; the more neurons there are, the more correlations can be detected and stored.

A large number of neurons and excitatory connections between them are also required for the development and maintenance of a train of thoughts. While it is still difficult to imagine the details of long-lasting time-structured events in the cortex such as a coherent train of thoughts, it is even more difficult or almost impossible to imagine such events in other parts of the mammalian brain that are either small or

Table 16.1: Requirements for Cell Assemblies and Structure of the Cortex

Requirements	Structure
Many neurons of the same kind	About 85% pyramidal cells
Connected with each other	Most synapses are between pyramidal cells
Excitatory connections	About 89% type I synapses
Modifiable connections	About 75% synapses on spines
Individual neurons connected to as many others as possible	About 8000 synapses/neuron
Connections between distant regions of the network	Large amount of white matter

characterized by inhibitory interactions. An approach to long-lasting dynamic aspects of cognitive functions is provided by the theory of synfire chains (Abeles, 1991), which is also based on the particular connectivity of the cerebral cortex and which can be well combined with the theory of cell assemblies.

Another important requirement would be that the network, despite its large size, should be richly connected within itself. Connections should also be possible over long distances. Each part of the network should be able to easily communicate with other parts of the network in order to be prepared for all possible constellations of common activity that might appear in the particular environment to which an individual is exposed. A highly specific prewiring between individual neurons is unlikely and would actually defeat the purpose of a learning device. A prewiring that enables individual elements to interact with a large number of other elements seems to be more advantageous.

Although the cerebral cortex is far from being a fully connected network in which each element is connected to every other one, one of the really unique features of the cortex is its rich connectivity within itself. This is evident from the large amount of white matter in larger brains, as well as from the fact that most pyramidal cells connect to thousands of others, both in their vicinity and at a distant place. In the isocortex of the mouse, the connectivity is such that each region is connected to every other by one or a few synaptic steps (Palm, 1984).

In conclusion, the cerebral cortex, like no other part of the brain, has the connectivity required for storing and handling a large number of correlations. It can be assumed to be a particularly efficient learning device in which memory items can be retrieved and combined in ever new ways, allowing for the detection of further and more complex correlations.

COMPARATIVE ASPECTS

Brain Size and Connectivity

The striving for a high degree of connectivity also becomes evident when comparing small and large mammalian brains. A large cortex has the advantage of having a large storage capacity, but it may be difficult for it to maintain the same degree of connectivity of a network with a smaller number of neurons. The attempt to uphold connectivity can be deduced from the following trends:

1. The volume of the cortical white matter increases much more than the volume of the gray matter. In some basal insectivores, the white matter amounts to only 6% of the isocortical volume, whereas in apes and humans it is around 40% (Frahm et al., 1982).

2. In brains with a larger cortex, individual neurons make more synapses on average. This can be deduced from the facts that the density of neurons per cubic millimeter decreases in larger brains (for review, see Jerison, 1973) and

that the density of synapses per cubic millimeter seems to stay constant, as has been shown for hedgehog and monkey (Schüz and Demianenko, 1995).

3. In addition, the average thickness of fibers increases, partially compensating for the longer conduction times that come with the larger distances in larger brains.

All of this cannot, however, fully compensate for the larger size of the cortex. For example, the average number of synapses per neuron may differ by a factor of at most 10 across mammalian species (Schüz and Demianenko, 1995), while the number of neurons in the cortex may differ by a factor of more than 1000. Furthermore, the average thickness of fibers does not increase sufficiently either to compensate for the longer conduction times that come with the increased distances (Jerison, 1991; Schüz and Preißl, 1996). This is suggested by measurements of the thickness of myelinated fibers in the corpus callosum of mouse and monkey (Jerison, 1991; Schüz and Preißl, 1996), as well as by calculations by Ringo et al. (1994), who show that otherwise large brains would need to be much larger than they are. Although individual fibers can become very thick in the monkey (Fig. 16. 4), the bulk of (myelinated) fibers has a quite similar diameter in small and large brains (between 0.5 and 1 μm in mouse and monkey). As pointed out by Ringo (1991), this should lead to a higher degree of local specialization in larger mammalian brains.

Allocortex and Reptilian Cortex

Both the mammalian allocortex and the reptilian cortex differ architectonically from the mammalian isocortex, and a lack of quantitative data on these structures makes it difficult to compare their connectivity with that of the isocortex. There is evidence, however, that both allocortex and reptilian cortex share important properties with the

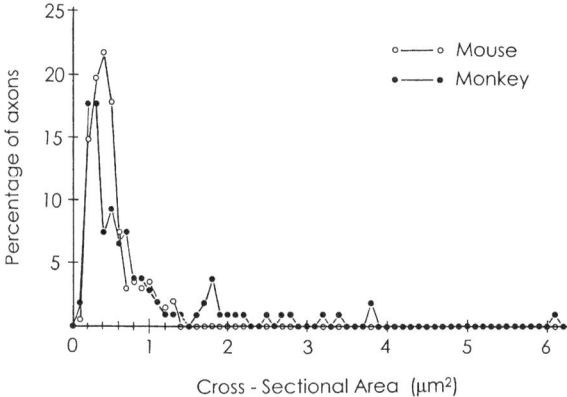

Figure 16.4. Thickness of myelinated axons in the corpus callosum of mouse and monkey. Each symbol corresponds to the relative frequency of axons of a given cross-sectional area. Bin width: 0.1 μm². (Same data as in Jerison, 1991; modified from Schüz and Preißl, 1996.)

mammalian isocortex. For example, in the mammalian hippocampus, excitatory connections between pyramidal cells also constitute a large proportion of the connectivity (Braitenberg and Schüz, 1983). In the reptilian cortex, it has been shown that there too the various parts of the cortex connect to each other (Halpern, 1980; Desan, 1988; Hoogland and Vermeulen-Van der Zee, 1988), and there are also cells that resemble the pyramidal cells of the mammalian cortex. They carry spines, and there is evidence for mutual excitation of these neurons (Kriegstein and Connors, 1986; Reiner, 1993).

Thus, the basic requirements for storing correlations in a Hebbian manner are also there in the reptilian cortex. With the elaboration of the acoustic and olfactory system in mammals, which can be assumed to be the result of the invasion of the nocturnal niche by the early mammals (Jerison, 1973), a more detailed picture of the environment reached the cortex. A larger and more elaborated learning device was certainly advantageous. The most important improvement may have been the introduction of the elaborated system of long-range connections (Miller, in press) that is so typical of the mammalian isocortex. The long-range connections are mainly made by the pyramidal cells from the upper cortical layers, and it is that layers which seem to be lacking in the reptilian cortex (Reiner, 1993).

REFERENCES

Abeles, M. (1991) *Corticonics. Neural Circuits of the Cerebral Cortex.* Cambridge University Press, Cambridge.

Blinkov, S.M., and Glezer, I.I. (1968) *Das Zentralnervensystem in Zahlen und Tabellen.* VEB Gustav Fischer, Jena.

Braak, H., and E. Braak, (1986) Ratio of pyramidal cells versus non-pyramidal cells in the human frontal isocortex and changes in ratio with ageing and Alzheimer's disease. In D.F. Swaab et al., (eds.): *Progress in Brain Research.* Elsevier Science, Amsterdam, pp. 185–212.

Braitenberg, V. (1977) On the *Texture of Brains*, Springer-Verlag, Berlin.

Braitenberg, V. (1978a) Cortical architectonics: general and areal. In M.A.B Brazier et al. (eds.): *Architectonics of the cerebral Cortex.* Raven Press, New York.

Braitenberg, V. (1978b) Cell assemblies in the cerebral cortex. In R. Heim et al. (eds.):Lecture Notes in Biomathematics, 21, *Theoretical Approaches to Complex Systems.* Springer-Verlag, Berlin, pp. 171–188.

Braitenberg, V. (1985) Charting the visual cortex. In A. Peters et al. (eds.): *Cerebral Cortex*, vol. 3, Plenum, New York, pp. 379–414.

Braitenberg, V. (1986) Two views of the cerebral cortex. In G. Palm et al. (eds.): *Brain Theory*. Springer-Verlag, Berlin, pp. 81–96.

Braitenberg, V., D. Heck, and F. Sultan, (1997) The detection and generation of sequences as a key to cerebellar function. Experiments and theory. *Behav. Brain Sci.* 20(2):229–245.

Braitenberg, V., and F. Pulvermüller, (1992) Entwurf einer neurologischen Theorie der Sprache. *Naturwissenschaften* 79:103–117.

Braitenberg, V., and A. Schüz, (1983): Some anatomical comments on the hippocampus. In W. Seifert. (ed.,): *Neurobiology of the Hippocampus*, Academic Press, London, pp. 21–37.

Braitenberg, V. and A. Schüz, (1991) *Anatomy of the Cortex. Statistics and Geometry.* Springer-Verlag, Berlin. (2nd revised edition 1998)

Desan, P.H. (1988) Organization of the cerebral cortex in turtle. In W.K. Schwerdtfeger and W.J.A.J. Smeets (eds.): *The forebrain of Reptiles. Current Concepts of Structure and Function*, Karger, Basel, pp. 1–11.

Frahm, H.D., Stephan, H., and M. Stephan, (1982) Comparison of brain structure volumes in Insectivora and Primates. I. Neocortex. *J. Hirnforsch.* 23:375–389.
Halpern, M. (1980) The telencephalon of snakes. In S.O.E. Ebbesson. (ed.,): *Comparative Neurology of the Telencephalon.* Plenum Press, New York, pp. 257–295.
Hebb, D.O. (1949) *Organization of Behavior. A Neuropsychological Theory*, 2nd ed. Wiley and Sons, Inc., New York.
Hoogland, P.V., and E. Vermeulen-Van der Zee, (1988) Intrinsic and extrinsic connections of the cerebral cortex of lizards. In W.K. Schwerdtfeger and W.J.A.J. Smeets (eds.): *The Forebrain of reptiles. Current Concepts of Structure and Function.* Karger, Basel, pp. 20–29.
Horner, C.H. (1993) Plasticity of the dendritic spine. *Progr. Neurobiol.* 41:281–321.
Houser, C.R., J.E., Vaughn, S.H.C., Hendry, E.G. Jones, and A. Peters, (1984) GABA neurons in the cerebral cortex. In E.G. Jones and A.Peters (eds.): *Cerebral Cortex, vol. 2, Functional Properties of Cortical Cells.* Plenum Press, New York, pp. 63–89.
Jerison, H.J. (1973) *Evolution of the Brain and Intelligence.* Academic Press, New York.
Jerison, H.J. (1991) *Brain Size and the Evolution of Mind.* American Museum of Natural History, New York.
Kriegstein, A.R., and B.W. Connors, (1986) Cellular physiology of the turtle visual cortex: synaptic properties and intrinsic circuitry. *J. Neurosci.* 6(1):178–191.
Miller, R. (1996) Cortico-thalamic interplay and the security of operation of neural assemblies and temporal chains in the cerebral cortex. *Biol. Cybernet.* 75:263–275.
Miller, R. (in press) Laminar continuity between neo- and mesocortex. In R. Miller and A. Schüz (eds.): Cortical Areas: Unity and Diversity. Harwood. Academic Publishers, Amsterdam.
Miller, R., and J.R. Wickens, (1991) Corticostriatal cell assemblies in selective attention and in representation of predictable and controllable events. A general statement of corticostriatal interplay and the role of striatal dopamine. *Concepts Neurosci.* 2(1):65–95.
Nieuwenhuys, R. (1994) The neocortex. An overview of its evolutionary development, structural organization and synaptology. *Anat. Embryol.* 190:307–337.
Palm, G. (1982) *Neural Assemblies. An Alternative Approach to AI Springer-Verlag.* Berlin.
Palm, G. (1984) Associative networks and cell assemblies. In G. Palm and A. Aertsen (eds.): *Brain Theory.* Springer-Verlag, Berlin. pp. 211–230 (1984).
Palm, G. (1990) Cell assemblies as a guideline for brain research. *Concepts Neurosci.* 1:133–147.
Peters, A., and E.G. Jones, (1984) Classification of cortical neurons. In A. Peters and E.G. Jones (eds.): *Cerebral Cortex, vol. 1, Cellular Components of the Cerebral Cortex.* Plenum Press, New York, pp. 107–121.
Peters, A., and D.A. Kara, (1985) The neuronal composition of area 17 of rat visual cortex. I. The pyramidal cells. *J. Comp. Neurol.* 234:218–241.
Plenz, D., and A. Aertsen, (1996) Neural dynamics in cortex-striatum co-cultures. 1. Anatomy and electrophysiology of neural cell types. *Neuroscience* 70:861–891.
Pulvermüller, F. (1992) Constituents of a neurological theory of language. *Concepts Neurosci.* 3:157–200.
Ringo, J.L. (1991) Neuronal interconnection as a function of brain size. *Brain Behav. Evol.* 38:1–6.
Ringo, J.L., R.W. Doty, S. Demeter, and P.Y. Simard, (1994) Time is of the essence: a conjecture that hemispheric specialization arises from interhemispheric conduction delay. *Cerebral Cortex* 4:331–343.
Rockel, A.J., R.W. Hiorns, and T.P.S. Powell, (1980) The basic uniformity in structure of the neocortex. *Brain* 103:221–244.
Schüz, A. and G.P. Demianenko, (1995) Constancy and variability in cortical structure. A study on synapses and dendritic spines in hedgehog and monkey. *J. Brain Res.* 36:113–122.
Schüz, A. and Palm, G. (1989) Density of neurons and synapses in the cerebral cortex of the mouse. *J. Comp. Neurol.* 286: 442–455.
Schüz, A. and H. Preißl, (1996) Basic connectivity of the cerebral cortex and some considerations on the corpus callosum. *Neurosci. Biobehav. Rev.* 20:567–570.
Steriade, M., E.G. Jones, and R.R. Llinás, (1990) *Thalamic Oscillations and Signaling.* John Wiley and Sons, New York.
White, E.L. (1989) *Cortical Circuits. Synaptic Organization of the Cerebral Cortex. Structure, Function, and Theory.* Birkhäuser, Boston.
Wickelgren, W.A. (1992) Webs, cell assemblies, and chunking in neural nets. *Concepts Neurosci.* 3:1–53.
Wickens, J. (1993) *A Theory of the Striatum.* Pergamon Press, Oxford.

Chapter 17

EVOLUTION AND COMPLEXITY OF THE HUMAN BRAIN: SOME ORGANIZING PRINCIPLES

Michel A. Hofman, Netherlands Institute for Brain Research

Seltsamer Zufall, das alle die Menschen, deren Schädel man geöffnet hat, ein Gehirn hatten. (L. Wittgenstein, Über Gewissheit)

INTRODUCTION

The explicit recognition of the brain as the seat of sensation and thought probably originated with the Greek philosopher Alcmaeon of Croton in the late fifth century BC. The present view is that of the brain as the receiver and integrator of information from the senses and as the organ through which an organism can explore and communicate with the outside world (Hodos and Campbell, 1990; Jerison, 1991). Therefore, functionally significant changes in the internal organization of the brain during evolution would be a sufficient condition to enable species to cope with the ecological demands of newly invaded niches. Such a pattern of brain evolution is indeed a phenomenon found in many groups of vertebrates. Major variations in gross brain size are found as well, however, and are often even more prominent than the differences in organization (Fig. 17.1).

During the past two decades considerable progress has been made in explaining the evolution of (relative) brain size in terms of physical and adaptive principles (see Pirlot, 1987; Deacon, 1990; Harvey and Krebs, 1990; Aboitiz, 1996). In addition, a quantitative approach to the comparative morphology of the brain has made it possible to identify and formalize regularities in the apparent diversity of brain design, especially in the development and evolution of the mammalian brain (e.g., Haug, 1987; Hofman, 1989; Welker, 1990; Finlay and Darlington, 1995).

Although many aspects of brain evolution remain unexplained, these comparative investigations, using scaling methods and mathematical models, have provided new insights into the evolutionary dynamics of the brain and its morphological constraints. The object of this review is to present current perspectives on brain evolution, especially in humans, and to examine some hypothetical organizing principles that may underlie the brain's complex organization.

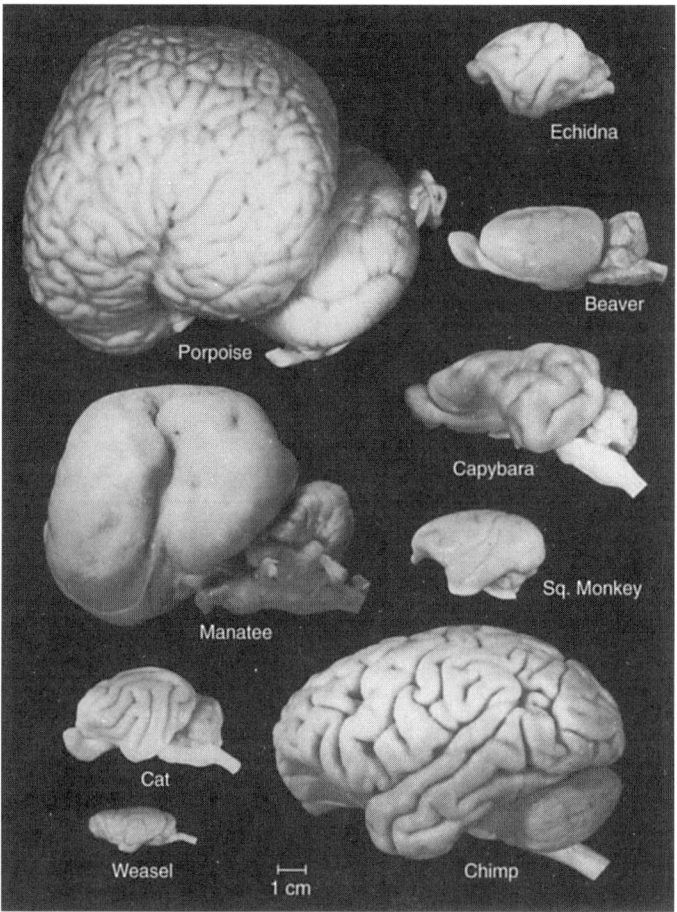

Figure 17.1. Diverse brain conformations and gyral and sulcal patterns in nine different mammals. Note the large, but lissencephalic, cerebrum of manatee. Specimens are from the Wisconsin Comparative Mammalian Brain Collection. (From Welker, 1990, by permission of Plenum Press, New York.)

EVOLUTION OF BRAIN SIZE

The human brain contains about 100 billion neurons, more than 100,000 km of interconnections, and has an estimated storage capacity of 1.25 terabytes (Cherniak, 1990). Yet the energy consumption of this massive neural system is extremely low (~15 W). Although these extraordinary numbers make our brain one of the most complex and efficient structures in the known universe, it is by no means unrivaled either in size or in computational power.

Absolute brain size, however, is not the most appropriate measure for determining the evolutionary level of encephalization reached by a species, because brain size in vertebrates is also a function of the size of the animal according to the power function

$Y = kX^\alpha$, where Y is brain weight and X is body weight. Logarithmic transformation yields the linear equation $\log Y = \alpha \log X + \log k$, with α being the slope of the regression line and k the scaling coefficient. A graphic representation of brain versus body size across species of different mammalian orders (Fig. 17.2) indeed shows that the two variables are highly correlated, explaining more than 90% of the variance in brain size (Jerison, 1973; Harvey and Krebs, 1990). The rationale behind this

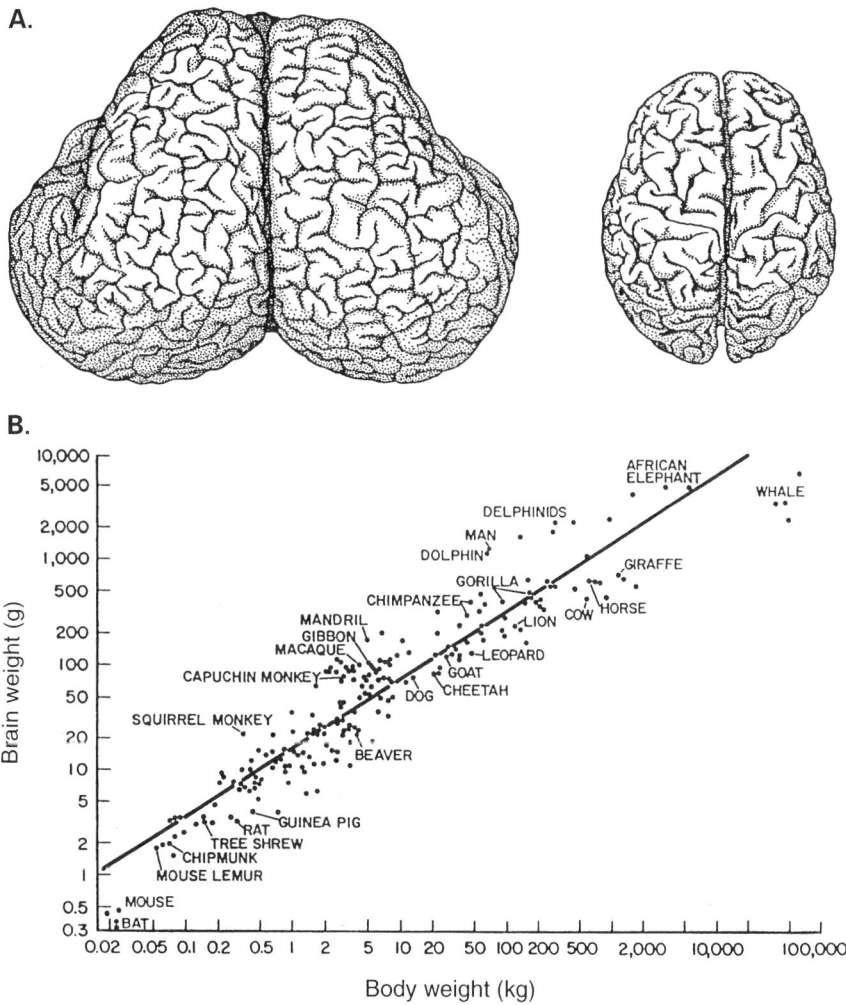

Figure 17.2. Brain size compared with body size in mammals. (A) Dorsal view of the brain of an adult fin whale (left) and an adult man (right). The scale of the pictures is the same. Although the body weight of a fin whale (*Balaenoptera physalus*, one of the largest cetaceans) is approximately 1000 times that of a man, the brain weights differ by a factor of only about 5. (B) The relationship between brain size and body size for a large number of mammalian species. Logarithmic scale. The straight line, representing the solution of the allometric equation, has a slope of about 3/4. (Modified and reproduced with permission from Purves, 1988.)

phenomenon is that larger animals need to have larger brains in order to control and service the increasing somatic and vegetative demands that are the inevitable consequences of increases in body size. This scaling factor is often referred to as the *somatic* component of brain size.

For interspecific sequences of mammals the parameters of the allometric equation have been determined, yielding an exponent of 0.75, which means that brain weight increases slower than body weight, resulting in smaller brains relative to body size in larger mammals. When the exponent was found to be 0.75, a relation was suggested with basal metabolic rate, which also scales with body weight with an exponent of 0.75. Recent studies, however, have shown that brain size and basal metabolic rate in mammals are not related (McNab and Eisenberg, 1989; Hofman, 1993). Another interpretation of the 0.75 exponent assumes that during prenatal life brain and body growth are genetically coupled and both variables grow at a fast rate (Riska and Atchley, 1985; Deacon, 1990). Shortly after birth the brain slows its growth, whereas the rest of the body keeps growing at a fast rate for a longer period. This results in postnatal decoupling in the growth of the respective parts. In other words, adult brain size is mainly determined by the prenatal period, whereas adult body size depends on both the prenatal and postnatal periods of growth (Fig. 17.3). In larger species, the postnatal component becomes increasingly important in specifying adult body size, leading to a decrease in the brain/body ratio.

Although the main axis in the brain–body weight graph gives information about an important part of brain size variance, there is still a notorious residual variation in this relationship. This dispersion is supposed to correspond with species differences in cognitive information capacity, or biological intelligence (Jerison, 1973, 1991), and can be referred to as the *nonsomatic* component of brain size. In short, current perspectives on brain evolution relate brain size variability to two main parameters: a scaling factor that corresponds to overall body size and a nonsomatic, ecological factor associated with processing capacity and cognition.

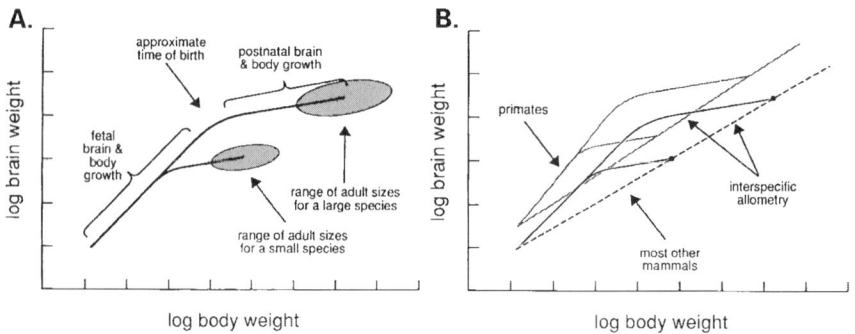

Figure 17.3. Allometric patterns of mammalian brain growth. (A) Ontogenetic developmental trajectory for brain and body growth in two typical mammals of different body size. The prenatal phase overlaps completely for most species. (B) Ontogenetic curves for different mammalian species and their relation to interspecific trends. Note the shift of ontogenetic curves that distinguishes primates from other mammals. (Modified and reproduced with permission from Deacon, 1990.)

Recently, Aboitiz (1996) argued that in evolution body weight and ecological conditions have different effects on brain structure, resulting in distinct differences in neural architecture, even if both factors may produce brain size increases. When the brain grows just following an overall size increase, it would do so by changing little of its neural organization. On the other hand, if the brain grows in response to ecological conditions, this would occur associated with important cellular and connectional rearrangements that result in increased perceptual and behavioral skills. This view emphasizes the role of connectional modifications in increasing brain capacity and contrasts with current ideas of a unitary process of evolutionary brain growth, where a larger brain size per se produces better processing capacity, regardless of the causal factor behind it. In other words, it would make a difference in terms of neural organization and function whether the brain grows following a body size increase or by selection of specific behavioral capacities.

ENCEPHALIZATION IN PRIMATES

Selection pressures toward enlargement of the brain beyond the requirements of large bodies were probably very strong when birds and mammals diverged from their different reptilian ancestral stocks. Particularly with the evolution of anthropoid primates (apes and monkeys) a progressive enlargement of the brain appears to have taken place, which can be associated with a dramatic increase in the functional and behavioral capacity of this group of mammals (Martin, 1983; Jerison, 1991). Indeed, some primates, such as humans and cebus monkeys, have considerably larger brains than would be expected for their body sizes (Fig. 17.4).

A large part of this residual variation in brain size among primates has to do with ecological differences and social organization. For example, both New World and Old World frugivorous primates (e.g., Cercopithecines) tend to have larger brains than folivorous species (e.g., Colobines) for a given body weight. In general, animals that have to search for their food in an extended area tend to have larger brains than do animals that have easy access to food in a small home range. Another determinant of encephalization is that the more well developed the senses, the larger the brain. This partly explains the high encephalization of species that live in a diverse and unpredictable environment, as most primates do. Furthermore, it has been found that relative brain size correlates with troop size in prosimians, with troop range in New World monkeys, and with individual home range in Old World monkeys (Sawaguchi, 1988). Similar findings were reported for polygonous and terrestrial primate species (Martin, 1983), indicating that ecological and behavioral factors may affect the amount of brain tissue beyond that relating to scaling of body size.

A further interesting finding is that fossil hominids are to be excluded from other anthropoid primates because of their relatively larger brains (Fig. 17.4). In that respect, australopithecines, the earliest known hominoid ancestors of the genus *Homo*, who lived about 4 to 1 million years ago, had already attained a higher level of encephalization than any of the living pongids. Regardless of what factors were

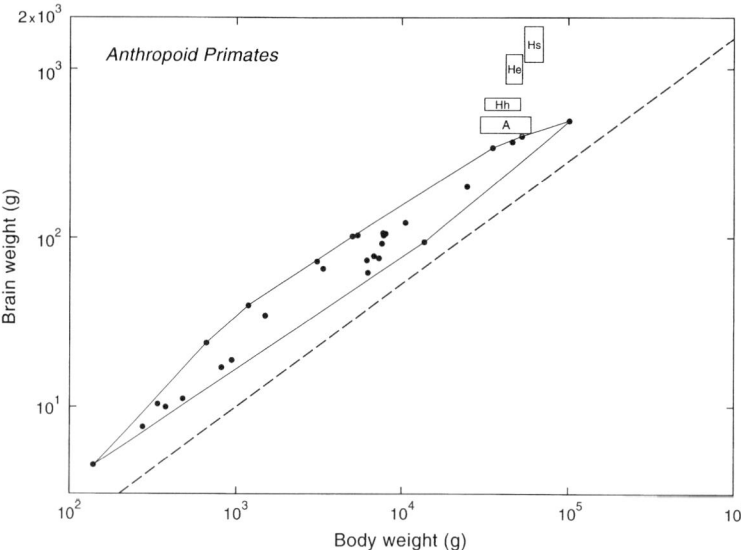

Figure 17.4. Brain weight as a function of body weight for 29 species of anthropoid primates (monkeys, apes, humans). Logarithmic scale. Hominids indicated are *Australopithecus* (A), *Homo habilis* (Hh), *Homo erectus* (He), and *Homo sapiens* (Hs). The dashed line indicates the regression for living mammals. Note that the fossil hominids are to be excluded from the extant primates for having larger brains for a given body size. (From Hofman, 1983, by permission of Karger, Basel.)

actually selected for encephalization in *Homo*, this process could only have occurred if the increase in relative brain size was not precluded by energetic constraints. Due to the extreme thermal sensitivity of the central nervous system, a large complex brain requires an elaborate cooling system both to remove the heat it generates, and to protect it from high environmental temperatures. It has been suggested that some of the more distinctive hominid features may have evolved as thermoregulatory adaptations to help stabilize body temperature in stressing environments. It has also been suggested, by Falk (1990) and others, that the evolution of a "cranial radiator" by hominids helped provide additional cooling to delicate and metabolically expensive parts of the brain, such as the isocortex. This vascular cooling mechanism would have served as a "prime releaser" that permitted brain size to increase dramatically during human evolution.

Another important aspect of human brain evolution is that the organism must be capable of supplying a larger brain with its increased energy requirements, a problem exacerbated by the high metabolic cost of this organ. Foley and Lee (1991) therefore proposed that the expansion in relative brain size that took place during the evolution of *Homo* could not have been achieved without an associated dietary shift to a higher quality diet: from folivorism to omnivorism. Consequently, a lower dietary quality not only directly restricted encephalization in australopithecines, but also precluded the development of the "cranial radiator" by these hominids for anatomical and physiological reasons. Although there may be something to these arguments, the possible contributions of energetic factors in determining encephalization still remain to be elucidated. It must be kept in mind that (1) the relationship between diet and metabolic rate in eutherian mammals has been seriously questioned when controlling for body size differences (Harvey et al., 1991), and (2) there is no correlation between relative brain size and basal metabolic rate (McNab and Eisenberg, 1989; Hofman, 1993).

Additional factors relating to brain size in primates have to do with aspects of the life history strategy, such as gestation time, age at sexual maturity, and reproductive rate (Harvey and Krebs, 1990). It means that natural selection operates on brain size at the expense of growth and reproduction, which could explain its correlation with life span (Hofman, 1993). Indeed, it has long been postulated that species with larger brains tend to live longer. Allman et al. (1993) have now found strong quantitative support for this position in anthropoid primates. They hypothesize that brain is a buffer against environmental variation. Animals that have longer life spans are likely to experience more extreme environmental fluctuations and thus be exposed during the course of their long lives to more severe crises (such as shortages in normally used food resources) than will animals with shorter life spans. Therefore the relative sizes of some brain structures, such as the cerebellum, hippocampus, and isocortex, that enable animals to store information about the environment and develop cognitive strategies, are especially well related to life span.

Although adaptive principles may explain the correlation between brain size and longevity to some extent, it could as well be that the prolonged phases of development and generation time found in anthropoid primates require a reduction of the mortality rate, and consequently an increase in longevity, to enable animals to produce enough offspring during their lives. It would mean that life span is not causally related to relative brain size but that it is simply a byproduct of the life history strategy adopted by the species (extreme K-selection in anthropoids). This evolutionary strategy is most obvious when considering the evolution of hominids, where there has been a presumed twofold increase in life span associated with a more than threefold increase in brain size in a mere 2 million years (Fig. 17.5).

GENERAL CONSTRAINTS ON BRAIN EVOLUTION

How is the organization of the brain as a whole affected when a species undergoes strong selection pressure for the optimization of a behavioral ability that depends on the size and functional capacity of a specific substem of the brain. The need for energetic efficiency suggests that it should result in the most localized possible increase in brain volume corresponding to the behavioral adaptation. Required computational structures or the nature of existing developmental programs could, however, severely constrain the range of local adaptations. We therefore have to consider the roles of both specific adaptations for particular behaviors and general organizing constraints in determining the paths of brain evolution.

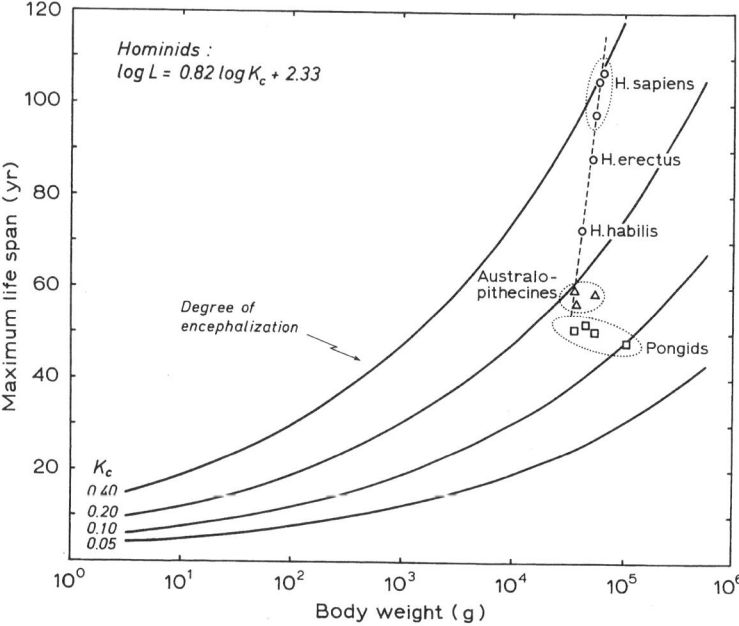

Figure 17.5. Maximum potential life span (L) as a function of body size and degree of encephalization (K_c) in pongids and fossil hominids. Semilogarithmic scale. Note the close association between the evolution of brain size and the progression in longevity in hominids. (Modified and reproduced with permission from Hofman, 1984.)

To explore the relative magnitude of changes in brain organization attributable to these two factors, Finlay and Darlington (1995) studied the major brain regions and patterns of neurogenesis in a wide variety of insectivores, bats, and primates, including humans. It was shown that the volumes of brain components from medulla to forebrain are highly predictable from absolute brain size by a nonlinear function. Thus, the original finding that there is a highly predictable relation between isocortex size and total brain size (Hofman, 1989) seems to apply to all major brain subdivisions. The nonlinear nature of these relations is emphasized by plotting the actual values of the volume of the structures as a function of total brain size (Fig. 17.6). This method of representation shows the difference in the rate of change of particular structures as brain size increases, as well as the progressive nature of corticalization in primates with large brains, most notably in humans. This observation may explain the multiple facets and rapid rate of human evolution and supports the idea of the isocortex as a general-purpose integrator that allows the organism to take advantage of the extra brain structure in ways not directly selected during evolution.

Principal component analysis, furthermore, showed that more than 99% of the total variance in volume of these brain structures is explained by two factors (Fig. 17.7). The first factor, which is most highly correlated with the isocortex, loads strongly on all structures but the olfactory bulb and accounts for 96.3% of the total variance. The

General Constraints on Brain Evolution 509

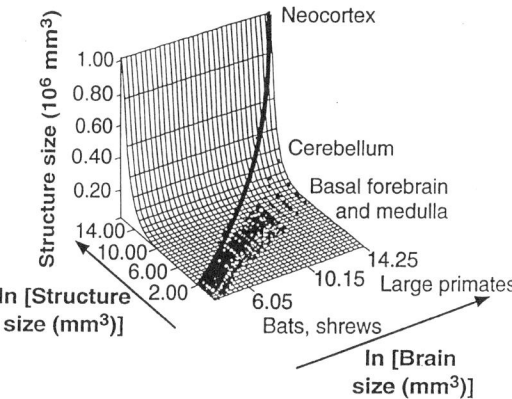

Figure 17.6. Volumes of 10 brain subdivisions as a function of total brain size for 131 mammalian species including *Homo sapiens*. The volumes of the brain divisions are plotted in actual values and on a logarithmic scale. This method of representation emphasizes the difference in the rate of change of particular structures as brain size increases, as well as the progressive nature of change in neocortex (= isocortex) volume across species. Structures and species listed along the horizontal and vertical axes are placed approximately to illustrate the dimensions scaled. (From Finlay and Darlington, 1995 by permission of AAAS, Washington.)

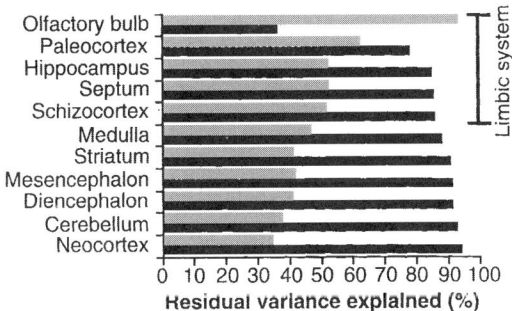

Figure 17.7. Relative loadings of the two factors of the principal component analysis on the 11 brain divisions, including the olfactory bulb. The first factor (black bars) loads strongly on all structures but the olfactory bulb, whereas the second factor (gray bars) loads more strongly on structures with a major limbic component. The diencephalon has both limbic and nonlimbic components. The terms *neocortex* and *paleocortex* refer to the isocortex and olfactory cortex, respectively. The schizocortex includes the entorhinal, perirhinal, and (pre)subicular cortices (Stephan et al., 1981). All cortices include the underlying white matter. For further details see text. (From Finlay and Darlington, 1995 by permission of AAAS, Washington.)

second factor, which is very small compared with the first, is most highly correlated with the olfactory bulb and loads more strongly on structures with a major limbic component; it accounts for 3.0% of the variance. This two-factor model provides a more accurate description of brain configuration than did the previous one-factor model. These findings suggest that simple across-species generalizations account for most of the variance in the size of brain components.

Finlay and Darlington (1995) also found that neurogenesis is highly conserved across a wide range of mammals and correlates with the relative enlargement of brain structures. For instance, structures that grow disproportionately large as brain size increases, such as the isocortex and cerebellum, have late birth dates and a prolonged cell division. The longer neurogenesis is delayed, the more precursor cells can be formed and the larger the structure that results (Kaas, 1993; Rakic, 1995). In fact, an additional 17 doublings of a structure's precursor cells can yield some 131,000 times the final number of neurons, which is roughly equivalent to the difference between the size of the human isocortex and that of the shrew. These observations are in accord with a developmental constraint hypothesis that suggests that it should be possible to predict the size of any neural structure in any species from a simple rule. Consequently, the most likely brain alteration resulting from selection for any behavioral ability may be a generalized enlargement of the entire nonolfactory brain.

How can we reconcile this evidence for cross-species conservatism in patterns of brain enlargement with the strong intuition and evidence that species-specific brain adaptations must exist? Finlay and Darlington (1995) came up with several answers to this question. First, the structures considered are rather broad brain divisions, and there may be reallocation of functions within these divisions. Second, brains vary on other dimensions, including connections, cell morphology, and neurotransmitter complements. Third, the enormous range of structure sizes across species may allow for noticeable amounts of species-specific variation in the size of those brain parts, despite the high cross-species correlations among them. The volume of individual brain structures may differ by a factor of as much as two to three, even when the two species being compared are very similar on the two major factors discussed above. Although specific adaptations of brain structures to behavior have indeed been reported (for reviews, see Pirlot, 1987; Aboitiz, 1996), they often involve developmental processes, such as neurogenesis or regressive events that are rare and difficult to accomplish, as they require a coordinated enlargement of many independent components of one functional system without enlargement of the rest of the brain. For human evolution in particular, theories that emphasize the highly conserved order but nonlinear scaling of neurogenesis provide an explanation why selection for any one ability, such as tool use, language, or aspects of social organization, might cause, in parallel, neural changes in the entire brain leading to the constellation of behavioral traits we now possess.

EVOLUTION AND GEOMETRY OF THE CEREBRAL CORTEX

Among the most distinctive morphological features of mammalian brains is the evolutionary expansion of the cerebral cortex. Particularly in species with large brains, and most notably in great apes, dolphins and whales, the brain becomes disproportionately composed of a cortical structure (Welker, 1990; Northcutt and Kaas, 1995). The evolutionary origin of the cerebral cortex is thought to result from the adaptation to nocturnal life, along with the development of olfactory-driven behavior in mesozoic mammals (Jerison, 1973).

A consequence of this evolutionary phenomenon is that the geometry of the brain, and especially its surface area, has changed notably since the late Cretaceous (Jerison, 1973). Comparisons among mammals show that the surface area of the cortical sheet varies by more than five orders of magnitude, while the thickness of the cortex varies by less than one order of magnitude (Fig. 17.8) (Hofman, 1989; Allman, 1990; Welker, 1990). Therefore, evolutionary changes in the cerebral cortex have occurred mainly parallel to the cortical surface (tangentially) and have been sharply constrained in the vertical (radial) dimension, which makes it especially well suited for the elaboration of multiple projections and mapping systems.

A mosaic of functionally specialized areas have indeed been found in the mammalian cortex, some of the functions being remarkably diverse (Kaas, 1993). At lower processing levels of the cortex, these maps bear a fairly simple topographical relationship to the world, but in higher areas precise topography may be sacrificed for the mapping of more abstract functions. Here, selected aspects of the sensory input are combined in ways that are likely to be relevant to the animal. Over the past 20 years the use of modern anatomical tracing methods and physiological recording has established that each sensory modality is mapped several times in different areas, with about a dozen representations of the visual world and half a dozen each of auditory inputs and somatosensory sensations. In fact, the maps differ in the attributes of the stimulus represented, in how the field is emphasized, and in the types of computations performed. Clearly, the specifications of all these representations means that functional maps can no longer be considered simply as hard-wired neural

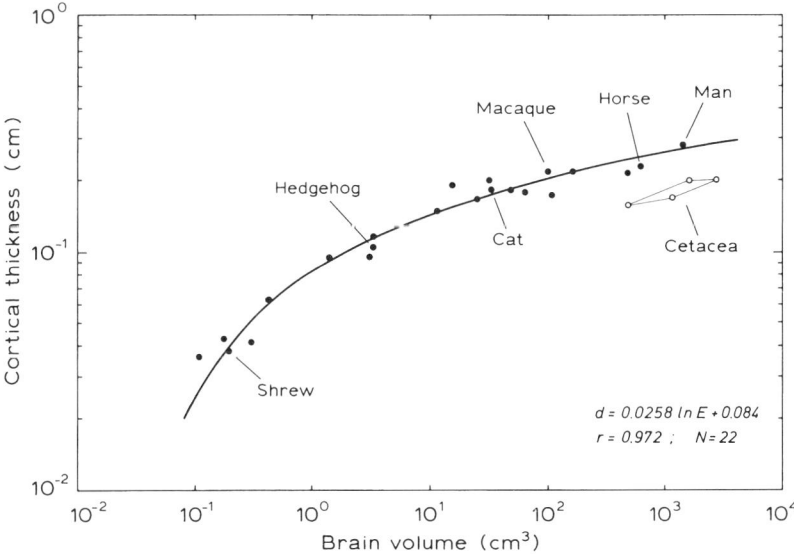

Figure 17.8. Mean cortical thickness as a function of brain volume. Logarithmic scale. The curve for terrestrial mammals is described by a semilogarithmic equation. The thickness of the cortex varies by less than one order of magnitude. Note that dolphins and whales are distinct from nonmarine mammals in that their cortices are relatively thin. (From Hofman, 1988, by permission of Karger, Basel.)

networks. They are much more flexible than previously thought and are continually modified by feedback and lateral interactions. These dynamic changes in maps, which seem likely to result from local interactions and modulations in the cortical circuits, provide the plasticity necessary for adaptive behavior and learning.

Although species vary in the number of cortical areas they possess, and in the patterns of connections within and between areas, the structural organization of the cerebral cortex is remarkably similar. It has been estimated, for example, that within 1 mm^3 of human cortex there are about 50,000 neurons that contain 150 m of dendrites and 100 m of axons and that these neurites have about 50×10^6 synapses (Cherniak, 1990). The basic structural uniformity of the isocortex suggests that there are general architectural principles governing its growth and evolutionary development. It is now well established that the cerebral cortex forms as a smooth sheet populated by neurons that proliferate at the ventricular surface and migrate outwards along radial glial fibers (Rakic, 1995). Why, then, does the cortex remain smooth (lissencephalic) in some species, particularly those with small brains, yet become highly convoluted (gyrencephalic) in others, particularly those with large brains? The primary reason is that, from a brain volume of about 3 to 4 cm^3 onward, the surface area of the cortex increases disproportionally with brain size.

In these animals, the cortical surface area, rather than being proportional to the 2/3 power of geometric similarity, is nearly a linear function of brain volume (Fig. 17.9). It means that if a mouse brain (E = 0.5 cm^3) were scaled up as the two-thirds power to the size of a human brain (E = 1400 cm^3) it would have a cortical surface of only

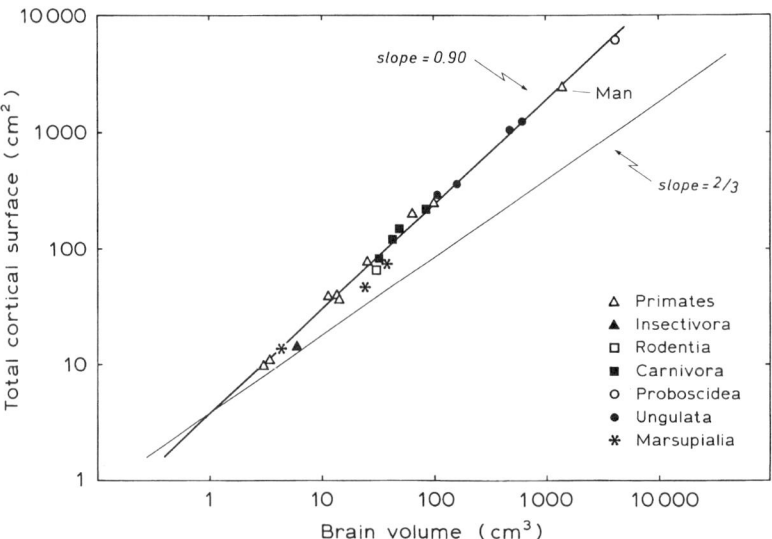

Figure 17.9. Total cortical surface area as a function of brain volume in terrestrial mammals. Logarithmic scale. The slope of the regression line is 0.90 ± 0.012, representing the surface-volume relation for convoluted brains. The dashed line represents the scaling of the cortical surface area according to the 2/3 power of geometric similarity. Note that the cortical surface area of species with convoluted brains (area >10 cm^2) is nearly a linear function of brain volume.

about 480 cm². The actual surface area of the human cerebral cortex, however, is about 2000 cm², which is more than four times larger than would be predicted assuming geometric similarity, indicating that mammalian brains change their shape by becoming folded as they increase in size (see Fig. 17.1). Most of this bias is attributable to the preference for tangential versus radial expansion. Differences in the duration of neurogenesis, which increases more rapidly with brain size for the cerebral cortex than for subcortical areas (Caviness et al., 1995; Finlay and Darlington, 1995; Rakic, 1995), lead to a systematic increase in the ratio of cortical to subcortical regions. The volume of gray matter expressed as a percentage of total brain volume increases from about 25% for insectivores to 50% for humans (Fig. 17.10).

When convolutions occur, what determines the spatial pattern of folding? Previous hypotheses about cortical folding have emphasized mechanisms intrinsic to the cortical gray matter (for review, see Hofman, 1989). Van Essen (1997) recently suggested that extrinsic factors are more important and that tension along axons in the white matter is the primary driving force for cortical folding. By keeping the aggregate length of axonal and dendritic wiring low, tension should contribute to the

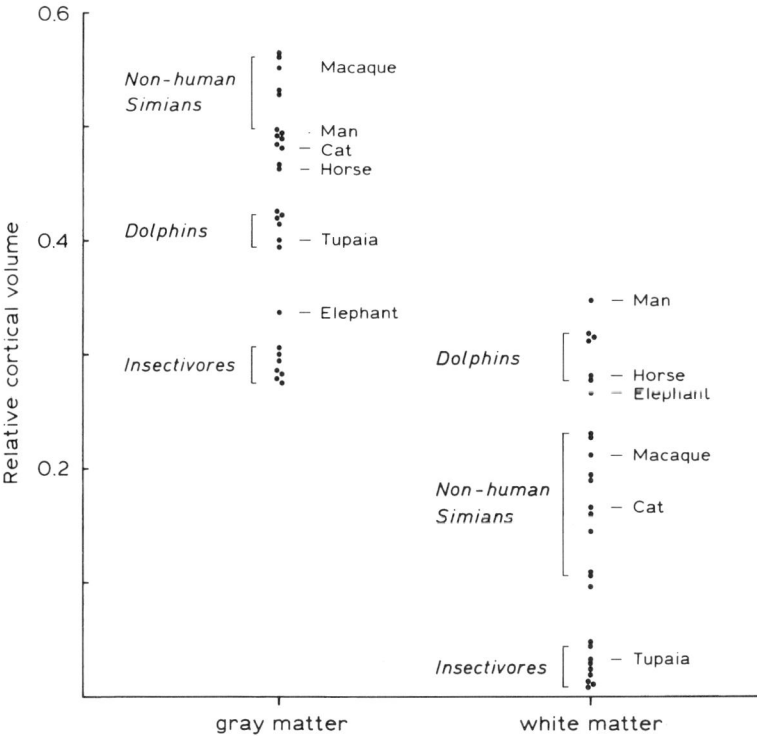

Figure 17.10. Volumes of cortical gray and white matter expressed as a percentage of total brain volume for 27 mammalian species. Note the relatively large amount of white matter in humans (From Hofman, 1988, by permission of Karger, Basel.)

compactness of neural circuitry throughout the cortex. Thus, local wiring and cortical folding is a simple strategy that helps to fit the large sheetlike cortex into a compact space and keeps cortical connections short. An important evolutionary advantage of this design principle is that it enables brains to be more compact and faster with increasing size.

DESIGN PRINCIPLES OF NEURONAL ORGANIZATION

Explaining how the brain works requires some information about how it is organized structurally. From anatomical studies we know that the mammalian cortex is made up of distinct neural networks that are organized in columnar arrays stretched out through the depth of the cortex (Leise, 1990; Malach, 1994; Krubitzer, 1995). It has been postulated that these modular units have spatial dimensions depending on the number of local circuit neurons (Hofman, 1985) and that both the number and size of modules increase with increasing brain size (Prothero, 1997). Scaling models, furthermore, indicate that the difference in modular diameter among mammals is only minor compared with the dramatic variation in overall cortex size (Hofman, 1985; Prothero, 1997). Thus it seems that the main cortical change during evolution has presumably been an increase in the number, rather than in the size, of these units.

Although the details of the interpretation of the columnar organization of the cortex are still controversial (Hofman, 1985; Crick, 1989), it is evident that the cerebral cortex is characterized by the hierarchical organization of groups of neurons. To group neurons into clusters interacting over relatively short distances allows these groups to inform as many adjacent clusters of neurons about the state of the "emitting" cluster with as little as possible redundancy of information. Figure 17.11 shows a simple schematic diagram illustrating the effect of increasing the number of functional units on the number of interconnections. When the modular units are connected to all others by separate fibers and when each additional unit becomes connected with each of the already existing ones, then the number of connections (C) is related to the number of units (U) according to the equation $C = U(U-1)$, which is nearly equivalent to $C = U^2$. In such a system the number of connections increases much faster than the number of units. Recently we showed that in species with convoluted brains the mass of interconnective nerve fibers, forming the underlying white matter, is proportional to the 1.5 power of cortical surface area (Hofman, 1991). In other words, the fraction of mass devoted to wiring seems to increase much slower than that needed to maintain a high degree of connectivity between the modular units.

These findings are in line with a model of neuronal connectivity (Deacon, 1990; Ringo, 1991) that says that as brain size increases there must be a corresponding fall in the fraction of neurons with which any neuron communicates directly. The reason for this is that if a fixed percentage of interconnections is to be maintained in the face of increased neuron number, then a large fraction of any brain size increase would be spent maintaining such degree of wiring while the increasing axon length would reduce neural computational speed (Ringo et al., 1994).

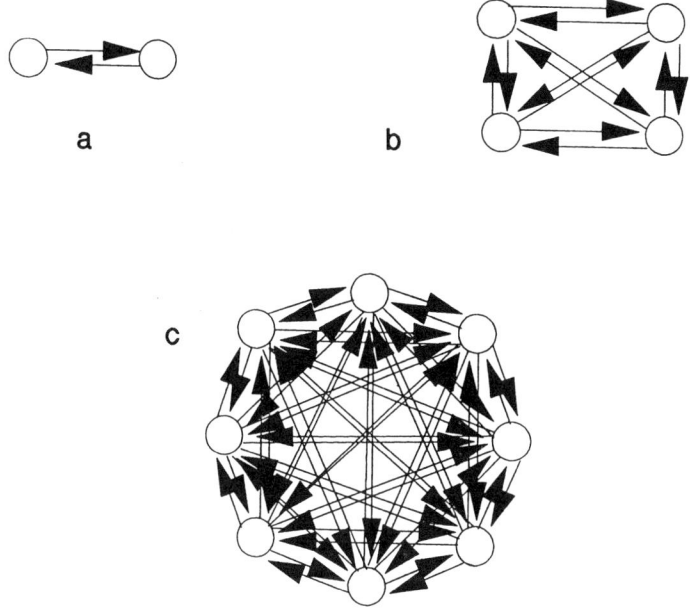

Figure 17.11. The problem of network allometry is represented by three neural circuits (a–c) that exhibit maximum connectivity. The diagrams depict that the number of connections (C) grows much faster than the number of units (U) in a fully connected network: $C = U(U-1)$. (From Ringo, 1991, by permission of Karger, Basel.)

Once the brain has grown to a point where the bulk of its mass is in the form of connections, then further increases (as long as the same ratio in interconnectivity is maintained) will be unproductive. Increases in number of units will be balanced by decreased performance of those units due to the increased conduction time. This implies that large brains may tend to show more specialization in order to maintain processing capacity. Indeed, an increase in the number of distinct cortical areas with increasing brain size has been reported (Kaas, 1987; Welker, 1990). It may even explain why large-brained species may develop some degree of brain lateralization as a direct consequence of size. If there is evolutionary pressure on certain functions that require a high degree of local processing and sequential control, such as linguistic communication in human brains, these will have a strong tendency to develop in one hemisphere (Aboitiz, 1996).

BIOLOGICAL LIMITS TO INFORMATION PROCESSING

The processing or transfer of information across cortical regions, rather than within regions, in large-brained mammals can only be achieved by reducing the length and number of the interconnective axons in order to set limits to the axonal mass. The *number* of interconnective fibers can be reduced, as we have seen, by compartmentalization of neurons into modular circuits in which each module, containing a large number of neurons, is connected to its neural environment by a small number of axons. The *length* of the interconnective fibers can be reduced by folding the cortical surface and thus shorten the radial and tangential distances between brain regions (Fig. 17.12). Local wiring—preferential connectivity between nearby areas of the cortex—is a simple strategy that helps keep cortical connections short. In principle, efficient cortical folding could further reduce connection length, in turn reducing white matter volume and conduction times (Young, 1993; Griffin, 1994; Scannell et al., 1995). Thus the development of the cortex does seem to coordinate folding with connectivity in a way that produces smaller and faster brains.

A major disadvantage of this strategy, however, is that an increase in the relative number of gyri can only be achieved by reducing the gyral width (Prothero and Sundsten, 1984; Todd, 1986). At the limit, the neurons in the gyri would be isolated from the remainder of the nervous system because there would no longer be any opening for direct contact with the underlying white matter. It follows that, under the assumption of constant design, this model predicts an upper limit to cortical folding. Without a radical change in the macroscopic organization of the brain, however, this hypothetical limit will never be approached, because the neurons in the gyri always have to receive direct fiber input from, or project to, the subcortical regions of the brain.

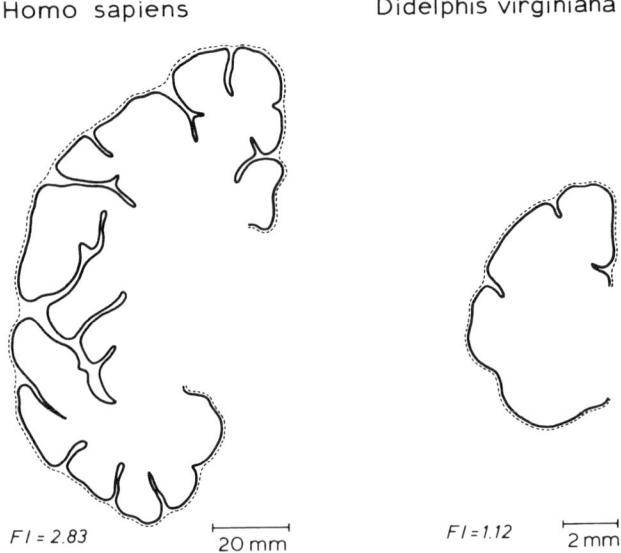

Figure 17.12. Transverse sections through the human brain and the brain of the opossum at the level of the anterior commissure. Folding of the cortical surface shortens the radial and tangential distances between brain regions and thus reduces the length of the interconnective nerve fibers. The folding index (FI), a measure of convolutedness, is the ratio between the total cortical surface area, including all gyri and sulci (continuous line), and the outer, exposed cortical surface area (dashed line) of the prosencephalon. (From Hofman, 1991, by permission of Akademie Verlag, Berlin.)

Prothero and Sundsten (1984) therefore introduced the concept of the gyral "window", which represents the hypothetical plane between a gyrus and the underlying white matter through which nerve fibers running to and from the gyral folds must pass (Fig. 17.13). According to this hypothesis, there would be a brain size where the gyral "window" area has an absolute maximum. A further increase in the size of the brain beyond that point would increase the cortical surface area, but the "window" would decrease. This implies that very large brains (e.g., over 5 kg as in

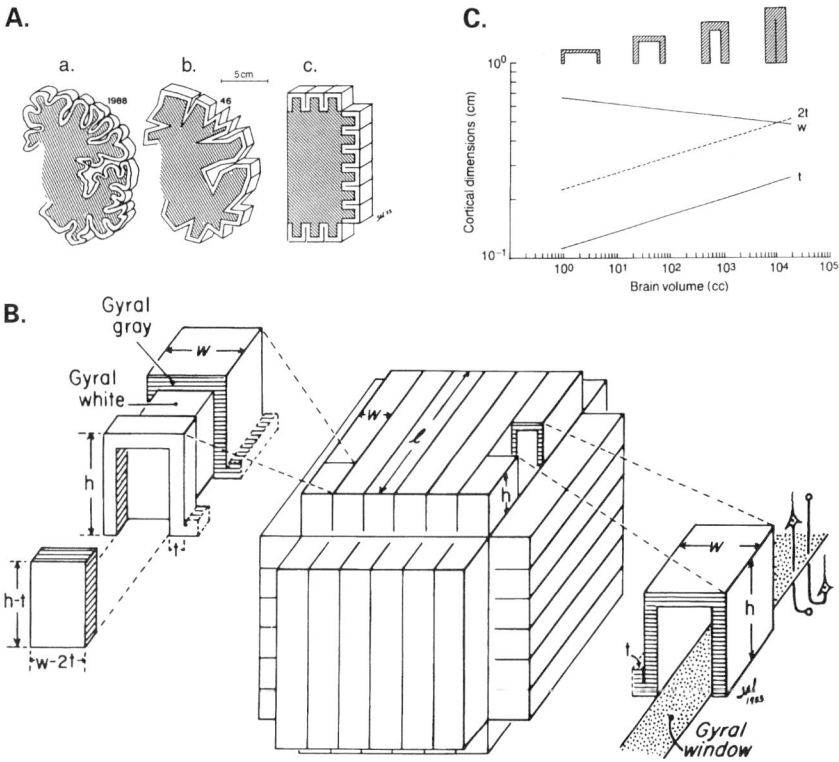

Figure 17.13. Prothero and Sundsten's illustrations (1984) of a model of cortical folding. (A) Macroscopic model showing (a) direct tracing of the cortical surface of a slab of human brain in frontal section; (b) low-resolution representation of figure a produced from digitized coordinates after omitting 98% of the points; (c) a section of an idealized model of the brain with the gyri represented by close-patterned slabs superimposed on the cut surface of a hemisected cube. (B) Dimensions of the full model. A model gyrus is defined by four parameters: length (l), width (w), height (h), and cortical thickness (t). A gyral "window" is shown in dots. It is the hypothetical plane at the base of each gyrus through which all the cortical fibers leaving and entering a gyrus must pass. (C) A maximum brain size predicted by the model. Because gyral width decreases (simulated) and cortical thickness increases (empirical) with increases in brain size, there is a hypothetical extrapolated brain size at which gyral width is equal to twice its cortical thickness. The lines in the graph representing cortical thickness (t), twice cortical thickness (2t), and gyral window (w) are shown as a function of brain size. The reduction in gyral width with increasing brain size is illustrated at the top. This scheme reveals that a gyrus must remain sufficiently broad to allow passage of afferent and efferent fibers to its cortex. (From Prothero and Sundsten, 1984, by permission of Karger, Basel.)

elephants), although containing increasing numbers of cortical neurons, may have a declining capability for integrating cortical with subcortical regions. In other words, the larger the brain grows beyond this critical size, the less efficient it will become, thus limiting any improvement in processing power.

Recently, Cochrane and his colleagues (1997) looked at the different ways in which the brain could evolve to process more information or work more efficiently. They claim that the human brain has (almost) reached the limits of information processing that a neuron-based system allows and that our evolutionary potential is constrained by the delicate balance maintained between the size and number of neurons and the associated blood vessels that nourish them.

It is unlikely, however, that the rate of blood flow or the increasing volume used by blood vessels constrain the potential size of a human-type brain. A bigger brain is physiologically possible, if only because our cardiovascular system could evolve to transport more blood at greater pressure to meet the increased demand. A far more serious problem is that there is a number of fundamental limits to the transmission and processing power of the brain. When the brain's geometry was considered in combination with the processing and transmission time of axons and dendrites (Ringo, 1991; Cochrane et al., 1997; Prothero, 1997), the degree of neuronal interconnectivity was found to be near optimal for processing performance. Once the brain has grown to a point where the bulk of its mass consists of connections, further increases will be unproductive due to the declining capability of neuronal integration and increased conduction time. At this point, corresponding to a brain size two to three times that of modern humans (i.e., at about 3500 cm^3), the brain reaches its maximum processing power (Hofman, 2000). The larger the brain grows beyond this critical size, the less efficient it will become.

One cannot exclude the possibility of new structures evolving in the brain or a higher degree of specialization of existing brain areas, but within the limits of the existing *Bauplan* there does not seem to be an incremental improvement path available to the human brain. This implies that, as a species, *Homo sapiens* is nearly at the end of the road as far as brain evolution is concerned. Any further steps in the evolution of intelligence will have to take place outside our nervous system, in a silicon world where the selection mechanisms and forces are radically different from those operating in nature.

CONCLUDING REMARKS

It is evident that the potential for brain evolution results not from the unorganized aggregations of neurons but from cooperative association by the self-similar compartmentalization and hierarchical organization of neural circuits and the invention of fractal folding, which reduces the interconnective axonal distances.

The design of the mammalian brain is such that it may perform a great number of complex functions with a minimum expenditure of energy and material both in the performance of the functions and in the construction of the system. According to this principle of adequate design, the shape of an object—whether it is a machine or an organism—will depend on the external conditions under which it will be used. In general there will be a number of adequate designs for an object, which, for practical purposes, will all be equivalent. The brains of birds and mammals, for example, differ quite considerably in their geometry and structural organization, but do not differ in the performance of their biological functions. The similarity in brain design among mammals, on the other hand, indicates that brain systems among related species are morphologically constrained and that the mammalian brain could evolve within the context of a limited number of potential forms. It means that internal factors of brain design may be the primary determinants directing the evolution of the brain and that geometric similarity among species may be derived from a common ancestor rather than being immediately evolved in response to environmental conditions.

The conservative design of the mammalian brain also appears from its intrinsic neural organization. Evolutionary scenarios have been formulated in which the evolution of brain size as well as overall differences in the complexity of brain organization are thought to be the results of alterations in specific developmental mechanisms. A significant implication of this basic plan of brain organization is that it can explain how changes in the information processing capacity of the brain during evolution and the extension and differentiation of brain functions could have come about without drastic changes in the original *Bauplan* of the brain. Apparently, a gradual, but disproportionate enlargement and specialization of particular neural systems, especially of the cerebral cortex, seem to have been sufficient to allow the evolution of unique behavioral and cognitive features in our species.

REFERENCES

Aboitiz, F. (1996) Does bigger mean better? Evolutionary determinants of brain size and structure. *Brain Behav. Evol.* 47:225–245.

Allman, J.M. (1990) Evolution of neocortex. In E.G. Jones and A. Peters (eds): *Cerebral Cortex*, vol. 8A. Plenum Press, New York, pp. 269–283.

Allman, J.M., T. McLaughlin, and A. Hakeem (1993) Brain structures and life span in primate species. *Proc. Natl. Acad. Sci. U.S.A.* 90:3559–3563.

Caviness, V.S., T. Takahashi, and R.S. Nowakowski (1995) Numbers, time and neocortical neurogenesis: a general developmental and evolutionary model. *Trends Neurosci.* 18:379–383.

Cherniak, C. (1990) The bounded brain: toward quantitative neuroanatomy. *J. Cogn. Neurosci.* 2:58–66.

Cochrane, P., C.S. Winter, and A. Hardwick (1997) Biological limits to information processing in the human brain. British Telecommunications Publications. (unpublished) http://www.labs.bt.com/papers/index.htm

Crick, F. (1989) Neural edelmanism. *Trends Neurosci.* 12:240–248.

Deacon, T.W. (1990) Rethinking mammalian brain evolution. *Amr. Zool.* 30:629–705.

Falk, D. (1990) Brain evolution in *Homo*: the "radiator" theory. *Behav. Brain Sci.* 13:333–381.

Finlay, B.L., and R.B. Darlington (1995) Linked regularities in the development and evolution of mammalian brains. *Science* 268:1578–1584.

Foley, R.A., and P.C. Lee (1991) Ecology and energetics of encephalization in hominid evolution. *Philos. Trans. R. Soc. Lond. [Biol.]* 334:223–232.

Griffin, L.D. (1994) The intrinsic geometry of the cerebral cortex. *J. Theor. Biol.* 166:261–273.

Harvey, P.H., and J.R. Krebs (1990) Comparing brains. *Science* 249:140–146.

Harvey, P.H., M.D. Pagel and J.A. Rees (1991) Mammalian metabolism and life histories. *Am. Nat.* 137:556–566.

Haug, H. (1987) Brain sizes, surfaces and neuronal sizes of the cortex cerebri. A stereological investigation of man and his variability and a comparison with some mammals. *Am. J. Anat.* 180:126–142.

Hodos, W., and C.B.G. Campbell (1990) Evolutionary scales and comparative studies of animal cognition. In R.P. Kesner and D.S. Olton (eds.): *Neurobiology and Comparative Cognition*, Lawrence Erlbaum, Hillsdale, N. J, pp. 1–20.

Hofman, M.A. (1983) Encephalization in hominids: evidence for the model of punctuationalism. *Brain Behav. Evol.* 22:102–117.

Hofman, M.A. (1984) On the presumed coevolution of brain size and longevity in hominids. *J. Hum. Evol.* 13:371–376.

Hofman, M.A. (1985) Neuronal correlates of corticalization in mammals: a theory. *J. Theor. Biol.* 112:77–95.

Hofman, M.A. (1988) Size and shape of the cerebral cortex in mammals. II. The cortical volume. *Brain Behav. Evol.* 32:17–26.

Hofman, M.A. (1989) On the evolution and geometry of the brain in mammals. *Prog. Neurobiol.* 32:137–158.

Hofman, M.A. (1991) The fractal geometry of convoluted brains. *J. Hirnforsch.* 32:103–111.

Hofman, M.A. (1993) Encephalization and the evolution of longevity in mammals. *J. Evol. Biol.* 6:209–227.

Hofman, M.A. (2000) Brain evolution in hominids: are we at the end of the road? In D. Falk and K. Gibson (eds.): Evolutionary Anatomy of the Primate Cerebral Cortex. Cambrige University Press, Cambridge, U.K. (in press).

Jerison, H.J. (1973) *Evolution of the Brain and Intelligence*. Academic Press, New York.

Jerison, H.J. (1991) Brain size and the evolution of mind. *Fifty-ninth James Arthur Lecture on the Evolution of the Human Brain*. Am. Mus. Nat. Hist., New York.

Kaas, J.H. (1987) The organization of neocortex in mammals: implications for theories of brain function. *Annu. Rev. Psychol.* 38:129–151.

Kaas, J.H. (1993) Evolution of multiple areas and modules within neocortex. *Perspect. Dev. Neurobiol.* 1:101–107.

Krubitzer, L. (1995) The organization of neocortex in mammals: are species differences really so different? *Trends Neurosci.* 18:408–417.

Leise, E.M. (1990) Modular construction of nervous systems: a basic principle of design for invertebrates and vertebrates. *Brain Res. Rev.* 15:1–23.

Malach, R. (1994) Cortical columns as devices for maximizing neuronal diversity. *Trends Neurosci.* 17:101–104.

Martin, R.D. (1983) Human brain evolution in an ecological context. *Fifty-second James Arthur Lecture on the Evolution of the Human Brain*. Am. Mus. Nat. Hist., New York.

McNab, B.K., and J.F. Eisenberg (1989) Brain size and its relations to the rate of metabolism in mammals. *Am. Nat.* 133:157–167.

Northcutt, R.G., and J.H. Kaas (1995) The emergence and evolution of mammalian cortex. *Trends Neurosci.* 18:373–379.

Pirlot, P. (1987) Contemporary brain morphology in ecological and ethological perspectives. *J. Hirnforsch.* 28:145–211.

Prothero, J.W. (1997) Cortical scaling in mammals: a repeating units model. *J. Brain Res.* 38:195–207.

Prothero, J.W., and J.W. Sundsten (1984) Folding of the cerebral cortex in mammals: a scaling model. *Brain Behav. Evol.* 24:152–167.

Purves, D. (1988) *Body and Brain. A Trophic Theory of Neural Connections*. Harvard University Press, Cambridge, MA.

Rakic, P. (1995) A small step for the cell, a giant leap for mankind: a hypothesis of neocortical expansion during evolution. *Trends Neurosci.* 18:383–388.

Ringo, J.L. (1991) Neuronal interconnection as a function of brain size. *Brain Behav. Evol.* 38:1–6.

Ringo, J.L., R.W. Doty, S. Demeter, and P.Y. Simard (1994) Time is of the essence: a conjecture that hemispheric specialization arises from interhemispheric conduction delay. *Cerebral Cortex* 4:331–343.

Riska, B. and W.R. Atchley (1985) Genetics of growth predict patterns of brain-size evolution. *Science* 229:1302–1304.

Sawaguchi, T. (1988) Correlations of cerebral indices for "extra" cortical parts and ecological variables in primates. *Brain Behav. Evol.* 32:129–140.

Scannell, J.W., M.P. Young, and C.J. Blakemore (1995) Analysis of connectivity in the rat cerebral cortex. *J. Neurosci.* 15:1463–1483.

Stephan, H., H. Frahm, and G. Baron (1981) New and revised data on volumes of brain structures in insectivores and primates. *Folia Primatol.* 35:1–29.

Todd, P.H. (1986) *Intrinsic Geometry of Biological Surface Growth. Lecture Notes in Biomathematics*, vol. 67. Springer Verlag, Berlin.

Van Essen, D.C. (1997) A tension based theory of morphogenesis and compact wiring in the central nervous system. *Nature* 385:313–318.

Welker, W. (1990) Why does cerebral cortex fissure and fold? A review of determinants of gyri and sulci. In E.G. Jones and A. Peters (eds.): *Cerebral Cortex*, vol. 8B. Plenum Press, New York, pp. 3–136.

Young, M.P. (1993) The organization of neural systems in the primate cerebral cortex. *Proc. R. Soc. Lond. Biol.* 252:13–18.

Chapter 18

THE EVOLUTION OF NEURAL AND BEHAVIORAL COMPLEXITY

Harry J. Jerison, Department of Psychiatry and Biobehavioral Sciences, University of California at Los Angeles

INTRODUCTION

The brain evolved under the constraint to minimize the use of energy for its work in processing information. That is my fundamental assumption. "Complexity" is an intuitively understood conventional characterization of aspects of the information. The evident differences among species in the complexity both of their behavior repertoires and of their brains have been the basis of an additional but false assumption of equivalence of neural and behavioral[*] complexity. It may be correct, nevertheless, that to generate complex information, neural or behavioral, is costly in some sense and that the evolution of complexity occurred only when the resulting adaptive gain offset the energetic cost. The neural costs and behavioral costs of complexity can be evaluated independently, and my objective in this Chapter is to analyze these costs in order to reach a clearer understanding of the nature of complexity and its evolution.

From the formal analysis of information as the number of changes of state in a system (Shannon and Weaver, 1949), it follows that neural complexity may be defined and measured by the number of synaptic connections that can be made in a brain. In mammals the number of both neurons and synapses is remarkably well estimated by gross brain size. Thus, as a first approximation, neural complexity may be measured by brain size. If we seek to relate this to behavioral complexity, it is useful to keep in mind that the amount of neural tissue that is actually devoted to controlling a behavior is probably determined by the minimum amount of tissue required to do it well. If a behavior requires a great deal of neural machinery, then enlarged brains had to evolve in species in which that behavior was to be part of the repertoire. If a behavior can be done well by relatively little neural machinery, however, there would be no selective advantage for an enlarged brain. The approach is fundamentally evolutionary in the implication that natural selection minimizes costs.

---

[1] I follow the conventional usage among psychologists of considering experience as a category of behavior, often measurable objectively by inference from behavior, but no less important for the cognitive sciences when it is known only personally and subjectively.

I believe that we can reduce some of the difficulties with theorizing about the neural control of complex behavior if we distinguish the neural from the behavioral. Intuition tells us, for example, that sensory perception is easy and simple and that abstract thought is difficult and complex. From a neural perspective, however, perception is behaviorally easy only because brains are built to do it, to handle information about the external world. Much of the enlargement of the brain in mammals resulted from the solution of the difficult computational problem of translating patterns of neural information into a form of information about the environment that is the basis of sensory perception (Jerison, 1991). When this pattern recognition problem is solved, animals can "perceive," or "know," a real world. I think of perception and cognition in this way—as based on information generated by pattern recognition programs that analyze neural information.

(The neural information to which I refer is available for scientific analysis as the information recorded from single neurons, as action potentials, trains of action potentials, membrane potentials, or other records of cellular events. That information can be related to environmental information only by performing additional analyses, usually requiring transformations of probabilistic data into deterministic data. The complete pattern recognition problem solved by brains includes such transformations, which have the effect of providing maps of real environments, as it were, constructed from distributions of various neural events. It may be important to keep in mind that, when we humans perform the analysis, our methods of recording neural information intervene to enable us to understand that information and certainly introduce artifacts about which we should be aware. The "maps" that are finally constructed by brains, perhaps analogously to the way we perform psychophysical analysis of recorded neural data, are what I have in mind as the data of sensory perception, and they may also be thought of as worlds that are experienced as I discuss these here.)

When we reflect on the nature of perception, we recognize that it involves a *representation* of a real world. The representation results from the work of sensory and brain systems, and these may differ in different species. We must all have been impressed by von Uexküll's classic discussion (1934) of perceptual worlds, or *Umwelten*, which provides a sense of the constructed, species-typical, nature of the experience of the real world. It is the difficult job of the brain to create a useful representation of reality. In that sense, the work of the brain can be to create a real world. For the human animal this is the reality that we know intuitively. Furthermore, our intuitive knowledge, or cognition, includes our knowledge of the nature of our own minds, and it is a feature of that knowledge that is behaviorally true but neurally false. We "know" that perceiving is easy work. It comes naturally. Only when we analyze it do we appreciate that it is, in fact, a very hard information-processing job, which seems easy only because our brains are designed to do it.

Abstract thought is intuitively recognized as difficult and complex. I believe that this is true, because, despite its size, the mammalian brain did not evolve as a specialized thinking machine. Hence the relatively simple computations required to solve problems in logic must be performed by neural systems that are better adapted for pattern recognition.

In short, perceiving and knowing a real world, which is easy and "cheap" behaviorally, involves difficult and costly activity by a brain. As a behavioral adaptation, it is performed so successfully that we are unaware of its neural costliness. Our intuition about its cost is appropriate for evaluating it as behavior but entirely inappropriate for evaluating it as an activity controlled by the brain. Solving problems in logic or mental arithmetic, which we think of as difficult and perhaps costly in neural terms, can be trivially easy for machines designed to handle the necessary information. A hand-held computer or calculator solves many of them, even though these machines may have a small fraction of the information-processing elements that are present in a brain. The elements and circuitry of a dedicated computer are however, different from those in the brain. The brain's circuitry is not normally adapted to handle those computations, whereas computations for pattern recognition, many of which are still beyond the capacity of the largest computers, are handled easily and routinely and unconsciously by the brain's very large and extensive neural networks.

I have defined neural complexity as measurable by counting the synaptic connections made in the brain. It is not as easy to measure behavioral complexity. There is a "new science of complexity," sometimes called chaos theory (Abraham and Gilgen, 1995), which I must mention in connection with my topic, but I have a few older ideas that I wish to develop here, which have remained inadequately resolved. The issue arose for me when I studied problems of vigilance, or sustained attention, in animals and undergraduates (Jerison, 1967, 1977). I discuss my experiments in some detail to provide examples of the complexity of the idea of complexity. I will conclude that rather than attempt a precise definition of behavioral complexity we would do better to confine our theorizing to neural complexity and discuss behavioral complexity in terms of the neural machinery that supports it.

VIGILANCE AND ATTENTION: AN OLD-FASHIONED VIEW

Before shifting to paleoneurology, I worked as an experimental psychologist studying human and animal vigilance. My subjects were mainly undergraduates, but also hedgehogs, rats, cats, and monkeys. I am proud of my past as a comparative cognitive psychologist, even though my work was early in the cognitive revolution. I have not kept up with the field and have little to tell you about its current concerns, but it was in my work on cognition that I first encountered problems of cost in the analysis of behavior. More or less accidentally, I performed a kind of behavioral cost/benefit analysis of sustained attention.

Vigilance, or sustained attention, experiments were part of the beginning of the cognitive revolution in psychology (Mackworth, 1950; Broadbent, 1958, 1971; Warm, 1984). They began as war research to find out what happens when an observer watches for an occasional signal embedded in a matrix of nonsignal events. The practical problem was that watch-keepers failed to report visual radar signals from submarines encountered during World War II reconnaissance. Such signals were rare and unpredictable but otherwise easily detectable, yet human watch-keepers missed many of them after only a few minutes of monitoring their instruments. For an operations research analysis of the problem, the task was successfully simulated in the laboratory, and the "decrement function" in detections could be reproduced. It was very orderly, and many of the factors that determine performance on such tasks are now well understood.

I began working with vigilance tasks after the war in a program to determine nonauditory effects of noise on human performance, because vigilance performance was found to be sensitive to effects of noise (Broadbent, 1958; Jerison, 1959). Among the factors that determined performance was a set described as "observing responses" (Holland, 1957). B.F. Skinner (1959) included this research when he reviewed various operant conditioning experiments to show their importance for the analysis of all behavior; he demonstrated a basic uniformity of performance across many animal species. I realized, therefore, that sustained attention could be studied in animals as easily as in humans using the paradigm of vigilance experiments (Jerison, 1965), which appealed to my interest in evolutionary issues. Partly with an animal research program in mind, but also for its intrinsic interest, Holland's procedure seemed worth adopting, and I undertook to work with the observing response paradigm.

COSTS AND ATTENTION

Skinner had defined observing responses as any responses that enable one to observe external stimuli. Holland's vigilance experiments were with undergraduates, who made such observing responses by pressing a lever to illuminate a screen on which a signal might appear. Very occasionally, easily detectable signals would appear on the screen, following a "schedule of reinforcements" as arranged by the experimenter. These signals were analyzed as the reinforcements for the observing responses. Under this regime, Holland was able to demonstrate that schedules of these reinforcements resulted in the same kind of response patterns as in operant conditioning experiments in other species with other responses and reinforcements. Vigilance appeared to be analyzable as a topic in Skinnerian psychology. Because I planned to use the basic paradigm, my first concern was to repeat the experiment. I failed.

A critical but unreported feature of the experiment turned out to be the tension on the response lever. My student subjects were required to report a signal as soon as they saw it. When I used an ordinary microswitch for their observing responses, the subjects pressed at a very regular rate faster than once in two seconds throughout the experiment, regardless of the schedule of signals that I presented. In this way, they kept the display continuously illuminated. By simply increasing the tension on the lever, to make it harder to depress, I found a tension at which I could get Skinner's effect, namely, that the rate of responding was determined by the schedule of reinforcement. The interpretation is obvious. The "cost" of pressing the lever had to be great enough for the "benefit" of the reinforcement to be effective. The cost/benefit feature was peripheral to the basic task of being attentive at the right time, but its appearance alerted me to its potential role in behavioral experiments.

I used the observing-response technique in only a few experiments because it turned out to be insensitive to signal presentation conditions to which engineering solutions could be applied (Jerison and Wing, 1961). My job as an engineering psychologist, or ergonomist, was to find such solutions. I found them in a second cost/benefit view of human vigilance that was more directly related to the cost of being attentive.

The laboratory setting on which I had settled involved repeated presentation of nonsignal stimuli (movement of a clock hand), replaced occasionally by a somewhat stronger stimulus (a double-step of the hand) that served as an easily detected signal. The subject had to observe every stimulus in order to determine whether it was nonsignal or signal. The probability that a stimulus was a signal was a major variable in the theory of signal detectability, which was being applied to the topic (Broadbent, 1971), and it was here that I made my most interesting discovery. I found that this probability was unimportant compared with the background rate at which all stimuli were presented in determining whether observers would actually detect signals.

To be specific, I presented signals at irregular intervals that averaged 30 times per hour. My measure of attention was whether these easily detectable signals were, in fact, reported correctly. All signals were reported correctly at the beginning of a vigil, but within a few minutes the performance decrement appeared, and the rate of correct reports dropped to an asymptotic level. I found that regardless of signal probability, when nonsignal stimuli were presented at 5 second intervals, the asymptotic performance of my undergraduate subjects was at about an 80% detection rate. Their performance fell to about 30% detections when the nonsignal stimuli were presented more rapidly, at 2 second intervals (Jerison, 1967). This was the basic result. Thus, my engineering solution to the vigilance decrement was to suggest that watch-keeping tasks be designed to require paced rather than continuous observations and to require observations no more frequently than once every 5 seconds (Jerison and Pickett, 1963). I have done little more with that problem. It has been developed especially by Joel Warm and his associates (see Warm, 1984) as studies of the "event-rate effect." It remained important for my scientific education, however, in alerting me to another aspect of the role of costs and benefits in determining behavior.

For our topic, the major lesson lies in significance of the cost of the "simple" behavior of being attentive. Because failures to detect these signals were due only to failures to attend to the stimuli that were being presented, being attentive to stimuli every 2 seconds was clearly more costly in behavioral terms than being attentive every 5 seconds. It was evidently harder for my subjects to maintain their attention to the display at the faster stimulus presentation rate than at the slower rate.

My most dramatic experience with a cost/benefit analysis of sustained attention was incidental to research with rhesus, spider, and squirrel monkeys on a task modeled after my human vigilance task (Jerison, 1965, 1967). I had trained monkeys in "Skinner boxes" to watch a steady stimulus light and to press a response lever when signaled by the repeated flashing of that light. If the monkey failed to press the lever within 8 seconds after the flashing signal began, it was shocked electrically (1.0 mA) through the grid bars of the floor of its cage. All monkeys learned to make the "conditioned avoidance" lever-pressing response relatively quickly, sitting oriented toward the light and responding as soon as the flashing began. I was surprised by several of my animals, however, when they discovered successful behavioral strategies that did not require that they attend to the light.

In Figure 18.1, I present Skinnerian performance curves produced by one squirrel monkey, which show its two response strategies. A word, first, about these curves, which may be unfamiliar. The cumulative curve is, in a sense, drawn by the animal as it behaves, a procedure invented by B.F. Skinner (1959). Recording paper in the machine moves at a constant rate, and when the animal presses its lever, a pen writing on the paper moves at right angles to the paper's movement. The ink record is then a cumulative response curve, line A in Figure 18.1, the slope of which is proportional to the animal's rate of responding. When responding is at a very regular rate, the

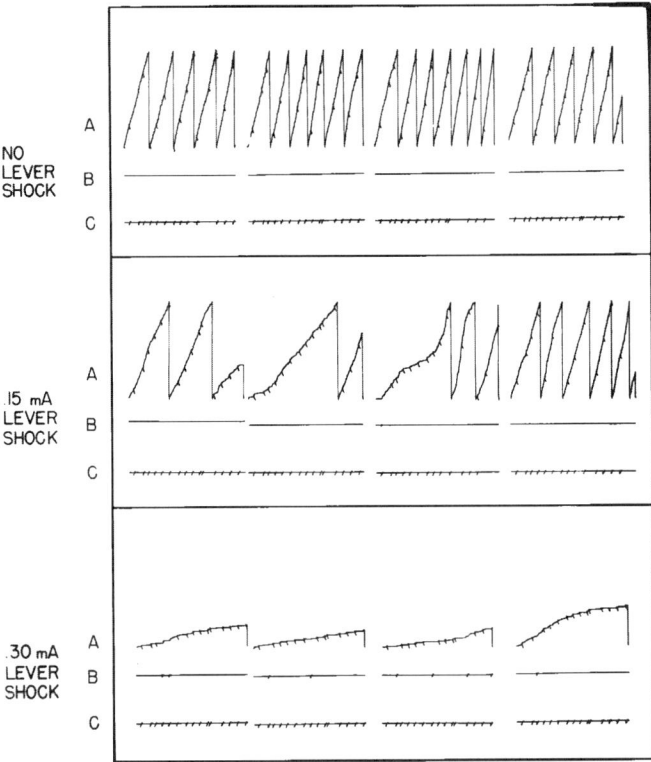

Figure 18.1. Effect of changing lever shock ("costs") on response strategies in a squirrel monkey. (A) Cumulative lever-pressing response curves (reset after 300 responses); (B) Avoidable grid shocks that were delivered when lever pressing did not occur within 8 seconds of signal presentation; (C) Signal (flashing light) presentations. Top record is "free-response" strategy discovered by this monkey after successful training to monitor the light, which resulted in occasional failures to respond correctly and 1 mA grid shock. Middle record shows partial shift from free response to attentive strategy when 0.15 mA shock was delivered through the response lever for free responses (when no signal was presented). Bottom record shows permanent shift to attentive strategy when lever shock was increased to 0.30 mA. Records from a total of 12 half-hour work sessions are shown.

resulting line is quite straight, and variations in rate are reflected by changes in the upward curvature of the line. In addition, when a reinforcement is delivered in connection with a response, a small tick mark is made by the pen. In this way the rate of responding can be correlated with reinforcements, and the effect of a schedule of reinforcements is made obvious. In my records the pen was reset automatically after 300 responses were recorded. The top record in Figure 18.1 is from four half-hour work periods, and one can see that about 6500 lever-pressing responses at a very regular rate were made during those 2 hours. Missed signals when the monkey received a grid shock are recorded on line B, and line C recorded the signals.

I had assumed correctly that all of my animals would learn to be attentive to the light and in that way avoid shocks. Signal detections then served as reinforcements under a Skinnerian "variable interval" schedule, and the performance curves were typically as in the bottom of Figure 18.1 (the "0.3 mA LEVER SHOCK" curves). The monkeys pressed the lever at a slow but steady rate, a typical pattern found in all species that have been studied in operant conditioning under either positive or negative reinforcement under a variable interval schedule. I was interested in failures of attention in these experiments, and expected to find that, like human observers, my monkeys would occasionally be inattentive and fail to respond in time to the signal.

After first learning the problem as expected, the squirrel monkey that produced the records in Figure 18.1 defeated me, showing me a way to solve its problem that did not involve attention at all. Instead of attentively observing the light, it learned to press the lever at a rapid regular rate (performance comparable with that of my human observers with the easy microswitch situation), and it always turned off the flashing whenever it occurred, that is, whenever I had scheduled a signal. When I watched the animal as it worked, I could see that it actually avoided even looking at the signal light, presumably a noxious element in its world. It evidently knew that the light presented signals and that the signals presaged electric shocks that it might receive. Its performance at this time is recorded in the top set of curves in Figure 18.1, labeled "NO LEVER SHOCK." During a 14 day period, when it worked in this way, it emitted over 25,000 lever presses and avoided every scheduled grid shock, without ever looking at the light as far as I could tell.

From my experience with undergraduates, in order to study attentiveness in this monkey I realized that I had to find a way to increase the cost of pressing the lever. I chose to electrify it. If it pressed the lever when no signal was presented (when the light was steady), the monkey received a very weak electric shock (0.15 mA) through the lever, an added cost for making "free responses." (In signal detectability theory these would be called *false alarms*, but it was clear that these responses had nothing to do with erroneous reports that a signal had been presented.) During the signal period, there was no lever shock. Although this at first disrupted the "free response" strategy that the monkey had adopted (the middle set of curves in Fig. 18.1), after a few days it evidently chose to suffer the very weak lever shock, which enabled it to avoid the stronger grid shock, rather than maintain a level of attention sufficient to detect signals. It returned to the "free response" strategy. I then increased the "cost" of pressing the lever to 0.30 mA, and the effect was immediate as shown in the lowest set of curves. The monkey returned to an "attentive strategy" in which it watched the light carefully. Despite the high cost of the 1.0 mA grid shock, which it suffered occasionally when it failed to attend properly to the signal light, the benefit to this squirrel monkey for avoiding most of the grid shocks was presumably greater than the cost it would have incurred with 0.3 mA lever shocks in its free-response strategy.

Being attentive was not a cheap or reliable activity for the squirrel monkey that wrote the records in Figure 18.1. Rather than rely on attentiveness, it chose to expend its energy on pressing a lever many thousands of times rather than simply to watch the light and press the lever when the easily detected signal appeared. Of course, the basic situation was highly artificial, but the monkey had previously learned and adapted to that situation quite well. This is evident from its quick shift back to an attentive strategy when the lever shock became stronger.

The costs of the components of this squirrel monkey's behavior were complex because, in addition to the intrinsic cost of being attentive, if attention failed there was the added cost of an electric shock through the grid. Although the difference between a steady and flashing light was quite dramatic and easily recognizable, the monkey simply could not rely on being attentive because under an attentive strategy it always missed at least one or two signals during a half hour vigil.

What lessons had I, the experimenter, learned? First, I verified the fact that attention and perception can be studied in many animal species. In other experiments, Skinner (1959) had shown that pigeons were actually much better than people at many kinds of watch keeping, and Herrnstein (1985) has shown that they can be more perceptive in recognizing objects and people than are humans. Second, it was clear that in both the human and the animal experiments I could affect performance by manipulating the costs of various responses and the benefits of making them. In my animals, I manipulated costs and benefits by shocking the animal and by enabling the animals to avoid shocks of various intensities, and I knew that I could have used positive reinforcement such as food pellets or candies in comparable situations. In my human subjects the only things I could manipulate were the load on behavior (how often an observing response had to be made) and the effort of a fairly trivial part of the situation (pressing a microswitch).

A third lesson was that although I could manipulate the costs, it would be difficult to specify them in a meaningful quantitative way. The benefits in the experiments with undergraduates were completely uncontrolled, depending primarily on a social contract with subjects who presumably tried to do as well as they could on their tests. Their benefits, if measurable, would be the personal and subjective satisfaction of doing a job right. Finally, thinking about the relationship between behavioral and neural dimensions of behavior, I retained my intuition that attention and perception are behaviorally simple activities. Furthermore, from the results of work with animals I recognized that there is no obvious advantage connected with having a complex human brain. A simple pigeon brain is good enough—or even better for some tasks. For my large-brained human subjects, however, the cost of being attentive continuously or at very short intervals was great enough for them to fail to detect easy signals.

We must conclude that our intuition about the complexity of a behavior is a poor guide for analysis and that it would be difficult to define and measure it objectively.

I have presented these several examples to indicate how varied behavioral costs may be and how difficult it can be to evaluate and quantify these costs with only intuition as a guide. For an understanding of the evolution of complexity, including the capacity for complex behavior, I believe that we will do best to be guided by the simpler measures of neural complexity.

COSTS AND BRAINS

The brain is an energetically expensive organ. Although a human brain's weight is less than 2% of that of the body, it accounts for about 15% of the total metabolic activity (Aiello and Wheeler, 1995). The amount of information that a brain can process is proportional to the number of connections that its neurons can make, and, in comparisons among species, the number of neurons and synapses in mammalian brains can be estimated surprisingly well from the overall size of the brain.

Figure 18.2 shows the relationship between cortical surface area and brain size in 50 species of mammals. The orderliness is typical of relationships of parts of the brain to the whole brain. From other sources (Rockel et al., 1980), we know that the number of neurons beneath a particular amount of cortical area is approximately constant, and

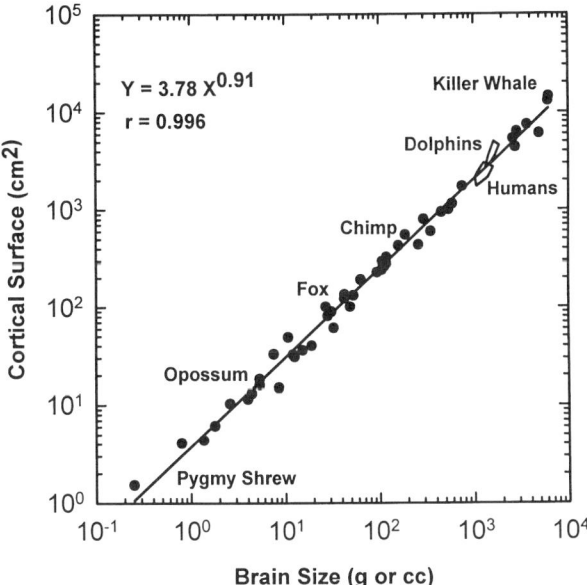

Figure 18.2. The relationship between cortical surface and gross brain size in 50 species of mammals. Each point represents a species. In addition, two labeled minimum convex polygons indicate within-species variability in humans (N = 23) and dolphins (*Tursiops truncatus*, N = 13). Several species are labeled by name to indicate the diversity of the sample. (From Jerison, 1991, by permission.)

surface area is, therefore, a valid estimator of the total number of neurons. We also know (Stephan et al., 1981) that the volume of the cerebral cortex is related in a very orderly way to gross brain size and that the average number of synapses per unit of cortical volume is approximately constant (Schüz and Demianenko, 1995). I will review this material again and in more detail in a later section, where I will also explain the exceptional situation in cetaceans, but for the present we can conclude that gross brain size can serve as a kind of statistic to estimate the total neural information-processing capacity of a mammalian brain.

The neural complexity of a process may be defined by the amount of neural machinery that is required for its control. This definition leads to occasional paradoxes, of course. For example, the control of bodily temperature by warm-blooded species is neurally less expensive, and in our sense less complex, than that by cold-blooded species. Lizards have to move bodily into and out of the shade, or raise and lower their bodies when on desert sand, as ways to cool off or warm up. Mammals can usually maintain a fixed body temperature by reflex control of the capillary bed and of their sweat glands, which involves only a small amount of neural tissue in the brain stem. In that sense, endothermy may be neurally less expensive and thus less complex than ectothermy. We need not be surprised. After all, if natural selection is toward minimizing neural work, as a later arrival on the adaptive landscape in vertebrate evolution, endothermy might have had, as one of its advantages, its demand of less neural energy expenditure than ectothermy.

My conclusion about the complexity of perceptual processing in mammals is more natural, because we know that perception involves very extensive neural circuits distributed through much of the brain (Goldman-Rakic, 1988). From the anatomical literature (Diamond, 1979; Jones and Powell, 1970), one may conclude that much of the surface of the isocortex is mappable "projection" cortex on which the sensory and motor surfaces of the body are represented in elaborate ways. (With the exception of the human language areas, "association" cortex is generally intercalated within these projection areas. Human language areas may be genuine association areas in the classic sense in that their inputs and outputs appear to involve only cortico-cortical pathways and do not involve "projections" via direct connections to thalamic and other subcortical structures.) The large amount of neural tissue involved in the cortical mapping of the external world is the feature of the brain's organization that leads to the view that perception and related cognitive activities are neurally very complex, even though they are subjectively simple and elementary.

Since brain size is a kind of statistic that estimates the number of synapses and neurons in brains, the evolution of neural complexity was a feature of the evolution of enlarged brains. The evidence of this evolution is available from the fossil record (Bauchot and Stephan, 1967; Edinger, 1929, 1948; Falk, 1987; Jerison, 1973, 1990; Piveteau, 1958, 1961; Radinsky, 1976, 1979; Tobias, 1967, 1990). Brains of fossil vertebrates can be studied from endocranial casts ("endocasts"), which are castings for which the cranial cavity is the mold. Brain size is, of course, related to body size, and postcranial fossilized skeletal remains enable one to estimate body size. To outline the evolutionary history of the brain, I begin with a quantitative overview of the present diversity of vertebrate brains and bodies (Fig. 18.3).

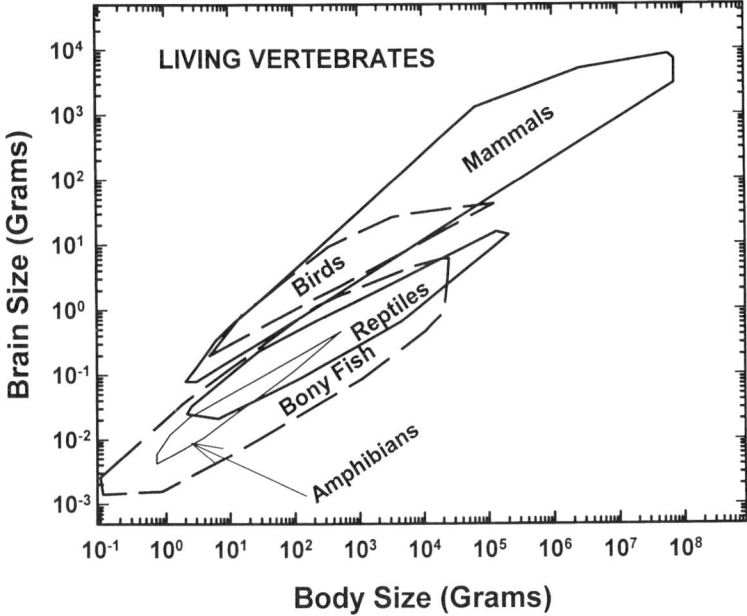

Figure 18.3. Brain–body relations in 1954 living vertebrate species enclosed in minimum convex polygons. The samples are 647 mammals, 180 birds, 1027 bony fishes, 41 amphibians, and 59 reptiles.

BRAIN SIZE IN LIVING VERTEBRATES: ALLOMETRY AND ENCEPHALIZATION

The "minimum convex polygons" in Figure 18.3 (external angles greater than 180°) are the smallest that can be drawn to contain most of the presently available data on the indicated classes of vertebrates. They summarize several important features about the evolution of brain size. First, the polygons are in a restricted region of "brain–body space," which indicates a general constraint on the size of the brain that could evolve in each group. Second, within each group the polygon is oriented upward, indicating a necessary relationship between brain size and body size. Larger bodied animals have to have larger brains. This is the "allometric" relationship. When lines rather than polygons are drawn to show it, the equation of the line tells us an expected brain size for a given body size within each group, and the residual from that line for each species is its encephalization "quotient." Third, the polygons are in two different clusters. Birds and mammals are literally higher vertebrates because they are in the higher cluster, and bony fishes (Osteichthyes), amphibians, and reptiles are lower vertebrates. The vertical shift is the effect of "encephalization." Higher vertebrates generally have several times as much brain as lower vertebrates per unit body weight. These three points can be read directly from the empirical relationships shown in Figure 18.3.

The data of Figure 18.3 are from several sources. Professor Roland Bauchot has generously allowed me to use his unpublished data on 1027 species of bony fish. The mammalian data are from Worthy and Hickie (1986) and are on 647 species. The amphibians are of 40 species of urodeles from Thireaux (1975) and a bullfrog from Crile and Quiring (1940). The reptiles are 59 species recorded by Platel (1979). The data on birds are from 180 species from Mlikovsky (1980) and my personal records (Jerison, 1987). In preparing the graphs I oriented the labels of the groups (within the polygons) at angles of 67° to indicate the orientation of a 2/3 exponent, the slope of a line (on logarithmic scales) that might be fitted to the data within a polygon. Although not part of my present concerns, I should note that empirically fitted regression lines to the mammalian data yield a 3/4 exponent, approximately. Exponents closer to 1/2 would fit the other data sets. The issue of applying regression analysis to determine allometric exponents and intercepts is considered in several places (Jerison, 1991; Martin, 1990).

Figure 18.3 presents the most significant *general* trends in the evolution of the information-processing capacity in vertebrates. Exceptions to these trends are reviewed in the section that follows, where I discuss data on two additional classes of fish: the jawless fish (class Agnatha) and the cartilaginous fish (class Chondrichthyes: sharks, rays, and skates). Other exceptions are large-brained dinosaurs and species of electric fish that were not in Bauchot's sample. I will, finally, also consider problems in the analysis of cetacean brain size, in which there are fewer nerve cells per unit cortical surface than in land mammals.

It is important for a general review to indicate something about the present diversity of vertebrate species. Here are some of the numbers, which I have assembled from personal communications with zoologists who have been concerned with such issues. About 50,000 living vertebrate species have been identified at this time. The consensus is that there are about 25,000 species of bony fishes, 800 species of cartilaginous fishes, and 70 species of agnathans. I have seen listings of 4184 species of amphibians, 6300 species of reptiles, 9198 species of birds, and 4629 species of mammals. The exact numbers need not be taken too seriously. They are important mainly to suggest the relative diversities of the groups and the extent to which they are adapted to different niches. In an evolutionary sense, the jawless and cartilaginous fishes are, thus, relatively unsuccessful in that they are much less diverse than the other classes of living vertebrates.

From the perspective of the evolution of complexity as defined by neural control, it is correct to recognize that size alone implies complexity. The control system for handling the body has to be larger in a larger bodied species than in a smaller bodied species. In other words, the allometric effect of evolving larger bodies demands the evolution of larger, and hence more complex, brains. These allometric increases in neural complexity are of relatively little interest, however, merely reflecting the obvious fact that larger bodies need larger control systems. I usually point out to nonbiologists concerned with "intelligent" machines that, unlike machines, in living systems size is determined by the number of cells in an organism. Neural control is, as a first approximation, effected by fixed ratios of controlling neurons relative to the sensory and motor cells in the body that are controlled. Furthermore, living animal cells are all approximately the same size—within about an order of magnitude from smallest to largest. This is a familiar fact related to the physics of cell membranes and cell metabolism (Schmidt-Nielsen, 1984). The allometric effect is, thus, an effect of the diversification of body sizes in vertebrate evolution, which the brain as control organ must track in order to do its work. The number of neurons in a brain bears a necessary minimum relationship to the number of cells in the body.

When species are encephalized beyond the expectations of allometry—the situation for all "higher" vertebrates—they are even more neurally complex, according to the usage of this chapter. Measurable as "encephalization quotients" by the residuals in a regression analysis, the enlargement of the brain beyond the expectation of body size is amenable to quantification. It is sufficient for the present chapter, however, to indicate all of the effects nonparametrically as in the graphic analysis of Figure 18.3, avoiding the theoretical baggage introduced by statistical regression analysis. Our concern is primarily with encephalization rather than allometry, because it is this feature that involved evolutionary selection that was specific for enlarged brains.

The mammals and birds are clearly encephalized relative to the reptiles from which they evolved. Within the birds, the most encephalized groups are the crows and parrots, species of which are well known for their good performance on animal "intelligence tests" (see Pepperberg, 1994). Within the mammals, we are most familiar with encephalization as a feature of primate evolution (Martin, 1990). When the hominoid ancestors of chimpanzees, gorillas, and humans branched into these three lineages between 5 and 8 million years ago all were already two or three times as large-brained as average mammals. The earliest evidence of hominids (the human lineage) from australopithecines of between 3 and 4 million years ago shows that in encephalization they were comparable to, or very slightly in advance of, living great apes. With the evolution of modern humans, there was approximately a further doubling or tripling of brain size, occurring in identifiable stages within the past 2 million years. Neural complexity as the evolution of encephalization evolved in all birds and mammals, however, a kind of plesiomorphy requiring an analysis of the selective advantage of the initial investment in neural machinery that it entailed.

Mammal brains are unique among vertebrate brains in the appearance of the cerebral cortex as an enormous expansion of forebrain. In birds there was comparable forebrain expansion related to the evolution of other neural systems quite different in construction from cortex but possibly functionally equivalent (Karten, 1969, 1991). These evolutionary developments in birds and mammals are measurable as the encephalization evident in Figure 18.3. The result is an impressively orderly picture that distinguishes "lower" from "higher" vertebrates. It is not, however, quite a true picture. Let me begin by introducing major exceptions, which complicate the analysis of encephalization and brain size.

EXCEPTIONS

Although the exceptions that I review here involve a small fraction of living species, as well as a few fossils, they are an important challenge for the analysis of the evolution of information-processing capacity. In terms of number of species, the most important exceptions are many of the living cartilaginous fishes, which are at a

18 The Evolution of Neural and Behavioral Complexity

mammalian grade of encephalization. As is evident in Figure 18.4, this class Chondrichthyes overlaps the lower and higher vertebrate polygons that were shown in Figure 18.3. Although they number relatively few species compared with the other living vertebrate classes, it is stretching things to describe them as evolutionarily unsuccessful. It is more useful to recognize that as a group they are a restraint on speculation about the role of brain power in successful adaptations.

When we encounter evidence of encephalization, it is natural to assume that natural selection was at work and that there was selection for additional-information processing capacity, beyond some minimal amount. I will suggest scenarios for such selection, especially in the mammals, and it is usually possible to develop appropriate scenarios for other encephalized groups. I have little idea, however, about the information that might have required so much additional neural tissue in chondrichthyans. There is one fossil Paleozoic shark, *Cobelodus*, which lived about 275 million years ago (Zangerl and Case, 1976). This animal's brain and body sizes were quite similar to those of living horned sharks (*Heterodontus*), and it was more encephalized than comparable bony fishes. This is actually the first instance in vertebrate history of encephalization beyond the "lower vertebrate" grade of Figure 18.3. Encephalization was, thus, a primitive trait—a plesiomorphy in evolutionary terms—in chondrichthyans, just as it can be shown to be in birds and mammals. There are avian and mammalian behavioral adaptations of the perceptual and cognitive systems,

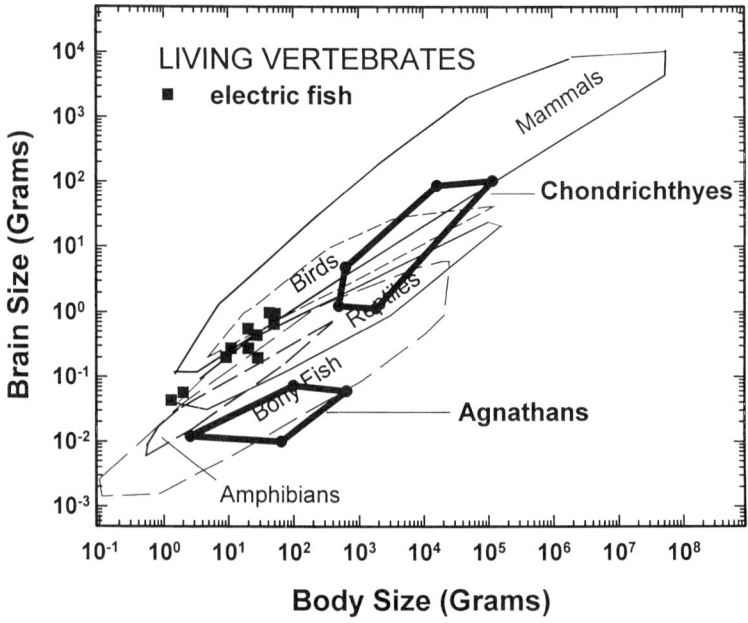

Figure 18.4. Exceptions: Polygons on class Chondrichthyes (sharks, rays, and skates) and class Agnatha (lampreys and hagfish), and previously unpublished data on 11 electric fish (Mormyridae) added to the polygons of Figure 18.3 to illustrate exceptional vertebrate brain–body adaptations. (Mormyrid data courtesy of A. Bass; other added data from Butler and Hodos, 1996, published by permission.)

however, that suggest a requirement for an enlarged brain. Too little is known about chondrichthyan behavior for analogous speculation. The required analysis remains a challenge to evolutionists and animal behaviorists.

The opposite evolutionary problem was assumed to have arisen in the data on the brains in living agnathans, which I present in Figure 18.4. The oldest fossil vertebrates were Paleozoic agnathans recovered from Spitzbergen, and these were about 450 million years old. From the perspective of evolutionary selection for information-processing capacity, it could, therefore, be true that the jawless fish represent the initial minimal vertebrate requirement for neural control and that the present "lower vertebrate" grade shown in Figure 18.3 involved some encephalization beyond that minimum. I had assumed that this was an issue on the basis of previously published graphs of the relationship between agnathans and other vertebrates (e.g., Butler and Hodos, 1996, Fig. 5–10). These indicated that agnathans were below the grade of encephalization of living bony fishes. With the very much larger sample of data on bony fishes provided by Bauchot and used in the polygon of Figure 18.3, however, it is clear that almost all agnathans are within that polygon. The slight extension of the agnathan polygon below that of bony fishes suggests that they represent a lower margin for a minimal grade of encephalization that characterizes all vertebrates but that there is no real need for scenarios unique to the agnathan niche. Nevertheless, such scenarios have been offered, and I review them presently.

There is another problem specific to the analysis of fossils. Although fossil agnathan endocasts are known, they provide marginal evidence on encephalization because the brain does not fill the braincase in lower vertebrates (Jerison, 1973). It may be that the small brains of living agnathans represent loss of tissue related to an adaptation for parasitism, the typical niche of adult lampreys, and to a cessile adaptation typical of the larval ammocoetes form. Hagfish, the other agnathan group, are not parasitic, however. As in my view of the sharks and their relatives, one knows too little about the behavioral adaptations and their neural control in jawless fish to offer a satisfactory scenario for their brain sizes. It is appropriate to recognize, also, that whatever scenario works for agnathans might also be applied to the least encephalized of living bony fishes.

Other examples of encephalization in "lower vertebrate" species, which complicate the picture in Figure 18.3, include hitherto unpublished data on mormyrid electric fish shown in Figure 18.4. These are on 11 species, measured by Professor Andrew Bass of Cornell University. The mormyrids have enlarged cerebellums, which are comparable in relative size to mammalian cerebral cortex. Although we have no information on why such analysis would require very large amounts of additional neural tissue, the enlargement appears to be related to the analysis of information from electric organs. If there is something peculiar about the analysis of electric data, which requires unusual encephalization, perhaps this could be related to the enlarged chondrichthyan brain illustrated in Figure 18.4. Although a full picture of the behavior of chondrichthyans remains to be developed, the role of electroreception within this vertebrate class may also help explain their encephalization. Electroreception is a relatively common vertebrate adaptation, however, perhaps too poorly understood to explain the presence or absence of encephalization in electroreceptive species (Bullock and Heiligenberg, 1986).

The final exceptional instance of brain enlargement may be in fossil "ostrich-dinosaurs" (struthiomimids and ornithomimids), which have been reported as comparable to ostriches in relative brain size (Hopson, 1979; Russell, 1972). The enlarged brains of these dinosaurs, and other fossil evidence from clustering of eggs and complex tracks, have inspired scenarios about birdlike dinosaur social behavior and care of the young (see Horner and Gorman, 1988), which might have required birdlike brain enlargement. The speculation is encouraged by the present almost unanimous opinion among paleontologists that birds are a surviving group of dinosaurs, which may justify adducing evidence of birdlike social behavior from the fossil remains of "other" dinosaurs (Novacek, 1996). Whether this is enough to explain brain enlargement is another question.

There are a number of problems with the scenarios explaining brain enlargement in these dinosaurs, although if we accept the dominant view of living birds as surviving dinosaurs we would find it easier to accept encephalization in at least some dinosaur groups. Among the problems, first, there is at present no evidence about brain size in the coelosaurians, the nearest relatives of birds among the dinosaurs. The brain of *Archaeopteryx*, the earliest of known birds, which is from the upper Jurassic (about 150 million years ago), was at the lower margin of the brain–body polygon of living birds and above a reptilian polygon that includes most dinosaurs. The large-brained ornithomimid dinosaurs were distant relatives of the immediate ancestors of birds and actually appeared later in time than the earliest birds. Second, one can be sceptical about the explanatory force of the scenarios that have been offered as explanations for the encephalization. These are behavioristic scenarios describing complex social behavior, but comparably complex behavior is known in many small-brained "lower vertebrates" as well as in invertebrates. We should appreciate that it is mainly in perceptual-cognitive adaptations identified in mammals that very large amounts of neural tissue appear to be required. Such neurobehavioral adaptations in living birds can be assumed from their performance in perceptual tasks that appear to require capacities comparable with those in mammals for pattern recognition. Finally, the basic data on this encephalization need to be examined more carefully, because brain size in these species may have been overstated. For what it is worth, when I have compared endocasts, that of *Struthiomimus* has seemed to me more nearly comparable with that of an albatros in my collection rather than that of an ostrich, and I plan to reexamine the reported data. The basic fact of some encephalization in dinosaurs appears to be correct, however, but one needs better measurements.

Allowing for these exceptions, it remains true that of the 45,000 or 50,000 living vertebrate species, only the 5000 or so mammals and the 9000 or so birds are encephalized to the extent that gross brain and body measurements put them in the upper classes, as it were. Selection for neural complexity was evidently rare in most vertebrate ecological niches. It was primarily a feature of the avian and mammalian adaptive zones.

Before discussing that selection, I have to consider another exceptional datum, which complicates the interpretation of brain size as a statistic that estimates neural information-processing capacity. This is on cortical thickness in dolphins. Although formal reports of quantitative data are presently lacking, from data of Rockel et al.

(1980) one can estimate cortical thickness to vary approximately with the 1/6 power of brain size. This was part of the evidence in that report for the uniformity among mammals in number of cortical neurons beneath a unit area of cortical surface, and it supports the results presented in Figure 18.2, above, as evidence for the appropriateness of brain size as a statistic. The uniformity in cortical thickness, however, is not applicable to cetaceans. Dolphin brains (and, very likely, other cetacean brains) are not like those of land mammals in this respect. The isocortex is thinner, its layers are less clearly defined, and it has only about 2/3 the number of neurons per unit surface area compared with that of land mammals (Garey and Leuba, 1986). Interestingly, these corrected numbers do not change our conclusion about the utility of gross brain size as a statistic. The surface area of dolphin cortex is about half-again as great as in the other species with a comparably large brain, namely, *Homo sapiens*, leading to the conclusion that we and the dolphins have about the same number of neurons, that is, about the same information-processing capacity. Brain size is an effective statistic for this estimation. The analysis of encephalization can continue to be accepted as an approach to the analysis of the evolution of information-processing capacity and of neural complexity.

EARLY AVIAN AND MAMMALIAN ENCEPHALIZATION

The fossil history of encephalization in birds is recorded in about a half-dozen specimens and is summarized by Jerison (1973). Definitely a bird, *Archaeopteryx* had a brain that completely filled the brain case and was at the lower edge of the avian polygon of Figure 18.3, but within the range of living birds. The only clearly nonavian feature of the brain of *Archaeopteryx* is the absence of a Wulst, an identifiable forebrain area in all living birds, which is associated with processing visual information. By the early Eocene, about 50 million years ago, a fossil shorebird, *Numenius gypsorum*, had appeared with a definite Wulst but with evidence that the rest of its forebrain was slightly smaller than that of its living relatives. By the Miocene, about 20 million years ago, bird brains were comparable with those of living species both in size and in shape. Mammals had a more varied record, as indicated in Figures 18.5 and 18.6, below.

Appearing at about the same time as the first dinosaurs, mammals are much more ancient vertebrates than birds, and they were probably more encephalized than any of their immediate ancestors among the reptiles (Jerison, 1990; Kielan-Jaworowska, 1986; but see Quiroga, 1980). The earliest mammals appeared late in the Triassic period of the Mesozoic era, about 225 million years ago. We first know their brains from an endocast from the upper Jurassic *Triconodon mordax*, which lived about 150 million years ago and is from an entirely extinct archaic group of early mammals. Both in brain size and in body size, however, *Triconodon* was comparable with many living insectivores. Skeletal remains of earlier mammals suggest that they were also comparable in every respect.

The Mesozoic mammals were about four times as encephalized as their relatives among the reptiles and were also much reduced in body size. I have estimated the body size of one near relative of the early mammals, the small mammal-like reptile *Thrinaxodon*, as about 500 g. The first mammals were much smaller and probably weighed no more than 50 g. Better evidence is available from much later strata, which are about 70 million years old (late Cretaceous period of the Mesozoic era). An extraordinary variety of fossil mammals have recently been discovered, and we have evidence about both their brains and their bodies (Kielan-Jaworowska, 1986; Novacek, 1996). At present, analysis of this material is underway, and though incomplete, it does not appear to challenge conclusions based on more fragmentary earlier available material (Jerison, 1973). All Mesozoic mammals were small, no larger than living house cats, and usually the size of small mice. Like living moles and shrews, their brains were about half the size of those of mice. Another important feature of the early evolution of mammals is that their level of encephalization remained approximately the same throughout their more than 150 million years of existence during the Mesozoic era.

The Mesozoic era probably ended with a great earthly catastrophe, when a comet or asteroid struck the area near Yucatan in what is now the Gulf of Mexico, about 65 million years ago. Many animal and plant species became extinct about then, including the large dinosaurs and other dominant vertebrates. During the Paleocene epoch at the beginning of the Cenozoic era, 55 to 65 million years ago, mammals became significantly diverse in size, with some species weighing several hundred kilograms. Presumably they had "discovered" some of the terrestrial niches left empty by the disappearance of dinosaurs. Their brains, however, remained relatively small, becoming complex only to the extent required by allometry. One might think of them as enlarged hedgehogs. Living rodents have larger brains, but the giant rodent, the living capybara, might suggest the pattern of brain evolution in archaic Mesozoic and Paleocene mammals. This South American rodent, which may weigh 50 kg or more, has a brain that appears to be organized as a simple allometric enlargement of the brain of a guinea pig (Welker, 1990).

Most of the mammals of the early Cenozoic were from "archaic" orders, that is, orders now entirely extinct. Data on their encephalization in Figure 18.5 are presented against a background of the polygons for living mammals and for living and fossil reptiles. The reptilian data include some dinosaurs to present a clearer picture of the status of the group from which mammals evolved. Within the polygon of living reptiles I also indicate how a minimum convex polygon is constructed. Let me discuss these points in reverse order.

If one imagines the living reptile points as a set of pegs, minimum convex polygons can be represented by the smallest possible string that can be pulled about the pegs. The outer pegs support the string. I use the polygons to indicate regions in brain–body space occupied by species grouped in appropriate ways. A parametric quantitative treatment of the space about the points is possible by using data from the bivariate normal distribution to determine the dimensions of an ellipse containing either all of the points or some fixed subset of them. The polygons are nonparametric, and, as drawn, encompass the entire range rather than some indication of central tendency such as the mean or standard deviation of the distribution of points.

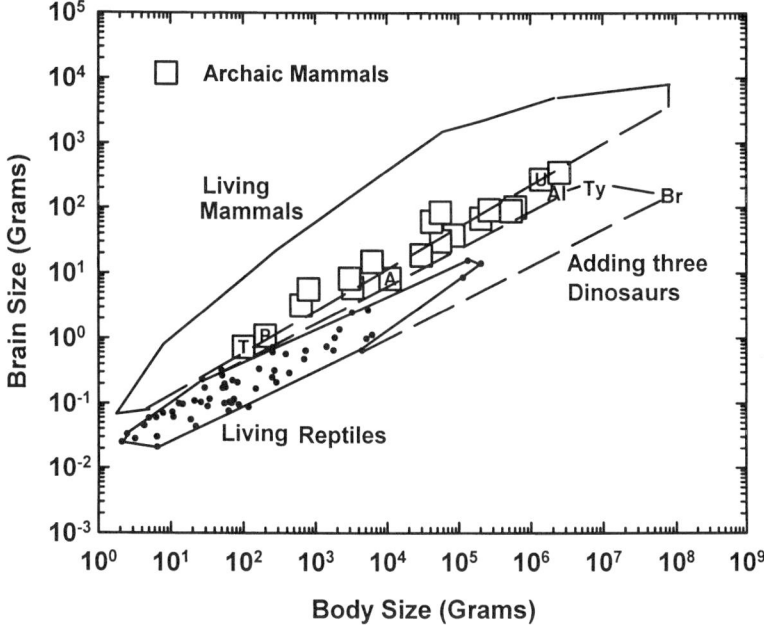

Figure 18.5. Brain–body relations in archaic fossil and living mammals and reptiles, each class enclosed in a minimum convex polygon. See text for further explanation.

In presenting the data on dinosaurs, I used the estimates in Jerison (1973) and Hopson (1979) of brain and body size. In adding them to living reptiles I also demonstrate the utility of the analysis of gross brain size and the adequacy of the polygons for a scientific analysis. If we pose the frequently asked question, "were dinosaurs unusually small brained?", we can answer with Figure 18.5. With respect to their brains, the three dinosaurs that I added to Figure 18.5 were normal reptiles. These dinosaur species, *Allosaurus* (Al), *Tyrannosaurus* (Ty), and *Brachiosaurus* (Br), were not small brained. With the exception of the large-brained ornithomimids mentioned earlier, all of the reptiles of the Mesozoic, including the flying reptiles (pterosaurs) and the mammal-like reptiles that were the immediate ancestors of the mammals fit within the extended reptilian polygon (Jerison, 1973; Hopson, 1979).

The data on archaic mammals demonstrate that in their first departure from the grade of encephalization of their reptilian ancestors the mammals had probably become more encephalized. The conclusion is based on a single point, *Triconodon*, marked "T," representing the earliest mammalian endocast as mentioned earlier. It may be that some of its immediate ancestors among the mammal-like reptiles had already evolved enlarged brains (Quiroga, 1980) or that the very earliest true mammals had not yet achieved a mammalian grade of encephalization. The evidence is equivocal. In one case (Kemp, 1979), a mammal-like reptile brain has been reported as mammalian in encephalization, but I judged the "brain" region of the endocast to be space for an olfactory tract rather than forebrain. The problem will undoubtedly be resolved when more fossils become available for analysis. The earliest evidence of mammal brains shows them as encephalized relative to reptiles, and the latest evidence of mammal-like reptile brains shows them as at a reptilian grade (Jerison, 1973; Hopson, 1979). The gap is, however, more that 75 million years. Specimens in which endocasts can be analyzed are available to close some of the gap, and their evidence will be available within the next few years.

The archaic mammal data in Figure 18.5 are the small square symbols. In addition to *Triconodon* (T), those with lettered markings are a multituberculate, *Ptilodus* (P, 60 ma), a creodont, *Arctocyonides* (A, 60 ma), and an amblypod, *Uintatherium* (U, 40 ma). It is clear that as a group the archaic mammals were not encephalized beyond the level achieved by the earliest mammals. They are very close to, and even slightly below, the lower margin of living mammals, although all are above a reptilian grade of encephalization. I have concluded that the earliest mammals had "discovered" an available adaptive zone early in their evolution, which required some enlargement of the brain relative to their reptilian ancestors, but that their further evolution involved adaptations other than those associated with encephalization. I speculate on that adaptive zone later, and indicate why it required additional neural complexity, after presenting the data on further encephalization in mammals.

In summary, the evidence in Figure 18.5 is that, early in their history, mammals became encephalized compared with their reptilian ancestors, and they then maintained that level of encephalization for the next 150 million years. That level persisted for an additional 10 million years, the Paleocene epoch of the Cenozoic era, after the extinction of other large land vertebrates and after they had evolved larger bodies in adapting for life in the available niches of the time. Then things changed.

PROGRESSIVE ENCEPHALIZATION IN MAMMALS

With the possible exception of encephalization in primates, which may have begun during the Paleocene, mammalian encephalization beyond the basal level is a phenomenon of the past 55 million years. It began at the transition from the Paleocene to the Eocene epoch, following 150 million years or more of equilibrium in relative brain size. The mammals began as encephalized species compared with other vertebrates, but they remained at their initial level until the beginning of the Eocene. The full picture is too complex to review in a few pages, but I use Figure 18.6 to suggest its general structure.

Maintaining the framework of the present diversity in brains and bodies in the mammals and their reptilian ancestors, I have added several data points on living mammals and all of the known fossil history of the horse brain. From Figure 18.6 one can read the fact that there exist living mammal species that are no more encephalized than the earliest mammals. The letter O on the graph represents the Virginia opossum, *Didelphis marsupialis*, well known on American highways throughout the United States. The opossum's ability to contribute so exuberantly to the population of road kills is clear evidence of the fitness of these small-brained animals as among the most successful of living mammals in an evolutionary sense. Animals do not live by brains alone.

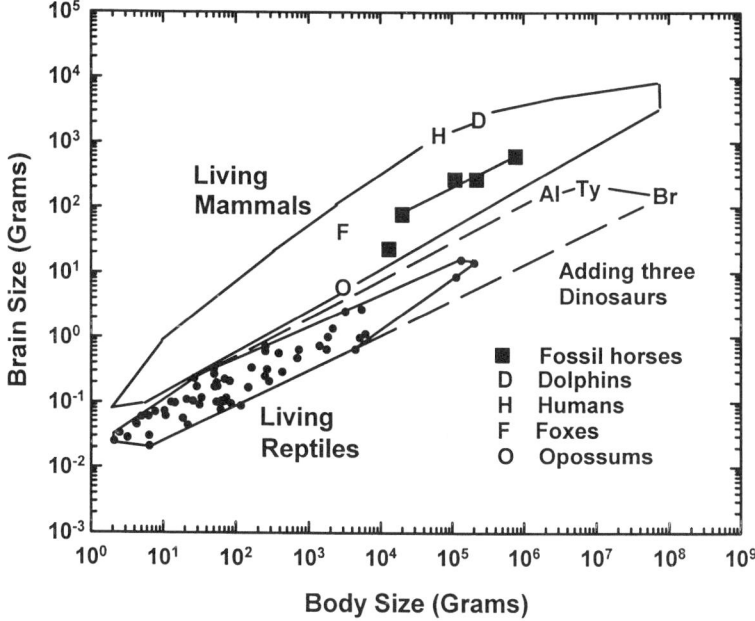

Figure 18.6. Brain–body polygons of Figure 18.5, with archaic mammal data removed and data on fossil equids (filled squares) added. Labeled living mammals: O, opossum; F, fox; H, human; D, dolphin. Regression line is through Oligocene and later equids. See text for further explanation.

We humans (H in Fig. 18.6) share the status of the most encephalized of living mammals with dolphins (*Tursiops truncatus*; D in Fig. 18.6). I indicated earlier that as primates we can trace the pattern of our encephalization to our australopithecine ancestors of about 3.5 million years ago. That grade of encephalization was about the same as in living great apes. If we trace the ancestry we share with the great apes back further in fossil history, we probably would meet the Oligocene *Aegyptopithecus*, perhaps the earliest species in the ape lineage. Its grade of encephalization was comparable with that of living lemurs and below the grade of living monkeys. The pattern that we would be able to detect is that of relatively rapid evolution of encephalization followed by a period of stasis. The living lemuroids are still with us and are at the same grade of encephalization that they had achieved during the Oligocene epoch. In any given encephalized group, the evidence is usually of a rapid period of evolution to a particular grade followed by a long period of equilibrium at that grade. The model is that of "punctuated equilibrium" (Eldredge and Gould, 1972).

The horse lineage, the large filled squares in Figure 18.6, is a simple example of the phenomenon. The species, reading from the left, are the lower Eocene eohippus (*Hyracotherium*), the Oligocene *Mesohippus*, the Miocene *Merychippus*, the Pliocene *Pliohippus*, and the Pleistocene La Brea horse, *Equus*. They are the evidence from 50, 30, 15, 5, and 0.1 million years ago, respectively. By inspection it is clear that the four species of horses, beginning with the Oligocene, were at the same grade of encephalization. The advance occurred between the time of *Hyracotherium* and the later species, with the equilibrium then maintained, beginning about 30 million years ago. By analogy with the evolution of hominoid primates, in which the earliest representative, *Aegyptopithecus*, was at a lower grade of encephalization compared with that of the descendant species, I excluded eohippus when calculating the regression line for fossil equids. As you see, the line runs through the middle of the mammalian polygon. Extended to the left, it would run through the datum on the living fox, and it represents an average degree of encephalization of living mammals. All living carnivores and ungulates would be well represented by such a line.

We must now return to the question of the why of it. What benefits were associated with the enlargement of the brain to make its energetic cost worthwhile? Why was the evolution of this costly organ system supported? What was being selected for when the various encephalized species evolved? To answer, we have to look more deeply into what a brain does for an animal.

MORE ON NEURAL INFORMATION

We began by learning more about what happens when brains vary in size among species. The first answer was in Figure 18.2, above, and the related discussion. I will elaborate now. Brain size is a superb statistic for estimating many interesting things the about brains of different mammalian species. We have inadequate data to be certain that it works as well in other vertebrates, but it is a reasonable conjecture that with suitable parametric adjustments it would, because the effect is basically a reflection of the efficient packing of neural material and supporting tissue in the brain. In mammals, brain size estimates total cortical surface area, between species, with an "error" of about 1% (Fig. 18.2). It estimates equally well the volume of the basal ganglia, of the cerebellum, and of the cerebral cortex with comparably small errors (Jerison, 1991, 1994). Although the sample of species is very small, it even appears to estimate the volume of the prefrontal cortex (Brodmann, 1913; Jerison, 1997; Semendeferi et al., 1997; Uylings and Van Eden, 1990).

In short, the brain hangs together. If we know one part, we can estimate many other parts surprisingly well. Gross brain size also estimates some functional properties. When properly analyzed, Figure 18.2 and the additional information that I cited demonstrate that brain size estimates the total information-processing capacity of a mammalian brain, or, in other words, mammalian neural complexity. Let me present some numbers on the enormous amount of information handled even by small mammalian brains.

The best data are on mice (Braitenberg and Schüz, 1991). A house mouse weighs about 40 g, and its brain weighs about 0.5 g. It contains a total of about 40 million neurons, about 10 million of which are cortical and most of the rest cerebellar. There are about 80,000,000,000 synapses in its isocortex alone. To relate these numbers to information-processing capacity, we note that a formal unit of information, a bit, is one yes–no event, and the typical unit for describing a computer's capacity, the byte, is eight bits. A synapse is a space at a junction between neurons at which a yes–no event can occur, and the number of synapses is, therefore, a measure of the information-carrying capacity of a brain. From the number of its synapses, a mouse's isocortex, thus, has an information-processing capacity of 10^{10} bytes (per unit time).

For a human perspective on neural information, here are some more numbers. As I indicated earlier, present evidence is that there are about the same number of synapses per unit volume of cerebral cortex in all mammals (Schüz and Demianenko, 1995). Because the volume of cortex is proportional to brain size, this means that the total number of synapses in a brain is approximately proportional to its size. The number of cortical synapses in humans would, therefore, be estimated as of the order of 10^{14}. These numbers show how brain size can function as a statistic that estimates complexity.

We have become accustomed to numbers as large as these. We have learned computerese in our time and are not overwhelmed by the information-processing capacity of very large computers, nor are we troubled by different processing procedures. It is sobering that we do not really know the brain's analogue for a byte, or for a microprocessor, or for information-storage capacity, as these words have been developed in computerese. Computer scientists confidently call the storage capacity "memory," borrowing freely from the psychologist. Although we have borrowed as freely from the computer scientist when we discuss "programs" and "scripts" as cognitive units, however, these are not confident borrowings. We do not have a vocabulary at that level of analysis for what brains do. In fact, even the ideas of the bit or byte may be questioned when applied to neural units. These ideas were appropriate when one accepted a strict "all-or-none" view of neural activity, but we recognize a real role for graded pre- and postsynaptic potentials, as well as complications from inhibitory as well as excitatory transmission, and the likelihood that information in the brain is processed by a system that is better modeled by a combination of analog and digital computation.

We have not created dictionaries that enable us to translate honestly from computers to brains. In addition, let us recognize that the very large numbers with which we deal so readily are themselves a problem in that when we think about them, it is probably by analogy to smaller numbers that are more manageable and more imaginable. Our problem may be comparable with that in the transition from classic to relativistic physics, when it was recognized that elementary ideas such as time, length, and distance depended on intuitions about simultaneity and the rigidity of perceivable rulers and measuring tapes and that these intuitions were misleading. We have to begin with our intuitions, of course, but we must also be sensitive to their limitations.

At this point in the discussion, we are safe with the analogy of a mouse's tiny brain and the recognition of how enormous an information processing system it is. Its tens of millions of nerve cells and tens of billions of connections may help our intuition about why a mouse can do the marvelous things it does: not only classic and instrumental conditioning, not only generalization, and contrast effects, but also learning in context and transferring training in sensible ways to new situations, learning cognitive maps, and surely doing much more, were we only clever enough to pressure it to demonstrate its abilities. In fact, it is difficult to be precise about any further advantage that may accrue from having a still larger brain.

NEURAL AND BEHAVIORAL COMPLEXITY

If language and language-like activities are omitted from behavioral measurements, it is surprisingly hard to distinguish among species with respect to objective measures of animal intelligence (Macphail, 1982). The tiny brain of the mouse is really not so tiny as an information-processing system. Does this system really have to be as big as it is to do its thing in controlling "higher mental processes" in mice? Given our recent knowledge, it would be hard to provide an unequivocally positive answer. When we categorize the behavioral repertoire in different animal species, we have few good ways to distinguish among species according to the complexity of the repertoire. Euan Macphail (1982, 1987, 1993) gave us this message, but few of us have really taken it to heart. I appreciated it much better when I heard M.E. Bitterman (1988) describe his experiments on "higher mental processes" in honeybees. There are important lessons for us in Macphail's review and critique of the comparative analysis of cognition and brain differentiation in living animals.

The lesson does not depend on whether Macphail was entirely right or wrong. He missed Duane Rumbaugh's elegant transfer index (Rumbaugh and Pate, 1984) to differentiate the behavioral capacities of primate species, for example, in which encephalization can be a useful guide (Rumbaugh, 1997). I can illustrate the problem with a few case histories. Bitterman (1988), working with methods developed as improved and elaborated versions of those originally devised by von Frisch (1950), has shown that honeybees learned essentially all of the various behaviors that Macphail has discussed as the categories of complex behavior that can define the intelligence of nonhuman mammals.

The lesson on neural complexity is from the honeybee's brain. Most invertebrates have concentrations of neurons that work the way a vertebrate brain does. In insects the analogues of the vertebrate cerebral hemispheres are the mushroom bodies. Honeybees have among the largest of all insect mushroom bodies, and the number of neurons has been counted. They have about 340,000 neurons in these structures (Erber et al., 1987). This is about 4% of those in a mouse's cortex. One must conclude that a mammalian grade of information-processing capacity (i.e., brain size) is not a prerequisite for the effective control of complex behavior, at least not for the control of the repertoire of social, communicational, and related behavior that has been demonstrated in honeybees.

The behavioral capacities of honeybees require a critical reassessment of measures of behavioral complexity. Behaviors describable by certain input–output relationships are controllable by much smaller nervous systems than seem to be required by mammals. I believe that this is evidence that one can fill the organic black box that connects input with output with a variety of systems. Mammals and insects that demonstrate the same capacities do it in experiments in which the data are response categories as output and stimulus categories as input. Experimenters then draw graphs showing that response is a function of stimulus, and these graphs look the same in different species. This does not mean that the transformation from input to output was effected in the same way. I ran into this issue earlier in my recognition that vigilance cannot be distinguished in pigeons, rats, monkeys, and people when analyzed by certain experimental procedures. The probability of "observing" as a function of various situational parameters varies in the same way in all of these species.

In evolutionary terms, this points to convergent evolution with respect to the behaviors that are to be controlled in the face of divergent evolution of the neural control systems. That argument cannot be maintained by a selectionist concerned with the energetics of the brain. If a behavioral solution is required for a particular environmental challenge, then the energetics of brain control should dictate that the smallest effective system should have evolved. We may allow for some differences in body plan (*bauplan*), but it is hard to assume that nervous systems as profligate as those of mammals in their use of energy would have evolved if such simple solutions had already been "discovered" in so many species of invertebrates. The answer must be in some feature of the body plan, but it cannot be a feature that is constrained only by the required input–output relationship connected by an empty black box.

The effectiveness of small brains for controlling complex behavior is demonstrable not only in invertebrates. Roth and his colleagues (Roth, 1987; Roth et al., 1990, 1993; Roth and Wake, this volume, Chapter 8) describe a miniaturized Mexican salamander, *Thorius narisovalis*, as a bit over 1 cm long, with a brain less than 2 mm^3 in volume. Its brain is just about the same size as the head of a pin. They report a total of about 250,000 neurons in its brain, which is significantly fewer than the number in the honeybee's mushroom bodies. Although I have seen only observational reports and no learning studies of this salamander's behavior, from the reports by Roth and his colleagues it is clearly an entirely normal salamander, displaying the characteristic tongue-capture capacities of salamanders associated with a well-integrated retino-tectal visual system and its operation. It is a challenge to be clever in stretching the behavioral capacities of amphibians, including this miniature species, to learn the limits of their capacity for "higher mental functions," at least in the way that von Frisch (1950) discovered the dance of the bees. One can anticipate, however, that we will find nothing about the behavior of *Thorius* to prove that its tiny brain constrains its behavior in ways that would surprise or disprove Macphail's contentions.

The basic conclusion remains. Complex behavior can be controlled by small (and perhaps simple) brains. What is wrong with this conclusion? I think it is mainly in the assertion about the complexity of behavior—the implication that we know when behavior is simple or complex and our association of its simplicity and complexity with a corresponding simplicity or complexity of brains and of brain mechanisms. I have indicated a resolution in the introduction to this chapter, and it requires a reintegration of the idea of neural and behavioral complexity.

WHY SOME BRAINS ARE BIG: WHAT DO BIG BRAINS DO?

Birds and mammals have really big brains, and only the mammalian brain is well enough understood to enable us to speculate about what a large brain provides compared with a small brain, although the speculations may help us understand the enlarged brains of birds. (Encephalization in cartilaginous fish and in electric fish remains an enigma from this perspective.) I have presented some of the conclusions of the following discussion in the introduction to this chapter but will repeat them to present an integrated account.

A large fraction of a mammal's brain (a person's or a mouse's) is taken up by cortex, and the rest of the brain makes intimate connections with the cortex. In fact, if we analyze the sizes of the parts of the brain in mammals, we find that we can "explain" about 90% of the variance among the sizes of all of the parts (excepting the olfactory bulbs) by a single "brain size" factor (Jerison, 1991). We can answer the question—why so big?—by looking at the work of the cortex, and at the relations between the size of the cortex as a whole and total brain size. For a quantitative sense, we may note some averages from Stephan et al. (1981). Cerebral cortex accounts for more than half of an average brain's weight, cerebellum for about 10%, diencephalon less than 5%, and midbrain for about 1%. It is an acceptable extension of the evidence about cortex to apply it to these other structures.

There are familiar brain maps shown as homunculi or animalculi as laid out across the expanse of the cortical surface. These are maps of receiving areas for sensory information from the periphery of the body and sense organs and of mapping of motor control areas in the cortex relative to the parts of the body that are controlled. We usually remember the somatosensory maps, but we should also recognize that sensory maps of the retina and of the cochlea are also extensive and that there are equivalent maps subcortically on tectal and dorsal thalamic tissue and on the cerebellum.

We may not have assimilated the major message from such mapping studies, however, which is that most of the mammalian brain is mappable in this way. Almost all of a mammal's brain may be considered as "projection area." The statement may sound odd, because at the level of the cortex we usually think of association cortex (what was once known as *silent* cortex) as taking up space between the projection areas. This is, however, a misconception. We now know that there are no truly "silent" areas in the brain. Nerve cells everywhere are active most of the time. Furthermore, almost all of the areas involve the projection of information in an orderly way from the external world via sensory surfaces and from other areas in the brain. Association areas defined anatomically or physiologically can be thought of as intercalated among the variously specified projection areas.

The basic idea that we are accustomed to is nineteenth-century mental chemistry that had the brain creating the equivalent of molecules out of atoms or compounds out of molecules. The idea may be fine, but the inference that the components for the "chemical" combination are in clearly delimited and different parts of the brain is wrong. The brain's work is based on systems distributed throughout its material (cf. Goldman-Rakic, 1988), and Lashley's discredited idea of mass action actually describes this work more correctly than a strict localization point of view.

Mapping is the critical feature, and we should treat it as more than a metaphor or convenient description of studies of localization of function. Rather, we should think of the brain (at least in mammals) as a mapping machine, which takes information about the external world that is in the form of neural events and converts it into sets of maps of the external world. The maps should sometimes be thought of in exactly the same way as geographers' maps, as partial representations of reality, but they should be given a broader meaning. The maps may have cognitive dimensions of the sort that Tolman (1948) discussed, providing solutions to various navigational problems that might arise, in addition to providing a passive representation of the world. One may really go much further and recognize that the mapping of the external world by the brain amounts to the creation of a real world. The representation from conscious experience, for example, is very different from the concatenation of data that are recorded when we measure the brain's activity. Let me emphasize the point. I believe that a literally correct conclusion about what big brains are up to is that they create real worlds, worlds full of objects and animals and people and so on, and, if the brain is up to it, worlds with projections of future states, attributions of feelings and emotions, and theories of mind in other animals: Mind is the reality created by very large working brains.

Do we really need the kinds of maps that I just described? The answer is "Yes, in mammals," and I have offered an elaborate scenario to explain that answer (Jerison, 1973, 1991). It begins with the fact that there are multiple sources of information about the external world, and this multiplicity was probably a feature of the environmental niche invaded by the reptiles that became the first mammals 225 or more million years ago. My scenario places these first mammals as only slightly modified reptiles, which survived because they had "invaded" the previously empty nocturnal adaptive zone. To succeed in that zone they required adaptations for handling distance information to supplement the normal visual adaptations of reptiles. These adaptations were for much improved night vision, hearing (and echolocation), and olfaction. Brain enlargement was related to the integration of information from the several modalities to identify the information as coming from a single "object." According to the scenario, the integration of information enabled the earliest mammals to respond to events in the external world as real events in a real world rather than as concatenations of neural signals that are correlated with sensory stimuli and motor responses.

The issue is, why do mammals have large brains? And the answer is: to pack the extensive neural machinery required to construct maps of the external world. The result of this adaptation is part of everyday experience, which we share with other mammals. We humans see, or know, that a coin remains a coin whether we see it head-on (circular) or in side view (elliptical). Processes of this kind, "pattern recognition," when simulated on computers, require much more computer power than simulations of the more usual candidates for examples of human intelligence, such as proving theorems in symbolic logic. Contrary to our intuition, perception may take more neural machinery than "pure thought," and this is the paradox of complexity.

To repeat my statement in the introduction, we are misled because we believe intuitively that things that are easy to do require little processing machinery. Perception, which is immediate and instinctive according to our intuition, would seem to require less brain tissue than complex thought. A more correct view, however, is that perception seems easy only because brains are built to do it, to handle information about the external world. Complex thought is hard, because, despite its size, the mammalian brain did not evolve as a specialized thinking machine. There are unlikely to be many fundamental neurobiological adaptations that are designed specifically for thinking hard about abstractions. The amount of tissue that is actually devoted to a process in a living brain should be determined by how much tissue is needed to do it well, and if it can only be done well by a lot of neural machinery, then it might be worth a heavy investment in the machinery to do the job right. If it can be done well by relatively little neural machinery, however, there would be no selective advantage to doing it by more.

We can now think once again about the work of small brains. We must recognize that mammals and birds may be unique in requiring the labeling of integrated information from the environment as objects and so forth. If reflex control (including the control of "fixed action patterns") is sufficient for behavior, as it may be in the tongue-flicking insect-catching activity of salamanders, there is no justification for the expenditure of energy on the work of an elaborate brain, and smaller would be better. This argument can be applied to insect adaptations. It may be stretching the analysis to lump all of the variety of behaviors of bees and wasps and ants into a system of reflex operations, but their small nervous systems argue that they may indeed behave as Cartesian reflex machines. There may not be enough machinery there for pattern recognition as it occurs in large-brained vertebrates.

I would also emphasize that certain categories of behavior that we think of as implying complexity are, in fact, not necessarily demanding with respect to neural control. Communication can be remarkably elaborate and complex in small-brained creatures. In fact, all animals communicate in some ways with one another. The same is true for social behavior. It is even true for learning. A strong argument can be made for the proposition that educability (or plasticity) can be a property of either single neurons or, at most, small networks of neurons.

When we study "higher order" learning we are probably usually studying learning in situations in which *knowledge* of reality—a constructed environment with objects, and so forth—is required to solve a problem, and the learning is about the nature of the problem. When we discover that very small-brained species can solve such a problem we might do well to examine the problem more carefully to try to identify alternate routes to its solution. Some of these may require the construction of a model of the environment, that is, a real world, which may be possible only with large, complex brains. It is normally a better solution in terms of energetic costs to use a reflex machine, as it were, to solve the learning, communication, or social problem.

We can safely assume that big brains are complex brains. We cannot assume that a particular kind of behavior is simple or complex. It is here that the assumption that I stated at the outset, equating complexity of behavior with complexity of brain control, fails.

I must emphasize that my last argument is two-faced. It may be true that a problem can be solved in a large-brained or in a small-brained way, in a reality-constrained or in a reflex-constrained way. In that case, however, we obviously make a serious mistake if we assume a priori that one or the other way is being used in a particular animal. It will remain a real problem to determine the mechanisms underlying any behavior that we describe only by its input and output. Comparative psychology has been in a straightjacket when it took Lloyd Morgan's canon, or Occam's razor, to heart. Uncritically, these assume that the simplest kind of information-processing system always controls behavior. In fact, in mammals it is very likely the energetically less efficient reality-building system that is often at work.

REFERENCES

Abraham, F.D., and A.R. Gilgen, (eds.) (1995) *Chaos Theory in Psychology*. Greenwood Press, Westport, CT.
Aiello, L.C., and P. Wheeler, (1995) The expensive-tissue hypothesis: the brain and the digestive system in human and primate evolution. *Curr. Anthropol.* 36:199–221.
Bauchot, R., and H. Stephan, (1967): Encéphales et moulages endocrâniens de quelques insectivores et primates actuels. In Problèmes Actuels de Paléontologie (Évolution des Vertébrés). *Colloq. Int. Cent. Nat. Rech. Sci.* 163:575–587.
Bitterman, M.E. (1988) Vertebrate–invertebrate comparisons. In H.J. Jerison, and I.L. Jerison, (eds.); *Intelligence and Evolutionary Biology*. Springer–Verlag, Berlin, pp. 251–276.
Braitenberg, V., and A. Schüz, (1991). *Anatomy of the Cortex: Statistics and Geometry*. New York, Berlin.
Broadbent, D.E. (1958) *Perception and Communication*. London, Pergamon.
Broadbent, D.E. (1971) *Decision and Stress*. New York, Academic Press.
Brodmann, K. (1913) Neue Forschungsergebnisse der Grosshirnrindenanatomie mit besonderer Berucksichtung anthropologischer Fragen. *Verhandlungen des 85ste Versammlung Deutscher Naturforscher und Aerzte in Wien*, pp. 200–240.
Bullock, T.H., and W. Heilingberg, (eds.) (1986). *Electroreception*. New York, Wiley-Interscience.
Butler, A.B., and W. Hodos, (1996) *Comparative Vertebrate Neuroanatomy*. Wiley-Liss, New York.
Crile, D.P., and D.P. Quiring, (1940) A record of the body weight and certain organ weights of 3690 animals. *Ohio J. Sci.* 40:219–259.
Diamond, I.T. (1979) The subdivisions of the neocortex: a proposal to revise the traditional view of sensory, motor, and association areas. *Prog. Psychobiol Physiol. Psychol.* 8:1–43.
Edinger, T. (1929) Die fossilen Gehirne. *Ergeb. Anat. Entwicklungsgesch.* 28:1–249.
Edinger, T. (1948) *Evolution of the Horse Brain. Geological Society of America*, Baltimore, Memoir 25.
Eldredge, N., and S.J. Gould, (1972) Punctuated equilibria: an alternative to phyletic gradualism. In T.J.M. Schopf, (ed.): *Models in Paleobiology*. Freeman, Cooper and Co., San Francisco.
Erber, J., U. Homberg, and W. Gronenberg, (1987) Functional roles of the mushroom bodies in insects. In A.P. Gupta, (ed.): *Arthropod Brain: Its Evolution, Development, Structure, and Functions*. Wiley-Interscience, New York, pp. 485–511.
Falk, D. (1987). Hominid paleoneurology. *Annu. Rev. Anthropol.* 16:13–30.
Garey, L.J. and G. Leuba (1986). A quantitative study of neuronal and glial numerical density in the visual cortex of the bottlenose dolphin: evidence for a specialized subarea and changes with age. *J. Comp. Neurol.* 247:491–496
Goldman-Rakic, P.S. (1988) Topography of cognition: parallel distributed networks in primate association cortex. *Annu. Rev. Neurosci.* 11:137–166.
Herrnstein, R.J. (1985) Riddles of natural categorization. *Philos. Trans. R.S. Lond.* [*Biol.*] 308:129–144.
Holland, J.G. (1957) Technique for behavioral analysis of human observing. *Science* 125:348–350.
Hopson, J.A. (1979) Paleoneurology. In C. Gans, R.G. Northcutt, and P. Ulinski, (eds.): *Biology of the Reptilia, vol. 9*. Academic Press, New York, pp. 39–146.
Horner, J.R., and J. Gorman, (1988). *Digging Dinosaurs*. Harper and Row, New York.
Jerison, H.J. (1959) Effects of noise on human performance. *J. Appl. Psychol.* 43:96–101.
Jerison, H.J. (1965) Human and animal vigilance. *Percept. Motor Skills* 21:580–582.
Jerison, H.J. (1967) Activation and long term performance. In A.F. Sanders, (ed.): *Attention and Performance I* (A Special Edition of Acta Psychologica, Vol. 27). North-Holland Publishing Company, Amsterdam, pp. 373–389.
Jerison, H.J. (1973) *Evolution of the Brain and Intelligence*. Academic Press, New York.
Jerison, H.J. (1977) Vigilance: biology, psychology, theory, and practice: keynote address. In R. R. Mackie, (ed.): *Vigilance: Theory, Operational Performance, and Physiological Correlates*. Plenum, New York, pp. 27–40.
Jerison, H.J. (1987) Brain size. In G. Adelman, (ed): *Encyclopedia of Neuroscience*. vol. 1. pp. 168–170.
Jerison, H.J., (1990) Fossil evidence on the evolution of the neocortex. In E.G. Jones, and A. Peters, (eds.): *Cerebral Cortex, vol. 8A*. Plenum, New York, pp. 285–309.
Jerison, H.J. (1991) *Brain Size and the Evolution of Mind: 59th James Arthur Lecture on the Evolution of the Human Brain*. American Museum of Natural History, New York.
Jerison, H.J. (1994) Evolution of the brain. In D. Zaidel, (ed): *Neuropsychology (Handbook of Perception and Cognition, 2nd ed.)* Academic Press, New York, pp. 53–82.

Jerison, H.J. (1997) Evolution of prefrontal cortex. In N. Krasnegor, R. Lyon, and P. Goldman-Rakic, (eds.): *Development of the Prefrontal Cortex: Evolution, Neurobiology, and Behavior*. Paul H. Brookes Company, Inc., Baltimore, pp. 9–26.

Jerison, H.J. and R.M. Pickett, (1963) Vigilance: a review and re-evaluation. *Hum. Factors* 5:211–238.

Jerison, H.J., and J.F. Wing, (1961) Human vigilance and operant behavior. *Science* 133:880–881.

Jones, E.G., and T.P.S. Powell, (1970) An anatomical study of converging sensory pathways within the cerebral cortex of the monkey. *Brain* 93:793–820.

Karten, H.J. (1969) The organization of the avian telencephalon and some speculations on the phylogeny of the amniote telencephalon. *Ann. N. Y. Acad. Sci.* 167:164–179.

Karten, H.J. (1991) Homology and evolutionary origins of the "neocortex." *Brain, Behav. Evol.* 38:264–272.

Kemp, T.S. (1979) The primitive cynodont *Procynosuchus*: functional anatomy of the skull and relationships. *Philos, Trans. R. Soc., Lond.* 285:73–122.

Kielan-Jaworowska, Z. (1986) Brain evolution in Mesozoic mammals. In J.A. Lillegraven, (ed.): G.G. Simpson Memorial Volume. *Contributions to Geology, University of Wyoming*, Special Paper 3:21–34.

Macphail, E.M. (1982) *Brain and Intelligence in Vertebrates*. Oxford, Clarendon, pp. ix + 413.

Macphail, E.M. (1993) *The Neuroscience of Animal Intelligence: From the Seahare to the Seahorse*. Columbia University Press, New York.

Macphail, E.M., et al. (1987) The comparative psychology of intelligence. *Behav. Brain Sci.* 10:645–695. (Also later commentary, e.g., 1989, 12:377–380.)

Mackworth, N.H. (1950) *Researches on the Measurement of Human Performance*. MRC Special Report 268. His Majesty's Stationery Office, London.

Martin, R.D. (1990) *Primate Origins and Evolution: A Phylogenetic Reconstruction*. Chapman and Hall, London.

Mlikovsky, J. (1980) Zwei Vogelgehirne aus dem Mizan Bohmens. *Casopis Miner. Geol.* 25:409–413.

Northcutt, R.G. (1987) The evolution of the vertebrate brain. In G. Adelman, (ed.): *Encyclopedia of Neuroscience, vol. 2*. Birkhauser, Stuttgart, pp. 415–418.

Novacek, M. (1996) *Dinosaurs of the Flaming Cliffs*. Doubleday, New York.

Pepperberg, I.M. (1994) Vocal learning in African grey parrots: effects of social interaction. *Auk* 111:300–313.

Piveteau, J. (ed.) (1958) *Traité de Paléontologie*, Tome VI, vol. 2. Masson, Paris.

Piveteau, J. (ed.) (1961) *Traité de Paléontologie*, Tome VI, vol. 1. Masson, Paris.

Platel, R. (1979) Brain weight–body weight relationships. In C. Gans, R.G. Northcutt, and P. Ulinski, (eds.): *Biology of the Reptilia, vol. 9*. Academic Press, New York, pp. 147–171.

Quiroga, J.C. (1980) The brain of the mammal-like reptile *Probainognathus jenseni* (Therapsida, Cynodontia). A correlative paleo-neurological approach to the neocortex at the reptile-mammals transition. *J. Hirnforsch.* 21:299–336.

Radinsky, L. (1976) Oldest horse brains: more advanced than previously realized. *Science* 194:626–627.

Radinsky, L. (1979) *The Fossil Record of Primate Brain Evolution*. The James Arthur Lecture. American Museum of Natural History, New York, 27 pp.

Rockel, A.J., R.W. Hiorns, and T.P.S. Powell, (1980) The basic uniformity in structure of the neocortex. *Brain* 103:221–244.

Roth, G. (1987) *Visual Behavior in Salamanders*. Springer-Verlag, New York.

Roth, G., et al. (1990) Miniaturization in plethodontid salamanders (Caudata: Plethodontidae) and its consequences for the brain and visual system. *Biol. J. Linn. Soc.* 40:165–190.

Roth, G,. et al. (1993) Paedomorphosis and simplification in the nervous system of salamanders. *Brain Behav. Evol.* 42:137–170.

Rumbaugh, D.M. (1997) Competence, cortex, and primate models: a comparative primate perspective. In N.A. Krasnegor, G.R. Lyon, and P.S. Goldman-Rakic, (eds.): *Development of the Prefrontal Cortex: Evolution, Neurobiology, and Behavior*. Paul H. Brookes Publishing Co., Baltimore, pp. 17–139.

Rumbaugh, D.M., and J. L. Pate, (1984) The evolution of cognition in primates: a comparative perspective. In H.L. Roitblat, T.G. Bever, and H.S. Terrace (eds.): *Animal Cognition*. Lawrence Erlbaum Associates, Hillsdale, N.J., pp. 569–585.

Russell, D.A. (1972) Ostrich dinosaurs from the Late Cretaceous of Western Canada. *Can. J. Earth Sci.* 9:375–402.

Schmidt-Nielsen, K. (1984) *Scaling: Why Is Animal Size so Important?* Cambridge University Press, Cambridge, England.

Schüz, A., and G.P. Demianenko, (1995) Constancy and variability in cortical structure: a study on synapses and dendritic spines in hedgehog and monkey. *J. Hirnforsch.* 36:113–122.

Semendeferi, K., H. Damasio, R. Frank, and G.W. Van Hoesen, (1997) The evolution of the frontal lobes: a volumetric analysis based on three dimensional reconstructions of magnetic resonance scans of human and ape brains. *J. Hum. Evol.* 32:375–388.

Shannon, C.E., and W. Weaver, (1949) *The Mathematical Theory of Communication.* University of Illinois Press, Urbana.

Skinner, B.F. (1959) *Cumulative Record.* Appleton-Century-Crofts, New York.

Stephan, H., H. Frahm, and G. Baron. (1981) New and revised data on volumes of brain structures in insectivores and primates. *Folia Primatol.* 35:1–29.

Thireau, M. (1975) L'allométrie pondérale encéphalo-somatique chez lez urodèles. II. Relations interspécifiques. *Bull. Mus. Nat. Hist. Nat.* 207:483–501.

Tobias, P.V. (1967) *The Cranium and Maxillary Dentition of Australopithecus (Zinjanthropus) boisei. Olduvai Gorge, vol. 2.* Cambridge University Press, London.

Tobias, P.V. (1990) *The Skulls, Endocasts, and Teeth of Homo habilis. Olduvai Gorge, vols. 4A and 4B.* Cambridge University Press, London.

Tolman, E.C. (1948) Cognitive maps in rats and men. *Psychol. Rev.* 55:189–208.

Uylings, H.B.M. and C.G. Van Eden, (1990) Qualitative and quantitative comparison of the prefrontal cortex in rat and in primates, including humans. In H.B.M. Uylings, C.G. Van Eden, J.P.C. De Bruin, M.A. Corner, and M.G.P. Feenstra (eds.): *Progress In Brain Research*, vol. 85. Elsevier, Amsterdam, pp. 31–62.

von Frisch, K. (1950) *Bees: Their Chemical Senses, Vision, and Language.* Cornell University Press, Ithaca.

von Uexküll, J. (1934) *Streifzüge durch die Umwelten von Teiren und Menschen.* Springer-Verlag, New York: [translated in Schiller, C.H. (ed.) (1957) *Instinctive Behavior: The Development of a Modern Concept.* International Universities Press, New York, pp. 5–80].

Warm, J.S. (ed.) (1984) *Sustained Attention in Human Performance.* Wiley, New York.

Welker, W.I. (1990) Why does cerebral cortex fissure and fold? A review of determinants of gyri and sulci. In E.G Jones, and A. Peters, (eds.): *Cerebral Cortex vol. 8B.* Plenum Press, New York, pp. 1–132.

Worthy, G.A.J., and J.P. Hickie (1986) Relative brain size in marine mammals. *Am. Nat.* 128:445–459.

Zangerl, R., and G.R. Case, (1976) *Cobelodus aculeatus* (Cope), an anacanthous shark from Pennsylvanian black shales of North America. *Palaeontographica A.* 154:107–157.

Chapter 19

THE EVOLUTION OF CONSCIOUSNESS

Gerhard Roth, Brain Research Institute, University of Bremen, and Hanse Institute for Advanced Study, Delmenhorst

Among neuroscientists and cognitive psychologists it is now largely accepted that consciousness is strictly bound to the activity of the human brain. At the same time, it is debated whether consciousness is unique to humans or whether at least *some* states of consciousness can be found in at least some animals, while others may be unique to humans. In the first case, neuroscientists should be able to identify unique features in the human brain the presence of which could explain the uniqueness of consciousness in humans; alternatively, one should be able to reconstruct the evolution of consciousness in vertebrates in parallel to the evolution of vertebrate brains.

Taxonomically and biologically we are mammals, and within the class Mammalia we are primates. Among the order Primates, we belong to the Old World primates (Catarrhini). Within this group we are members of the family Hominidae (or superfamily Hominoidea), which is composed of the "apes" (gibbons, orang-utans, gorillas, chimpanzees, and humans) as opposed to "monkeys," that is, the remaining Old World primates (family Cercopithecidae) and all New World primates (suborder Platyrrhini). Among the hominids/hominoids, we are members of the subfamily Homininae (or family Hominidae), which includes the gorilla (*Gorilla gorilla*), humans (*Homo sapiens*), the two chimpanzee species (common chimpanzee, *Pan troglodytes*, and bonobo, *Pan paniscus*), and the orang-utan (*Pongo pan*) and excludes the gibbon (*Hylobates*) (Fig. 19.1).

Traditionally, gibbons, orang-utans, gorillas, and chimpanzees were grouped together into the family Pongidae, while humans (with their extinct ancestors) were put into the separate family Hominidae. Such a distinction, although psychologically understandable, is unjustified in the light of modern taxonomy and evolutionary biology. Biologically, *Homo sapiens* and the two chimpanzee species are more closely related to each other than the chimpanzees to any other living primate; we share about 99% of our genes with them. Therefore, humans and the two species of chimpanzees should be placed together in a separate taxon, for which no name yet exists. The closest relative of this nameless group are the gorillas, and the closest relative of the African great apes is the orang-utan. The earliest primates originated at least 65 million years (my) ago, the separation between Old and New World primates took place about 40 my ago, and that between Old World monkeys (Cercopithecidae) and apes including humans about 30 my (or less) ago. Gibbons branched off at 19 to 17 my, the orang-utan 16 at my, and the gorilla at 9 to 7 my. Humans and chimpanzees separated from each other 6.7 to 6.2 my ago (Byrne, 1995). Thus, given the evolutionary age of about 65 my of the order Primates, the divergence between *Homo* and *Pan* is relatively recent.

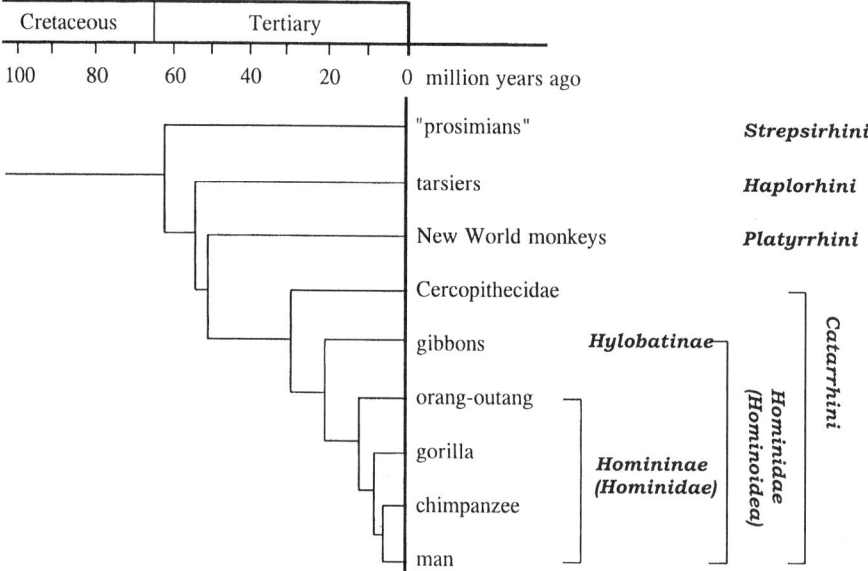

Figure 19.1. Taxonomic relationship (cladogram) of the primates. (Modified from Nieuwenhuys et al., 1998.)

Do these evolutionary relationships not only determine the structure and functions of our body, but likewise include consciousness as our "highest" cognitive ability, or is there a fundamental gap with respect to consciousness between humans and all other animals?

To prove directly the presence or absence of states of consciousness is impossible because we are uncertain about consciousness even in our conspecifics. There are, however, *indirect* ways to determine the presence of consciousness in animals as likely or unlikely. In essence, these are (1) to check in groups of animals for the presence of those cognitive functions that in humans can be exerted only consciously, (2) to examine which parts of the human brain are necessary for (and active during) the different states of consciousness, and (3) to examine which of these centers of the human brain are present (and active) in the brains of those animals that—based on behavioral evidence—show certain states of consciousness. Taken together, these pieces of evidence should give us a relatively reliable answer to the question of the way different states of consciousness have evolved in parallel to vertebrate, mammalian, primate, and human brain evolution.

PHENOMENOLOGY OF CONSCIOUSNESS

In humans, consciousness includes very different phenomena that only have in common the fact that we have subjective awareness of them. There are general states of consciousness without clear link to any content. The most prominent of this is *wakefulness* or *vigilance*. It is characterized by a general responsiveness to sensory stimuli. Other general states of consciousness are fatigue, dizziness, anxiousness, hunger, comfort, and the awareness of temporal duration and of spatial layout (Farber and Churchland, 1995; Knight and Grabowecky, 1995). These states form a background for more specific types of consciousness. These include *conscious perception* of events happening in the world around me and within my body, which differs in modality, submodality (quality), quantity, intensity, location in space and time, content, and meaning. *Mental activities* such as thinking, remembering, imagining, and planning are another class of specific states of consciousness and are usually felt differently from perceptions, as is the case with *emotions*. Even more special types of consciousness include *body-identity awareness*, that is, the belief that I belong to the body that apparently surrounds me; *autobiographic consciousness*, that is, the conviction that I am the one who existed yesterday; *reality awareness* of what was going on in the past and is happening in the world surrounding me; awareness of *voluntary control of movements and actions*, of *being the author of my thoughts and deeds*; and, finally, *self-awareness*, that is, the ability of self-recognition and self-reflection. *Attention* is a state of increased and focused consciousness. It can be driven externally or internally. In the latter case, it goes along with improved perceptual abilities (e.g., increased visual acuity or lowered auditory threshold).

There is strong evidence for a *modular* organization of consciousness. Different aspects of consciousness can dissociate, that is, they can be impaired selectively after damage of restricted parts of the brain (Kinsbourne, 1995; Knight and Grabowecky, 1995). There are patients who have normal states of cognition, consciousness, and intelligence except that they deny that this is their own body or who do not know *who* or *where* they are. Furthermore, different states of consciousness interfere only little with each other if they are dissimilar in their general nature (perceptions vs. thoughts vs. emotions) or in their modality or semantic content. We can have emotions or thoughts while perceiving something, and in the same way we can watch the traffic on the street while listening to a Mozart symphony. On the other hand, it is impossible for the untrained ear to listen to the details of two pieces of music simultaneously. This is, however, largely subject to training: An experienced conductor is capable of consciously following a large number of instruments. Generally, people can expand their conscious capacity either by increasing their efforts or by improving their perceptual and attentional skills (Hirst, 1995).

There are things that can and those that cannot be done without attention. Many if not most things of our daily life we execute in a relatively automatized way, for example, writing on a computer keyboard, riding a bicycle, or driving our car along a familiar route, which are at best accompanied by general consciousness. Most of these functions required attention when we started learning them, but with increasing exercise conscious attention became less and less necessary. There are ways of unconscious processing of sensory information, for example, identification of objects, but most psychologists state that such processing is "shallow," being based on physical features and excluding meaningful information (Broadbent, 1958; Hirst, 1995). There is "implicit", that is, unconscious, learning (e.g., of syntactical rules), but people typically remain unaware of what they have learned and how. On the other hand, it is impossible to handle meaningful, complex information that afterwards can be reported without being attentive (e.g., grasping the meaning of a hitherto unheard sentence or comparing two complex pictures), to plan a complicated sequence of actions, or to acquire a new complex motor skill (e.g., learning to play the piano or skating). In summary, everything that can be done effortlessly, does not require attention, while all effortful tasks need to be accompanied by awareness and attention. Also, unattended or poorly attended information is poorly recollected (Moscovitch, 1995).

THE NEUROBIOLOGICAL BASIS OF THE DIFFERENT STATES AND APPEARANCES OF CONSCIOUSNESS

It appears that we are only aware of those things that are bound to the activity of the so-called associative cortex, while the activity of all subcortical and extratelencephalic brain centers, regardless of how important they are for the emergence of consciousness, is never accompanied by consciousness. This is true, above all, for the reticular formation, because its destruction leads to a general loss of consciousness, that is, to coma (Hassler, 1978).

The reticular formation consists of three columns of nuclei, a median, medial, and lateral column, that extend from the anterior mesencephalon through the pons to the medulla oblongata and rostral spinal cord (Nieuwenhuys et al., 1988). The *medial* column receives input from all sensory modalities and the cerebellum as well as descending cortical input via the pyramidal tract. Its ascending projections form the so-called nonspecific afferent or "extralemniscal" system, also called the *ascending reticular activating system*. This system projects to the intralaminar thalamic nuclei, which, in turn, project (with some topography) in parallel and via different groups of neurons to the striatum and the cortex. The function of the medial reticular formation is the control of the wake–sleep cycle and of general cortical activity.

The *median* column is formed by the so-called raphe nuclei. These nuclei, predominantly the dorsal raphe nucleus, send serotonergic fibers to all parts of the limbic system that are involved in cognitive functions (e.g., the hippocampal formation, amygdala, basal forebrain, limbic thalamic nuclei, cingulate, frontal, parietal, and occipital cortex). The *lateral* column contains the noradrenergic locus coeruleus complex, which again projects to all parts of the limbic–cognitive system (Fig. 19.2). The locus coeruleus is supposed to exert a role in controlling attention and "monitoring" continuously the external and internal environment for important events. Its projection to the prefrontal cortex particularly may mediate information about the relevance of complex sensory events and situations (Robbins, 1997). The raphe nuclei are supposed to play a modulatory role in the context of behaviorally relevant events, apparently by counteracting and dampening the arousing effect of the other systems.

The next most important brain centers for the control of consciousness are the intralaminar and midline thalamic nuclei, because they are the most important relay station for the ascending projections of the reticular formation. These thalamic

The Neurobiological Basis of the Different States of Consciousness 559

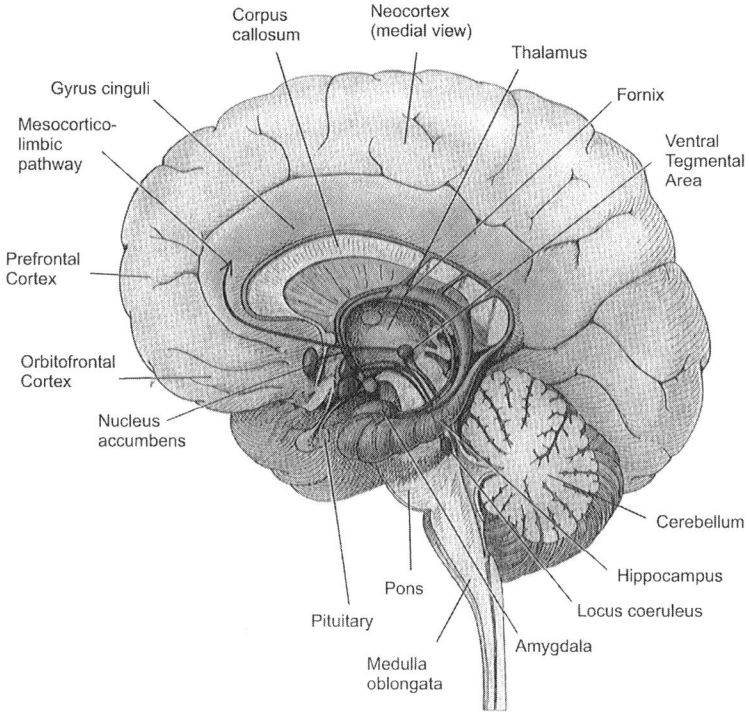

Figure 19.2. Medial view of the human brain showing major limbic centers. (Modified from Spektrum/Scientific American, 1994.)

centers receive input from the entire cortex and project, with some topography, back to it, predominantly to prefrontal cortex, and additionally to the striatum; they are likewise connected to the entire limbic system. Damage to these thalamic nuclei leads to impairment or loss of consciousness (Hassler, 1978; Smythies, 1997). Other thalamic nuclei important for the mediation of activity of the limbic system to the cerebral cortex are the anterior thalamic nucleus, which has reciprocal connections with the anterior cingulate gyrus (see below), and the medial thalamic nuclei (above all the dorsomedial nucleus), which connect limbic centers, above all the amygdala and the dorsal and ventral striatum/pallidum, with the prefrontal cortex (Alexander et al., 1990). Without these connections, emotions and other functions of the limbic system would not become conscious.

The nucleus reticularis thalami surrounds the entire lateral part of the thalamus in a bowl-like fashion. It receives collaterals from thalamocortical as well as corticothalamic tracts and has reciprocal connections with the sensory and limbic thalamic nuclei. It does not project to the cortex; rather, it exerts inhibitory control over most thalamic nuclei via GABAergic fibers. It is assumed to function as a "filter" for various kinds of information coming from the sensory periphery and brain stem, acting under the control of the cortex and the limbic system. It may, therefore, be involved in guidance of attention (Smythies, 1997; Guillery et al., 1998).

The brain centers mentioned thus far belong to the limbic system in a wider sense, which in the vertebrate brain is the system that subconsciously controls all aspects of cognitive and emotional states and accordingly voluntary behavior. The limbic system evaluates what the organism does and stores the result of this evaluation in the different kinds of memory. Other parts of the limbic centers discussed in the following contribute in more specific ways to the different states of consciousness (Fig. 19.2).

The amygdala is a complex of different nuclei and is reciprocally connected with the associative cortex, particularly with the orbitofrontal cortex (either directly or via the mediodorsal thalamic nucleus) and the hippocampal formation (Aggleton, 1992, 1993; Holland and Gallagher, 1999). It strongly influences the sensory (visual, auditory, gustatory) cortex. It receives subcortical input from the olfactory system, the limbic thalamic nuclei, and also from the rest of the limbic system. The amygdala is in control of so-called autonomic responses (via the hypothalamus); regarding cognitive and emotional functions, it is an important center (together with the anterior cingulate cortex; see below) for evaluation and perhaps storage of *negative* experience (e.g., in the context of fear conditioning and anxiety) (Aggleton, 1992; Davidson and Irwin, 1999). The involvement of the amygdala or parts of it in positive affect is still a matter of debate (Holland and Gallagher, 1999; Davidson and Irwin, 1999). There are close connections of the basolateral amygdala to the ventral striatal dopamine system and the orbitofrontal cortex that may play a role in food-motivated associative learning, while the central amygdaloid nucleus may contribute, via the basal forebrain and the dorsolateral striatum, to the control of attention (Holland and Gallagher, 1999).

The hippocampal formation (Ammon's horn, subiculum, dentate gyrus) and the surrounding parahippocampal and perirhinal (including entorhinal) cortices are important centers for the formation and the consolidation of traces of declarative memory inside the cortex (i.e., of those kinds of memory that in principle can be consciously retrieved and reported) (Squire, 1987; Markowitsch, 1992; Squire and Knowlton, 1995). It is presently debated whether the hippocampal formation is necessary for *retrieval* of traces of declarative memory as well (Markowitsch, 1999). According to Moscovitch (1995), the hippocampal system acts as an associative, episodic memory module that exclusively picks up information that is consciously apprehended. Consciousness thus becomes an inherent property of memories that are recollected. This work of the hippocampus, however, is considered "unintelligent"—as opposed to that of the prefrontal cortex—because events are encoded only by simple contiguity and by associations that memory traces form with each other and with cues. Whenever "strategic" episodic memory, (i.e., a search for the where and why) is required, the prefrontal cortex comes into play, and this happens in an effortful manner and under voluntary control. Other authors are skeptical about this idea of automatic production of consciousness by the corticohippocampal system.

The dorsal parts of the basal ganglia (i.e., the putamen, nucleus caudatus, globus pallidus, nucleus subthalamicus, and substantia nigra) are closely associated via the ventral lateral, ventral anterior, and dorsomedial thalamic nuclei with the prefrontal, premotor, and parietal cortex as well as with the entire limbic system. The dorsal basal ganglia deal with subconscious planning and final decisions to voluntary action under the influence of the limbic system (Passingham, 1993). The ventral striatum/nucleus accumbens, together with the ventral tegmental area, are involved in the prediction, processing and perhaps storage of reward and other pleasant aspects and consequences of behavior.

The basal forebrain–septal nuclei complex is connected reciprocally with the hippocampus and the amygdala as well as with the centers of the reticular formation already mentioned. Its cholinergic fibers project to all parts of the cortex. The basal forebrain is believed to be involved in the control of attention and of activity of neocortical neuronal networks, primarily in the context of earlier experience (Voitko, 1996). The so-called mesolimbic system (i.e., nucleus accumbens, lateral hypothalamus, ventral tegmental system)—like the substantia nigra—is characterized by the neuromodulator dopamine. This system has strong connections with the orbitofrontal cortex and is—apparently in cooperation with parts of the amygdala— involved in the formation of positive memories and pleasure and perhaps in the control of attention in the context of new events (Robbins and Everitt, 1995; Holland and Gallagher, 1999). Its impairment may be involved in cognitive misinterpretation and misevaluation in schizophrenics.

All these subcortical parts of the brain contribute substantially to consciousness, while their activities remain completely unconscious. Damage to these subcortical centers usually produces either complete loss of consciousness or profound impairment of conscious cognitive and emotional functions. This may include the inability to recognize positive or negative consequences of action, impairment of attention, and/or loss of declarative memory. Importantly, patients usually are unaware of these deficits.

While activity in the cortex is necessary for consciousness, we are similarly unaware of processes going on in the primary and secondary sensory and motor areas of the cortex, although these processes are necessary for the specific contents of awareness of events inside or outside our body. We are aware only of those processes bound to the activity of the cingulate and the associative cortex and even then of only some of those processes.

The *cingulate cortex* (Figs. 19.2 and 19.3A) is that part of the cortex that surrounds the subcortical parts of the telencephalon and the thalamus. It is tightly connected with the prefrontal and parahippocampal cortex, the basal forebrain–septal region, the amygdala, the limbic thalamic nuclei, and the reticular formation. The anterior part is involved in the sensation of pain (in combination with the somatosensory cortex, the medial thalamic nuclei, and the so-called central tegmental gray) and in memory of painful events. In this sense, it may be the conscious counterpart of the amygdala. It is always active for tasks requiring attention (Posner, 1995).

The associative cortex (Fig. 19.3B) is that portion of the cortex that contains no primary sensory or motor cortical areas, but is involved in higher order processing of information coming from these areas. It includes the *posterior parietal cortex* (PP). The left PP is involved in symbolic–analytic information processing, mathematics, language, and interpreting drawings and symbols. Lesions impair reading and writing

562 19 The Evolution of Consciousness

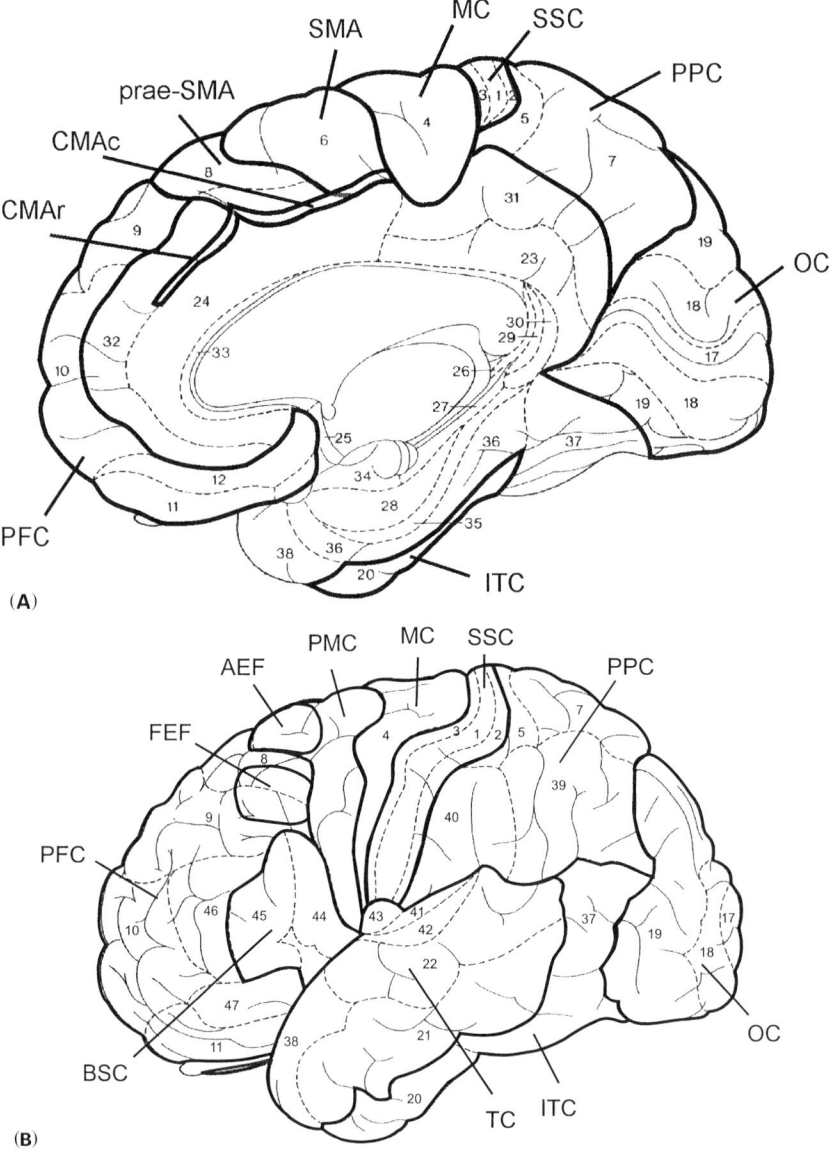

Figure 19.3. (A) A Medial view of the human cortex showing medial cortical areas. Numbers refer to cytoarchitectonic cortical fields according to Brodmann. CMAc, caudal cingulate motor area; CMAr, rostral cingulate motor area; ITC, inferotemporal cortex; MC, motor cortex; OC, occipital cortex; prae-SMA, presupplementary motor area; PFC, prefrontal cortex; PPC, posterior parietal cortex; SMA, supplementary motor area; SSC, somatosensory cortex. (Modified from Nieuwenhuys et al., 1989.) (B) Lateral view of the human cortex. Numbers refer to cytoarchitectonic cortical fields according to Brodmann. AEF, anterior eye field; BSC, Broca's speech center; FEF, frontal eye field; ITC, inferotemporal cortex; MC, primary motor cortex; OC, occipital cortex; PFC, prefrontal cortex; PMC, dorsolateral premotor cortex; PPC, posterior parietal cortex; SSC, somatosensory cortex; TC, temporal cortex. (Modified from Nieuwenhuys et al., 1989.)

and respective memory functions. The right PP deals with real and mental spatial orientation, the control of hand and eye movement, change of perspective, and control of spatial attention. Lesions of inferior right PP produce neglect (e.g., ignoring the contralateral half of the body or events in the contralateral visual hemifield) or anosognosia (i.e., lack of insight or denial of disturbances).

The associative *superior* and *middle temporal cortex* houses perception of complex auditory stimuli, including (generally left side) Wernicke's semantic speech center, which is crucial for the understanding and the production of meaningful written and spoken language. Perception of music usually involves the right medial temporal cortex. The *inferior* temporal cortex (IT) is decisive for complex visual information regarding nonspatial properties of visual objects and scenes along with their meaning and correct interpretation. Lesions in IT produce object agnosia (left IT), color agnosia (right IT), prosopagnosia, that is, inability to recognize faces (right or bilateral IT), deficits in categorization, changes in personality and emotionality, and deficits in the use of contextual information.

The *prefrontal cortex* (PFC) represents the largest portion of the human cortex (about 30%) and has been viewed by many neuroscientists as the "highest brain center." In contrast to all other parts of the cortex, its anatomical and functional substructures are still a matter of debate (cf. Roberts et al., 1998; Petrides and Pandya, 1999). Usually, two major parts are distinguished in the primate, including human, brain: a dorsolateral and a ventral-orbitofrontal portion. The *dorsolateral* PFC (including Brodman areas 9, 10, 44, 45, 46) receives cortical input mostly from the parietal and the anterior cingulate cortex and subcortical limbic input via the medial thalamic nuclei.

The dorsolateral PFC appears to be involved in (1) attention and selective control of sensory experience; (2) action planning and decision making; (3) temporal coding of events; (4) judgement and insight, particularly with respect to reality; (5) spontaneity of behavior; (6) strategic thinking; (7) associative thinking; and (8) working memory. Thus, the dorsolateral PFC is predominantly, although not exclusively, oriented toward the external world and its demands, including short-term or working memory. It is viewed to monitor and adjust one's behavior confidently and to be aware of one's consciousness, thus exerting supervisory functions (Knight and Grabowecky (1995). Lesions of the dorsolateral PFC result in perseveration and impairment of making appropriate cognitive or behavioral switches.

Of special importance for consciousness is the immediate or working memory, which most experts locate in areas 9 and 46 of the dorsolateral prefrontal cortex. The working memory (Baddeley, 1974) is that center that for a short period of a few seconds integrates all pieces of cortical information that are relevant in order to cope with the present situation and problems in the immediate future and particularly with the exact temporal order of events. The working memory is highly limited in its information-processing capacity, but has access to long-term memories in the parietal and temporal cortex. It is the primary source of attention and the "stream of consciousness."

The *orbitofrontal* PFC includes Brodmann areas 11 to 14 and 47. It receives cortical input mostly from the inferior temporal, anterior cingulate, entorhinal, and parahippocampal cortices and from subcortical limbic centers, above all from the amygdala. The orbitofrontal cortex is involved in social and emotional aspects of behavior, ethical considerations, divergent thinking, risk assessment, awareness of consequences of behavior, emotional life, and emotional control of behavior. Accordingly, damage to the orbitofrontal PFC results in loss of interest in important life events, loss of self, in "immoral" behavior, disregard of negative consequences of one's own behavior (Damasio, 1994). Thus, the orbitofrontal PFC is predominantly oriented toward the internal emotional and social aspects of life.

The *supplementary motor area* (SMA, prae-SMA) (Fig. 19.3A) is situated between the medial aspect of the motor cortex and the dorsomedial PFC and represents sort of an associative motor cortex. The prae-SMA is active during the preparation and planning of complex movements and even during imagined movements (Roland et al., 1980). Together with the PFC, it apparently contributes to the awareness of being the author of one's own deeds.

In summary, there is neither *consciousness* per se nor *a highest brain center* producing consciousness. Rather, different parts of the associative cortex contribute in different ways to the high diversity and content of consciousness, including awareness of external and internal sensory events; consequences of one's own behavior; autobiographic, body, and ego identity; action planning; and authorship of one's own deeds. The associative cortex does this under the strong influence of the primary and secondary sensory and motor cortices as well as of the subcortical centers mentioned.

COGNITION AND CONSCIOUSNESS IN ANIMALS

After the brief summary of the neural basis of higher cognitive functions and states of consciousness, I now turn to the question what kind of cognitive abilities can be found in the different groups of vertebrates and particularly mammals. Checking recent reviews on the "animal mind" (Stamp Dawkins, 1993; Parker et al., 1994; Byrne, 1995; Pearce, 1997; for criticism, see MacPhail, 1998), it seems that all vertebrates and probably also invertebrates with large brains (e.g., cephalopods) display sensory or focused attention, extended memory, categorization, and the formation of cognitive maps. Whether this is accompanied by some kind of consciousness is difficult to determine in fishes, amphibians, or reptiles. Many of the so-called higher cognitive functions such as concept learning, knowledge representation, analogical thinking, the formation of abstract representations, and imitation in the sense of copying a behavior are found at least among birds and mammals, and even in humans these higher cognitive functions are not necessarily accompanied by consciousness.

There are, however, cognitive functions that in humans require at least some states or levels of consciousness. These functions include

1. Imitation in the sense of task structure or task principle learning and tool learning. This is found in macaque and capuchin monkeys, in apes, and maybe in some other mammals (e.g., otter).

2. Taking the perspective of the other in deception and counterdeception. This is found in monkeys (e.g., baboons) and great apes.

3. Anticipation of future events (e.g., the preparation of tools in advance). This has been found in the great apes and may be present in some monkeys (Fig. 19.4A).

4. Comprehension of underlying mechanisms, for example, in the use of tools. This has been reported only in great apes (Fig. 19.4B).

5. Knowledge attribution/theory of mind. This is found in great apes, particularly chimpanzees.

6. Self-recognition in a mirror. This is present in great apes and perhaps in dolphins.

7. Teaching. This is again found only in chimpanzees.

8. Understanding and use of simple syntactical language (up to three-word sentences). This is found in great apes and dolphins and probably in parrots.

9. Use of complex syntactical language. This is found only in humans.

Functions 4, 5, 6, and 8 have been studied extensively in the recent past and are of special interest because they might draw a borderline between monkeys and great apes among the primates. Such a borderline is less emotionally laden than that between humans and nonhuman apes. Primatologists agree almost unanimously that monkeys (e.g., capuchins) exhibit the use of tools (as many other animals do), but without an understanding of the underlying mechanism. They do not seem to "know" why one tool is effective and another is not (Visalberghi and Limongelli, 1994). Even more telling are the experiments concerning mirror self-recognition (cf. Parker et al., 1994). Monkeys are capable of making use of mirrors, for example, to look behind objects that otherwise are inaccessible (Byrne, 1995). Kummer reports that baboons recognize a group member on a slide and identify themselves as mother or child on slides without difficulty. Yet, primatologists agree that monkeys show no sign of mirror self-recognition. Among apes, chimpanzees and orang-utans definitely show mirror self-recognition, while among gorillas only Koko does (it is assumed that gorillas often are too shy to pass the test). Chimpanzees show great interest in their mirror image and pass the marking test (i.e., removing marks of paint from face or body using the mirror image) well. Interestingly, at least some dolphins are reported to show mirror self-recognition, too, but their behavior appears to be very different from that of apes in front of a mirror. They show no natural interest in their mirror image and dislike the marking test (Marten and Psakaros, 1994). The reasons for these differences are unclear, irrespective of the many methodological and conceptual problems. There are dolphin specialists who doubt that dolphins really recognize themselves in the mirror (Marino et al., 1994).

The presence of knowledge attribution or theory of mind to others (Baron-Cohen et al., 1985) is difficult to distinguish from the capability of taking the perspective of the other. For most animals with complex behavior, it is important to guess what the

19 The Evolution of Consciousness

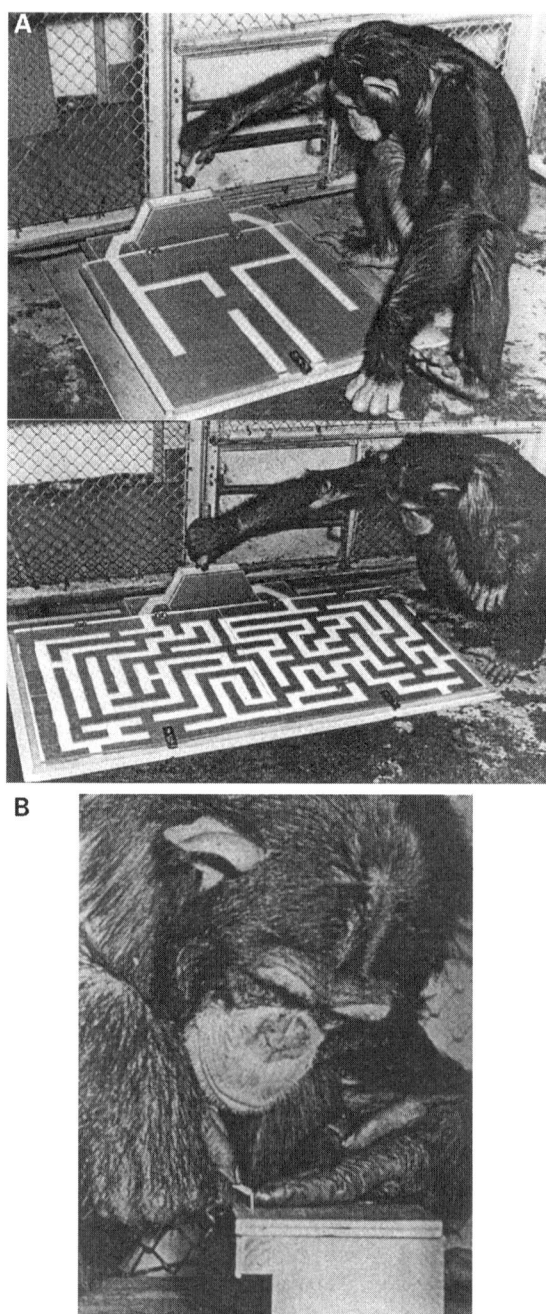

Figure 19.4. (A) The chimpanzee Julia from the Zoological Institute of the University of Muenster mastering mazes of different complexity. (B) Julia handling a screwdriver and guiding it with the nail of the left index finger. (From Rensch, 1968.)

other is going to do, for example, in agonistic behavior (cf. Stamp Dawkins, 1993). However, primatologists (e.g., Kummer) state definitely that monkeys (e.g., baboons) do not take into account what the other is *thinking*. Important in this context is the performance of very young children. According to Mitchell (1993), self-detection in children starts at 3 months, and mirror self-recognition is shown at an age of 18 months on average. Little children, however, show embarrassment and coy reactions earlier than that. Self-recognition in photos starts at 24 months, followed by signs of self-evaluative emotions (e.g., shame and pride). A true "theory of mind" are assumed by Meltzoff and Gopnik (1993) to emerge at 4 years. These authors stress that these events occur in the same sequence in apes, although at a much slower rate.

Much has been written about the presence or absence of "true," that is, syntactically complex, language in nonhuman primates (and other animals). Monkeys have complex systems for intraspecific vocal communication that are able to express relatively complicated meaning, including symbolic information (i.e., about objects and events that are not present) or about relationships between events (e.g., parental relationships). Many of these calls have to be learned by the infant monkey, and—as in songbirds—dialects exist (cf. Zimmermann et al., 1995). Most authors agree that sentences consisting of up to three words are understood and used by chimpanzees, gorillas, and dolphins. Whether this is a sign for a "simple" syntax is a matter of debate. Most authors agree that nonhuman primates are unable to infer differences in the meanings of a phrase or sentence from differences in the sequence of words. Chimpanzees do combine "words" to form new words (Gardner et al., 1989), but they do not go beyond the linguistic capabilities of a 3-year-old child, even after intense training (Savage-Rumbaugh, 1984).

Of great interest in this context is the development of language in human children (Locke, 1995). In humans, language learning starts long before speaking (viz., in utero). Vocal learning of the mother's voice begins prenatally; 3-day-old neonates show a preference for the maternal voice the way it is transmitted to the fetal auditory system prenatally. Facial learning starts immediately after birth; babies seem to be preadapted to it. At 6 months after birth, children show a preference for familiar over foreign language. First voweling sounds are produced around 4 to 6 months, when "babbling" starts; first consonant-like sounds occur at 9 to 12 months. Children seem to have great pleasure at producing sounds and speaking. First reproduction of maternal intonation contours takes place around 6 months or even earlier, and first words are produced between 8 and 20 months (average 12 months). Around 18 to 23 months, children begin to combine words and form two-word utterances. Then, they gradually begin to use sentences longer than two words, but typically in a "telegraphic" style similar to that found in patients with lesions of Broca's speech area (Stromswold, 1995). Children use two to three word sentences without conjugation and declination, and they say little that they have not heard before. In the third year, children start distinguishing singular and plural and asking the famous question "what's that?" From this point on, their language syntactically becomes rapidly more elaborate. Between 3 and 4 years, utterances are completely grammatical.

Passive vocabulary is larger than active from the very beginning: At 8 months, infants understand an average of 36 words, but produce fewer than 2, and at 10 months they understand 67 words on average, but they will not produce that many words until at least 6 months later. At 16 to 18 months, there is a rapid acceleration in the rate at which new words and phrases are comprehended (7 to 9 words per day until an age of 6 years). Around the end of the second year, the vocabulary of the child consists of 150 to 200 words. At an age of 3 to 4 years, children have a vocabulary of 1500 and understand an additional 3000 to 4000 words in addition. While apes after 4 to 6 years of intense training may use some hundred words in a meaningful manner, a child of the same age has an active vocabulary of 4500 words. The average adult has an active vocabulary of about 10,000 words and a passive vocabulary that is about ten times larger. It has been estimated that during speaking more than 1000 grammatical rules are applied (Corballis, 1991). Thus, it seems that apes have simple linguistic capabilities comparable to a human child of 2 to 3 years, but from then on humans rapidly develop a fully syntactical language that is far superior to any communicative system known in animals.

In conclusion, based on the experimental evidence reported above, we may—with some caution—identify several evolutionary steps among tetrapod vertebrates regarding cognitive abilities; (1) Among tetrapods from amphibians and "reptiles" (i.e., turtles, snakes, and lizards) to birds and mammals; (2) among mammals from nonprimate mammals to primates (a similar step might have occurred toward cetaceans); (3) among primates from prosimians and monkeys to apes; (4) among apes from gibbon, orang-utan, and gorilla to chimpanzee and human, and (5) from chimpanzee to human. This scenario does not take into consideration large-sized and big-brained land mammals such as elephants because the abovementioned experiments on cognitive abilities have not been carried out in these animals.

ANIMAL BRAINS AND HUMAN BRAIN

Are we able to correlate the above differences in higher cognitive functions including consciousness among groups of tetrapods and more specifically mammals with properties of their brains? To answer this question, we first have to clarify what kind of differences we need to look for. First of all, differences in cognitive abilities among animals could be simply the result of the presence or absence of major brain structures relevant for cognition (e.g., it could be that some animals are less intelligent because their brains have no cortex or hippocampus). Second, assuming—as most neurobiologists now do—that all brain functions including cognition and consciousness are the result of the anatomy and physiology of networks formed by neurons and their synapses, differences in higher cognitive functions should result from structural and physiological differences within these networks. Thus—given the same overall organization of brains—what should count for cognition including consciousness is (1) the number of neurons in the entire brain or in those brain centers that are necessary for a particular cognitive function or state of consciousness; (2) the number of synapses per neuron in the brain or specific brain centers; (3) short-term plasticity of synapses (i.e., how quickly synapses can change their properties relevant for fast transmission of neuronal activity); (4) plasticity of synapses in the context of memory formation; and (5) the ontogenetic dynamics of synapses (i.e., how long synapses retain a high degree of plasticity during their lifetime). If the packing density of neurons and the number of synapses per neuron remained roughly constant, then an increase in brain size would mean a proportional increase in number of neurons and synapses and consequently an increase in the performance of neuronal networks.

Thus, what we have to look for are differences in (1) overall organization of brains, (2) absolute or relative brain size, (3) absolute or relative size of those parts of the brain relevant for higher cognitive abilities, (4) size of the associative cortex and the prefrontal cortex in particular, and (5) differences in physiological properties of the brains under consideration (e.g., synaptic plasticity).

All tetrapod vertebrates (amphibians, "reptiles", birds, mammals) have brains that—despite enormous differences in outer appearance, overall size, and relative size of major parts of the brain—are very similar in their general organization and even in many details (Roth and Wullimann, 1996). More specifically, all tetrapod brains possess a median, medial, and lateral reticular formation inside the medulla oblongata and the ventral mesencephalon. There is a corpus striatum, globus pallidus, nucleus accumbens, basal forebrain/septum, and amygdala within the ventral telencephalon, a lateral pallium, homologous to the olfactory cortex of mammals, and a medial pallium, homologous to the hippocampal formation (at least Ammon's horn and subiculum). This means that all structures required for attention, declarative memory (or its equivalents in animals), motivation, guidance of voluntary actions, and evaluation of actions are present in the tetrapod brain. These structures essentially have the same connectivity and distribution of transmitters, neuromodulators, and neuropeptides in the different groups of tetrapods.

A more difficult problem is the presence of structures homologous to the mammalian isocortex in the telencephalon of other tetrapods. Amphibians possess a dorsal pallium, turtles and diapsid reptiles have a dorsal cortex plus a dorsal ventricular ridge (DVR), birds have a Wulst and a DVR, and these structures- or at least the Wulst- are believed by many comparative neurobiologists to be homologous to the isocortex—and not to the basal ganglia—of mammals (Karten, 1991; Northcutt and Kaas, 1995; Striedter, 1997; Macphail, this volume, Chapter 13; Shimizu, this volume Chapter 5). Major differences exist, however, between these structures with regard to cytoarchitecture and size. In amphibians, the dorsal pallium is small and unlaminated; in lizards it is relatively larger, and in turtles and some diapsid reptiles it shows a three-layered structure. In birds, those parts assumed to be homologous to the mammalian cortex (i.e., the DVR and Wulst) are large, but unlaminated. In mammals, with the exception of insectivores and cetaceans, the dorsal pallium or cortex shows the characteristic six-layered structure. When we compare birds such as pigeons or parrots with roughly equally intelligent mammals such as dogs, then it becomes apparent that the same or very similar cognitive functions are performed by anatomically very different kinds of pallium/cortex.

Let us now turn to the relevance of absolute and relative brain size, because large brains have been correlated with *intelligence* or *higher cognitive abilities* (Jerison, 1973; this volume, Chapter 18). Among mammals, very large brains are found in primates (1.4 kg in *Homo sapiens*), in elephants (up to 5.7 kg), and in whales and dolphins (up to 10 kg), (Fig. 19.5). The reasons for increase in brain size are unclear; body size appears to be the single most important factor influencing brain size, that is, large animals generally have large brains in absolute terms. Increase in brain size does not, however, strictly parallel the increase in body size, but follows only to the power of 0.66 to 0.75 (i.e., 2/3 or 3/4, depending on the statistics used; Jerison, 1991)—a phenomenon called *negative brain allometry* (Jerison, 1973) (Fig. 19.6). Consequently, small animals of a given taxon have *relatively* larger brains and large animals of this group *relatively* smaller brains. Among mammals, this is reflected by the fact that in very small rodents brains occupy up to 10% of body mass, in pigs 0.1%, and in the blue whale, the largest living animal, 0.01% (Fig. 19.7).

In addition, the different groups of vertebrates, while satisfying the principle of negative brain allometry, exhibit considerable differences in their fundamental brain–body relationship. Among tetrapods, mammals and birds generally have larger brains relative to body volume/weight than amphibians and "reptiles," and among mammals, cetaceans and primates have relatively larger brains than other orders. Thus, during the evolution of birds and mammals and more specifically of cetaceans and primates, genetic and epigenetic systems controlling brain size have undergone substantial changes in favor of relatively larger brains. These changes resulted in enlargements of brains beyond that associated with body size (Jerison, 1991; this volume, Chapter 18).

Thus, contrary to a common belief, humans do not have the largest brain in either absolute or relative terms. Unless we accept that cetaceans and elephants are more intelligent than humans and/or have states of consciousness not present in humans, the absolute or relative size of the human brain per se cannot account for our factual or alleged superior cognitive abilities. Among relatively large animals, however, humans stands out with a brain that constitutes 2% of body mass. We can quantify this fact by determining the so-called encephalization quotient (EQ), which indicates the ratio between the actual relative brain size of a group of animals to the relative brain size as expected on the basis of brain allometry determined by body size alone. Calculating the EQ for the human brain, it turns out that it is about seven times larger than that of an average mammal and about three times larger than that of a chimpanzee if they had the size of a human being (Jerison, 1973, 1991). Apparently, during the evolution of *Homo sapiens*, over a period of 3 to 4 million years, additional genetic and epigenetic processes led to a constant further increase in relative (and absolute) brain size. Although humans stand out in this respect among primates, similar processes must have taken place among cetaceans. Toothed whales, particularly members of the family Delphinidae, exhibit EQs that are far superior to all primates except *Homo sapiens* (Marino, 1998). Although humans have an EQ of about 7, the dolphins *Sotalia fluviatilis*, *Delphinus delphis*, and *Tursiops truncatus* have EQs of 3.2, and the great apes (except humans) have EQs around 2. Thus, humans have a much larger brain than expected among primates, but even in this respect their brain is by no means unique, as the example of dolphins shows.

What about the absolute or relative size of the human cortex? There are enormous differences both in absolute and relative brain and pallial/cortical sizes among

Animal Brains and Human Brain 571

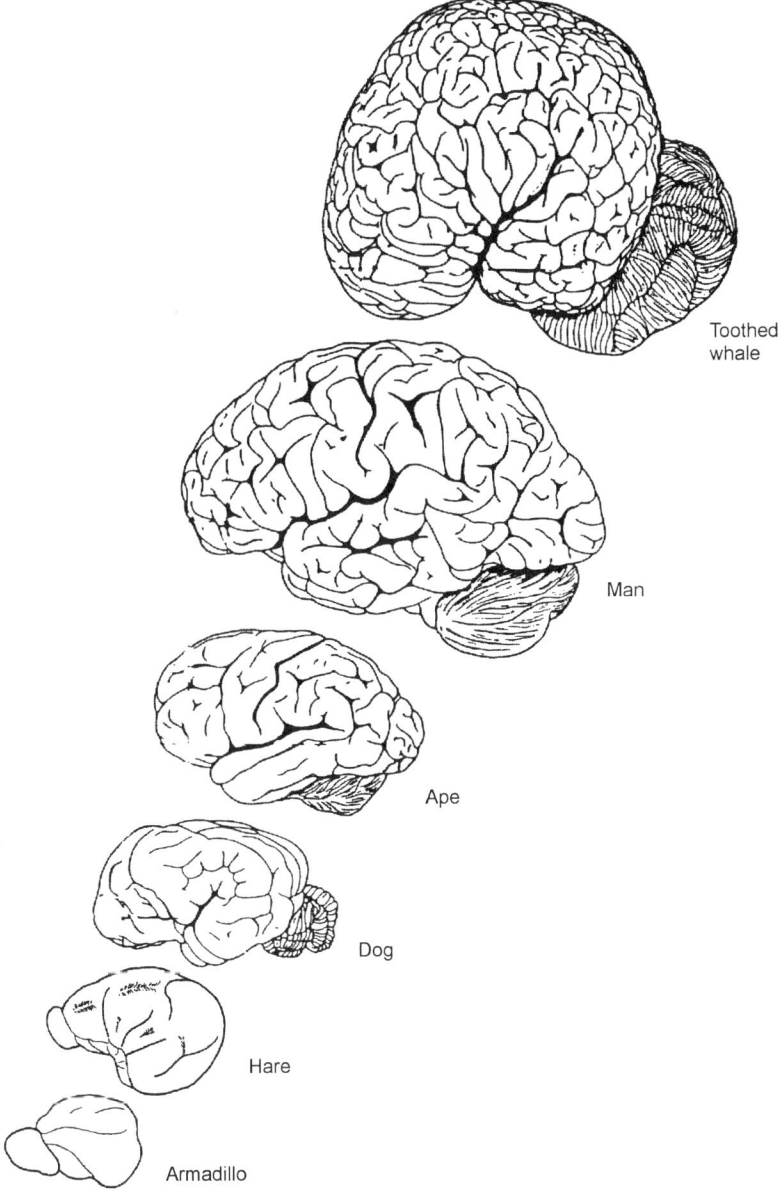

Figure 19.5. Series of mammalian brains, all drawn to the same scale. Evidently, humans have neither the largest brain nor the most convoluted cortex. With rare exceptions, convolution of the cortex as well as of the cerebellum increases monotonically with an increase in brain size.

572   19 The Evolution of Consciousness

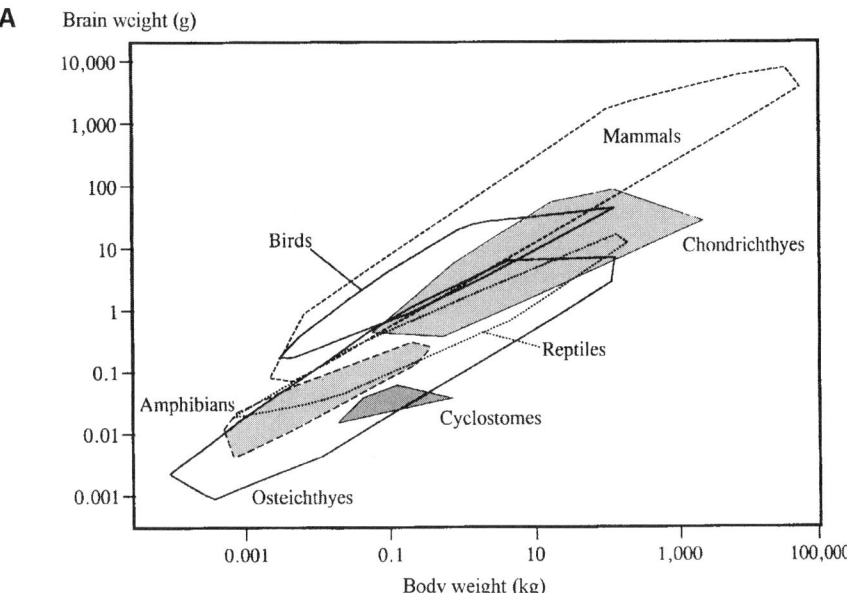

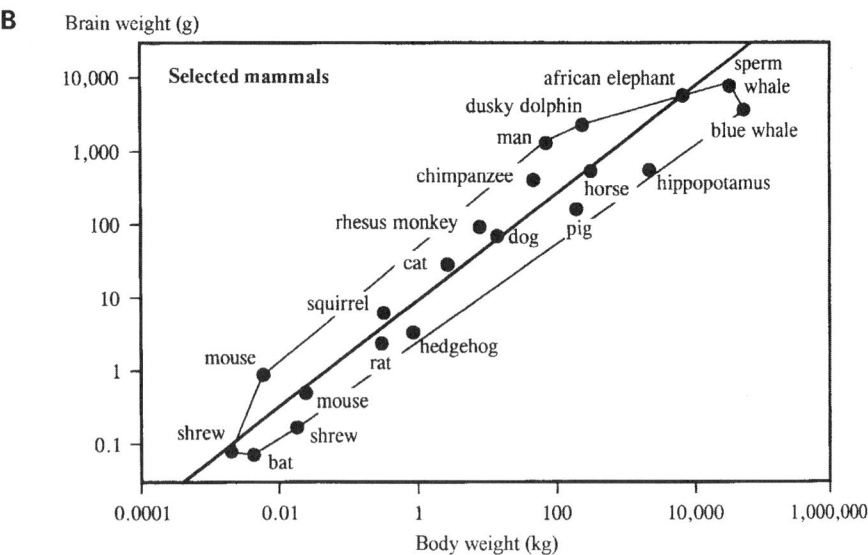

Figure 19.6. Diagrams showing the relationship between body weight and brain weight in a double logarithmic graph (A) Convex polygons for brain sizes of the main vertebrate groups. (B) Data from 20 mammalian species. (Modified from Nieuwenhuys et al., 1998).

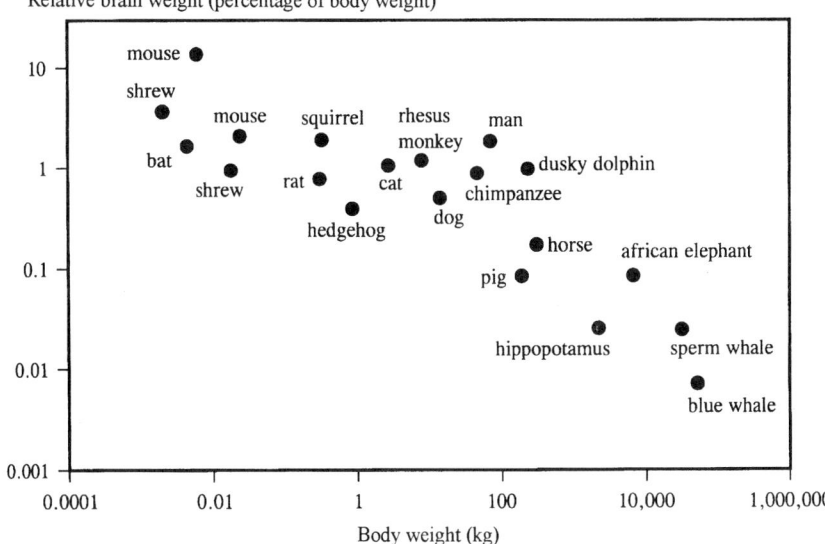

Figure 19.7. Brain weight as a percentage of body weight for the same 20 mammalian species as in Figure 19.6B Double logarithmic graph. (Modified from Nieuwenhuys et al., 1998.)

tetrapods and among mammals in particular. For example, humans have a brain and a cortex that are roughly 3000 times larger in volume than those of a mouse. This implies that changes in *relative* size of cortex are inconspicuous, because in mammals cortical size rather strictly follows changes in brain size, but, again, there are differences within mammalian groups. Apes (including humans) have somewhat larger isocortices than other primates and other mammals because their forebrains (telencephalon plus diencephalon) are generally somewhat larger, constituting 74% of the entire brain as opposed to about 60% in other mammals including mice. At 40% of brain mass the human cortex has the size expected in a great ape (Jerison, 1991).

The enormous increase in cortical volume is partly the result of an increase in brain volume and consequently in cortical surface (which is related to an increase in brain volume by exactly the power of 2/3; Jerison, 1973) and partly the result of an increase in the thickness of the cortex. The cortex is about 0.8 mm thick in mice and 2.5 mm in humans. The number of neurons per unit cortical volume, however, decreases with an increase in cortical thickness and brain size. While about 100,000 (or more) neurons are found in 1 mm^3 of motor cortex in mice, "only" 10,000 neurons are found in the motor cortex of humans (Jerison, 1991). This decrease in the number of cortical neurons per unit volume is a consequence of a roughly equal increase in the length of axonal and dendritic appendages of neurons, in the number of glial cells, and in the number of small blood vessels. Without such an increase in glial cells and blood vessels, large isocortices would probably be both architecturally and metabolically impossible.

Thus, the dramatic decrease in nerve cell packing density is at least partly compensated for by an increase in cortical thickness. This could explain why all mammals have a roughly equal number of neurons contained in a cortical column below a given surface area (e.g., 1 mm^2) (Rockel et al., 1980). Furthermore, as explained above, what should count for the performance of neuronal networks is not so much the number of neurons per se but the number of synapses their axons and dendrites form or carry, plus the degree of plasticity of synapses. An increase in length of axons and dendrites paralleling a decrease in nerve cell packing density should lead to more synapses, and such an increase in the number of synapses could additionally compensate for the strong decrease in nerve cell packing density as well. It has been estimated that the mouse cortex contains about 10 million (10^7) neurons and 80 billion (8×10^{10}) synapses and the human cortex about 100 billion (10^{11}) neurons and a quadrillion (10^{15}) synapses, ten thousand times more than the mouse cortex (Schüz and Palm, 1989; Jerison, 1991). These differences certainly have important consequences for differences in the performances of the respective cortices.

What about animals with brains and cortices that are much larger than those of humans, (e.g., elephants or most cetaceans)? Should they not be much more intelligent than humans or have some superior states of consciousness (a popular assumption for whales and dolphins)? As to cetaceans, there is currently a debate on how many neurons their cortices really contain. Their cortex is unusually thin compared with large-sized land mammals and shows a different cytoarchitecture (e.g., lacking a distinct cortical layer IV). Accordingly, experts report a lower number of nerve cells contained in a standard cortical column than in land mammals. While Garey and Leuba (1986) report that in dolphins the number of cortical neurons per standard column is 2/3 that of land mammals. However, recently Güntürkün and von Fersen (1998), after examining the brains of three species of dolphins, recently reported that this value amounted only to one fourth. Accepting this latter lower value, then—given a cortical surface of about 6,000 cm^2 in dolphins (three times that of humans)—the cortex of the bottlenose dolphin (*Tursiops truncatus*) should contain three fourths of the corresponding number of neurons found in humans (i.e., 6×10^{10}), which is about equal to the number of cortical neurons estimated for chimpanzees. Calculations of the number of cortical neurons in cetaceans with much larger brains and cortices (e.g., in the sperm whale with a cortical surface of more than 10,000 cm^2) are difficult, because precise data on cortical nerve cell number per standard cortical column are lacking. Even assuming that—due to enormous expansion of the cortex—the respective value is only one eighth of that found in land mammals, however, a sperm whale cortex should contain approximately the same number of cortical neurons as dolphins. Based on these calculations, we should expect cetaceans to be roughly as intelligent as nonhuman great apes, which is what cognitive behaviorists have found out about these animals.

The case of elephants remains, with a similarly enormously large brain (around 4 kg) and cortical surface of about 8000 cm^2, which at the same time is thicker than that of cetaceans but also possesses a typical six-layered structure. Assuming that the number of cortical neurons is two thirds the value found in primates, elephants should have at least as many cortical neurons and cortical synapses as humans. Again, we do not know enough about the organization of the elephant's cortex, but elephants should come close to the cognitive and mental capabilities of humans, if it were only the number of cortical neurons and synapses that counted.

Perhaps it might be safer to restrict our consideration to the size of the associative cortex, because, as I mentioned at the outset, different kinds of consciousness are necessarily bound to the activities of specific parts of the associative cortex. There is a common belief that the associative cortex had increased dramatically in both absolute and relative terms during hominid brain evolution and that this was the basis for the uniqueness of human mind. Such an increase is difficult to assess, however, as there are no precise criteria for distinguishing primary and secondary sensory cortical areas from true association areas. Recently, Kaas (1995) argued that the number of cortical areas increased dramatically from about 20 such areas in the hypothetical insectivore-like ancestor to more than 60 in primates. What has increased, however, according to Kaas, was the number of functionally intermediate areas (such as V3 or MT), but neither the primary nor the highly associative areas. Kaas is right to warn about the danger of greatly underestimating the number of functionally different cortical areas in small-brained mammals.

Available data suggest that, contrary to common belief, the associative cortex has increased roughly in proportion to an increase in brain and cortical size. This apparently is the case for the prefrontal cortex, which is regarded by many neuroscientists and neurophilosophers as the true seat of consciousness. Anatomically, the prefrontal cortex is defined as the cortical area with major (although not exclusive) input from the mediodorsal thalamic nucleus (Uylings et al., 1990; Roberts et al., 1998). Using this definition, it turns out that the PFC has increased isometrically with an increase in cortical and overall brain volume within groups of mammals, but here again we find an additional increase in relative PFC size with an increase in absolute brain size across mammalian orders: in rats, PFC constitutes 6.5%; in dogs, 8.7%; in cows 9.8%; and in humans 10.6% of brain mass (Jerison, 1997). The human PFC has exactly the size expected according to primate brain allometry. Of course, cetaceans as well as elephants have prefrontal cortices that are much larger in absolute terms than the human PFC, but what they do with this massive "highest" brain center remains a mystery so far.

We have not yet found anything in brain anatomy that would explain the factual or alleged superiority of humans regarding cognition and consciousness. Given the fact that *Homo sapiens* has an absolutely and relatively large brain and cortex, it appears to be the animal with the highest number of cortical neurons and/or synapses, probably with the exception of the elephant. Thus, in this respect humans are not truly exceptional. What remains is the question whether there are any anatomical or physiological specializations in the human cortex that could be correlated with the higher cognitive abilities and states of consciousness attributed to humans. As to the general cytoarchitecture of the human cortex, it is indistinguishable from that of other primates and most other mammals. Likewise, no differences have been discovered thus far between humans and nonhuman mammals with respect to short-term or long-term plasticity of cortical neurons, the action of neuromodulators, and so forth. Only two traits have been discovered that could drastically distinguish the human cortex from that of other primates: (1) differences in growth rate and length of growth period and (2) the presence of the Broca speech center.

As to the first trait, maturation of the brain is more or less completed at 2 years after birth in prosimians and 6 to 7 years in monkeys and nonhuman apes, but the human brain still continues to mature until the age of 20 years, which is much longer than in any other primate (Pilbeam and Gould, 1974). A critical phase in the development of the human brain seems to occur around the age of 2.5 years. At this time, major anatomical rearrangements in the associative cortex have come to a stop, and the period of fine-wiring appears to start, particularly in layer 3 of the prefrontal cortex (Mrzljak et al., 1990). As mentioned above, at this time, human children "take off" cognitively compared with nonhuman primates. Without any doubt, the drastically prolonged period of brain development constitutes one important basis for an increased capability of learning and memory formation.

The other trait concerns the presence of the Broca speech center in the frontal lobe (cf. Fig. 19.3B) responsible for temporal aspects of language, including syntax, along with the Wernicke speech center in the temporal lobe, which is responsible for the meaning of words and sentences (although meaning is likewise dependent on syntax and grammar). It is to date unclear whether these speech centers are true evolutionary novelties. All mammals studied thus far have a center for intraspecific communication within the temporal lobe (mostly left side), which may be homologous to the Wernicke center for semantics. It has been reported that destruction of these areas leads to deficits in intraspecific vocal communication (Heffner and Heffner, 1995). In addition, it has long been argued that the posterior part (A 44) of the Broca speech center in humans and the ventral premotor area of nonhuman primates probably are homologous (Preuss, 1995). The ventral premotor area controls the movement of forelimbs, face, and mouth, which is likewise the case for the posterior portion of the Broca area.

According to a number of primatologists, nonhuman primates lack a direct connection between the motor cortex and the nucleus ambiguus, where the laryngeal motor neurons are situated. In humans, bilateral destruction of the facial motor cortex abolishes the capacity to produce learned vocalization, including speech or humming a melody, while a similar destruction in monkeys has no such consequences (Jürgens, 1995). According to a number of experts, the evolutionary basis for human language was an emotionally driven stereotyped language typical of nonhuman primates. During hominid evolution, the cortex gained control over this system such that beyond the initiation of hard-wired, innate sounds a flexible production of sounds and their sequences became possible (Deacon, 1990; Jürgens, 1995). Such an interpretation, however, contrasts with recent evidence of a high degree of sound learning in monkeys (Zimmermann, 1995) and the mentioned consequences of destruction of left-hemispheric, Wernicke-like temporal areas in all mammals.

Be that as it may, nonhuman primates including the great apes are strongly limited even in nonvocal speech based on the use of sign language or symbols, and these limitations seem to concern mostly syntax. Accordingly, if anything concerning language in the human brain developed relatively recently or underwent substantial modifications, it was probably the Broca center rather than the Wernicke center. Such an assumption is consistent with the fact that the most clear-cut differences between humans and nonhuman primates concern syntactical complexity of language. Thus, during hominid evolution a reorganization of the frontal–prefrontal cortex appears to have been organized such that the facial and oral motor cortices and the related subcortical speech centers came under the control of a kind of cortex that is specialized in all aspects of temporal sequence of events, including the sequence of action (Deacon, 1990).

CONSCIOUSNESS AND LANGUAGE

In his book *The Evolution of Consciousness* published in 1998, Euan MacPhail argues that only humans have consciousness because only they have language. All animals and all young children before developing language are unconscious, regardless of how complex their behaviors and achievements are. After having reviewed the relevant literature supporting the idea of the existence of at least some states of consciousness in at least some animals, he finds this idea unconvincing and argues that all achievements of animals that indicate consciousness can be explained more parsimoniously by unconscious associative learning. He assumes a big leap in the evolution of humans that consists in a fundamental reorganization of the corticohippocampal system leading from merely implicit associative learning and memory ("knowing how") to explicit-declarative learning and memory (knowing that") as the basis of introspection, self-consciousness, and feeling-consciousness. For MacPhail, "true" syntactical language and consciousness are two sides of the same coin; one cannot exist without the other.

Although many of MacPhail's critical comments to the relevant literature on animal consciousness are worth considering, I find his conception intrinsically inconsistent. There is no neuroanatomical or neurophysiological evidence for a fundamental reorganization of the corticohippocampal system from nonhuman primate ancestors to humans; rather, our hippocampus and its connections with the isocortex are very much like those of other primates. Furthermore, if we accept MacPhail's view, we should expect that patients without a hippocampus (like H.M.) should be unconscious and unable to speak; similarly, humans without language should have no consciousness, and autistic children believed by some psychologists to lack self-consciousness should have neither language nor consciousness. Apparently, both are not the case.

Most importantly, we would be forced to assume that animals (e.g., monkeys or apes) are capable of unconsciously mastering cognitive tasks that in humans require the highest concentration (e.g., following the track of a tiny spot of light on a screen), while at the same time their brains show the same activation pattern. It is highly implausible that the famous chimpanzee Julia from Bernhard Rensch's laboratory could have mastered the complicated maze better than students from the Zoological Institute of the University of Muenster or carefully manipulate a screw driver (as shown in Fig. 19.4) without a comparable human state of consciousness and attention. No human being is known for being capable of doing so unconsciously.

There can be no doubt, however, that in humans many aspects of consciousness are intimately connected to language. Of particular importance in this respect are the experiments by Gazzaniga and co-workers carried out in so-called split-brain patients (i.e., in patients where most or all of the corpus callosum was sectioned and the two cortical hemispheres are active largely independently of each other except for some common functions that are mediated by the undivided subcortical areas and the brain stem) (Gazzaniga, 1995). Because in most persons only the left hemisphere contains the speech centers, patients can report only on functions exerted by this hemisphere. In addition, the two hemispheres are said to possess very different kinds and degrees of intelligence and consciousness. Although the "talking" left hemisphere appears to have normal intelligence, including discrimination abilities and complex judgements and normal states of consciousness, the right, "mute" hemisphere appears to have very limited cognitive capabilities, barely being able to carry out simple same–difference judgements. In some patients of Gazzaniga and co-workers, the right hemisphere understood verbal or written commands, but again was poor at making simple inferences, and it seemed to have only raw feelings. Although there were signs of superiority of the right hemisphere over the left one (e.g., in visuospatial tasks), the overall impression is that the right hemisphere, besides being mute, is unable to exert complex cognitive functions and has only reduced states of awareness.

According to Gazzaniga, the left, "talking" hemisphere is the *great interpreter*. It monitors and synthesizes mental as well as behavioral activites; it acts in the formation of beliefs, plans, expectations; it gives "reasonable" explanations and forms the "story line of our lives" (Gazzaniga, 1995, 1998). Particularly interesting are those cases where the right hemisphere does something the reasons for which the left hemisphere is completely unaware of. In those cases, the left hemisphere starts confabulating in the absence of information about what was going on in the inaccessable, mute right hemisphere.

If these findings are not simply the result of overinterpretation of split-brain data by Gazzaniga and colleagues, they would nicely fit with MacPhail's central argument that only humans have consciousness, because only they have language: The left hemisphere is much more intelligent than the right one, because it has language. In this sense, the right hemisphere of the human brain would be simply equivalent to the entire isocortex of nonhuman primates, which are said to lack consciousness as all other animals do. There are difficulties, however, with such a conception. First, birds and mammals, and among them particularly parrots, primates, and cetaceans, exhibit forms of intelligence that are far superior to the alleged low intellectual capabilities of the right hemisphere of split-brain patients, such as logical inference, action planning, insight into mechanisms, and complex problem solving, provided that language is not involved (see above). MacPhail himself stated repeatedly that it is remarkably difficult to show that genuine differences in intelligence exist among vertebrate species and that there are no signs for qualitative differences in intelligence except the one connected to the presence of language in humans (MacPhail, 1982; this volume, Chapter 13). If the reports by Gazzaniga and colleagues about the poor performance of the right human hemisphere are reliable, then we have to conclude that it became intellectually impoverished while the left hemisphere developed language centers. This may have happened during the evolution of the human brain or may regularly happen during its early ontogeny. Linguistic intelligence could become so powerful that it dominates all or most of speechless intelligence present in the right hemisphere as well as in the entire primate brain. A strong argument for this view are those cases in which humans very early in life develop speech centers in the right hemisphere and are later indistinguishable in intelligence from people with language centers in the left hemisphere.

CONCLUSIONS

Among all features of vertebrate brains, the size of cortex or structures homologous to the mammalian cortex as well as the number of neurons and synapses contained in these structures correlate most clearly with the complexity of cognitive functions including states of consciousness. This would explain the observed differences in cognition between birds and mammals on the one hand and other tetrapod vertebrates on the other. Furthermore, with the exception of elephants, which have not been sufficiently tested cognitively, apes (at least gorillas and chimpanzees) and cetaceans with large cortices containing ten to hundreds of billion (10^{10} to 10^{11}) neurons apparently have superior cognitive abilities compared with other mammals. This does not, however, explain the alleged superiority of chimpanzees over the gorilla because gorillas have larger brains and cortices than chimpanzees. The superiority of humans over all other animals probably results from a very high number of cortical neurons, a drastically prolonged period of ontogenetic plasticity of cortical synapses, and the presence of centers underlying syntactical language.

Thus, it is fair to assume that all vertebrates with larger cortexlike structures, particularly those with cortices showing cross-modality information transfer, have awareness about what is going on around them. This does not necessarily imply a continuous stream of consciousness, because this may be bound to the existence of an autobiographic memory. Self-recognition as evidenced by the mirror test apparently requires a large associative, including prefrontal, cortex. The evolution of a syntactical language may have favored strongly the highest states of consciousness such self-reflection, thinking, and action planning. Although thinking is not necessarily bound to language, most people think verbally. Furthermore, many concepts typical of the human mind exist only linguistically, because we can *talk* about them (e.g., future events or abstract entities such as society, freedom, and so forth). It may well be that the evolution of a special type of prefrontal cortex (viz., a cortex dealing with the analysis of the temporal sequence of events) was at the basis of increased capability for action planning, syntactical language, imitation, and understanding the behavior of others.

ACKNOWLEDGMENTS

I am grateful to Prof. Jerison, UCLA/Hanse Institute for Advanced Study, and Prof. Wullimann, Brain Research Institute, University of Bremen, for helpful criticism.

REFERENCES

Aggleton, J.P. (1992) *The Amygdala: Neurobiological Aspects of Emotion, Memory, and Mental Dysfunction.* Wiley-Liss, New York.
Aggleton, J.P. (1993) The contribution of the amygdala to normal and abnormal emotional states. *Trends Neurosci.* 16:328–333.
Alexander, G.E., M.D. Crutcher, and M.R. DeLong (1990) Basal ganglia–thalamocortical circuits: parallel substrates for motor, oculomotor, "prefrontal" and "limbic" functions. In H.B.M. Uylings, C.G. van Eden, J.P.C. de Bruin, M.A. Corner and M.G.P. Feenstra (eds.): *The Prefrontal Cortex. Its Structure, Function and Pathology.* Elsevier, Amsterdam, pp. 119–146.
Baron-Cohen, S., A.M. Leslie, and U. Frith (1985) Does the autistic child have a "theory of mind"? *Cognition* 21:37–46.
Broadbent, D.E. (1958) *Perception and Communication.* Pergamon, London.
Byrne, R. (1995) *The Thinking Ape. Evolutionary Origins of Intelligence.* Oxford University Press, Oxford.
Corballis, M.C. (1991) *The Lopsided Ape. Evolution of the Generative Mind.* Oxford University Press. New York.
Damasio, A.R. (1994) *Descartes' Error. Emotion, Reasons and the Human Brain.* G.P. Putnam's Son, New York.
Davidson, R.J., and W. Irwin (1999) The functional neuroanatomy of emotional and affective style. *Trends Cogn. Sci.* 3:11–21.
Deacon, T.W. (1990) Rethinking mammalian brain evolution. *Am. Zool.* 30:629–705.
Farber, I.B., and P.S. Churchland (1995) Consciousness and the neurosciences: philosophical and theoretical issues. In M.S. Gazzaniga et al. (eds.): *The Cognitive Neurosciences.* MIT Press, Cambridge, 1295–1306.
Gardner, R.A., T.B. Gardner, and T.E. van Cantfort (1989) *Teaching Sign Language to Chimpanzees.* State University of New York Press, New York.
Garey, L.J., and G. Leuba (1986) A quantitative study of neuronal and glial numerical density in the visual cortex of the bottlenose dolphin: evidence for a specialized subarea and changes with age. *J. Comp. Neurol.* 247:491–496.
Gazzaniga, M.S. (1995) Consciousness and the cerebral hemispheres. In M.S. Gazzaniga, et al., (eds.): The Cognitive Neurosciences. MIT Press, Cambridge, MA, pp. 1391–1400.
Güntürkün, O., and L. von Fersen (1998) Of whales and myths: numerics of cetacean cortex. In N. Elsner and R. Wehner (eds.): *New Neuroethology on the Move.* Proceedings of the 26th Göttingen Neurobiology Conference, vol. II. Thieme, Stuttgart, p. 493.
Guillery, R.W., S.L. Feig, and D.A. Lozsádi (1998) Paying attention to the thalamic reticular nucleis. *Trends Neurosci.* 21:28–32.
Hassler, R. (1978) Interaction of reticular activating system for vigilance and the truncothalamic and pallidal systems fro directing awareness and attention under striatal control. In P.A. Buser and A. Rougeul-Buser (eds.): *Cerebral Correlates of Conscious Experience.* Elsevier/North-Holland, Amsterdam, pp. 111–129.
Heffner, H.E., and R.S. Heffner (1995) Role of auditory cortex in the perception of vocalization by Japanese macaques. In E. Zimmermann, J.D. Newman, and U. Jürgens (eds.): *Current Topics in Primate Vocal Communication.* Plenum Press, New York, pp. 207–219.
Hirst, W. (1995) Cognitive aspects of consciousness. In M.S. Gazzaniga, et al. (eds.): *The Cognitive Neurosciences.* MIT Press, Cambridge, MA, pp. 1307–1321.
Holland, P.C., and M. Gallagher (1999) Amygdala circuitry in attentional and representational processes. *Trends Cogn. Sci.* 3:65–73.
Jerison, H.J. (1973) *Evolution of the Brain and Intelligence.* Academic Press, New York.
Jerison, H.J. (1991) *Brain Size and the Evolution of Mind.* American Museum of Natural History, New York.
Jerison, H.J. (1997) Evolution of prefrontal cortex. In: N.A. Krasnegor, G.R Lyon, and P.S. Goldman-Rakic, (eds.): *Development of the Prefrontal Cortex: Evolution, Neurobiology, and Behavior.* Brookes, Baltimore, pp. 9–26.
Jürgens, U. (1995) Neuronal control of vocal production in non–human and human primates. In E. Zimmermann, J.D. Newman, and U. Jürgens (eds.): *Current Topics in Primate Vocal Communication.* Plenum Press, New York, pp. 199–206.

Kaas, J.H. (1995) The evolution of isocortex. *Brain Behav. Evol.* 46:187–196.
Karten, H.J. (1991) Homology and evolutionary origins of the "neocortex." *Brain Behav. Evol.* 38:264–272.
Kinsbourne, M. (1995) Models of consciousness: serial or parallel in the brain? In M.S. Gazzaniga, et al. (eds.): *The Cognitive Neurosciences.* MIT Press, Cambridge, MA, pp. 1321–1329.
Knight, R.T., and M. Grabowecky (1995) Escape from linear time: prefrontal cortex and conscious experience. In M.S. Gazzaniga, et al. (eds.): *The Cognitive Neurosciences.* MIT Press, Cambridge, MA, pp. 1357–1371.
Locke, J.L. (1995) Linguistic capacity: an ontogenetic theory with evolutionary implications. In E. Zimmermann, J.D. Newman, and U. Jürgens (eds.): *Current Topics in Primate Vocal Communication.* Plenum Press, New York, 253–272.
Marino, L. (1998) A comparison of encephalization between odontocete cetaceans and anthropoid primates. *Brain Behav. Evol.* 51:230–238.
MacPhail, E.M. (1982) *Brain and Intelligence in Vertebrates.* Clarendon Press, Oxford.
MacPhail, E.M. (1998) *The Evolution of Consciousness.* Oxford University Press, Oxford.
Markowitsch, H.J. (1992) Neuropsychologie des Gedächtnisses. Hogrefe, Göttingen.
Markowitsch, H.J. (1999) Gedächtnisstörungen. Kohlhammer, Stuttgart.
Marten, K., and S. Psakaros (1994) Evidence of self-awarenes in the bottlenose dolphin (*Tursiops truncatus*). In T. Parker, R.W. Mitchell, and M.L. Boccia (eds.): *Self-Awareness in Animals and Humans: Developmental Perspectives.* Cambridge University Press, Cambridge, pp. 361–379.
Meltzoff, A., and A. Gopnik (1993) The role of imitation in understanding persons and developing a theory of mind. In S.Baron-Cohen, H. Tager-Flusberg, and D.J. Cohen (eds.): *Understanding Other Minds: Perspectives from Autism.* Oxford University Press, Oxford, pp. 335–366.
Mitchell, R.W. (1994) Mental models of mirror-self-recognition: Two theories. *New Ideas Psychol.* 11:295–325.
Moscovitch, M. (1995) Models of consciousness and memory. In M.S. Gazzaniga, et al. (eds.): *The Cognitive Neurosciences.* MIT Press, Cambridge, MA, pp. 1341–1356.
Mrzljak, L., H.B.M. Uylings, C.G. van Eden, and M. Judás (1990) Neuronal development in human prefrontal cortex in prenatal and postnatal stages. In H.B.M. Uylings, C.G. van Eden, J.P.C. de Bruin, M.A. Corner, and M.G.P. Feenstra. (eds.): *The Prefrontal Cortex. Its Structure, Function and Pathology.* Elsevier, Amsterdam, pp. 185–222.
Nieuwenhuys, R., J. Voogd, and Chr. van Huijzen (1988) *The Human Central Nervous System.* Springer, Berlin. (German edition: Nieuwenhuys, R., J. Voogd, and Chr. van Huijzen [1991] *Das Zentralnervensystem des Menschen.* Springer, Berlin.)
Nieuwenhuys, R., H.J. ten Donkelaar, and C. Nicholson (1998) *The Central Nervous System of Vertebrates,* vol. 3. Springer, Berlin.
Northcutt, R.G., and J.H. Kaas (1995) The emergence and evolution of mammalian isocortex. *Trends Neurosci.* 18:373–379.
Parker, S.T., R.W. Mitchell, and M.L.. Boccia (eds.) (1994) *Self-awareness in Animals and Humans*: *Developmental Perspectives.* Cambridge University Press, Cambridge, MA.
Passingham, R. (1993) *The frontal lobes and voluntary action.* Oxford University Press, Oxford.
Pearce, J.M. (1997) *Animal Learning and Cognition.* Psychology Press, Exeter.
Petrides, M., and D.N. Pandya (1999) Dorsolateral prefrontal cortex: comparative cytoarchitectonic analysis in the human and macaque brain and corticocortical connection patterns. *Eur. J. Neurosci.* 11:1011–1036.
Pilbeam, D., and S.J. Gould (1974) Size and scaling in human evolution. *Science* 186:892–901.
Posner, M.I. (1994) Seeing the mind. *Science* 262; 673–674.
Preuss, T.M. (1995) Do rats have a prefrontal cortex? The Rose-Woolsey-Akert program reconsidered. *J. Cogn. Neurosci.* 7:1–24.
Rensch, B. (1968) Manipulierfähigkeit und Komplikation von Handlungsketten bei Menschenaffen. In B. Rensch (ed.): *Handlungsgebrauch und Verständigung bei Affen und Frühmenschen.* Hans Huber, Bern, pp. 103–126.
Robbins, T.W. (1997) Arousal systems and attentional processes. *Biol. Psychol.* 45:57–71.
Robbins, T.M., and B.J. Everitt, (1995) Arousal systems and attention. In M. Gazzaniga, et al. (eds.): *The Cognitive Neurosciences.* MIT Press, Cambridge, MA, pp. 243–262.

Roberts, A.C., T.W. Robbins, and L. Weiskrantz (1998) *The Prefrontal Cortex. Executive and Cognitive Functions*. Oxford University Press, Oxford.

Rockel, A.J., W. Hiorns, and T.P.S. Powell (1980) The basic uniformity in structure of the neocortex. *Brain* 103:221–244.

Roland, P.E., B. Larsen, N.A. Lassen, and E. Skinhut (1980) Supplementary motor area and other cortical areas in organization of voluntary movements in man. *J. Neurophysiol.* 43:118–136.

Roth, G., and M.F. Wullimann (1996) Die Evolution des Nervensystems und der Sinnesorgane. In J. Dudel, R. Menzel, and R.F. Schmidt (eds.): Lehrbuch der Neurowissenschaft, VCH Weinheim, pp. 1–31.

Savage-Rumbaugh, S. (1984) Acquisition of functional symbol usage in apes and children. In H.L. Roitblat, T.G. Bever, and H.S Terrace (eds.): *Animal Cognition*. Earlbaum, Hillsdale, N.J., pp. 291–310.

Schüz, A., and G. Palm (1989) Density of neurons and synapses in the cerebral cortex of the mouse. *J. Comp. Neurol.* 286:442–455.

Smythies, J. (1997) The functional neuroanatomy of awareness: with a focus on the role of various anatomical systems in the control of intermodal atttention. *Consciousness Cogn.* 6:455–481.

Squire, L.R. (1987) *Memory and Brain*. Oxford University Press, New York.

Squire, L.R., and B. Knowlton (1995) Memory, hippocampus, and brain systems. In M.S. Gazzaniga, et al. (eds): *The Cognitive Neurosciences*. MIT Press, Cambridge, MA, pp. 825–836.

Stamp Dawkins, M. (1993) *Through Our Eyes Only? The Search for Animal Consciousness*. W.H. Freeman/Spektrum, Oxford, New York, Heidelberg.

Striedter, G. F. (1997) The telencephalon of tetrapods in evolution. *Brain Behav. Evol.* 49:179–213.

Stromswold, K. (1995) The cognitive and neural bases of language acquisition. In M.S. Gazzaniga, et al. (eds.): *The Cognitive Neurosciences*. MIT Press, Cambridge, MA, pp. 855–870.

Uylings, H.B.M., and C.G. van Eden (1990) Qualitative and quantitative comparison of the prefrontal cortex in rat and in primates, including humans. In H.B.M. Uylings, C.G. van Eden, J.P.C. de Bruin, M.A. Corner, and M.G.P. Feenstra (eds.): *The Prefrontal Cortex. Its Structure, Function and Pathology*. Elsevier, Amsterdam, pp. 31–62.

Visalberghi, E., and L. Limongelli (1994) Lack of comprehension of cause–effect relationships in tool-using capuchin monkeys (*Cebus apella*). *J. Comp. Psychol.* 108:15–22.

Voitko, M.L. (1996) Cognitive functions of the basal forebrain cholinergic system in monkeys: memory or attention? *Behav. Brain Res.* 75:13–25.

Zimmermann, E., J.D. Newman and U. Jürgens (1995): *Current Topics in Primate Vocal Communication*. Plenum Press, New York.

Zimmermann, E. (1995) Loud calls in nocturnal prosimians: structure, evolution and ontogeny. In E. Zimmermann, J.D. Newman, and U. Jürgens (eds.): *Current Topics in Primate Vocal Communication*. Plenum Press, New York, pp. 47–72.

Index

A

aboral nervous system 43
abstraction 348
acanthocephalan 15
Acanthurus bahianus 311
Acanthurus coeruleus 311
accessory olfactory bulb 147
acetylcholinesterase 406
across-frequency integration 220
actinopterygian fishes 318
active memory 347
actualistic strategy 286
adaptation 271
African gray parrot 3
agnathans 534
alar plate 31
alignment of visual and auditory maps 226
allocortex 491, 498
allogeny 130
allometric 534
   approach 267
   effect 535
   relationship 533
Allosaurus 541
alternation 407
ambiguous code 225
ambulacral epithelium 49
γ-aminobutyric acid 406
amniotes 4, 139
amphibian 4, 136, 534
Amphioxus 86
amphisbaenians 82
amygdala 4, 148, 155, 319, 404, 558, 559, 560, 561, 564, 569
amygdala hypothesis 166, 169
anaerobic (fermentative) metabolism 174
anagenesis 452, 478
analogies 288
anamniotes 4
anapsid 140
Anas 280
ancestral descending motor system 79
ancestral motor system 90
animal intelligence 546
animal mind 564

annelids 17, 19, 21, 22, 24, 34, 367
Anoptichtys jordani 299
Antedon bifida 52
antennal lobes 336 f
   odortopic representation 379
   structure and connections 379
antennapedia-ultrabithorax complex 33, 35
anterior cingulate cortex 560, 563
anterior cingulate gyrus 559
anterior commissure 321, 411
anterior end of the brain 31
anterior lateral nucleus 150
anteroposterior axis 12
anteroposterior patterning 32
anteroposterior specification 36
Anthropoidea 84
anthropoid primates 505
anticipation of future events 565
Apis mellifera 334 ff
Apogon 311
apomorphy 13, 14, 162
appearance of extremities 79
aquatic environments 298
arachnids 24
Archaeopteryx 145, 538
archistriatum 160, 404
Archosauromorpha 142
archosaurs 142
area dorsalis telencephali 311
   pars centralis 317
   pars lateralis 313
   pars medialis 319
   pars medialis superficialis 321
area tegmentalis ventralis 195
Arius felis 299
arousal 320
arthropod 15, 17, 19, 21, 22, 24, 26, 335
ascending reticular system 192
associations 408
associative cortex 548, 558, 561, 564, 569, 575, 576
associative learning 359
Asterias rubens 52
asteroids 41, 52
Astyanax mexicanus 299, 306

Ateles 84
attention 6, 227, 334, 343, 359, 530
attentive strategy 529
auditory 254
auditory association cortex 187
auditory system 253
auricle feathers 210
Auricularia hypothesis 28
auricularia-larva 27
autapomorphy 14
autoshaping 407
avian brain 282
avian pyramidal tract 106
avoidance learning 300
avoidance responding 303
axonal guidance system 124
axons 512

B

backward pairing 342
Balistes vetula 311
barn owl 423
basal forebrain 558, 560, 569
basal forebrain-septal nuclei complex 561
basal ganglia 3, 4, 146, 189, 404, 544, 560
basal plate 31
basic cognition 354, 359, 360
basic features in motor control 79
basiepithelial
 nervous system 43
 neurons 44
basolateral amygdala 409
bat 12
Bathygobius soporator 298
bats 288, 508
Bauplan 11, 275, 449
 bilaterian 15
beak of birds 104
behavior 2, 3, 5, 7, 297
behavioral
 capacities 505
 complexity 523
 studies 322
benefit 526
Beryciformes 308, 311
Bessel detectors 460
Betta splendens 299
biconditional discrimination 345
bilateral symmetry 356
bilaterian bauplan 15, 20, 24
binaural process 221
binding 218, 225

binocular vision 215
biological intelligence 504
bipolar neuron 117
birds 3, 4, 12, 104, 136, 403, 451, 452, 455
bird song 421
bivalvians 22
blind and sighted characins 306
blocking 343, 354, 415
bluegill sunfish 311, 312, 318, 320
body plans, commonality of 393
body size 503
body weight 2
Bolitoglossini 238, 240, 241, 243, 248, 249, 250, 254, 255, 256, 257, 258, 259, 260
bony fish 297, 534
brachiation 83
brachiopods 17
Brachiosaurus 541
brachium conjunctivum 98
brain 483
 antennal lobes 369
 central complex 369
 deutocerebrum 367
 Diptera 370
 genetic equivalence 392, 394
 Hymenoptera 370
 mushroom bodies 369
 mushroom bodies and hippocampus 394
 of insects 372
 optic lobes 369
 protocerebrum 367, 372
  multimodal convergence 373
  organization of 373
 regions compared, central complex and cerebellum 391, 394
  insect mammalian analogues 391, 393
  mushroom bodies and hippocampus 391
 segmentation 372
 segments 367
  evolution of 373
 suboesophageal ganglion 368
 tritocerebrum 367
brain allometry 575
brain-body relationship 570
brain-body size 304, 456
brain evolution 1, 501
brain lesions 298, 300
brain lesion studies 323
brain size 427, 497, 502
 as a statistic 545
 reduction 283
brain stem locomotor region 89

Index 585

brain volumes 308
brain weight 266
brain weight/body weight 2
Branchiostoma lanceolatum 80, 86
breeding strategies 480
brittle stars 41
Broca speech center 576
bryozoans 17
budgerigars 422
butterfly fishes 299

C

cache recovery 413
cadherins 125
calcichordates 28
Captorhinida 140
Carassius auratus 96
carnivores 275
carp 302, 318
categorization 229, 354 ff, 359, 456
 music 457
 objects 457
 pictures 457
 symmetry 458
category 356
catfish 299, 305, 318, 320
caudate nucleus 404
caudatoputamen 4, 151
Cebuella 287
cell adhesion molecules 124
cell assemblies 495
cell migration 246, 254
cell size 255, 256, 257, 258
central complex
 components of 383
 connections to/from 386
 evolution 383
 function 385
 in *Macroglossum* 387
 location of 369
 neurons 386
 organization 384, 386 f
 phyletic comparisons, arachnids 390 f
  crustaceans 390 f
  onychophorans 390 f
  primitive insects 390 f
 sensory integration 388
 species differences 387
  in *Notonecta* 387
  in *Polistes* 387 f
central nucleus 150
central pattern generator 87

ceolenterates 15
cephalization index 333
cephalochordates 27
cephalopods 21, 22
cerebellar association system 199
cerebellar cognitive affective syndrome 200
cerebellar cortex 495
cerebellar extirpation 303
cerebellar lesions 302
cerebellar nuclei 100
cerebellorubrospinal circuit 101
cerebellorubrospinal limb control system 98
cerebellum 98, 189, 278, 302, 305, 306, 319, 323, 453, 494, 548
cerebral cortex 5, 510, 535, 548
cerebral ganglion 15, 20, 22, 23, 27, 35
cetacean 539, 570
Chabos chickens 284
chambered organ 51
chaos theory 525
characteristic delay 224
Cheilotrema saturnum 322
chelicerates 23, 24
chemical interoreceptors 113
chemical senses 113
chicken 218, 410
chimpanzee 555, 565, 567, 568, 570, 574, 577, 579
choice-dependent learning 300
choice process 349
cholinergic modulatory systems 194
Chondrichthyes 536
chordate larva 27
chordates 15, 27
Cichlasoma cyanoguttatum 311
cichlid 302, 323
 of the african great lakes 306
ciliary bands 28
cingulate cortex 558, 561
cladistics 3, 11, 13
cladogenesis 478
cladogram 13, 14, 15
classical conditioning 300, 323, 338, 407
claustrum 4, 155
claustrum hypothesis 166, 168
clawed hand 84
climbing vertebrates 83
clonal restriction 30
clustered 226
Cobelodus 536
coelenterates 14, 20, 25
coelom 21

coelosaurians 538
cognition 1, 2, 5, 6, 7, 266, 451, 494, 504
cognition in fishes 298
cognition-like concepts 359
cognition-like processes 345
cognitive
  abilities 5
  abilities of birds 3
  brain 193
  deficits 199
  functions 491, 492
    in nonhuman animals 6
  map 301, 350, 352, 360, 548
  neuroscience 6
  psychology 6
coincidence-detecting neurons 229
coincidence detection 218
collar ganglion 27
collothalamic 146
collothalamo-telencephalic pathways 150
collothalamus 119
color opponencey 355
color space 355
color vision 113, 334, 455, 458
comparative morphology 501
comparative neuroanatomy 2
compass direction 350
compass flight 347
complex human brain 530
complex thought 549
concept 356, 461
concept formation 334 f, 354 ff, 359, 360, 420
conchiferans 22
conditioned reflexes 302
conditioning process 303
conduction times 498
configural
  association 342, 346, 359
  conditioning 345
  learning 335, 349
  unit 346
connectivity of cortex 492
consciousness 5, 6, 7
consolidation 340
context-dependent learning 354
context learning 346
contour feathers 210
control of locomotion 77
convergence 12
co-option 121
coral reef 298, 303, 318, 323
coral reef fishes 301, 325
coral reef percomorphs 307

coral-reef teleosts 300
corpus callosum 498
correlated activity 496
cortex 411, 491
cortical circuits 512
cortical folding 516
cortical gray matter 513
corticalization 508
cortical surface area 531
corticohippocampal system 577
corticomedial amygdala 409
corticospinal tract 97
cortico-subcortico-cortical association
  systems 195
corvid 455, 475, 478, 479
Coryphopterus nicholsi 298
cost/benefit analysis 527
counting 348, 475, 476
cowbirds 415
cranial nerves 115
craniate brain 22, 30
craniates 25, 27, 35
crinoids 41, 51
crow 465, 475
crustaceans 24
Cryptosyringida 54
ctenophores 14, 15
cue-directed choice 301
cumulative curve 528

D

D1-receptor 433, 437, 438, 439, 440, 441
damselfishes 299, 307, 313
Darwin 265, 403
Darwinian fitness 454, 478
declarative memory 560
deductive thinking 467
delayed spatial alternation 424
delay lines 219
dendrites 512
dendritic spine 494
dendritic tree 219
dentate gyrus 413
descending supraspinal pathways 93
design principles 514
deuterostome 15, 17, 18, 25
deuterostome ancestor 27
deuterostome nervous systems 25
deutocerebrum 23, 34, 35
developmental neurogenetics 11
development of language 567
Diadectes 163

diapsids 140
Didelphis virginiana 92
diencephalon 31, 145, 317
digging vertebrates 83
dinosaurs 142
dipleurula larva 27
direct development 240, 258
displacement theory 286
dissociation 121
distance estimation 348
distance measurement 208
divergence 121
dogs 285
dolphin 539
domestication 283, 455
dominance of vision 306
dopamine 406, 433, 434, 437, 438, 447, 449
dopaminergic 433, 434, 437, 438, 439, 444, 449
dorsal and ventral striatum 559
dorsal cortex 156
dorsal pallium 148, 452, 569
dorsal thalamus 31
    anterior group 153
    dorsal lateral geniculate nucleus 152
    dorsal lateral optic nucleus 157
    dorsomedialis 157
    intralaminar group 153
    lateral posterior and/or pulvinar complex 153
    medial geniculate nucleus 153
    medial group 153
    nucleus dorsalis intermedius ventralis anterior 157
    nucleus dorsolateralis anterior 157
    nucleus reuniens pars compacta 158
    nucleus rotundus 158
    ventral nuclear group 153
dorsal ventricular ridge 156, 569
dorsolateral PFC 563
dorsolateral striatum 560
dorsoventricular ridge 3, 4
Drosophila 30, 34, 36
    central complex mutants 385
    learning mutants of 382
dual-expansion hypothesis 166, 167
duplication 121
dysmetria of thought 200

E

ear asymmetry 211, 228
ecdysozoan 17, 18, 19, 26, 367, 394

echinoderms 25, 27, 41
    basement membrane 49
    bilateral symmetry 61
    glia 49
    homeotic genes 62
    larval nervous system 44
    locomotion 66
    pentaradial symmetry 61
    photoreceptors 57
    postmetamorphotic nervous system 45
    sensory cells 48
    statocysts 59
echinoids 41, 58
ecological niche 360
ectoneural nerve cord 50
ectoneural nervous system 43
ectostriatum 158, 404
ectotherms 174
ectothermy 532
Eigenmannia 322
electrical stimulation 310, 319, 320
electric fishes 325
electric organs 299
electromagnetic radiation sense 113
electroreceptors 122
electrosensory information 303, 322
elementary association 335, 342
elephant shrew 274
Eleutherozoa 41
ems 34, 36
Emx 32, 36
encephalization 237, 267, 502, 533, 535
encephalization index 307, 309
encephalization quotient 533, 570
endocast 2, 163, 532
endopiriform nucleus 169
endotherms 174
endothermy 532
engrailed 35, 68
enlarged telencephalon of percomorphs 321
enteropneusts 27
entopeduncular nucleus 405
environmental maps 300
Epinephelus cruentatus 311
Epinephelus fulvus 311
epineural canals 54, 56
episodic memory 560
equivalence concepts 464
equivalencies 464
equivalent-cell hypothesis 166
Eutheria 142
even rate effect 527
evolutionary changes in the ancestral motor system 90

evolutionary polarity 14
evolutionary strategy 507
excessive phenotypes 127
excitatory input 495
excitatory synapse 494
expectancy 354
expectation 334, 335, 345, 348, 354, 359
exploratory flights 350
external fertilization 171
extinction 453
extrapyramidal systems 421
eye morphogenesis 11
eye movements 421

F

false-target problem 220, 221
familiarity-novelty 466
fear 409
feather specializations 228
feather stars 41
feature additivity 460
feedback loop 316
feeding 421
feeding strategy 243, 260
Field L 158, 417
filefishes 307
first-order multipolar neurons 117
fixed action patterns 550
flatworms 14, 367
flexibility 208
flight 478
flying 478
food storers 270
food-storing birds 413
foraging 334
forebrain 4, 136
forebrain gene expression pattern 4
forkhead 68
free response strategy 529
freshwater teleosts 304
frontal eye field 423
frontally oriented eyes 211
fruit fly 11, 32
functional equivalence 462
functional morphology 265
fusion of ventral cord ganglia 34

G

Gabor detectors 460
galliform birds 278

ganglia
　abdominal 368
　central pattern generator 372
　chelicerates 370
　evolutionary traits 369
　insects 368
　local interneurons 372
　motor axons 371
　protocerebrum 368
　Pycnogonida 370
　sea spiders 370
　sensory axons 371
　sensory maps 371
　sensory representation 371
Garstang's hypothesis 68
gastropods 21, 22
gastrotrich 15
gaze control 423
gene expression 11, 12, 30
generalization 354 ff
genome size 256, 257, 258, 260, 270
genomic coadaptation 454
Geogale 273
geometric representation 350
geometry of the brain 511
"giant" axons 54
giant neurons 56
Ginglymostoma cirratum 97
globus pallidus 151, 404
Gnathonemus petersii 299
gnostic sensibility 186
goal-directed limb movements 98
goldfish 298, 299, 300, 301, 302, 303, 304,
　320, 321, 323
granular layer 152
grasping vertebrates 83
gray matter 492, 497, 513
great apes 5
greater limbic system 193
growth rate 576
gustatory mapping 299
gustatory stimulation 320
gustatory systems 305
gyral windows 517

H

habituation 298, 300, 321, 341
Haemulon plumieri 311
hagfish 537
Hebbian mechanisms 219
hemichordates 27
Heterodontus 536

hexapods 24
higher brain functions 205
high-frequency 217
high vocal center 421
hippocampal formation 558, 560, 569
hippocampus 4, 272, 319, 404, 499, 561, 568, 577
hippuritacean bivalve reefs 307
Holocentrus ascensionis 311
Holocentrus rufus 311, 321
holothuroids 41, 59
homeobox genes 68, 169
hominids 506
Homo 506
homoeothermy 453
homologues 424
homology 12, 162
homoplasy 12, 162
Homo sapiens 5, 518
honeybee 333 ff, 546
horizontal disparities 215
Hox 12, 35
Hox-B 32, 33, 35
human brain 502
human cortex 570
human intelligence 6
hummingbirds 288
hunting 206
hunting strategies 207
hydrocoel 49
hydrozoans 14
hyobranchial apparatus 241, 242, 243, 258
hyperstriatum 404
hyperstriatum accessorium 156
hyperstriatum ventrale 158, 281
hypertrophied pallial areas 315
hypertrophy of nuclei 213
hypoglossus nucleus 422
hyponeural ganglia 56
hyponeural nervous system 43
hyponeural plexus 50
hypothalamus 31, 306, 319, 409
hypothetical ancestor of vertebrates and insects 35
Hyracotherium 543

implicit learning 557
imprinting 301, 480
incentive learning 360
index of dexterity 86
individual neuron 335 f
inferior colliculus 146, 215
inferior lobe 320
inferior temporal cortex (IT) 563
information processing 492, 515, 519
infrared
    detectors 123
    radiation 114
    reception 116
inhibitory learning 341, 342
inhibitory synapse 494
innate predispositions 480
insect brain 335
insect CNS 32, 33, 34
insect compound eye 12
insectivore 272, 508
insight 403
instinct 483
instinctive behavior 3
instructive signal 226
instrumental conditioning 298, 300, 323, 408
integrated telencephalic-tectal-cerebellar systems 310
integrative functions 319
intelligence 286, 401, 452, 482
intensity pathway 214
interaural amplitude difference 210
interaural time difference 211
internal fertilization 172
intersexual selection 172
intralaminar thalamic nuclei 558
intrasexual selection 172
invariant code 225
invariant mapping 229
invertebrate brains 4, 333
invertebrate CNS 16
in vitro preparations 101
ion channels 217
isocortex 3, 4, 152, 275, 403, 452, 491, 492, 508, 569
isometry hypothesis 285
isomorphic representation 127

I

Ichthyophis kohtaoensis 96
ichthyostegids 81, 137
identity concept 465
imitation 564

J

Jeffress model 222
jumping vertebrates 83
juxtaligamental cell 45
juxtaligamental ganglia 57

K

Kamin effect 340
kangaroo rat 273
kinorhynchs 17, 18
knowledge attribution 565
knowledge of reality 550
koniocortex 186
Krox-20 32

L

laboratory rat 277
labyrinthodonts 137
Lagodon rhomboides 311
Lagothrix 84
laminar organization 246, 247
lamination 246, 248, 249, 252, 254, 259
lampreys 86, 537
landmark learning 334
landmarks 348 f
Lange's nerve 53
language 6, 563, 565, 567, 568, 576, 577, 578, 579
language acquisition 403
latent inhibition 415
lateral descending systems 96, 97
lateral geniculate body 191
lateralization 5, 480, 515
lateral magnocellular nucleus 421
lateral pallium 148
lateral undulation 77
Latimeria chalumnae 91
learning 268, 297, 335, 405, 451, 453, 483, 495, 496
learning and memory 303
learning deficits 303
learning models 470
learning-set formation 403
leech 34, 36
lemnothalamo-telencephalic pathways 148
lemnothalamus 119, 146
Lepidosauromorpha 142
Lepisosteus 318
Lepomis macrochirus 311, 312
lepospondyls 139
lesions 407
lesions in one hemisphere 321
life history 26
life span 507
limbic cortex 152
limbic system 558, 559, 560, 561

limbless locomotion 81
limb-moving generators 91
lobus parolfactorius 405
local circuit neurons 514
localization 207
locomotion on land 91
locomotor patterns 77
locus coeruleus 319, 558
logic 470
logical concepts 465
logic rules 470
longitudinal brain axis 31
longitudinal torus 321
long-range connections 499
long-term depression (LTD) 443, 444
long-term memory 6, 340, 347
long-term memory of learned entities before ablation 300
long-term potentiation (LTP) 415, 443, 444
long-term retention 340
lophotrochozoan 17, 18, 26, 367, 394
loss of lungs 239
loss of vision 306
LTD 443, 444
LTP 415, 443, 444
lunglessness 239, 240, 258

M

magnetoreception 116
main olfactory bulb 147
mallard ducks 410
mammalian brains 510
mammalian cortex 511
mammal-like reptiles 140, 541
mammals 4, 5, 136
mandibulates 23
mandibulation 79
manipulation 77
maplike representation 350
mapping 548
matching performance 349
matching-to-sample 464, 467
Mauthner cells 89
mazes 413
mechanical senses 113
medial descending systems 96, 97
medialis complex 159
medial nucleus of the dorsolateral thalamus 421
medial pallium 148, 319
medial septal nucleus 413
medullary cords 15, 16, 20, 21, 23, 35

memorizing 466
memorizing sounds 207
memory 6, 227, 297, 323, 324, 335, 340, 451, 453, 459, 466, 561, 563, 564, 569, 576, 577, 579
    consolidation 340
    content 340
    dynamics 340
    formation 340
    for sequences 349
    phases 340
    retrieval 346
    trace 340f
mental activities 557
mental model 452
Merychippus 543
mesencephalic tectum 247
mesencephalon 30
Mesohippus 543
mesolimbic system 561
Mesozoic 540
metabolic rate 172, 269, 504
metamorphosis 27, 129
Metatheria 142
metazoan 15, 16, 17
metazoan brain 12
metazoan central nervous system 11
microcircuitry of teleostean telencephalon 311
microsecond range 218
midbrain 317, 548
midbrain-hindbrain boundary 32
migration 257, 478
mind 5
minimum convex polygons 531, 533, 540
minnows 304
modular circuits 516
modular organization of consciousness 557
modular units 514
modules 121
mollusc 17, 20, 22, 24
monkey 267, 546
monoaminergic modulatory system 194
mormyrid 301, 303, 320, 537
morphological specializations for hearing 210
motion direction 226
motivation 347, 350
motor cortex 276, 421
mouse 11, 544
movement feedback 89
Müller larva 28
multimodal association area 188, 281
multimodal sensory integration 320

multiple memories 347
multisensory function 319
muscle tails 53
mushroom bodies 336, 361
    calyces, afferent supply 375, 376
        zones of 376
    cells of 374
    context-dependent-memory 383
    defects of 382
    discovery of 382
    GABAergic neurons 376
    globuli cells 375
    Kenyon cells 375
    lobes 375
        inputs to 376
        outputs from 376
        parallel organization 377
    multimodal integration 382
    outputs 382
    physiology 381
    place memory 383
    relationships to optic lobes 380
    relation to antennal lobes 379f
    roles in
        learning and memory 382
        olfactory processing 383
    short-term memory 383
    social insects 382
    structure 375
mushroom body evolution
    insects 377
        neopteran type, palaeopteran type 378
    lobes, local circuits 378
    phyletic comparisons
        chelicerates 389
        crustacean 389
        onychophoran 390
music 457
mutable connective tissue 45
mutation 454
myelination, optic nerve 249
myomeric musculature 86
myriapod 24
myxinoid 25

N

natural selection 523
navigation 298, 302, 335, 346f, 350, 359, 412, 479
negative brain allometry 570
negative patterning 345
nemathelminths 14, 15, 18

nematode 15, 17, 18
nematomorph 15, 17, 18
nemertine 14, 15, 17, 35
neocortex 186, 509
Neopilina galathea 21
neostriatum 158, 280, 404
neostriatum caudolaterale (NCL) 434, 436, 437, 438, 439, 440, 442, 447, 449
neoteny 27
nerve plexus 15
network allometry 515
neural 335, 359, 512
   algorithms 231
   architecture 505
   circuits 518
   complexity 523
   complexity of a process 532
   computations 205
   information 524
   network 454, 455, 461, 466, 476, 477, 511 f
   organization 505
   plasticity 453
   plate 62
   substrates of spatial representation 297
   tube 27, 56, 63
neuroethology 232
neurogenesis 287, 510
neurogenetics 483
neuromeres 30
neuromeric model 4, 29, 31
neuromery 30
neuromorphology 266
neuronal interconnectivity 518
neuronal network 464, 470
neurons
   reiterative 371
   uniquely identifiable 371
neurulation 27
NMDA receptors 415
nonolfactory pallium 308
nonolfactory telencephalon 311
nonspatial learning 300
nonvisual sensory input 315
noradrenergic coerulospinal 95
noradrenergic nucleus locus coerulus 194
notochord 27, 65
novel routes 350
nucleus
   accumbens 151, 405, 561, 569
   anterior 148
   basalis 104, 158, 422
   dorsalis intermedius ventralis
     anterior 417
   dorsolateralis anterior 416
   dorsolateralis posterior 159, 417
   glomerulosus 307, 320
   laminaris 213
   lateralis valvulae 324
   mesencephalicus pars dorsalis 417
   ovoidalis 159, 416
   paracommissuralis 318, 322
   prethalamicus 313, 316, 319, 324
   reticularis thalami 559
   robustus 421
   rotundus 416
   sphericus 159
   tectalis 316, 317, 318, 324
number of neurons 568
number of synapses 568
Numenius 539
numerical symbols 474
numerosity discrimination 472, 473, 474
nutrition 269
nutritional groups 287

O

objects 457
observatory learning 360
observing responses 526
occipitomesencephalic tract 105, 421
Octopus eye 11, 12
oddity-from-sample 465
odor learning 334
olfaction 301, 412, 479
olfactory
   bulb 272, 409
   conditioning 335
   cortex 4, 152
   pallium 148
   structures 279
   system 253
   tract 541
   tubercle 405
ontogenesis 270
ontogeny 482
onychophorans 15, 17, 19, 24
Ophiura opiura 57
ophiuroids 41, 54
optic lobes, structure 380
optic tectum 146, 243, 306
optic tectum/superior colliculus 417
orbitofrontal cortex 560, 561, 564
orbitofrontal PFC 563
Oreochromis (Tilapia) niloticus 299
organizing principles 501

orientation 298, 302, 479
orienting response 466
orthodenticle 68
orthologous genes 391, 392
Osteichthyes 136, 533
osteoglossomorph 318, 325
Osteoglossomorpha 307
osteolepiform rhipidistians 81
ostrich dinosaurs 538
otd 34, 36
Otx 32, 36
outgroup comparison 4, 14
outgroup hypothesis 166, 167
outgroups 14
overshadowing 408

P

paedomorphic 4, 13, 256
paedomorphosis 254, 255
paleobotany 1
paleoclimatology 1
paleoecology 1
paleoneurology 525
paleostriatal complex 160
paleostriatum 404
Paleozoic 537
Paleozoic amphibians 139
paleozoology 1
pallidum 4
pallium 3, 145, 491
paradox of complexity 549
parahippocampal 560
parahippocampal area 412
paralimbic cortical areas 193
parallelism 12, 288
parental investment 172, 453
parietal cortex 558, 561, 563
parieto-occipito-temporal association cortex 185
parrot 3, 455, 465, 475, 478, 481
passeriform birds 278
path integration 352
pattern recognition 6
pattern vision 355
pax-6 11, 12
Pelmatozoa 41
pelycosaurs 140
pentadactyl limbs 81
pentaradial symmetry 41
PER 339
perception 530, 549
perceptual category 357

perceptual concepts 465
Perciformes 311
percomorph teleosts 307, 323
periamygdaloid cortex 411
period histogram 216
Periophthalmus koelreuter 96
perirhinal 560
PFC 432, 433, 434, 436, 437, 438, 439, 440, 445, 447, 449, 564
   see also prefrontal cortex
phase ambiguities 221
phase-locking 216, 217
phenomenology of consciousness 556
phenotype 12
phoronids 17
photic environment 310
phyletic method 2
phylogenetic tree 13
phylogeny 452, 454, 482
physiogeny 482
pigeon 3, 282, 410, 454, 455, 458, 546
pigeon homing 413
piriform 148
piriform cortex 411
pit organs 122
place learning 301
planktonic larvae 26
plasticity 550
plathelminth 14, 15, 17, 18, 25, 28, 35
plesiomorphy 13, 162, 536
pleurovisceral cords 20
Pliohippus 543
pogonophorans 15
polarized light navigation 334
polysensory input 491
Pomacentrus 311
positive patterning 345
postcommissural fornix 413
posterior lateral nucleus 150
posterior parietal cortex 561
posterior tubercle complex 315
power grip 84
precision grip 84
predictedness 343
prediction 334, 345
prefrontal 433, 436, 437
   association cortex 185
   cortex/neostriatum caudolaterale 442
   cortex (PFC) 4, 5, 188, 424, 432, 442, 482, 544, 559, 560, 561, 563, 569, 575, 576, 577, 579
   see also PFC
preglomerular complex 319
prehensile extremities 84

premotor interneurons 88
prepiriform cortex 411
pretectum 31, 306, 320
priapulids 17
primary swimmers 80
primates 5, 508, 542, 555, 565, 567, 568, 570, 573, 574, 575, 576, 577, 578
principal optic nucleus 417
Pristigenys serula 311
proboscis extension reflex 338, 339
processing capacity 505
projectile tongue 241, 243, 259
projection area 548
projection cortex 532
prosencephalon 30
prosimians 84
prosomeres 29, 31
prosomeric organisation 31
prostomium 23, 25, 34, 35
protocerebral bridge, roles, and walking 386
   structure 384 f
protocerebrum 23, 34, 35, 336
protocounting 349
Protopterus amphibians 96
protostomes 15, 17, 36
Prototheria 141
Pseudemys scripta elegans 92
Pseudobarbus afer 305
Pseudobarbus asper 305
pterobranchs 27
putamen 404
pyramidal cell 492, 493, 494
pyramidal system 421

Q

quintofrontal tract 104

R

radial maze 403
Raja clavata 96
raphe 319
raphe nuclei 558
rats 546
reciprocal inhibition 89
rectilinear locomotion 82
recurrent pathways 471
red nucleus 95, 421
reduction or loss of limbs 81
reef teleosts 321
regression 503, 534

regulatory gene expression 33
regulatory genes 3, 4, 11, 32, 34
reinforcement 337
reinforcement processing 343
reinforcement reversal 462
reinforcing stimuli 343
relative and absolute numerosity 474
relative brain size 5
representation 451, 524
reptiles 136
reptilian 12, 413
reptilian cortex 498
Rescorla-Wagner model 346
reticular formation 421, 558, 561, 569
reticulospinal pathways 89
reticulospinal projections 95
retinofugal fibers 243, 249
retinotectal 243, 260
retinotectal projections 244
retinotopic pattern 314
retrieval 350
retrieval cues 352
retrobulbar cortex 411
retrograde degeneration 416
reversal 436
reversal learning 300, 323, 357, 433
reward 337
rewarded preexposure 415
rhombencephalon 30
rhombomeres 30, 32, 33
rodents 268
rostral preglomerular nucleus 315
rotiferan 15, 17
rubrocerebellar loops 103
ruff feather 210
rules 470

S

salamanders 91
Salamandra salamandra 96
SALMFamide 52, 55
saurian extinction 453
sauropsid 4, 136
scala naturae 2, 13, 135, 269
scaling 503
scaphopods 22
schedule of reinforcements 526
scleractinian coral reefs 307, 320
scyphozoans 14
sea cucumbers 41
sea lilies 41
sea stars 41

sea urchins 41
Sebastiscus 318
Sebastiscus marmoratus 312
secondary simplification 13, 17, 20, 237, 238, 254, 255, 256
secondary swimmers 80
second-order conditioning 344
segmental locomotor interneurons 88
segmentation 11, 21
selection 268, 538
selection pressures 454
self-recognition 557, 565, 567, 579
sensory
   invasion 129
   maps 126
   receptors 113
   specialist 122, 123
septomesencephalic tract 105, 421
septum 4, 148
sequential landmarks 348
serotonergic raphespinal 95
serotoninergic mesencephalic raphe nuclei 195
Serrasalmus nattereri 304
sexual selection 480
shortcut 350
short memory 6
short-term plasticity 568
Siamese fighting fish 320
signal probability 527
silent flight 210
Silky hens 284
simple pigeon brain 530
simplification 254, 258
single neurons 333, 359
single unit 461
siphonophores 14
sipunculids 17
size of hippocampus 413
skilled purposive movements 190
small brains 547
social learning 307
social systems 285
socioecological niches 453
soldierfishes 307, 308
Solenodon 287
somatosensory
   association cortex 187
   cortex 276
   system 253, 417
song 480
songbirds 480
sound-localization 207
space constancy 301

Spalax 276
spatial
   cognition 279
   learning 301, 307, 323
   map 413
   memory 349, 350, 479
   orientation 297
   representation 299, 348
spatiotemporal memories 348
speech center 5, 563, 578
spinal and supraspinal networks 87
spinal motoneurons 87
sponges 14
squirrelfish 307, 308, 313, 315, 317, 318, 319, 321, 324
stereo vision 212
sticklebacks 320
stimulus
   configurations 342
   equivalencies 464
   features 459
   generalization 459, 460, 463
stretch receptors 171
striatal association system 198
striatum 151, 278, 319, 494, 495, 569
strickleiter Bauplan 16
strickleiter nervous system 15, 19, 22, 23, 24, 26, 34, 36
Struthiomimus 538
subiculum 413
suboesophageal ganglion 24, 35, 336
subpallium 3, 145
substantia innominata 195, 405
substantia nigra 151
sulcus principalis 424
sunfishes 312
superior colliculus 146
supplementary motor area (SMA) 564
supraoesophageal ganglion 15, 20, 23, 24, 34, 336
supraspinal control 93
surgeonfish 307, 308, 313, 319
sustained attention 525
symmetrical 458
symmetry 356
symmetry categorization 357
synapomorphy 14, 15
synapses 544
synapses per unit of cortical volume 532
synapsids 140
synaptic connections 455
synchronization 220
synfire chains 497
syngeny 129

syntactical language 565
systems, distributed 548

T

taste pathways 320
taxonomy 206
tectal ablation 304
tectal-telencephalic connection 315
tectofugal visual system 417
tectum 243, 246, 248, 249, 250, 252, 256, 303, 305, 318, 323
tectum opticum 452, 461
tegmentum 407
telencephalic output channel 105
telencephalic projections spinal cord 97
telencephalic-tectal-cerebellar neural associations 307
telencephalon 145, 271, 300, 301, 306, 317, 323, 402
teleost fishes 297, 298
temporal cortex 563
temporal lobe 576
tentaculates 15, 17, 25
terrestriality 240, 253
terrestrial locomotion 81
tetraneural 21, 22
tetraneural Bauplan 16
Tetraodontiformes 308, 311
tetrapod 13, 136
tetrapod augmentation 95
thalamic association systems 196
thalamic relay 495
thalamic reticular nucleus 191
thalamofugal visual system 417
thalamus 404, 494
theoretical analysis 224
theory of meaning 6
theory of mind 565, 567
therapsids 140
Theria 141
theta rhythm 413
thickness of fibers 498
Thorius narisovalis 547
three-dimensional coordinate systems 208
Thrinaxodon 540
through-conducting fibers 56
Tilapia macrocephla 302
time pathways 214
timing 476
tongue-projecting salamanders 238, 244
tongue-projection 242
topography 511

torus longitudinalis 324
torus semicircularis 146, 325
transcortical pathways 189
transfer index 546
transitional cortex 152
transitive inference 403, 467
transitive responding 469, 471
transitivity 467
traplining 349
tree shrew 84
Triconodon 539, 541
trigeminal nucleus 422
triggerfishes 307, 308, 319, 320
tritocerebrum 23, 34, 35, 367
Triturus cristatus 92
tunicate 27
Tupaia glis 84
Tursiops truncatus 543
Tyrannosaurus 541

U

unconscious 561, 577
unconscious processing 557
unimodal association areas 186
urodeles 13, 534

V

vagal lobes 305
value-transfer 471
valvula of the cerebellum 303, 321
Varanus exanthematicus 92
variable interval schedule 529
ventral cord ganglia 15, 23, 24, 34, 35
ventral striatum 561
ventral substrate response 322
ventral thalamus 31
ventromedial nucleus of the thalamus 319
vertebrate eye 12
vigilance 525
vision specialists 310
visual
  association area 188
  discrimination 354 ff, 420
  landmarks 298
  learning 335
  pathways 302
  streaks 307
  system 249, 252, 455, 456
    insect, motion pathways 380
    insect, spectral pathways 380

visually based spatial maps 321
vocalization circuit 105
vomeronasal amygdala 159
von Uexküll 524
VUMmx1 335 f

W

waggle dance 334, 346 f
Weberian apparatus 305
Wernicke speech center 576
white matter 492, 497, 513
wings 12

working memory 347, 352, 353, 432, 434, 437, 439, 440, 446, 449, 482, 563
wrasses 307
Wulst 3, 156, 213, 417, 569

X

Xenopus embryo model 88
Xenopus laevis 96

Z

zootype 36